WITHDRAWN
FROM THE LIBRARY
UNIVERSITY OF ULST

for O. Duffy

D0492699

100572932

CASES

Introducing Communication Disorders Across the Life Span

CASES

Introducing Communication Disorders Across the Lifespan

John W. Oller, Jr., Ph.D.
Stephen D. Oller, Ph.D.
Linda C. Badon, CCC-SLP, Ph.D.

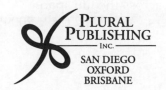

PLURAL
PUBLISHING
INC.
SAN DIEGO
OXFORD
BRISBANE

100572932
616.855
OLL

PLURAL PUBLISHING
INC.

5521 Ruffin Road
San Diego, CA 92123

e-mail: info@pluralpublishing.com
Web site: http://www.pluralpublishing.com

49 Bath Street
Abingdon, Oxfordshire OX14 1EA
United Kingdom

Copyright © by Plural Publishing, Inc. 2010

Typeset in 11/13 Palatino by Flanagan's Publishing Services, Inc.
Printed in Malaysia by Four Colour Imports

All rights, including that of translation, reserved. No part of this publication may be reproduced, stored in a retrieval system, or transmitted in any form or by any means, electronic, mechanical, recording, or otherwise, including photocopying, recording, taping, Web distribution, or information storage and retrieval systems without the prior written consent of the publisher.

For permission to use material from this text, contact us by
Telephone: (866) 758-7251
Fax: (888) 758-7255
e-mail: permissions@pluralpublishing.com

Every attempt has been made to contact the copyright holders for material originally printed in another source. If any have been inadvertently overlooked, the publishers will gladly make the necessary arrangements at the first opportunity.

Library of Congress Cataloging-in-Publication Data

Oller, John W.
  Cases : introducing communication disorders across the life span / John W. Oller, Stephen D. Oller, and Linda C. Badon.
       p. ; cm.
  Includes bibliographical references and index.
  ISBN-13: 978-1-59756-035-1 (alk. paper)
  ISBN-10: 1-59756-035-9 (alk. paper)
  1. Communicative disorders. I. Oller, Stephen D. II. Badon, Linda C. III. Title. IV. Title: Introducing communication disorders across the life span.
  [DNLM: 1. Communication Disorders. WL 340.2 O49c 2009]
  RC423.O475 2009
  616.85'5—dc22
                                                                        2009007739

CONTENTS

Preface   ix
Acknowledgments   xi

1 WHAT ARE COMMUNICATION DISORDERS?   1
Objectives   1
Key Terms   2
Success in Linguistic Communication Is the Norm   3
Communication   10
The Distinctly Human Language Capacity   17
Multiple Layers of Representation: Genome to Brain   20
The Anatomy of the Major Systems of Representation   22
Valid Representations Are Foundational   38
Resources for the Course   43
Summing Up and Looking Ahead   48
Study and Discussion Questions   49

2 GENETICS TO ANATOMY: CRANIOFACIAL ANOMALIES   51
Objectives   51
Key Terms   52
Bodily Disorders   54
When Things Go Wrong   68
The Case of Samuel Armas   71
4D Ultrasound: Moving Pictures of the Baby in the Womb   78
Sensory Disorders   87
Sensory-Motor Disorders   90
Sensory-Motor-Linguistic Disorders   96
Summing Up and Looking Ahead   99
Study and Discussion Questions   100

3 AUDITORY AND OTHER SENSORY DISORDERS   103
Objectives   103
Key Terms   104
Freedom of the Body and the Mind   105
Valentin Haüy and Louis Braille   109
How Can We Test the Authenticity of Communication?   115
Deafness Without Blindness   122
Spoken Languages, Manual Signed Languages, and Literacy   128
Freeing the Imprisoned Self   131
Summing Up and Looking Ahead   139
Study and Discussion Questions   139

4 SYSTEMS INTEGRATION AND HEARING DISORDERS   141
    Objectives   141
    Key Terms   142
    Integration of the Senses   143
    Layers and Ranks of Senses and Sensory Integration   151
    Meaningful Representations   159
    Central Auditory Processing Disorders   162
    Abstract Meaning, Anatomy, and Physiology   174
    The Dynamic Anatomy of Hearing   176
    Distinct Meaning Related Physiological Functions   181
    Connections Above, Through, and Below the Cochlear Nuclei   192
    Summing Up and Looking Ahead   194
    Study and Discussion Questions   195

5 CHILDHOOD DISORDERS   197
    Objectives   197
    Key Terms   198
    The Strange Puzzle   199
    Pervasive Developmental Disorders: Autism at the Center   204
    Theories to Explain the Increasing Number of Diagnoses   210
    Such Dramatic Change Cannot Be Uncaused   215
    The Role of Oxidative Stress   219
    Separating the Toxicology of Mercury from the Politics   225
    The Links to Autism Spectrum and Other Disorders Reconsidered   229
    Treating the Worst Problem First   235
    Behavioral Interventions for Developmental Disorders   242
    Summing Up and Looking Ahead   248
    Study and Discussion Questions   249

6 SWALLOWING, VOICE, AND "MOTOR" SPEECH   251
    Objectives   251
    Key Terms   252
    Swallowing Disorders Treated by Speech-Language Pathologists   254
    Anatomy—Form: The Mouth as "Grand Central Station"   256
    Physiology—Function: Accidents at the Crossroads   260
    Neurology—Control: Voluntary and Involuntary Systems   261
    Voice from the Producer's Position   271
    Diagnostic Voice and Speech Qualities   279
    Differentiating the Dysarthrias   286
    Treatment of Motor Disorders   300
    Summing Up and Looking Ahead   308
    Study and Discussion Questions   309

7 ARTICULATION DISORDERS   311
    Objectives   311
    Key Terms   312
    What Is the Articulation of Surface Forms?   313

Articulation and the Positions of Discourse 314
Getting Down to the Distinct Segments (Phonemes) of Speech 323
The Hierarchical Structure of Skilled Movements 334
The Articulation of Surface Forms 338
Different Writing Systems 344
Why Meaning Is Crucial to Articulation 353
Disorders of Articulation and Their Treatment 357
Therapeutic Interventions 360
Summing Up and Looking Ahead 363
Study and Discussion Questions 364

8   FLUENCY DISORDERS   367
Objectives 367
Key Terms 368
The Mystery of Stuttering 369
The World Health Organization Classification Criteria 371
The Genetic Factor 374
Loss of Control of the Speech Signal 377
Facilitating Contexts 380
Artificially Induced Stuttering 383
Theories and Findings About the Causes of Stuttering 390
Testing the Theories 398
Treatment of Stuttering 404
How Important Is Surface Form? 409
Treatment for Adults and Adolescents 412
Other Fluency Disorders 417
Summing Up and Looking Ahead 419
Study and Discussion Questions 419

9   LITERACY AND DYSLEXIA   423
Objectives 423
Key Terms 424
Acquiring Literacy 425
What Is "Dyslexia"? 434
Varieties of Dyslexia and Disorders in General 438
Causing Dyslexia 440
Elaborated Phonics: Phonological and Phonemic Awareness 450
Curing Instructional Dyslexia 456
Acquiring Multiple Modalities and Languages 464
Summing Up and Looking Ahead 472
Study and Discussion Questions 473

10   ADULT AND NEUROLOGICAL DISORDERS   475
Objectives 475
Key Terms 476
Communication Disorders of Adults 477
Mapping Brain Functions 481

Refining the Images of the Brain 487
Gross Relations Brains, Signs, and Functions 497
Sign Systems, Ranks, and Integration 509
Understanding Aphasias and Other Disorders 517
Across the Hemispheres: Indexing and Motor Functions 531
Commissurotomy: Disconnecting the Hemispheres 536
Abrupt Causes of Adult Neurological Disorders 539
Cumulative Causes of Adult Neurological Disorders 542
Treatment of Adult Diseases and Neurological Disorders 548
Summing Up and Looking Ahead 550
Study and Discussion Questions 551

11 ASSESSMENT, DIAGNOSIS, AND LANGUAGE/DIALECT 553

Objectives 553
Key Terms 554
Understanding Disproportionate Representation 555
The Role of Language/Dialect in Assessment 566
Three Proposed "Processing Dependent Measures" 570
The American Eugenics Records Office 573
What the IQ Tests Measure Best 576
Verbal Reasoning in Nonverbal/Performance Assessment 578
Development Versus Effects of Intervention 583
Summing Up and Looking Ahead 590
Study and Discussion Questions 591

12 ADVOCACY, LAW, AND ETHICS 593

Objectives 593
Key Terms 594
Freedom from Mental and Physical Bondage 595
The Long Road Toward Equality Under the Law 604
Disabilities in the Background 606
The Language/Dialect Factor in IQ Tests 621
Justice and Freedom in America 625
National Childhood Vaccine Injury Act of 1986 631
Into the New Millennium 639
The Highest Principles of Law and Ethics 655
Summing Up and Looking Beyond This Course 668
Study and Discussion Questions 669

Glossary of Terms 671
References 703
Index 743

PREFACE

This book introduces and reclassifies disorders across the board from the vantage point of a more dynamic, comprehensive, consistent, and coherent theory of sign systems. In doing so, it presents newly discovered theoretical connections along with up-to-date published empirical and experimental demonstrations.

It is becoming increasingly evident that disorders and disease conditions, especially the unexpectedly persistent ones singled out as "communication disorders," invariably involve problems in representation. Such problems range from difficulties at the deepest levels of genetics to the highest levels of human emotion and intelligence manifested in experience, actions, language, and reasoning. More than ever before it is clear that health depends profoundly on dynamic representations, especially true ones, of the way things really are and how they are changing over time.

Disease conditions and disorders invariably involve mistaking fictional or deliberately false representations for true ones. Disease agents, it is clear, can falsely represent themselves to the body's defenses. Toxins can disrupt the capacity of the body and its immune systems to represent things correctly from genetics upward through metabolism and on to the highest levels of emotion, cognition, language, and reasoning. When fictions are mistaken for true representations, as when deliberate deceptions or mere fictions are taken to be true representations of actual facts, problems result. Such communication problems at the deepest levels from genetics and metabolism right on up to the most general forms of language and thought, form the underlying basis for disease, disorder, and mortality.

Without exception, disorders of communication and disease conditions in general, are the consequence of breakdowns and failures in systems of representation. At the core of the distinctly human capacities of communication are the dynamic pragmatic mapping relations by which sensory impressions of the physical world are linked through actions to abstract concepts of the linguistic kind. The simplest examples involve naming: For instance, if we refer to one of our editors as "Sandy," we aim to map the surface form of the name onto a certain person. If we succeed, our representation qualifies, as far as it is intended to qualify, as a true and valid representation. Another simple example of the pragmatic mapping relation would be a baby waving goodbye when someone else is actually taking leave of that baby, or vice versa. In that case the waving would be appropriately associated by way of reference or signification with the act of taking leave.

Such pragmatic mapping relations, as well demonstrated in the study of communication disorders, are fundamentally programmed into our neurological systems. It is not too much to say that they are dynamically built-in to the architecture of the brain. With that in mind as the basis for the dynamic connection between abstract ideas and concrete things through intelligence, it is also becoming increasingly evident, as our readers and students are discovering, that the many fields of study concerned with human communication and its disorders are undergoing a paradigm shift from static theories of distinct bits and pieces, surface forms, and independent components, toward theories taking account of dynamic, interconnected, systems that communicate with each other.

The dynamic systems-oriented approaches to human experience are central to the paradigm shift that we believe is already underway in the health sciences. The shift is bringing with it a better understanding of the central role of valid communications to well-being. It is ultimately the dissolution of representations themselves, or we could say the development of communication disorders, that leads to diseases and disordered conditions. This book chronicles the initial stages of the paradigm shift that we believe is underway and it anticipates some of the ways in which the systems orientation must continue to develop in the coming months and years. Teachers who adopt the book and course, and their students, are assured of a cutting-edge introduction to the best of current theories and ongoing empirical research being applied to test them. No other introduction offers as much historical depth or experimental currency concerning well-researched cases. Nor does any other course provide a simpler, more coherent, or more intelligible theoretical perspective.

John W. Oller, Jr., Ph.D.
Stephen D. Oller, Ph.D.
Linda C. Badon, CCC-SLP, Ph.D.

ACKNOWLEDGMENTS

A project of this scope could only be carried out as a team effort. As many of our readers and friends will recognize, this *Cases* book and its accompanying DVD are companions (really prequels) to our *Milestones* course published by Plural 2006. However, we have more individuals and groups to acknowledge now than then because of the increased scope and depth of the *Cases* book and DVD.

In *Cases* we deal not only with the unfolding development of communication abilities and skills, but also with the causation, diagnosis, and treatment of disorders of communication, as well as the laws and history behind the study of those disorders. As in *Milestones* we work from a deep and rich semiotic perspective—one that takes dynamic sign systems as foundational. In *Cases* we have consolidated, extended, and enriched partnerships, collaborations, and commitments that were made in completing the prior project. We are especially grateful for the commitment of our forward-looking publisher and the insightful and scholarly individuals at Plural Publishing, Inc. Our colleagues there have all worked long, diligently, and enthusiastically to bring this project to fruition. We also thank our supportive administrators at the University of Louisiana, Lafayette, including Dr. Ray Authement, President Emeritus; Dr. T. Joseph Savoie, our current President; Dr. Steve P. Landry, Academic Vice President and Provost; Dr. C. E. Palmer, Dean of our Graduate School; and Dr. A. David Barry, Dean of the College of Liberal Arts; and at Texas A&M in Kingsville we thank Tom Fields, Interim Vice President for Academic Affairs and Graduate Studies.

Along with all the foregoing, we thank the many other researchers, publishers, and colleagues who have generously shared their findings, theories, diagrams, videos, and photographs, as well as clinical, historical, and legal knowledge with us. Although we cannot mention all of them by name, there are some whom we must not overlook. We are especially grateful to Dr. Stuart Campbell, M.D., of Create Health Clinic in London. Again, he has allowed us to use his pioneering work with 4D video of unborn babies. His research and findings have enormously advanced understanding of prenatal human development. We also thank the talented professional photographer and journalist Michael Clancy and the family of Samuel Armas for providing pictures and background on the surgery to repair Samuel's spina bifida at just 21 weeks of gestation. When the tiny unborn baby Samuel, whose whole body would have comfortably fit in the surgeon's hand, reached out and grasped the finger of Dr. Bruner, the whole world was touched. We thank Michael Clancy and the Armas family for sharing their experience with us and the world. We also thank Dr. Thomas G. R. Bower who has shared his wisdom, research findings, and experimental data concerning early development and Dr. Robert C. Titzer for his contributions to the understanding and teaching of literacy.

We thank Gene Mills, Judge Russell White, and all their colleagues at the Louisiana Family Forum for putting us on to the story of Ota Benga and various facets of the law and the interesting history pertaining to that immortal proposition that "all men are created equal, and endowed by their Creator with certain unalienable rights." We thank the Sertoma Club of Lafayette and Sertoma International for a small grant to the first author that helped to purchase technology used in developing certain aspects of this project. Sertoma also provided a broader and deeper support base for many aspects of the ongoing research in medical treatments of spectrum disorders. We must mention among the key Sertoma leaders, Steve Broussard, Ron Chauffe, Paul George, Gerald Domingue, Joey LeRouge, John Nugent, Burnie Smith, and Jimmy Thomas. We also thank those families associated with our local branch of the Autism Society of America—the Autism Society of Acadiana

(ASAC, an affiliate of Sertoma International) among whom we must name Theron, Terry, and Ethan Pitre, Charlie, Vickie, and Katherine Nettles, and Carolyn, Jamie, Lauren, and Chris Tate. We also thank all the ASAC families. We extend our gratitude to all the courageous parents, grandparents, and individuals who have patiently sought to enable all human beings everywhere—including persons with disabilities and persons in all races and ethnicities—to enjoy the fullest benefits of life, liberty, and the pursuit of happiness.

We thank our own families and above all the Creator God who gave all of us our unalienable rights. We also thank the individuals who pledged their lives, fortunes, and sacred honor to inscribe those rights in blood well before and long after the ink had dried on the the American Constitution and our Bill of Rights. We thank God for all those men and women who continue to defend our unalienable rights around the world. We recall what Lincoln said at Gettysberg during the most costly war of history. We document that it was fought not only to preserve the unity of the United States but also to guarantee rights under American law to all human beings including Africans brought here initially as slaves. We show how the troubles of those slaves paved the way for rights that would eventually be more fully guaranteed to persons with disorders and disabilities. We acknowledge the hundreds of thousands of persons with disorders, diseases, and disabilities who were exterminated by the Nazis prior to and during World War II. We document and acknowledge here the historical, legal, and practial *identity of the moral rights of the unborn, of helpless babies, of persons with disabilities, and of persons with minority status as well as of racial and ethnic diversity.*

The response to this project has been nothing short of amazing and we thank all those who have already participated in it as well as those who are yet to make common cause with us in the ongoing struggle to improve prospects for all persons with communication disorders, disabilities, and related conditions. We have been heartened by the enthusiasm with which our colleagues, often at a distance, have opened wide the doors of learning and have extended a warm welcome to us, to our students, and to our many collaborators. All of them, but especially our own students, have contributed to this project in uncountable ways. We thank them for their help and encouragement as we have worked side by side in prepublication uses of the material in this book and in its accompanying DVD.

In the text that follows, and on the DVD, we have explicitly thanked many individuals who have permitted us to use their names and to quote their words. Here we must mention Clint Andrus, Liang Chen, Jane Colette, Emily Ensminger, Melissa Fowlkes, Mallory Gauthier, Raquelle Horton, Heidi Kidder, Nicole Langlinais, Candice Nele, Ning Pan, Cheryl Sinner, Sarah Stutes, Sharon Williams, and Rachel Yan. We thank our introductory students and the graduate students who participated in the pretesting, rewriting, retesting, and final workup of the 600 multiple-choice items that are provided in the *Cases DVD*-Rom. We thank every person who attended classes, read the text, wrote comments, asked questions, made suggestions, and contributed to the inspiration and energy necessary to the completion of the *Cases* project. Thanks to all those who have shared the road with us thus far and to all those who will join us and continue the journey in years and decades to come.

Finally, we also thank those who generously provided materials for the text and/or the DVD, in the form of video recordings, photographs, diagrams, and illustrations. We especially acknowledge the following sources for material included in the figures mentioned:

Figure 1–1. Baby smiling in the womb. Retrieved March 20, 2009, from London's Create Health Clinic, http://www.createhealth.org/. Copyright 2004 by Dr. Stuart Campbell. Reprinted with permission. All rights reserved.

Figure 1–6. The mapping of the sensory and sensory-motor strips of the cortex onto the body. Retrieved March 20, 2009, from http://www.mie.utoronto.ca/labs/lcdlab/biopic/fig/46.09.jpg. Reprinted with permission. All rights reserved.

Figure 2–9. Mother Teresa at a meeting of the American Family Institute. Copyright ©1984 by the Human Life Foundation, Inc. From *Abortion and the conscience of the nation* (p. 37), by R. Reagan, 1984, Nashville, TN: Thomas

Nelson Publishers. Copyright 1984 by the Human Life Foundation, Inc. Reprinted with permission. All rights reserved.

Figure 2–10. The spina bifida surgery on Samuel Armas by Dr. Joseph Bruner. Copyright © 2005 by Michael Clancy. Retrieved February 16, 2009, from http://www.michaelclancy.com/story.html. Reprinted with permission. All rights reserved.

Figure 2–11. Samuel Armas at about four years. Copyright © 2003 by Jonathan Imbody. Retrieved February 16, 2009, from http://freerepublic.com/focus/f-news/1012548/posts. Reprinted by permission. All rights reserved.

Figure 2–12. Joanna Jepson today after surgery for a congenital craniofacial anomaly. Retrieved February 16, 2009, from http://web.archive.org/web/20060115213036/www.jjepson.org/index.php. Copyright © 2007, Joanna Jepson, St. Michael's Church in Chester. Reprinted by permission. All rights reserved.

Figure 2–13. Photos on the left side represent the condition and appearance prior to surgery and on the right after surgical repair of cleft lip and/or palate. Retrieved February 16, 2009, from http://www.chsd.org/12293.cfm. Copyright © n.d. by Rady Children's Hospital of San Diego. Reprinted by permission. All rights reserved.

Figure 2–16. The destruction of extremities due to current day biblical leprosy. Retrieved February 16, 2009, from http://www.leprosy.ca/site/c.anKKIPNrEqG/b.2012733/k.8C01/The_Disease.htm. Reprinted with permission. Copyright © 2009 by the Leprosy Mission Canada. All rights reserved.

Figure 2–17. Digits lost to leprosy. The destruction of extremities due to current day biblical leprosy. Retrieved February 16, 2009, from http://www.leprosy.ca/site/c.anKKIPNrEqG/b.2012733/k.8C01/The_Disease.htm. Reprinted with permission. Copyright © 2009 by the Leprosy Mission Canada. All rights reserved.

Figure 3–2. The Braille code as applied to the English alphabet. Copyright © 1995–2009 by the Royal National Institute of Blind People (RNIB). Retrieved February 16, 2009, from http://www.rnib.org.uk/xpedio/groups/public/documents/publicwebsite/public_braille.hcsp. Reprinted with permission. All rights reserved.

Figure 3–3. Helen Keller at age 7 years and two months, just five months after she met Annie Sullivan and began to acquire language. A photo in the public domain from the American Foundation for the Blind, retrieved February 23, 2009, from http://www.afb.org/Section.asp?SectionID=1&TopicID=194&SubTopicID=6&DocumentID=144.

Figure 3–4. A re-enactment of Helen Keller acquiring her first word with the help of Annie Sullivan. From *The Miracle Worker* (p. 34), by W. Gibson, 1956, New York: Doubleday. Copyright © 1956 by Doubleday. In the public domain because of expired copyright.

Figure 4–2. Redrawn images of Kaye and Bower (1994) to illustrate the pacifier experiment. Permission to modify and use the material granted by Dr. T. G. R. Bower.

Figure 4–6. The semicircular canals and the cochlea of the inner ear. Retrieved February 25, 2009, from http://pcbunn.cacr.caltech.edu/Cochlea/default.htm. Reprinted with permission. All rights reserved.

Figure 6–3. The epiglottis as seen in a radiographic image. Retrieved February 27, 2009, from http://www.rad.msu.edu/Education/CourseInfo/CHM_domain/ID/Morgan/default.html. Copyright © n.d. by the Department of Radiology at Michigan State University. Adapted and reprinted with permission. All rights reserved.

Figure 6–5. Regions of brain activity during pointing in contrast to eye movement. From "Parietal and Superior Frontal Visuospatial Maps Activated by Pointing and Saccades," by D. J. Hagler, Jr., L. Riecke, & M. L. Sereno, 2007, *Neuroimage, 35*(4), p. 1566. Copyright ©

2007 Elsevier Inc. Adapted and reprinted with permission from Elsevier. All rights reserved.

Figure 6–10. Contact ulcers on the vocal folds. Retrieved February 28, 2009, from http://www.gbmc.org/voice/disorders.cfm. Copyright © 1999 by The Milton J. Dance, Jr. Head & Neck Rehabilitation Center. Reprinted with permission. All rights reserved.

Figure 6–13. Electron micrograph of Helicobacter pylori. Retrieved February 28, 2009, from http://info.fujita-hu.ac.jp/~tsutsumi/photo/photo002-6.htm. Contributed with full permission from: Yutaka Tsutsumi, M.D. Professor Department of Pathology Fujita Health University School of Medicine.

Figure 6–15. An astrocyte, glial cell. Retrieved February 28, 2009, from http://www.sfn.org/index.cfm?pagename=brainBriefings_astrocytes. Photo by Vladimir Parpura, M.D., Ph.D., Iowa State University and University of California at Riverside. Copyright © 2000. Reprinted with permission. All rights reserved.

Figure 6–17. A schematic of the main afferent and efferent cranial nerves associated with sensory and motor systems. Retrieved February 28, 2009, from http://www.neurophys.com/EMG/Cranial_Nerves/CranialNerves.jpg. Copyright © 1997–2003 by Neurophys.com. Reprinted with permission. All rights reserved.

Figure 6–21. The interactions of UMN with LMN as mediated by the cerebellum and the basal ganglia (also known as the extrapyramidal tract). Retrieved February 28, 2009, from http://thalamus.wustl.edu/course/cerebell.html. Created by Diana Weedman Molavi, Ph.D., at the Washington University School of Medicine, Department of Anatomy and Neurobiology. Copyright © 1997 by the Washington University Program in Neuroscience http://neuroscience.wustl.edu. Adapted with permission. All rights reserved.

Figure 8–1. An inside (MRI) view of Wernicke's area divided between Heschl's gyrus (the cortical fold) just above and in front of the planum temporale (PT) and the PT itself in a healthy individual. From Y. Hirayasu et al., 2000, Planum temporale and Heschl gyrus volume reduction in schizophrenia: A magnetic resonance imaging study of first-episode patients. *Archives of General Psychiatry, 57*(7), Figure 1. Retrieved September 17, 2008, from http://www.spl.harvard.edu/pages/Special:PubDB_View?dspaceid=406. Copyright 2008 by Surgical Planning Laboratory. Adapted and reprinted with permission. All rights reserved.

Figure 10–4. Colorized diagrams of Brodmann's areas. Retrieved March 7, 2009, from at http://spot.colorado.edu/~dubin/talks/brodmann/brodmann.html. Copyright © 2007 by Professor Mark Dubin. Reprinted by permission. All rights reserved.

Figure 10–14. "Lichtheim's House." A diagram expanded from Brain 7(4), 436. Retrieved March 7, 2009, from http://www.smithsrisca.demon.co.uk/PSYlichtheim1885.html. Adapted and reprinted with permission from Derek Smith. Original image is in the public domain due to expired copyright.

Figure 10–15. Four views of the arcuate fasciculus connecting Wernicke's with Broca's area—the area damaged in conduction (sensory reception-to-motor production) aphasia. Retrieved March 7, 2009, from http://www9.biostr.washington.edu/cgi-bin/DA/imageform. Copyright © 1995 by the Digital Anatomist Project, University of Washington. Adapted and reprinted with permission. All rights reserved.

Figure 10–16. Pragmatic mapping of words (such as a name) onto their objects (such as the person named) and the major classes of communication disorders. Photograph of Cecilia Burman (at the right side of the figure) retrieved March 7, 2009, from http://www.prosopagnosia.com/. Reprinted with permission.

Figure 10–17. Differentiating the planes of motion relative to views of the brain created with MRI. Retrieved March 7, 2009, from http://www.med.wayne.edu/diagRadiology/Anatomy_Modules/brain/brain.html. Copyright © 1999 by J. E. Zapawa, A. L. Alcantara, and H. Nguyen. Adapted and reprinted with permission. All rights reserved.

Figure 10–20. An MRI of the corpus callosum (dotted outline) and the splenium (in the transparent oval). Retrieved March 7, 2009, from http://www.indiana.edu/~pietsch/callosum.html. Copyright 2008 by Paul A. Pietsch. Adapted and reprinted with permission. All rights reserved.

Figure 11–1. Dr. Roger Bannister breaking the four minute mile. Retrieved March 7, 2009, from at http://www.achievement.org/autodoc/photocredit/achievers/ban0-013. Copyright ©1996–2009 by the American Academy of Achievement. Reprinted with permission. All rights reserved.

*To the individuals and families affected by
the chronic disease conditions and disorders that interfere with
and disrupt the blessings of ordinary human communication*

1

What Are Communication Disorders?

OBJECTIVES

In this chapter, we:

1. Define communication and its disorders;
2. Consider why disorders are so costly;
3. Present an overview of the course and the DVD-ROM;
4. Begin to see disorders as they are seen by persons affected by them;
5. Discuss the systems of signs on which communication depends;
6. See how abilities come to light when things go wrong; and
7. Discuss how major classes of disorders are differentiated.

KEY TERMS

Here are some key terms of this chapter. Many you may already know, but it may help to review them. These terms are explained in the text and they are defined in the Glossary at the end of the book. They appear in **bold print** on their first appearance in the text.

abstractness	epidemiology	pathological lying
ADD/ADHD	etiology	phylogenetic speculation
adrenoleukodystrophy	fissure of Rolando	pragmatic mapping
afferent nerves	frontal lobes	pseudologia fantastica
Alzheimer's disease	gas theory of smiling	pseudologue
articulation	generality	reflex
autism	genome	reliability
autonomic nervous system	glial cells	semantic function
central sulcus	grammar	sensory cortex
cerebellum	hallucinations	sensory strip
cerebral palsy	hierarchy	sensory systems
cleft palate	illusions	somatic (bodily) systems
codon	immune systems	somatosensory cortex
communication disorder	infrasystems	startle response
conventional	instructional utility	surface forms
cortex	interneurons	symptomology
cortical functions	intonation	syntax
delusional pathology	manual signs	temporal lobes
dental amalgam	metabolism	toxins
detoxification systems	motor cortex	trauma
developmental regression	motor strip	traumatic injury
Duchenne-type smile	multiple sclerosis	validity
efferent nerves	mythomania	vegetative
emphysema	neurotransmitter	volitional control
entrainment	parietal lobes	

Communication systems are not static, unchanging "structures." For this reason, we use the term "systems" to call attention to the dynamic, changing, adaptive nature of all our bodily communication systems.

John Dewey said, "Of all affairs, communication is the most wonderful" (1925, p. 265). This chapter is about what communication is and why its disorders can be very costly. We introduce the sign systems on which communication depends and give a comprehensive overview of the full range of problems that can cause communication difficulties. At the outset, we should take notice of the fact that communication systems are not static, unchanging "structures." For this reason, we use the term "systems" to call attention to the dynamic, changing, adaptive nature of all our bodily communication systems.

Some of the critical systems, such as speech, writing, manual signing, and language, come under our voluntary control to a very high degree. Other communication systems that are essential to our survival, well-being, and the normal functioning of our language abilities, are outside of our conscious control. Systems that are partially or completely beyond conscious control may be referred to as communication **infrasystems**. As we will see throughout this book and its accompanying materials, the infrasystems are essential to the health and well-being of all our higher communication systems including language. An infection, disease, or injury from poisonous chemicals can set up a metabolic imbalance that affects multiple other systems including the brain and our language capacity. In the medical jargon, any persistent undesirable disorder, disease, or condition is referred to as **morbidity**. If it results in death, the corresponding term is—mortality.

As an instance of system interactions, although it actually surprises some specialists, we now know for a certainty that disease in the intestines can affect the body's production of biochemicals that are essential to normal brain functions.

The Recovery of Ethan Kurtz

Ethan Kurtz, for example, began to show unmistakable symptoms of the most severe form of nonverbal **autism** at the age of two. Ethan stopped responding to his name, quit talking, and showed no interest in or awareness of social relations. These are the classic symptoms of severe autism. Many treatment regimens were tried over the next two years with only slight improvements in Ethan's evident abilities. However, a change in diet and a course of antifungal medications to kill an infestation in his small intestine resulted in a return to normal language abilities within a period of 21 days. Without discounting the impact of other therapies, such as behavioral and physical work by speech-language pathologists and physical therapists, it was evident that clearing up the disease in the gut was the principal source of Ethan's amazing improvement. See the video documentation of Ethan's recovery on the DVD by clicking on Ethan Kurtz.

If communication is wonderful, any loss or failure to develop any aspect of even one of our systems of communication, must be a genuine loss. The more severe the disorder, the greater the loss. By the same reasoning, the restoration of lost communication abilities must also be wonderful.

If communication is wonderful, any loss or failure to develop any aspect of even one of our systems of communication, must be a genuine loss.

SUCCESS IN LINGUISTIC COMMUNICATION IS THE NORM

When things are going smoothly, we take our abilities to know what is going on around us and to communicate with each other through language for granted. When things are going well, we are like fish in water. But take the fish out of the water and we get an inkling of what it is like for a human being deprived of the ability to communicate.

Telling Disorders from Mere Difficulties of Communication

We define communication disorders *as* unexpectedly long-lasting, persistent, or recurrent difficulties that interfere with normal, successful, ordinary communication.

When any problem, difficulty, or interference with communication has an effect that unexpectedly persists or recurs over time, it can be referred to as a **communication disorder**. What distinguishes disorders from the most common ordinary breakdowns in communication—such as failures to comprehend, inability to get a particular idea across, and the like—is that *disorders are unexpectedly long-lasting, recurrent, and/or chronic difficulties*. They involve losses or failures to advance in development that are not normally expected to occur. Among them are many that have been traditionally recognized and treated as speech, language, and hearing problems. Surprisingly, some of the traditionally recognized disorders of swallowing—that are dealt with in speech-language pathology, for instance—do not on the surface involve speech, language, or communication. However, they are regarded as communication disorders and are treated by speech-language pathologists for reasons we consider in detail in Chapter 5.

In addition, many injuries and disease conditions that indirectly impact human communication abilities result in disorders, sometimes severe ones. All the things that can and sometimes do go wrong are impacted by our genetic makeup and some of the things that go wrong change our genes. As more and more details of human genetics are becoming known, deeper and more pervasive relations across all of the body's many systems of communication are also becoming known and better understood. Our bodily systems and even our social connections and relations interact.

By the standard definition of communication disorders—the one set off in italics just three paragraphs before this one—a temporary setback in development, for instance, such as the loss that may occur because of a childhood illness, is not necessarily indicative of a communication disorder. However, some problems should not be ignored. For instance, if a child suddenly and persistently—over a period of hours and days—stops responding to his or her own name, this is probably a sign of a deeper problem.

Defining Communication Disorders

Perhaps the most common and characteristic sign of the onset of a disorder is some sort of a **developmental regression**—a loss of previous gains where the individual seems to reach a higher level of development and then slip back to an earlier level. A dramatic loss of prior gains, for example, when a child such as Ethan Kurtz stops responding to his own name, is often the first sign of a serious problem.

In disorders such as autism, the triggering event may involve infection, poisoning, or some combination of factors affecting **metabolism** in a genetically susceptible individual (D. B. Campbell et al., 2006). Metabolism is the whole complex of processes that are involved in the uptake of nutrients and disposal of wastes, but especially it involves the processes that occur at the biochemical level.

In disorders such as autism, the triggering event may involve infection, poisoning, or some combination of factors affecting **metabolism** in a genetically susceptible individual (D. B. Campbell et al., 2006).

Parent Reports

Parents of children with autism often note that a series of vaccinations, antibiotics, an illness, or some combination of these has pushed their normally developing child over the edge (McCarthy, 2007). Dr. Bryan Jepson (see Jepson & J. Johnson, 2007) refers to such a series of events as leading to the "toxic tipping point" after which a cascade of problems begins (p. 46). Also see the Foreword to Jepson and J. Johnson (2007) by Katie Wright telling about her son's descent into autism. According to a recent study (Woo et al., 2007) of 31 adverse vaccine reactions reported according to guidelines laid down by law, 87% were diagnosed with autism and 61% showed the sort of regression described by parents of children with autism such as Jon Shestack, Jenny McCarthy, Stan Kurtz, and thousands of others.

As more is understood about our systems of metabolism as they interact with our genetics, digestion, bodily defenses, and disposal of poisons, figuring out communication disorders seems to be crucial to understanding how our bodies work in general at a biochemical level. Communication disorders are especially indicative of and susceptible to injuries that impact and are impacted by our biochemistry.

Many metabolic diseases are linked to environmental **toxins**—that is, to poisons that injure the body at the atomic and molecular level of the infrasystems that support and sustain our normal communication abilities. In this introduction we will see why it is essential to recognize that environmental toxins are a major part of the upsurge in communication disorders and neurological disease conditions that continue to rise exponentially in the 21st century (e.g., see J. W. Oller, & S. D. Oller, 2009). Among the worst offenders, in fact, as we have shown elsewhere, and as we will also see in this book, are certain known toxins that are being injected and/or ingested into our bodies through medicines, vaccines, dental fillings, food preservatives, and pesticides. Among the toxins contributing to the upsurge especially in diseases and disorders is the

To see how damaging that mercury can be, see the video titled How Mercury Damages Nerve Fibrils on the DVD (Leong, Syed, & Lorscheider, 2001).

heavy metal mercury in all its forms. Although there is considerable political controversy about mercury in vaccines, medicines, and **dental amalgam** (International Academy of Oral Medicine and Toxicology, n.d.), the toxicology is unambiguous and the research evidence is clear—mercury is a potent neurotoxin in parts per billion and is lethal in parts per million (U.S. EPA, "Mercury Compounds," 2000, retrieved March 20, 2009, from http://www.epa.gov/ttn/atw/hlthef/mercury.html).

The damage done by mercury in minute quantities at the molecular level results in the causation and/or worsening of many metabolic diseases and disorders. Interestingly, over half of the world's industrial mercury is in the mouths of human beings put there by well-meaning dentists who used it to fill cavities (Barr, 2004, retrieved March 20, 2009, from http://www.epa.gov/region5/air/mercury/meetings/Nov04/barr.pdf). On average, dental mercury accounts for well over half of the body burden of mercury in the human population (Aposhian et al., 1992). We will have a great deal more to say about the role of toxins in general, and mercury in particular, throughout the rest of the book.

Contrary to some theories of development that try to make disorders out to be normal, they would not be called "disorders" if they were the expected norm. Multiple bodily systems are out of balance in communication disorders and the disease conditions that produce them. Autism, **Alzheimer's disease (AD)**, **Parkinson's disease (PD)**, and so forth are examples. Jepson says that it makes about as much sense to call autism "a developmental disorder" as to call "a brain tumor a headache" (p. 44). It is important to differentiate the causes and nature of the various diseases, injuries, and disorders that produce communication disorders in order to get the diagnosis right and to provide effective treatment.

Disorders Show That Communication Normally Succeeds

Studies of communication disorders invariably begin from the underlying assumption that successful communication is usual, typical, normal, and desirable. By contrast, disorders are *neither* expected *nor* desired. In ordinary communication, things go well. We promise to meet people for coffee at a particular location and the various parties show up as agreed. We offer our credit or debit card to the clerk and the transaction goes through as expected. We put the letter in the mail on one side of the world, or we launch it through the Internet, and the intended person receives it miles away. We dial a series of numbers on our phone and we get connected with the person, or the voice mail of the person we wanted to talk to. We click on a URL and the link often takes us to the site we wanted to visit. We board a taxi, boat, train, or plane for a distant destination and, usually, we arrive there safe and sound. We tell someone what we experienced or what we are thinking and usually the other person understands much, if not all, of what we mean. Even when communication becomes difficult, because of noise, or disagreements, quarrels, and the like, the people involved often, though not always, understand whatever it is that they are in disagreement about. Even in difficult situations, success in communication is common.

We often understand what is going on in the world and we often communicate successfully with each other. The physicist Albert Einstein [1879–1955] agreed with the philosopher Immanuel Kant [1724–1804] that our ability to understand the universe is "a miracle" (1936/1956, p. 61). C. S. Peirce [1839–1906] stated the essential implication of that "miracle" in 1908 by insisting that the comprehensibility of the universe is evidence of the existence of an Almighty God. Some disagree with Peirce's conclusion, but even in disagreeing they demonstrate that *communication usually succeeds*. That is, disagreeing with any argument implies that we understand it at least to some extent. In fact, disagreement presupposes that communication can and often does succeed.

> When we consider how many things can go wrong, it is unsurprising that communication sometimes fails. In the light of all the things that can go wrong, what is surprising is that *communication usually succeeds*.

When Lives Hang in the Balance

To see just how common successful communication is, consider air transportation as an example. (see Boeing, 2007, retrieved March 20, 2009, from http://www.boeing.com/news/techissues/pdf/statsum.pdf). Extrapolating to the present year, 2009, the Boeing research shows that on the average about 50,000 jet aircraft of more than 60,000 pounds in weight (excluding only military planes) are departing from some airport every day. The vast majority of them arrive safely at their intended destinations. The same source shows that from 1970 to 2004 there were about 35,800 flights per day of the big nonmilitary jets. During that time, there were a total of 1,402 accidents with damage to the aircraft and 517 accidents that involved one or more fatalities. If we estimate that each flight depends on, say, about 100 successful exchanges of information between flight crews and ground personnel—an exceedingly low estimate for commercial jets carrying passengers and freight—there were about 43,435,000,000 communications of which fewer than one in 10 million resulted in an accident with damage to the plane and only about 1 in 100 million resulted in a fatal accident. We must suppose that all the rest of the communications on which flight safety depends were more or less successful. This means that billions of specific communications on which successful flights depend are successful every day, or at least they do not lead to any noteworthy incidents or accidents.

Communication Problems Cause Accidents

Continuing with international aviation as an example, when we consider the cases where a difficulty, near miss, or a fatal accident does occur, it also comes out, unsurprisingly, that unsuccessful communications are the most common cause. The reported difficulties were much less often due to lack of skill of those flying the plane, the crew's knowledge of procedures and equipment, or the reliability of the equipment including the aircraft, the runway, and so on. Rather, in the vast majority of cases, the difficulties were caused by failures to understand ordinary communications (R. Yan, 2007). In 28,000 incidents reported between 1982 and 1991, more than 70% of losses in property, injuries, and fatalities could be attributed to communication problems (Ritter, 1996; Tajima, 2004). The most vulnerable link, according to the International Civil Aviation Organization (2004), is the one between the pilots in the air and air traffic controllers on the ground. Lives throughout the whole of the aviation industry, and in all other high-risk industries, depend on successful communication.

It is reassuring to air travelers that data from 1959 to 2004 show a dramatic decline in accidents in spite of the fact that the number of flights of the big jets was steadily increasing. Daily departures nearly tripled during the study period (R. Yan, 2007). The downward trend of accidents combined with the upward trend of numbers of flights shows that communication in the air transportation industries is becoming more and more reliable worldwide. All of this shows that communication is important, that it usually succeeds, and that it can be improved by focusing our attention on communication itself and on the ways that communication sometimes goes awry.

Early Diagnosis and Timely Intervention

Sometimes a wait-and-see attitude is advisable, but in many cases—for example, where poisoning is known to be a factor, the wait and see approach can be a sure method of worsening, prolonging, or even causing communication disorders. Because of the inevitable costs—physical, emotional, social, and material—getting the diagnosis early and getting it right are high priorities.

As we will see throughout this book, early diagnosis and timely intervention are key factors in minimizing the severity and in some cases altogether preventing or curing a problem. Sometimes a wait-and-see attitude is advisable, but in many cases—for example, where poisoning is known to be a factor, the wait-and-see approach can be a sure method of worsening, prolonging, or even causing communication disorders.

If communication is wonderful, it follows that its loss is not good. In fact, any loss or difficulty that threatens our ability to share experience is undesirable. An individual's disability not only affects that one person, but because of the social nature of communication, it also impacts the persons who interact with the person affected. Communication disorders tend to reach out in spreading waves to touch those who study alongside, who work with, who teach, or otherwise normally communicate with anyone affected by one or more communication disorders. Ultimately, communication disorders affect the whole community of human beings. A loss to one of us is a loss to all just as the success of one of us is of benefit to all of us. The normal response is to try to restore, or perhaps to establish for the first time, what John Locke (2001) has termed "communion."

The loss of any ability to see, hear, feel, taste, and smell the world around us, or the loss of any ability to share experiences and emotions with others, is potentially a great loss. The loss of ability to move or carry out sequences of movements or the loss of any ability to use language, to think, talk, or write, or to understand others, is a great loss. We depend on communication with others through language to learn who we are, to discover our own names, the names of our family members, and to find out the identities of our parents and grandparents, our children, and grandchildren. We depend on communication to succeed in school, to get a job, to buy and sell, to own property, to get a driver's license, to use a credit card or a checkbook. In the case of fundamental communication disorders that interfere with the abilities we usually take for granted, the loss can be emotionally, financially, and physically draining.

Classification and Diagnosis of Disorders

Four major classes of communication disorders can be discerned on the basis of the sign systems affected: (1) bodily, (2) sensory, (3) sensory-motor, and (4) sensory-motor-linguistic. We will discuss these four classes of disorders in this order here and in following chapters.

Disorders are diagnosed and classified in three main ways. First, difficulties are noticed, diagnosed, and classified by their **symptomology**. How does the disorder in question affect the appearance, behavior, and/or abilities of the individual affected? Symptoms can be roughly divided into those that mainly affect the body in terms of its appearance and structure, sensations, movements, and its genetics and neurophysiology, feelings, moods, and behavior, and language, cognition, and mental abilities.

Second, difficulties can be classified with respect to recommended therapy. What is commonly done, if anything, to prevent, lessen, halt, or possibly cure the problem? Treatments are typically undertaken by different professionals or sometimes teams of them. They may include surgery in some cases, medicines aimed at improving body chemistry and/or removal of toxins, dietary regimens with a similar purpose, and physical or behavioral therapies aimed at improving range of motion, swallowing, **articulation**, gesturing, comprehension, intelligibility, and so forth. In some cases, the goal is merely to keep the condition from getting worse.

Third, difficulties may be classified by their supposed **etiology**. What are the suspected or known causes of the condition or problem? In fact, all the major ways of classifying communication disorders look ultimately to their causes. Underlying all of our discussion of such disorders is the presupposition that communication is both possible and desirable.

Major classes of communication disorders can be discerned on the basis of the sign systems affected: (1) bodily, (2) sensory, (3) sensory-motor, and (4) sensory-motor linguistic.

The associations that enable language to work are **conventional**. They depend on the way linguistic signs are used. Conventions of use link arbitrary symbols to whatever they may represent—just as a name, for instance, is associated with whatever it is used to name.

COMMUNICATION

We define communication as any interaction where information is transferred or exchanged between persons, organisms, or the parts of a system (even a computer, or a single person's mind or body) that relies on sign systems, or representations of any kind. Representations themselves are signs that are used to stand for things, persons, events, or relations between any of these. They may include sensations, actions, words, or sequences and combinations of any and all of these. Information is the abstract meaning that is validly associated with any representation. Of course, it is possible to associate anything with any representation whatever, but random associations cannot be informative or meaningful. With sign systems, the only kind of associations that count are those that are reliable and valid.

Conventional signs depend for their meaning on how ever they may be commonly used. This is all that is meant by the term "conventional" and it is the key distinctive quality of the signs of a particular language. In this book, we use the terms "representation" and "sign" almost interchangeably except that a representation is a sign that is applied to represent some particular meaning whereas a sign can be a sign without being applied—for example, the word "the" in quotes here in this sentence is just a sign and in this case represents only itself.

The Book in Your Hand as a Representation

This book is a representation and it consists almost exclusively of other representations. By writing this book, the authors communicate with other persons whom we cannot see, hear, or perceive in any way at this moment. By reading it, you make contact with us though you cannot perceive us just now. Our connection is only through abstract representations—words, diagrams, pictures, and other marks—that we present to you through these pages. That is how we are communicating even now as you read these words.

Except for its material pages and the accompanying plastic DVD-ROM, the book you are reading (and its DVD) only consist of three kinds of representations: (1) First, there are the words that refer to persons, research papers, theories, methods, diagrams, pictures, videos, the DVD itself, and one or more copies of the book itself. (2) Second, the book and the DVD consist of diagrams, lists (the References, the Glossary, the Index, this list), and illustrations that show complex relations between words and bodily persons, things, events, research papers, journals, other books, other authors, and combinations of all these. (3) Third, the book also consists of Web sites, still and moving pictures, and sounds that represent bodily persons, things, events, and their relations. Some of the pictures and sounds are contained in the pages of the book or on the DVD. Others will only be imagined by the reader, and yet the whole interaction between us is dependent almost completely on representations plus a little bit of paper, plastic, a few computers, and our separate material bodies.

The book itself with the accompanying DVD *is* a representation and consists *almost exclusively* of representations. Without the particular representations that its authors have created, this particular book would not exist at all. Paper pages and plastic disks by themselves could not constitute the book you are reading. A hundred million copies of blank pages and the blank disks could not make this particular book. To be the book that it is, it must contain the words that its authors wrote and that you are now reading. But representations alone do not result in communication. In order to result in communication, the representations have to be connected to things—persons, event sequences, and experiences—other than themselves. Printed words are representations but they do not produce communication unless someone interprets them. An unreadable inscription in an unknown language that is never deciphered cannot be said to communicate anything in particular. It may be about particular persons, events, and experiences, but until the writing is interpreted (correctly) by someone, the inscription might as well be a random sequence of empty syllables or random marks.

To communicate through a particular language, we have to acquire the conventions of that language. We cannot understand a language by merely perceiving its **surface forms**. Strings of syllables, printed words, or manual signs are useless unless we know how they connect through conventions with their deeper meanings. The surface forms alone tell us very little.

Making Sense of Impressions

What Einstein Had to Say

Einstein argued that it is only through abstract relations between sensory impressions that we understand the world and communications about it. He argued that we understand sensory impressions (seeing, hearing, smelling, touching, and tasting) through "the creation of general concepts, relations between these concepts, and by relations between the concepts and sense experience" (1936/1956, p. 61). If Einstein was right, it follows that *all experience is itself a form of communication*.

Normal human experience involves interactions between representational systems of various kinds. Those systems of representation include the *senses*, also our abilities to act and move, and our social interactions through language. Even the communications among other species now appear to involve interactions that mirror, to

To communicate through a particular language, we have to acquire the conventions of that language. We cannot understand a language by merely perceiving its **surface forms**.

some extent, the social interactions of human beings (Hogan & Bolhuis, 2005). Of course, humans are far more adept at understanding even simple demonstrations of tool use, for example, than other species such as macaques (Rigamonti, Custance, Previde, & Spiezio, 2005) or even chimpanzees (Penn & Povinelli, 2007).

When Does Communication Begin?

If our bodies and our senses are working properly, and if our abilities to move and think are intact, we live in a world of shared voices, words, stories, knowledge, purposes, and emotions. When things are going along normally, we are always in a common world shared with other persons. Although we have memories of the past, we generally are unaware of when we came to be in the world as we know it. By studying the development of human babies, however, we can learn more about ourselves and about how and when social interaction begins to take place. Interestingly, it begins soon after conception and long before birth.

Among the early signs of social awareness, and the natural human interest in communication, is the baby's first social (genuine) smile (Figure 1–1). Commonly, this kind of smile is regarded

Among the early signs of social awareness, and the natural human interest in communication, is the baby's first social (genuine) smile (Figure 1–1).

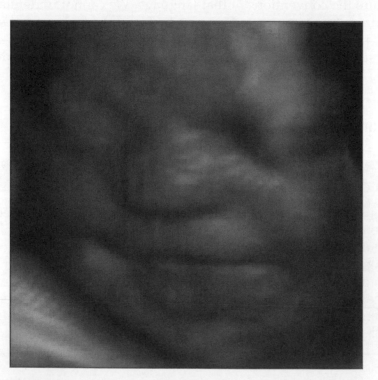

FIGURE 1–1. Baby smiling in the womb. Retrieved March 20, 2009, from London's Create Health Clinic, http://www.createhealth.org/. Copyright 2004 by Dr. Stuart Campbell. Reprinted with permission. All rights reserved.

by parents, casual observers, and communities around the world as having special significance. Social smiling is also linked, in normal cases, with an intensified interest in speech, language, and communication.

Smiling and Language as Social Actions

From early infancy, and even before birth, the human baby (see Figure 1–1) shows a clear **Duchenne-type smile**. The smile is named after Guillaume Duchenne [1806–1875] the French neurologist who became famous in part because of his descriptions of and experiments in producing facial expressions with electrical stimulation as shown in Figure 1–2. The smile of Figure 1–1 is the universal social smile with corners of the mouth upturned and eyes crinkled. It is found across all cultures, ages, and languages (Schmidt, Cohn, &

Compare the baby's smile with the artificially produced expression, perhaps of unmitigated pain, in the eyes of Dr. Duchenne's poor patient. Which of those expressions is more likely to be associated with pain?

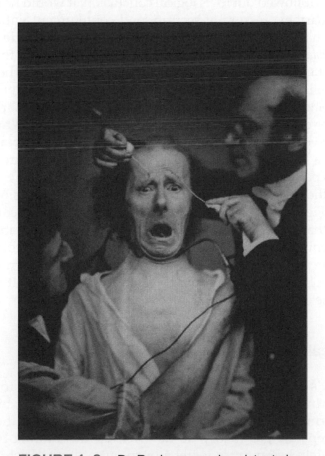

FIGURE 1–2.   Dr. Duchenne and assistant electrically stimulate the face of a patient circa 1833. Retrieved March 20, 2009, from http://en.wikipedia.org/wiki/Image:Duchenne_de_Boulogne_3.jpg. This image is in the public domain because its copyright has expired.

Tian, 2003). Before its birth the baby will not only smile but will also show its social nature by expressing special interest and enjoyment at the sound of happy voices.

Oddly, it has been widely claimed in the pediatric literature that the smile of a human infant was caused by gas pains. For a critique of that theory, see Sullivan and Lewis (2003) as well as J. W. Oller, S. D. Oller, and Badon (2006). The gas theory of infant smiling is charmingly embraced by Dr. David Feinberg, the Medical Director of the Resnick Neuropsychiatric Hospital at UCLA. In the Foreword to McCarthy (2007), he writes that babies smile "likely because they have gas" (p. xi). Let's examine that idea critically.

The "Gas Theory of Smiling"

It is amazing, if you think about it, that the **gas theory of smiling** was ever accepted and promoted by so many pediatricians. If it had only been followed out to its logical conclusion, it would have linked the ordinary expression of security and contentment with pain. It ought to have caused pediatricians and others to conclude that *pain causes babies to smile* though as they grow up they learn to grimace at pain. But, of course, neither of these statements is true. Such a conclusion would make nonsense of any reasonable understanding of how emotions normally work. Gas pains do not ordinarily cause babies, or children, or adolescents, or adults to smile. Why should anyone ever have believed that gas pains would cause a baby to produce a Duchenne-type smile—the kind seen in Figure 1–1?

Gas pain would be more likely to produce a facial expression such as the one seen in Figure 1–2. About all the expressions of the baby in Figure 1–1 and the adult in Figure 1–2 have in common is the fact that Duchenne described them both in considerable detail. In the genuine smile, he noted, the eyes crinkle at the corners, the cheeks are raised, and the lips spread and corners turn upward. In Figure 1–1 the smile dimples the baby's right cheek. It is clearly a genuine smile.

Empirically Testing the Theory

If a baby's smile were a sign of gas pains adults ought to comfort the baby by trying to get him or her to burp or pass gas, but that is not a normal reaction of adults to a baby's smile. Even those folks who accept the gas theory do not pick up the smiling baby and immediately begin to try to get a burp out of it or to get it to pass gas because it is smiling. Even the pediatricians who suggested the idea and helped to promote the gas pains theory never suggested that to get babies to smile you should give them gas producing foods, or that when they smile you should immediately hold them upright and pat them on the back.

You can see that same smile in a moving picture on the DVD by clicking on the Video of an Unborn Baby.

It is amazing, if you think about it, that the **gas theory of smiling** was ever accepted and promoted by so many pediatricians.

However, there is one good thing to be learned from the gas pains theory of smiling. It is that some theories, although often repeated by a great many people over a very long period of time, can still be very false no matter how many people believe them to be true. For that reason, it is best to examine the facts and think through the implications of every theory. With the gas theory of smiling as the test case, consider some relevant facts that you can assess by observation.

When adults see a baby smile, what do they actually do in response? Even if the baby is a total stranger, or say, a baby still in its mother's womb (as in Figure 1–1), one that we only see in a photograph, we tend to smile back at the baby. Why is this? Is it because, for instance, we identify with the baby's gas pains? Hardly. When a real live baby smiles at us, we almost invariably smile back and we do so almost immediately. By smiling we reassure one another of our humanity, of our common understanding, and of our shared existence. The adult shows recognition of the infant's innocence, friendliness, and dependence on the good will of others for its own well-being. The returned smile, supposing only that it is genuine, is a social reassurance of sharing and of consideration for the other person. By smiling at the baby, we indicate something like, "Hey! I see you smiling at me! I'm smiling back at you! I see you're a little helpless human being! I recognize you as one of us! I am like you! I will not hurt you! I am your friend! I will be gentle with you and you are safe with me!"

> By smiling at the baby, we indicate something like, "Hey! I see you smiling at me! I'm smiling back at you! I see you're a little helpless human being! I recognize you as one of us! I am like you! I will not hurt you! I am your friend! I will be gentle with you and you are safe with me!"

Smiling as a Social Act

Smiling is a distinctly social act. When the adult naturally smiles back at an infant's smile, the reaction might *almost* be a **reflex**, a kind of action that does not normally come under conscious control. Reflexes include such involuntary movements as the knee jerk caused by tapping the knee when the leg is bent and dangling in a relaxed way; the **startle response**, laughter, or vomiting.

Smiling is different. It is certainly not a mere reflex. It involves consciousness and is commonly connected with voluntary social interaction. The research shows that it takes just long enough for an adult to smile back at an infant for conscious recognition of the social act of the baby's smile to have occurred in the mind of the adult (D. K. Oller, Eilers, & Basinger, 2001, p. 50). Also, with effort, an adult can just barely stifle the tendency to smile back at the infant (if the adult is ornery enough to attempt this; we ourselves have not attempted it).

Ordinarily, we sense the friendliness, security, and trust in the baby's smile, and when we reciprocate the smile, we indicate that the baby's acceptance of us as human beings is not misplaced trust. We say something like, "Yep! You're okay with me and I'm okay with you." We acknowledge the existence and the humanity of the

Moms or other caregivers are more apt to speak or sign to a baby when the baby is smiling, and vice versa (D'Entremont, B., & Muir, D., 1999; Masataka, 2003).

baby by smiling back. We agree with the baby that we are both human and that all is well between the two of us.

Smiling, Imitation, and Language Are Linked

Relevant research shows that smiling in humans, and all our distinctly social forms of imitative behavior, are intrinsically involved with speech and/or with other forms of social signing. Moms or other caregivers are more apt to speak or sign to a baby when the baby is smiling, and vice versa (D'Entremont, B., & Muir, D., 1999; Masataka, 2003). Also, from before birth and by all accounts after birth (Condon & Sander, 1974), human babies have a special interest in speech (Nazzi, Bertoncini, & Mehler, 1998).

Condon and his colleagues claimed that infants at birth begin to match the rhythms in the speech of the adults that they happen to hear speaking. That is, the human baby moves its body in cadence with the rhythms of the speech of adults that it hears somewhat as if the infant and the speaking adult were on the same train and on the same track being pulled by the same engine. For all these reasons, the term **entrainment** has been widely adopted to refer to the coordination of the baby's rhythms with adult speech ever since Condon and Sander (1974) first published their findings about this phenomenon. With high resolution motion pictures and a sound track, they showed a tendency for infants to move their bodies in rhythm with the speech sounds and syllables of adults the baby could hear. Although their results were not easy to replicate, sound theory and research show beyond any reasonable doubt that coordination of movements is crucial to the acquisition of any language, including the sign systems of the Deaf[1] (Petitto & Marentette, 1991).

Language as the Highest Form of Imitation

What is more, speech, or other forms of language (including writing and **manual signs**), are obviously the most advanced and distinctive forms of imitative behaviors in any species. The research shows that infants direct more visual attention and smile more when adults imitate the baby's actions. The baby responds with less interest when the adult invents a new action rather than imitating the one performed by the baby (Meltzoff & C. A. Moore, 1997). If the baby sticks out its tongue and the adult does the same,

[1]When the word "Deaf" is written with a capital letter as it is here, we intend to refer to the whole community, or the communities in general of individuals who are deaf. Similarly, when we use the terms "White" or "Black" with capitalization, we intend to refer to whole communities of persons in the sense of ethnicity or race. We aim to follow this principle as consistently as possible throughout the book.

for instance, the baby is more apt to smile than if the adult does something different such as opening the eyes wide, blinking, or opening the mouth. Babies are more responsive when the adult enters the social game of imitation by smiling, making faces, sticking out the tongue, opening the mouth wide, protruding the lower lip, widening the eyes, and so on.

Similarly, the research also shows that adults are more apt to interact verbally with a babbling infant that produces speech-like sounds than one that merely burps or coughs or produces no sound at all (Masataka, 1995; Masataka & Bloom, 1994). As the child becomes more adept at imitating and producing the surface forms of language—whether in speech, manual signs, or written ones—intentional and volitional linguistic acts with the child increase (Gutierrez & Lopez, 2005). People talk more and interact more when mutual understanding is achieved.

From the very beginning and throughout life, human experience is essentially social, communicative, linguistic, and imitative. We tend to accommodate the expressions, moods, and gestures of the people we are with (Chartrand & Bargh, 1999). In fact, normal human experience depends greatly if not entirely on our abilities to communicate with each other.

> From the very beginning and throughout life, human experience is essentially social, communicative, linguistic, and imitative.

THE DISTINCTLY HUMAN LANGUAGE CAPACITY

We share the world with each other mainly through our words, signs, symbols, and stories. Our experience is essentially social and its foundations are anchored in the human language capacity. So far, *only humans* have shown the ability not only to invent, understand, and use arbitrary systems of symbols (words, phrases, sentences, and so on) that are completely general and fully abstract, but to pass them on to their offspring (Fitch, 2005; Kako, 1999; J. W. Oller, 2002; Shanker, Savage-Rumbaugh, & Taylor, 1999). Although complex systems of signals are used by many species and humans can teach some species of apes, monkeys, dolphins, and birds systems of arbitrary symbols, only human beings seem to have the capacity to teach arbitrary symbols to their offspring and, to a lesser extent, to other species.

Birds Can Do Surface Forms

Parrots, such as the now famous Grey Parrot, Alex, trained by Irene Pepperberg, can acquire a high degree of accuracy in producing the surface-forms of speech in one or more languages (Pepperberg, 1999). Alex's trainers have even claimed that he not only understands numbers but abstract concepts such as zero (Pepperberg & Gordon, 2005). There is no doubt that parrots and mynah birds and a few other species can produce the surface forms of speech—that is, the sounds, syllables, rhythms, and **intonations**, with considerable accuracy. They can also imitate vocal sounds that have little to do with speech, such as coughing, wheezing, burping, and other so-called **vegetative** sounds.

One of our students had a parrot that imitated her grandfather's coughing and wheezing from **emphysema**—a chronic obstructive lung disease that is tobacco linked, see Figure 5–9. The parrot was so accurate in its imitation that visiting friends and relatives sometimes thought grandpa was still in the back bedroom, long after grandpa had departed this world. Research suggests that, in the imitation of speech sounds, birds rely on a different region of the brain than is used for their songs (Bolhuis & Gahr, 2006). It is interesting to ask, therefore, as those authors do, whether the speech of parrots and other talking birds primarily involves the equivalent of the hearing **cortex**, or whether it involves that portion of the brain used for songs. The latter, in birds, is believed by some to parallel to the human cortex devoted to language and speech (or manual sign) production. Interestingly, however, birds don't try to communicate with each other by imitating human speech and they don't teach it to baby birds. They just sing their usual songs or make their usual bird calls.

Substantial Understanding of Meaning?

Species and Speech

By contrast to birds, dolphins, chimps, and gorillas do not do so well in producing the surface-forms of speech—but, like elephants, dolphins, some dogs, and other intelligent mammals—they can be taught to understand many complex speech forms and gestural signs (Kako, 1999; Savage-Rumbaugh & Lewin, 1994.

Gorillas, chimps, and bonobos in particular are able to acquire some meaningful signs similar to those used in so-called manual languages or signed languages. Bonobos, according to some researchers, notably Savage-Rumbaugh and colleagues, can produce recognizable vocalizations of words. Although the signs of such highly intelligent animals are similar in form to those used by the Deaf or possibly by very young children, the signs used by "great apes" taught by humans are simpler, less general, less abstract, and less reliable in their applications than the linguistic signs applied by normal human children (Goldin-Meadow, 1996; F. Patterson &

Linden, 1981; Penn & Povinelli, 2007; Povinelli, 1994; Premack & Woodruff, 1978; Sebeok & Umiker-Sebeok, 1980; Visetti & Rosenthal, 2002). They also seem to lack the critical quality of being shared by a community through language.

Claims made on behalf of Kanzi, the bonobo (Savage-Rumbaugh & Lewin, 1994), suggest that great apes can learn to understand and use more of a human language than previously thought. Kanzi and other apes, according to the homepage of the Great Ape Trust of Iowa (retrieved March 20, 2009 from, http://www.greatapetrust .com/research/index.php), "have the capacity to learn language." However, the most recently published research on the subject shows bonobos demonstrating abilities well short of the human language capacity. We are reminded of Chomsky's remark in the Managua Lectures that it would be amazing if there is a species of ape that has had the capacity to acquire and use human languages all along "but has never thought to use it until instructed by humans" (1988, p. 38). For this reason, Chomsky says the attempts to teach language to chimpanzees and gorillas "have failed" (p. 38). Butofskaya (2005)—among others—seems more hopeful in saying that "at least, some apes (Kanzi, Panbanisha, and others) are able to rate symbols by **semantic function** and possess some rudiments of **grammar**. Apes can associate concepts with arbitrary symbols but they have a limited mastery of **syntax**. Their linguistic abilities are comparable to those in very young children who [are] begin[ning] to acquire language" (p. 149).

Taglialatela, Savage-Rumbaugh, and Baker (2003) are bolder in claiming that bonobos—Kanzi in particular in addition to the "raspberry" or "the extended grunt" (Hopkins, Taglialatela, & Leavens, 2007, p. 281) used to attract human attention—are also able to produce vocalizations that resemble those of a human being speaking English. At any rate, it is true that humans can produce raspberries and extended grunts. Benson et al. (2004) followed up with additional analysis claiming that "an English speaking human interpreter" is able "to recognize English words in the distinctly non-human sounds emitted by a language competent bonobo engaged in discourse with the human" (p. 643). But so far, a bonobo's history of his parents or grandparents, or a monologue about a day in the life of an ape, or any similar discourse, is still in the realm of science fiction.

The apes come up well short of what is expected of a normal 3-year-old human child.

What Only Humans Do with Language

The child can ask questions, make comments on comments, understand a story about a story about a story, and so forth, negate, disagree, and talk about events past and future. The apes don't do any of these things.

A distinctive quality of human languages is that they are evidently applicable to any meaning in any context whatever—whether in experience, imagination, or impossible fantasy. For example, we cannot really construct a good concrete image of "a true square that is also a circle," or "a contradiction that doesn't contradict," and so on. Such things, if they exist at all, are unimaginable even though we can create phrases to refer to them. As remarkable as the achievements of other species may be, there are no known systems of representation other than human languages that enable such a high degree of **abstractness** and **generality**.

When we say languages are general, we mean that they can be applied to refer to anything at all, to nothing, to imaginable things, and to unimaginable ones. Languages are by an infinite margin the most abstract and generally applicable systems of representation that are known. When we say they are abstract, we emphasize the fact that we don't have to carry objects around to display representations of them. We can use words to refer to objects. We don't have to produce an explosion to talk about one. Words are abstract as contrasted with concrete entities that have mass and that are sensible in some way. We can say, write, or otherwise create a surface form of a word to make it perceivable, but the words "star" and "light" are the same words with the same meaning even when we are not producing any surface forms of them at all. For all these reasons, the generality and abstractness of language are, without any reasonable dispute, the most distinctive aspects of human communication.

MULTIPLE LAYERS OF REPRESENTATION: GENOME TO BRAIN

Disorders provide a natural laboratory for the study of the representational systems undergirding our abilities and processes of communication.

Although communication does commonly succeed, in those instances where it fails the invisible layers of representational systems on which normal communication depends often become evident. As a result, communication disorders—including all those caused by toxins, disease, physical injuries, emotional distress, or any other source—can reveal important facts about how representational systems normally work.

Four Major Systems

There are at least four major divisions of representational systems out of which human experience is constructed. These are diagramed in Figure 1–3. Successful human communication normally depends on all four systems working together. They are (1) *the bodily systems* from our genetics up to the brain—the whole material body itself; (2) *our sensory systems*—enabling us to see, hear, smell, touch, and taste; (3) *our motor systems* that enable us to move and act on the external world; and (4) *our higher cognitive systems* that integrate and

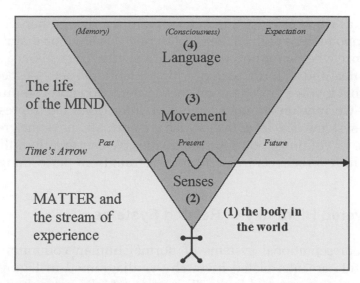

FIGURE 1–3. A diagram of our representational systems: (1) The body, (2) senses, (3) movement, and (4) language.

make sense of all the other systems under the guidance of language and the reasoning abilities that come with it. As we move upward in the layers of interrelated sign systems, each higher system includes the lower one(s) and, as we will see, is very well integrated with them. As we progress up through the levels, the systems increasingly come under **volitional control**. That is, we are able to choose to do them or not to do them on our whim. They come under the control of our own free will.

Free Will—Volition—Is Back

As we move upward in the layers of interrelated sign systems, each higher system includes the lower one(s) and, as we will see, is very well integrated with them. As we progress up through the levels, the systems increasingly come under **volitional control**.

A Nobel Laureate's View

As Roger W. Sperry [1913-1994] put it in his lecture of 1981 on receiving the Nobel Prize for Medicine, we must assign our intentions "an integral causal control role in brain function and behavior" (retrieved March 20, 2009, from http://nobel prize.org/nobel_prizes/medicine/laureates/1981/sperry-lecture.html).

In other words, we learn from studies of language and the human brain that we do have something that must be called "free will."

Although there are some processes of which we have no knowledge—for example, in our genes and metabolism which we cannot consciously influence by willing them to be other than however they may be—we can normally influence to a very high degree, such things as whether we get up at 6 AM or 10 AM, or whether we keep that appointment with Dr. Bernard or not. It is obvious that we can influence whether or not we flip a light switch, or swallow a sip of hot coffee, and so forth. In performing intentional acts—especially ones that involve or depend on social interaction and communication—we rely on multiple layers of interconnected representational systems. The layer over which we normally have the greatest degree of volitional control is language. We can greatly influence just which verbal acts we perform or refrain from performing.

A Layered Hierarchy of Related Systems

> The representational systems of normal human communication constitute an interrelated **hierarchy** as diagramed in Figure 1–3.

The representational systems of normal human communication constitute an interrelated **hierarchy** as diagramed in Figure 1–3. Each system portrayed in the diagram is actually a deeply layered system of systems. At the bottom of the triangle, contained within the schematic that represents the body, are the representational systems known as the senses. The next system of systems consists of movement abilities, followed by mental capacities and language at the top. Just below the center of the diagram running across from left to right is what Isaac Asimov, the famed scientist and fiction author, called "time's arrow."

It has commonly been observed that time seems to flow like a river going downhill. Both time and the river tend to go only in one direction. Time, unlike some rivers, can never (not in our world at least), flow backward. Time, as the diagram shows, is roughly divisible into the past—to the left of the triangle; the present—represented by the wavy line within the triangle; and the future—represented by the continuation of time's arrow to the right of the triangle. This flow of time is important in many different ways, and it forms the basis for our experience unfolding like a story where one thing follows another. We will see that this temporal unfolding is crucial to language, to planning, and to every kind of skilled movement as seen in speaking, writing, or manual signing.

THE ANATOMY OF THE MAJOR SYSTEMS OF REPRESENTATION

In discussing the anatomy of sign systems, we begin with the body itself. It is curious that the anatomy of signs, like the anatomy of the whole body, is contained within the deepest and most abstract sign system other than human language that we know of so far. The distinct human language capacity and all of the physiological systems on which it depends, especially the human brain and nervous system, must be prespecified to a very high degree within our genetic material.

Bodily Systems

In recent years we have learned much at the limits of the representational systems grounded in our bodies. At one pole of the universe of representations, we have the atoms and molecules that form the basic biochemicals of our own genetic systems. At the opposite pole we find the fully developed bodies of human beings in all of our diversity with all of our unique behavioral, cognitive, social, and especially linguistic abilities. We also find within living human beings a neurological system that is presided over by a brain that is known to be the center of control of voluntary movements, reasoning, social interactions, and especially of the acquisition and use of language.

Genetics and Biochemical Systems.

The human **genome** is common to all human beings although it is expressed differently in the individuals of our species. It provides for all the bodily systems and their higher functions. It consists of a sequence of molecular words called **codons** arranged in a highly compacted format, which allows the entire library of specifications for an individual organism—we human beings ourselves being the organisms of greatest interest to ourselves—into a space that is much tinier than the visible eye of a needle. The entire genome is packed into every cell in our bodies with most of the genetic material being found in the nucleus of each cell.

If we look into the system of representations contained in the genome, we find layer upon layer of embedded representations of astonishing depth, complexity, and articulate organization. As science has continued to penetrate more and more deeply into the physical universe of bodily systems of representation, the range of what is known and what can be actually viewed has greatly increased.

Bodily systems include the vast and intensive representational systems involved in genetics, the molecular biochemical systems of ordinary metabolism, the bodily defenses found in our **immune systems**, tissue maintenance and repair systems (both preventing and healing injuries), and the **autonomic nervous system** that controls many aspects of the beating of our hearts, breathing, swallowing, digestion, and elimination. Bodily systems also include the biological electrochemical processes that integrate the communications between molecular systems, cells, tissues, and all the organs of the whole body. They include the **detoxification systems** that normally remove poisonous substances from our bodies. As we will see throughout this book, damage to any of these systems can lead to and/or exacerbate communication breakdowns and disorders.

If the damage is caused by a sudden and shocking injury it is commonly referred to as **trauma** or a **traumatic injury**. A traumatic event, of course, is one where physical, emotional, or psychological distress or harm is caused. However, injuries to the bodily systems of communication can occur gradually as well and are inevitably

If we look into the system of representations contained in the genome, we find layer upon layer of embedded representations of astonishing depth, complexity, and articulate organization.

Regulatory processes that are controlled by our brains and our glandular systems can influence the functioning of every organ in the body.

Bodily representational systems are manifested in material chemical elements and structures of great physical complexity, for example, in the long and complex molecules of DNA, RNA, and the protein structures that constitute our cells, organs, brains, and our bodies.

cumulative over time. The interactions between the basic bodily systems are astonishingly complex. The balances are delicate and so completely interconnected that an imbalance in a protein that is not properly digested or manufactured by the body, for example, can impact our brains and our whole outlook, even our mental capabilities and social relations (Rodriguez et al., 2005). The reverse is also true. Regulatory processes that are controlled by our brains and our glandular systems can influence the functioning of every organ in the body. The lack or absence of a **neurotransmitter**—an element at the molecular level—in the nervous system can impact all the other bodily systems (see Conti-Fine, Milani, & Kaminski, 2006; also see Figure 5–3 and discussion there). The regulatory processes of metabolism and communication are dependent on interactions at the atomic level.

Bodily representational systems are manifested in material chemical elements and structures of great physical complexity, for example, in the long and complex molecules of DNA, RNA, and the protein structures that constitute our cells, organs, brains, and our bodies. The molecular representational systems not only consist of long strings of what may be thought of as words, phrases, and sentences of distinct interrelated language systems, but the strings of complex representations also are folded and arranged in dynamic three-dimensional structures that are mapped onto other structures. The layered systems of representation are structured much the way the words, phrases, and sentences of a language are fitted together with changing facial expressions, gestures, and other intentional actions to make sense of the stream of experience.

Logically, we must suppose that the representational systems specifying the molecules, cells, tissues, and organs of the whole human body together with all its amazing capacities, cannot be less complex than the body itself. It follows, then, that the full complexities of all the human capacities must first be contained in the genome. Fitch, Hauser, and Chomsky (2005) have offered some speculations as to how the special design of the language faculty could come about by random mutations and natural selection. In responding to their critics, they complain about the "the adaptive storytelling and **phylogenetic speculation** [hypothetical relations between man and apes] that has traditionally characterized the field" (p. 179).

Figure 1–4 is a diagram from the Human Genome Project showing a glimpse of the human DNA molecule (retrieved March 20, 2009, from http://www.ornl.gov/sci/techresources/Human_Genome/project/info.shtml#basics). The figure summarizes the processes beginning prior to conception and leading upward from the genome itself to the protein structures that form the basis for our cells, organs, and our whole bodies. The genome is a long molecule consisting of approximately 3 billion pairs of just four chemical bases—adenine, cytosine, guanine, and thymine. These are abbreviated simply as A, C, G, and T. The pairs in DNA consist of adenine with thymine (AT) and guanine with cytosine (GC). The 3 billion

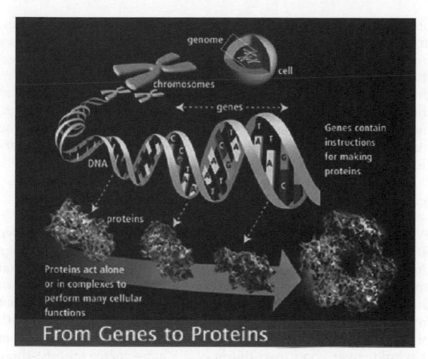

FIGURE 1–4. A diagram of our genetic basis. Retrieved March 20, 2009 from the Human GenomeProject, http://www.ornl.gov/sci/techresources/ Human_Genome/project/info.shtl_basics. U.S. Department of Energy Office of Science. Publication in the public domain.

pairs making up our genome are arranged in a linear sequence along the double spiral of DNA as shown in Figure 1–4. Recently, it has been shown that the sequence produces different results depending on whether the genome is read in one direction or the other, so the genome, in effect, consists of 6 billion base pairs (Sanford, 2005). What is more important, a huge amount of the material thought previously to be "junk DNA" has turned out to specify functional RNA molecules.

Cutting the summary of the process to its bare bones, in the construction of our bodily systems, the genes in the DNA are translated into RNA which in turn is used to build proteins. All of the complex molecules of DNA, RNA, and the proteins can be thought of as tiny but highly complex molecular engines. They are involved in such processes as communication between cells, transportation of supplies, military defenses against attackers, quarantine systems to eliminate poisons, maintenance and transportation systems to resupply healthy cells, and to repair or dismantle and dispose of dead ones.

Most of these physical systems of representation contained in those tiny engines seem to be well beyond our conscious control. They are foundational to the higher "automatic" systems that run without our conscious control. These automatic processes include what is called the autonomic nervous system. The autonomic system provides for the beating of our hearts, the involuntary functioning

It comes out that accurate and valid systems of representation are essential to our very existence all the way from the atoms at the molecular level to the highest mental functions of the human brain.

of our digestive processes, metabolism, waking and sleeping cycles, and a great deal more. However, it is known that higher cognitive processes, for example, persistent worry about a real or imagined threat, or desiring to be or accomplish something unattainable, can produce dramatic and sweeping adjustments in bodily functions at the molecular level. Thoughts and feelings can influence digestion, heart rate, blood pressure, and the overall health of the body. In some instances, they also can lead to serious communication disorders (for instance, see the story about John Forbes Nash in Chapter 10).

The Human Brain

When the genome is fully expressed in a mature human being, we find that the remarkable communication abilities of human beings depend largely volitional acts that are controlled by intentions that are most directly associated with our brains. At the highest level of the brain, we find the layer of tissue known as the "cortex." That layer is only about 4 millimeters thick—a little more than an eighth of an inch, but if it were stretched out into a two-dimensional sheet it would cover about two thirds of a square meter (almost three quarters of a square yard). To fit inside the confining space inside the skull the cortex is folded around the distinct sections of the brain in what are called convolutions. As shown in Figure 1–5, the brain is

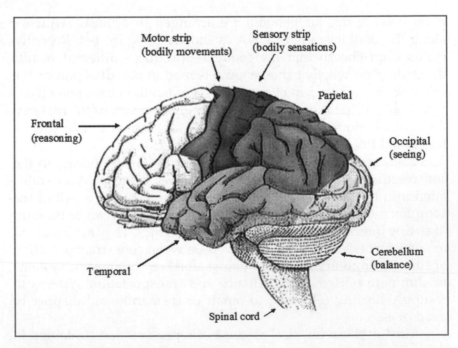

FIGURE 1–5. The major sections (lobes) of the left half of human brain along with the sensory and motor strips (viewed from the left side with the back of the brain to your right as you face the page, and the front to your left).

roughly divided into sections, or lobes, that can be associated to some extent, with different mental and representational functions.

The **frontal lobes** are known to be involved in reasoning, planning sequences of movements, higher functions of language, socialization, and, especially, abstract thinking; the **temporal lobes** are critically involved with hearing and the comprehension of language; the **parietal lobes** are involved in integrating visual information with the other sensory and motor systems; the occipital lobes are crucial to vision; and the **cerebellum** to balance, motor coordination, and the integration of information about movements flowing to and from the rest of the body through the spinal cord and its systematic branches out to the periphery. The **sensory strip**—also known as **somatosensory cortex**—and the **motor strip** are seen at the top and center of Figure 1–5. They are found at the major boundary between the frontal and parietal lobes known as the **fissure of Rolando** or more commonly today as the **central sulcus**—where "sulcus" is the Latin word meaning "trench, furrow, ditch, or wrinkle" (according to the *Oxford English Dictionary*, 1989). Luigi Rolando [1773–1831] was an Italian anatomist who supposed that distinct regions of the brain had different neurological and behavioral functions (Caputi, Spaziante, de Divitiis, & Nashold, 1995).

As shown in Figure 1–6, the sensory and motor strips of the cortex are systematically mapped onto the body. In fact, they map mostly (about 80 to 90% of their fibers) to the opposite side of the body from the hemisphere where the strips are located in the brain. That is, the strips on the left side of the brain map to the right side of the body and the strips on the right side of the brain map to the left side of the body.

In Chapter 2 we deal with disorders that affect the body itself. We see there that it is inevitable that bodily disorders, although they are commonly caused by problems in representational systems that are well below any levels over which we have conscious control, are nonetheless important to communication disorders. The body is the essential residence of the brain and the mind. As a result, bodily disorders are foundational and affect communication in an extremely general way. Also, injuries to the body even at an atomic level can impact every kind of representational system throughout the entire hierarchy shown in Figure 1–3. As we will see in the following chapters of this book, normal communication is necessarily situated in our bodies and in the real, material (physical) world of space and time.

Sensory Systems

At the first major representational level just above the body itself— a level of representation that is decidedly above the physical systems of the body itself, its metabolism, defenses, and so forth—we find the **sensory systems**. The senses, of course, consist of sight,

The sensory and motor strips of the cortex are systematically mapped onto the body. In fact, they map mostly (about 80 to 90% of their fibers) to the opposite side of the body from the hemisphere where the strips are located in the brain.

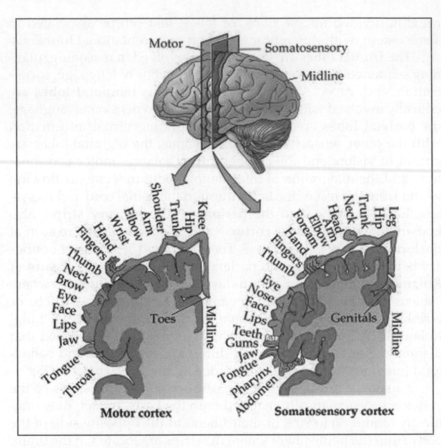

FIGURE 1–6. The mapping of the sensory and sensory-motor strips of the cortex onto the body. From Life—*The science of biology* (6th ed., Figure 49.6, p. 820) by W. K. Purves, D. Sadava, G. H. Orians, and H. C. Heller, 2001, Sunderland, MA: Sinauer Associates. Copyright © 2001. Reprinted with permission. All rights reserved.

The senses are often referred to as the **somatic (bodily) sensory systems** (or the "somatosensory cortex") insofar as they inform us of what our bodies are experiencing while the **motor cortex** plays major role in what our bodies are doing.

hearing, smell, touch, and taste. We deal with these sensory systems and major disorders of them such as blindness and deafness in Chapter 3. Especially in studying disorders of the senses, we see that sensory representational systems are intensely integrated with each other. Also, through the connections between hearing, touch, and our sense of balance, we also discover that the senses are deeply connected with our higher representational systems of movement and language. We develop and demonstrate many amazing interactions between the various layers of the sign hierarchy in Chapter 4.

The senses are often referred to as the **somatic (bodily) sensory systems** (or the "somatosensory cortex") insofar as they inform us of what our bodies are experiencing while the **motor cortex** plays major role in what our bodies are doing. Figure 1–6 shows roughly how these distinct systems are mapped onto the distinct parts of the body. Although sensation does not entirely come under conscious control, nonetheless, by choosing to attend or not to attend to certain sensations, we can voluntarily control our senses to a considerable extent. The senses, in spite of the fact that they are our first line of defense in a world that is not always friendly to us, are nevertheless higher **cortical functions**. That is, they are represented in the cortex—the outermost layer of the human brain, as shown in Figures 1–5 and 1–6. As we see in those figures, right next to the strip of tissue that controls our bodily sensations is another strip of cortical matter that is associated with voluntary movements.

Motor Systems

Systems of intentional voluntary and regular movement provide our abilities to move our bodies and body parts to negotiate space and to produce distinctive meaningful gestures, facial expressions, and voluntary vocalizations of all sorts. As we will see in Chapters 5 through 10, a great deal more than just the motor strip of the cortex is involved in volitional movements. Such movements include sucking, following a moving object with movements of the eyes and/or head, crawling, walking, running, speaking, manual signing, writing, drawing pictures or diagrams, dancing, playing a musical instrument, and so on.

The Afferent and Efferent Distinction

Just as systems for representing movement depend on the senses, and especially the sense of touch, the systems encompassed under the scope of the language capacity also depend on lower systems of representation. Without the ability to engage in voluntary intentional movements, it would be impossible for anyone to acquire the systems of speech, manual signing, or writing. It should be noted, however, that each of the interrelated systems of representation is more complex than a simple diagram can show. The senses, for example, not only involve distinct organs, but also all the interconnected neurocircuits linking seeing, hearing, smelling, touching, and tasting to each other and to other neurological systems.

The systems of the senses are not only intensively connected with each other but also with the systems involved in movement and in linguistic representation. Although it is true that **afferent nerves** of the **sensory cortex** are distinct from **efferent nerves** of the **motor cortex** (Figure 1–7), there are intricate interactions between and within these different systems through a vast system of what are loosely called **interneurons** and also through less well understood **glial cells** of the brain (Banerjee & Bhat, 2008; Halassa et al., 2007).

Also, setting the glial cells aside, the interneurons by themselves are evidently much more differentiated and are richly connected with the entire nervous system. What is more, as Einstein, Piaget, Luria, and Vygotsky all correctly argued, in normal humans at least, all these systems depend on abstract and general representations that are closely tied to our language abilities. Those language abilities, it turns out, also form the main basis for the control not only of the body but also the planning, sequencing, and major control functions of the brain.

The number of the interneurons exceeds the number of sensory and motor neurons combined (Mohler, 2007) and the glial cells exceed them all by about 10 to 1.

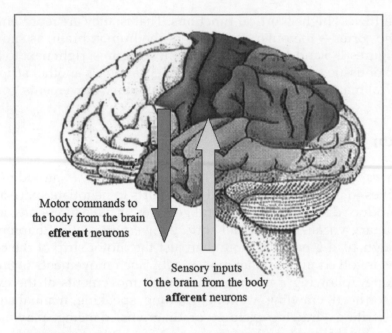

FIGURE 1–7. The system of afferent (sensory neurons) bringing information to the brain from the body and efferent (motor neurons) taking information from the brain to the body and vice versa.

Who's in Charge Here?

There has been a long-standing debate about the extent to which it is possible to associate particular functions with distinct regions of the brain.

There has been a long-standing debate about the extent to which it is possible to associate particular functions with distinct regions of the brain. Part of the debate has been about whether or not there might be a little man or woman inside the brain at some set of controls. Some critics spoofed the idea as reminiscent of the "man behind the curtain" in the *Wizard of Oz* talking into a microphone and operating switches and levers. But Figure 1–6 actually shows how those sensory and motor strips of cortical tissue separating the parietal and frontal lobes are mapped onto distinct areas of the body.

As can be seen in Figure 1–6, the mapping is such that there seem to be, not one, but two, miniature little humans located in brain tissue. In fact, the two *homunculi*—the plural Latin noun meaning "little humans"—have been immortalized in grotesque three-dimensional models that can be seen at the Natural History Museum in London (Figure 1–8). A close examination of the functions as mapped onto cortical tissue in Figure 1–6 shows that the two little humans can almost be overlaid one on top of the other. That is, the sensory and motor homunculi are almost side by side as if the two little distorted humans were standing shoulder to shoulder and operating hand in hand. At any rate, it seems that they often do so.

Figure 1–8 is interesting as a curiosity, more of art than science. In fact, the hands are too large in the models and the head and face

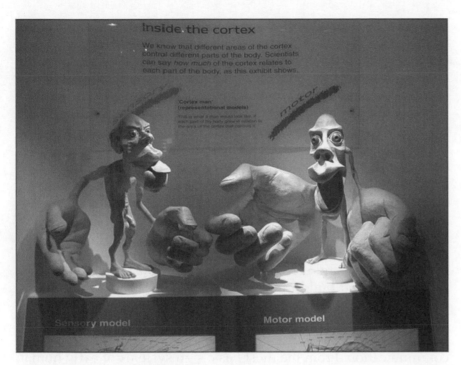

FIGURE 1–8. Photograph of the brain's homunculi in the Natural History Museum in London. Retrieved March 20, 2009, from http://en.wikipedia .org/wiki/Image:Sensory_and_motor_homunculi.jpg. Image in the public domain.

too small. In the mapping of the sensory and motor strips of the cortex as shown in Figure 1–6, the face actually gets more cortical tissue than do the hands. More importantly still, however, is the fact that the body, brain, and all of its sign systems from top to bottom normally work as a whole. Ordinarily, the sign systems of human experience are not much like two grotesque little naked men with huge hands reaching out to see, hear, smell, touch, and taste the world.

In fact, we see a remarkable kind of language—at least genetic —control from the beginning and throughout the development of the body. As sign systems develop from before birth, through infancy, and on to maturity, the normal development of sign systems progress from the body itself to the senses, movements, and language. Referring back to Figure 1–3, language development seems to be from the lowest level upward, bottom to top. However, even from before birth, human babies have a very special interest in the language spoken (or signed) by their mother and her interlocutors (Belin, Fecteau, & Bédard, 2004). They evidently learn to discriminate it from other languages and they know mom's voice before birth (J. W. Oller, S. D. Oller, & Badon, 2006). There seem to be, in other words, top-down influences as well.

Looking at the whole picture, it is clear that the genetic system specifies the whole from the beginning. The unfolding development

As sign systems develop from before birth, through infancy, and on to maturity, the normal development of sign systems progresses from the body itself to the senses, movements, and language.

is guided by a deep and abstract language in the genome to the development of general and abstract language abilities at the highest level of human communication abilities. Let us see how the process unfolds with respect to sign systems as the baby matures. In doing so, we can see where things can go wrong along the way. Normal development, as we will show, provides the basis for understanding and classifying disorders.

Unpacking the System

From early infancy, we use signs provided to us through our senses. With those signs we are able to understand and build up richer systems of signs that involve intentional movements. With the aid of both sensory and sensory-motor signs, we are able to unpack, understand, and build up sensory-motor-linguistic sign relations. Through combinations of these basic systems of signs—sensory signs, sensory-motor signs, and sensory-motor-linguistic signs—we are able to engage in the rich complexities of ordinary human communication. From the most basic sign systems of early human infancy, countless higher systems can be constructed.

> With the aid of both sensory and sensory-motor signs, we are able to unpack, understand, and build up sensory-motor-linguistic sign relations.

Developing Sign Systems

As Figure 1–9 suggests, the development of sign systems is constructive. It begins with complexes of sensory impressions that can be thought of as atoms of experience. They turn out to be things that the infant experiences through seeing, hearing, touching, tasting, and smelling. These atoms are the significant "things" of experience. Here we use the word "things" in the ordinary way. We intend the term "things" to include the significant persons, objects, events, states of affairs, as well as complex sequences of such atoms, and relations between them.

We might be tempted to say that things begin very simply and become very complex. Certainly, it is true that the sign systems the baby can handle become more complex as the baby matures, but this does not mean that the starting point is not already complex from the very beginning. In fact, sensory signs are already complex at the beginning. To get an inkling of just how amazingly complex a remembered visual image can be, see the panoramic drawing of Rome by Stephen Wiltshire (2009)—an individual who is diagnosed with autism. Stephen has the sort of autism that defines him as an amazing savant. His sensory-motor memory is astonishing. See "Beautiful Minds" at http://video.stumbleupon.com/#p=0k4lsi1dql and "About Stephen" (2009) both retrieved March 20, 2009 from http://www.stephenwiltshire.co.uk/.

The initial atoms, shown as the bottom layer in Figure 1–9 come to be linked through movements that connect them with each other in meaningful ways—like complex molecules built up from individual atoms. Complex connections between the atoms of experience are suggested in Figure 1–9 by the second layer of sensory-motor signs, just above the sensory signs. The third layer of signs consists of sensory-motor-linguistic signs. To continue the atomic and molecular metaphor, these higher sensory-motor-linguistic systems would be comparable to the kinds of relations we see between genes, proteins, and bodily functions in biochemistry.

Complex Language: Solved by Infants

Normal human communication capacities presuppose the most complex systems of language that are known to exist. On the one hand, this fact should cause us to realize that very simple explanations of human communication disorders are certain to be wrong. On the other hand, the complexity of normal human communication is somehow conquered by the resources available to a human infant. If babies can acquire systems as complex as those that undergird the use of human languages, surely it ought to be possible for intelligent adults to understand how they do it. In doing so, we can also set the stage for all that is to follow in this course and in the study, diagnosis, and treatment of communication disorders.

We can think of the increasing area of the triangle of sign systems in Figure 1–3 as dipping into the stream of experience. We begin with the moment when the triangle barely touches the stream

> If babies can acquire systems as complex as those that undergird the use of human languages, surely it ought to be possible for intelligent adults to understand how they do it.

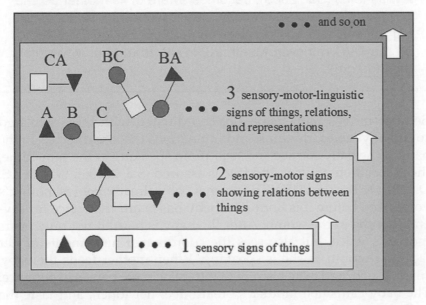

FIGURE 1–9. A diagram of the sign hierarchy showing how it is built up in layers.

of experience, when the baby in the womb begins to be conscious of its own experience. As development progresses, the triangle dips deeper into the stream. As higher and more powerful systems of representation are acquired and applied to the material stream of experience, our capacity to represent the present and to link it with the past and the future increases. Development of our ability to represent experience perceptually, emotionally, and cognitively increases from conception to birth and as we increase in experience over time. The wavy line gets longer and covers more ground. Our memory expands, our consciousness of what is going on is broadened, and our ability to anticipate what is likely to happen next also expands as we grow to maturity.

Sign Systems: Dynamic and Abstract from the Start

The normal baby begins to master many movements and to differentiate its own body parts through its actions within the first few weeks of gestation. From 4-dimensional video—provided by Dr. Stuart Campbell of London's Create Health Clinic —of the baby in the womb (see the British Broadcasting Company, story retrieved March 20, 2009, from http://news.bbc .co.uk/2/hi/health/3846525.stm; also see Video of an Unborn Baby on the DVD and S. Campbell, 2004), we know that the developing infant can make stepping movements, leap off the wall of the womb, suck its thumb, scratch body parts, stretch, rub its eyes, and even smile (as seen in Figure 1–1).

By sight and sound, the newborn, usually within its first few minutes (Sai, 2005), becomes aware of its mother as she holds and speaks to the baby (see National Center for Hearing Assessment and Management, 2004, Sound Beginnings on the DVD retrieved March 20, 2009, from http://www.infan thearing.org).

Because mom's movements are coordinated with the articulated sounds, syllables, rhythms, and intonations that are directed to the baby, if the baby can see and hear mom speaking at the same time, the association of voice and face is assured (Sai, 2005; J. W. Oller, S. D. Oller, & Badon, 2006). The normal baby already knows mother's voice from before it is born. The baby has heard that voice for several months in the womb. After the baby is born, it not only hears mother's voice, but also sees the coordinated movements of her face and mouth as she is speaking. When mother feeds the baby, smell, touch, and taste also come into play in the baby's experience. The baby can smell mother's breath, feel her touch, and taste the milk from her breast, or the bottle. At birth, the normal baby will be able to associate its mother's voice with her face within the first few minutes of life (Blass & Camp, 2001; Kaye & Bower, 1994; Walton & Bower, 1993).

Within a couple of days of birth, newborns also can distinguish pictures of different faces after about one minute of exposure (Walton & Bower, 1993; also see Bushnell, Sai, & Mullin, 1989). The baby can also distinguish emotions in its mother's language within its first two days of life and even before it is born (Mastropieri & Turkewitz, 1999). It can distinguish its mother's language from a foreign language through rhythms and intonations at least within its first couple of days of life (Moon, Cooper, & Fifer, 1993; Nazzi, Bertoncini, & Mehler, 1998).

Through the baby's senses and the baby's own movements and those of others, the remarkable world of experience is differentiated into distinct things (the bottom layer of Figure 1–9). As the things move around and interact—by being seen, heard, smelled, touched, and tasted by the baby—they are noticed and increasingly differentiated (the middle layer of Figure 1–9). Through the senses, a vocabulary of significant things comes to be represented in sensory signs. The things represented in distinct sensory signs will include persons such as mom and the baby itself. They will include the baby's hands, mom's hands, the breast, the bottle, the pacifier, the blankets, the crib, diapers, and so forth (the bottom layer of signs in Figure 1–9).

Talking and Signing Attract Interest

Some of the bodily entities that are being noticed and differentiated are also moving around in relation to each other, and some of them are talking or signing. The baby is sucking the bottle; mother is talking to the baby, picking up the baby, holding, feeding, and changing the baby, and so on. As these interactions occur, the baby also begins to form a repertoire of dynamic relations—ones that involve movement of one or both entities—between highly significant things (the middle layer of Figure 1–9).

As the relations between different things are noticed and taken into account through the sensory signs combined with movement, sensory-motor signs come into play (the middle layer of Figure 1–9). It is interesting that movements cannot be noticed or represented without also representing the things that move. It is strictly necessary for relations between things to be noticed to somehow represent the things that are dynamically related through their movements relative to each other. We cannot notice dancing without something that dances. Falling requires something that falls. A collision between two objects requires both of the objects that collide. Giving something to someone requires the giver, the thing given, and the recipient.

All *material* relations—ones that involve physical matter in some way, even ones that may seem to be static—require movement to be represented or noticed. To notice that the lamp is to the

Even before birth, space-time relations between moving things are noticed and begin to be differentiated by the baby. For instance, we know that the baby gains articulate control of its own movements in the womb. As this occurs the second layer of signs begins to come into view.

right of the computer, for example, requires an implicit movement rightward from the computer to the lamp or leftward from the lamp to the computer. It also suggests, in using the terms "right" and "left" the viewpoint of a person (possibly looking through a camera lens or at some representational device) that is somehow perceiving or noticing the computer relative to the lamp. All this may be done with the eyes, it is true, or even just by noticing the scene with the computer at the center and the lamp off to the right, but to get into a position to do this noticing always and without exception requires prior movement. Just as the baby cannot link mom's face with her voice without exiting the womb and coming into the larger world (Sai, 2005), we could not notice the relation between a lamp and a laptop without in some way—perhaps with the benefit of a camera or video recording device—entering the space where those objects are located. However, even a camera, a bug, or a recording device must be moved into range and within the right context in order to represent even static relations between, say, a lamp and a computer. Therefore, movement is involved in representing even what seem to be static relations that do not involve any movement. Stephen Wiltshire needed the helicopter ride to get the panoramic view of Rome that he would later put on a huge, very wide sheet of paper.

The Logical Progression

As Figure 1–9 suggests, each level of the hierarchy of signs forms the necessary basis for climbing up to the next level. In Figure 1–9 we take the body for granted as essential to the functioning of the senses. If the body were not there, or were defective, the senses could be entirely missing or defective. The senses are crucial to the regulation of intentional movements, and both the senses and the capacity for intentional movement are needed for language to develop normally. The senses and the body are needed for language comprehension to be initiated and for language to develop and continue to function normally.

Although movement is involved in forming sensory signs of any bodily thing, say, the baby's noticing of its own hand or head, the movement of the baby's hand to the baby's head cannot happen if the baby does not have both its hand and its head. Objects are necessary to movements.

Later, however, distinct movements, actions, interactions, and relations will be associated with distinct things—that is, with things that move besides the hand. When relations between distinct moving things come to be represented, very early in the unborn infant's repertoire of sign systems the child graduates from merely sensory signs to the higher level of sensory-motor signs. However, neither sensations of things nor movement of things are the most interesting to the normal baby.

Because the layer of sensory-motor signs cannot be formed without the prior existence of sensory signs for things, there is an order of progression. What is distinctive about the second layer of signs (see Figure 1–9) is that it involves the sorts of interactions between things where movement is crucial.

The Rhythms of Language

Even before birth, the entities that the normal baby takes the most interest in are the ones that both move and talk, or that use meaningful manual signs. Babies are intrinsically interested in other persons from the start—well before birth. Babies with all their senses are intensely interested in the syllables, rhythms, and intonations of speech or manual signing (Condon & Sander, 1974; Feldman, 2007; Kimura & Daibo, 2006; Masataka, 1992). Very soon after birth, the typical newborn hears its mother's familiar voice. Upon inspection it turns out that the familiar sounds, syllables, rhythms, and intonations are coming from a bodily person (MOTHER) who is looking at and speaking to the infant.

The baby is already aware of its own body through sensations. As a result, the atom consisting of MOTHER comes to be noticed in relation to the atom consisting of the INFANT. Linking the two are the sounds, the rhythmic movements of mom's body and mouth, and any other sensations that may be present from the baby's point of view. For instance, the baby may be able to smell mom's familiar breath, hair, and skin. The baby may also be able to smell, mom while the baby can also feel her touch and taste her milk. All these sensations link the MOTHER and the INFANT and enable the mapping of mom's familiar voice to her, until now, unfamiliar face, which is associated with all of the other familiar representations of her through the senses of sight, hearing, smell, touch, and taste.

We follow the simple convention of using CAPITALS to refer to the bodily object or person rather than to its name or a referring term or phrase.

The Simplest Pragmatic Mapping

Even in the simplest mapping of the mom's face to her voice (and vice versa), we also can see the emerging basis for referring relations that form the basis for all language acquisition (J. W. Oller, 2005; S. D. Oller, 2005). The voice functions as a symbol which refers to mom—that is, it is about her and directs the infant's attention to her. After that mapping is completed, the voice normally will cause the baby to think of the face even when the baby cannot see its mother, and seeing mother will enable the baby to think of the sound of her voice.

Even in the simplest mapping of the mom's face to her voice (and vice versa), we also can see the emerging basis for referring relations that form the basis for all language acquisition (J. W. Oller, 2005; S. D. Oller, 2005).

Sign Mapping

For the generalized mapping of signs onto the stream of experience we have used the term **pragmatic mapping** (J. W. Oller, 1975, 1993; J. W. Oller & L. Chen, 2007; J. W. Oller, S. D. Oller, & Badon, 2006; S. D. Oller, 2005). Also, this usage has become quite general (J. S. Damico, 1985a, 1985b, 2003; J. S. Damico & S. K. Damico, 1993; Krashen, 1980; Naremore,

1985; Richard-Amato, 2003). There is also a stream of research in theoretical linguistics that is using the phrase with essentially the same meaning (Ward, 2004). This mapping at a minimum involves a referring relation between a sign, such as a name, and an object, such as, for example, the person named. Such a relation can be summed up as: *Symbol—mapped-through-action-onto—OBJECT*.

It is noteworthy that the central element in such a mapping—that is, the action that connects a symbol to its object, and vice versa—invariably involves indexical operations that can only be done in the present tense. That is, pragmatic mapping operations are intrinsically actions in the here and now. Even if those actions are covert in the sense of only involving thought—as in thinking of someone by name—they are nonetheless present, indexical, and active rather than passive. As a result, motor activity in the expression of language plays a more critical role in its development and in its deployment in comprehension, speaking, listening, reading, writing, and thinking than is commonly realized. It is useful to note that successful pragmatic mappings constitute well-formed true representations in the most mundane and common sense of "truth" as we explain in greater detail in the immediately following sections.

In Figure 1–9 such pragmatic mapping relations are shown in the association of some linguistic sign—say, A, or B, or C—with a bodily thing such as a circle, square, or triangle. Such mappings when they are completed must contain at least three elements: There is (1) the abstract symbol, (2) the association, and (3) the object symbolized. We argue that successful therapies for language disorders must take the pragmatic mapping process into account (S. D. Oller, 2005). Any method that fails to do so will come up short of enabling ordinary communication. To get an idea of the surprising complexity of this simple mapping relation, see DeLeon et al. (2007) who studied the underlying neurological systems involved in brain-damaged patients attempting this naming relation (the simplest of pragmatic maps) either orally or in writing. Also see the analysis of the pragmatic mapping relation especially in Chapters 3, 4, 5, 9, and 10.

VALID REPRESENTATIONS ARE FOUNDATIONAL

It is necessary to keep in mind that language acquisition, according to sound theoretical arguments (see Bruner, 1975; Macnamara, 1972; J. W. Oller, 1970, 1993, 2005; J. W. Oller, Sales, & Harrington,

1969) and a multitude of empirical results (for summaries, see J. W. Oller, S. D. Oller, & Badon, 2006; J. W. Oller, L. Chen, Pan, & S. D. Oller, 2005) depends on the sort of pragmatic mapping process that is exemplified in ordinary true representations. Language acquisition and use ultimately depend entirely on representations that happen to be true of whatever they refer to, in the same way that a name is applied to the person who goes by that name. Of course, there are other kinds of representations including all kinds of fictions, errors, deliberate lies, and many gradations of nonsense. However, all of those other forms, as shown in strict logicomathematical proofs, must get whatever meaning they may have from ordinary true representations. So, it is important to think about what an ordinary true representation consists of and why babies have to start with them to begin to unravel the conventional sign systems of any language.

Truth in the Simplest, Most Ordinary, Mundane Sense

Here is an illustration of an ordinary true representation. If we say, "This is a book about communication disorders" and it is in fact such a book, then our statement is true in the mundane and ordinary sense of "true." Otherwise, if what we are pointing out is not a book, or is not about communication disorders, then our statement is not true. The idea of "truth" is simple enough for a child of about five to understand in this form, and this is the form of language with which every child unlocks and begins to unpack the language acquisition process. Philosophers such as Davidson (1996) have tried to make "truth" to be an exceedingly difficult concept. It is not as difficult as adult philosophers sometimes make out.

It turns out that ordinary referring expressions in experience, the kind that the child deciphers to figure out the meanings of the child's "first words," are true in precisely this simple sense. That is, the representation fits what it represents in much the way that a name fits its object, or that a glove fits a hand, or that the lower teeth fit the uppers with the mouth closed and the teeth clenched, or that Stephen Wiltshire's panoramic sketch can be recognized as a sketch of what he saw on a helicopter ride over Rome.

Keep in mind that for a name to fit its object, as, say, the name Bill fits a person by that name, is not a lofty and difficult philosophical problem. It is just a matter of convention. If THE-GUY-BILL is conventionally called *Bill*, then the name is as true of good old BILL as it can be expected to be. If the name doesn't claim to be anything other than his name (what he is called), then it is true of him at least to that extent. But being true in that conventional way is all that a name can do, so it is as true as it needs to be. It is also just as true as it can be. It cannot be any truer than it is if it is correctly applied to BILL.

Truth may be profound, but it must be simple enough to enable babies to figure out simple pragmatic mappings, as they do.

In language acquisition, the child must begin with ordinary true representations that fit the known facts of a given situation.

In language acquisition, the child must begin with ordinary true representations that fit the known facts of a given situation. At a significant remove from there we find representations that are fictional and that concern imagined facts, possibilities, or fantasies. Moving a little further from ordinary true representations of known facts, if we confuse an imagined fact for an actual one, we commit an error. This is the sort of thing that happens with an ordinary illusion. We think we see water ahead on the road but it is a shimmering illusion—a fiction that might be taken for a fact. Or we may think we see a friend, but it turns out to be a stranger. Or we may remember something we were told about our early childhood, or someone else's, and imagine that we can remember the event itself. An error involves mistaking a fictional possibility for a fact. A step farther away from ordinary true representations is possible if the known falsehood is embellished and presented as a true representation to someone else. The latter possibility is what we call lying. It involves representing a known falsehood as an ordinary true representation. Thus, we can define three meaningful grades of distance from ordinary truth telling. First, there is the level of fiction, then error, then lying. If we keep going one more step farther away from ordinary truth telling—that is, if we go beyond lying—we come to meaningless nonsense. Of course, there are gradations within each of the levels just defined, but the main categories are these: *truth > fiction > error > lie*. It is also interesting that children acquire the distinctions in exactly this order (see J. W. Oller, S. D. Oller, & Badon, 2006).

Falsehoods: Dreams, Fantasies, Errors, and Lies

Of course, memories, perceptions (consciousness of what is going on), and anticipations of the future are all fallible. They are not always true. Representations are not always true of what they purport to represent. We make mistakes and sometimes we think we are perceiving one thing when it is something else. When we are asleep, dreaming is normal but seems to be somewhat out of our control. When we are awake, if we remember the dream, we gain some volitional control and can examine and even embellish it in the retelling. But, normally, in recalling dreams and in dealing with fictions and fantasies in general, we don't actually suppose that they are true. It is normal when we are awake, rarely, to experience certain **illusions** where things seem different than they really are. We may think we see water in the distance on a hot dry stretch of road, but it may be a mirage—a shimmering illusion. The representation is not true. With drugs and extreme physical stress anyone can be caused to experience **hallucinations**. In the case of hallucinations, the confusion is more severe. People think they perceive things that are not present at all. If the hallucinations persist or recur spontaneously, without the drugs or external causes, a disorder may be involved. If we mistake a dream for reality while we are asleep, we make a minor error of judgment, but if the same mistake occurs repeatedly while awake, we enter the strange world of **delusional pathology**.

Certain disorders of that kind can be produced, it seems, by metabolic imbalances in the body that fail to fully shut down such normal processes as dreaming when the individual appears to be awake.

> ### The Case of Dr. John Forbes Nash
>
> In some cases, delusions may be produced by desires, not necessarily fully conscious ones, that seem to overwhelm reality. Take, for instance, the case of Dr. John Forbes Nash (2002, 2008), concerning whom the movie *A Beautiful Mind* was made (see Universal Studios and DreamWorks, 2001, retrieved March 20, 2009, from http://www.abeautifulmind.com/). We consider his case further in Chapter 10 (also Figure 10–13). He experienced vivid delusions of voices speaking to him (rather different than the coherent visual and auditory delusions portrayed in the movie). According to his own account, Dr. J. F. Nash (2002) reports that he wanted to be more famous and successful than he was, and his desire, by his own assessment, contributed to his pathology.

It seems that delusional tendencies also underlie what is popularly called **pathological lying** where the liar, at some point, may become unable without prodding to tell the difference between actual memories and the vivid recollections of invented falsehoods. When that kind of confusion occurs, the lying becomes pathological. It is also referred to as **mythomania** or **pseudologia fantastica** (Abe, Suzuki, Mori, Itoh, & Fujii, 2007; Dike, Baranoski, & Griffith, 2005; Langleblen et al., 2002; Y. Yang et al., 2007) and the person affected is called a **pseudologue**. The deceiver is captured in his or her own web of deception and the capacity to discern the difference between invented fiction and reality is muddled in the mind of its creator.

In Chapter 10, we will deal with several cases of this kind of disorder. There we will also see that it is possible with modern technologies to sharply distinguish brain activity involved in constructing a true report of known facts as contrasted with a deliberately deceptive representation (see Abe et al., 2007, for a review of that research). But unlike imagined representations and dreams, in ordinary experience perceptions are usually more or less correct.

If we mistake a dream for reality while we are asleep, we make a minor error of judgment, but if the same mistake occurs repeatedly while awake, we enter the strange world of **delusional pathology**.

It seems that delusional tendencies also underlie what is popularly called **pathological lying** where the liar, at some point, may become unable without prodding to tell the difference between actual memories and the vivid recollections of invented falsehoods.

What Is Versus What Is Only Represented

Do Our Senses Deceive Us?

Our senses normally do not deceive us. In the vast majority of instances, the representations of our senses agree with the way things really are. We perceive things the way that we do because, to a great extent, things really are the way they seem to be. We think we are awake and sitting at the computer, that someone is mowing the yard outside, and so forth, because these things are really happening just as they seem to be. That is, to a great extent, our perceptions are valid, and true. What is actually happening, agrees in many instances, with our representations of what is going on.

To consider an example at hand, we think this is a book about communication disorders. If it is, we are right in thinking this and if you agree, so are you. Our thoughts often are correctly informed by our senses. We think it is daylight outside because we can see the light coming in from the window. We think that the air conditioner just went off because we heard it running and then we heard it turn off. Such representations of the world often can also be checked.

Testing the Agreement

One of the ways that we can be relatively certain that our perceptions, memory, and expectancies are on the right track is that we often agree with other communicators. The chances of that happening by accident are so slim that, as soon as two or more representations come into relatively perfect agreement, the likelihood that such a coincidence (such agreement) could be owed to pure accidents, to mere chance, diminishes toward a vanishing point. As soon as experience becomes just a little complex—way before birth—the chance of distinct representations agreeing with each other by accident can be ruled out entirely.

In the material world, things change from one occasion to the next. The chance of complete agreement between two rapidly changing states of affairs is effectively nil. As a result, when multiple representations produce the same meaning repeatedly, the likelihood of their doing so because of material facts just happening to align themselves perfectly by accident, is effectively zero. So, any agreement in communication itself shows that we are justified in supposing that we are correct in our representations of what is going on much of the time.

To get an idea of just how unlikely it is that representations of different persons, or the same person at different times, should

> As soon as experience becomes just a little complex—way before birth—the chance of distinct representations agreeing with each other by accident can be ruled out entirely.

align themselves quite perfectly by accident, the reader might consider the following series of questions: How is it possible for the authors, publishers, and readers of this book to agree that it is about communication disorders? What kinds of accidents would have to happen in order for this agreement to come about by chance? Or what kinds of errors would produce so much agreement? What kind of chance or randomness can produce the same result on every occasion? Or, consider the many facts contained in the book that readers will also agree on: Who are the authors of the book? Does the book deal with autism? Does it discuss poisons that cause disorders? Is it published by Plural?

As soon as the number of details concerning any common experience exceeds 1, the likelihood of accidental agreement on those details rapidly drops to just about exactly zero. We are compelled to infer that something other than chance is at work. In fact, we must infer shared language and abilities of representers in a common world that agree about known and truly represented facts, for example, this really is a book about communication disorders, and so forth, and the people who agree on this do so because of common access to and shared understanding of the same actual world of experience.

In fact, disagreements, disorders, and confusions could not be known at all, as what they are, if it were not possible for us normally to understand experience validly and to understand communications about it. If we have no idea about how things really are, we cannot tell any difference between what is and what is not; what is normal versus what is disordered. If there were no true representations, we could not discriminate at all between them and ones that are fictional, in error, or intended to deceive. Ordinary true representations must exist before we become able to represent anything about fictions, fantasies, errors, lies, jokes, metaphors, and so on.

If there were no true representations, we could not discriminate at all between them and ones that are fictional, in error, or intended to deceive. Ordinary true representations must exist before we become able to represent anything about fictions, fantasies, errors, lies, jokes, metaphors, and so on.

RESOURCES FOR THE COURSE

In this section, we provide an overview of the teaching/learning resources that accompany this book, then we conclude this chapter with a discussion of the reasons commonly given for studying communication disorders. We especially want to encourage our readers to consider what we believe are the highest and best reasons for pursuing this field of study. We have been greatly encouraged by our students, readers, and colleagues in the work that we present to you here. We thank you in advance for being there and we assure you that we are eager to hear from you concerning any part of this course. On the back jacket, we quote some of the comments we have received from our students and we invite yours as well especially on the new resources and material offered here for the first time.

The DVD

The DVD that comes with this book contains an expanded Table of Contents with the introductions and summaries of each chapter along with working hyperlinks to URLs (Uniform Resource Locators on the Internet) referred to in every chapter. It also contains all of the figures, illustrations, and media files referred to in the text, and a searchable version of all the open-ended Discussion Questions, References, Glossary, Index, and the Multiple Choice Questions (600 of them) that are systematically linked page-by-page to the unfolding story told chapter-by-chapter. There is also a PowerPoint summary on the DVD for each chapter highlighting key points.

The Multiple-Choice Questions

The multiple-choice questions appear in the same order in which the material comes up in the textbook and each of the questions is cross-referenced to the text by one or more page numbers to show where the answer for it may be found. In the DVD, we explain each item so that it is possible to see why how each of the choices, except for the correct one, can be ruled out. We also give an item analysis for each question based on the performance of the student samples from universities where the book and accompanying materials were pretested.

Each question focuses on one or more key points from the course. Together, the questions provide the basis for a point-by-point review on a chapter-by-chapter basis throughout the course. They show in detail how multiple-choice items in standardized tests are constructed by professional test writers and they provide important teaching/learning/testing/review options throughout the course. From the questions concerning any given chapter, instructors can construct multiple-choice tests including midterm and final examinations, or the questions may be used as study-guides that are thoroughly grounded in the course material. We use the test items in three ways—as study materials, review guides, and as tests.

Our students routinely comment that the intensive study of our multiple choice test items has helped them to prepare for standardized tests in general. Students who were not good at taking multiple-choice tests comment that they have become good at it. The key is understanding how such items are constructed. It helps students prepare, for instance, for the PRAXIS test that is required nationally in the United States for licensing of **speech-language pathologists**. For instructors and students who prefer essay-type discussion questions, we provide lots of those too at the end of each chapter.

Should Students Study the Test Items?

Our research on this book—and also on our companion volume, *Milestones*, for the course on normal speech and language develop-

> Our students routinely comment that the intensive study of our multiple choice test items has helped them to prepare for standardized tests in general. Students who were not good at taking multiple-choice tests comment that they have become good at it.

ment—shows that allowing students to study the items in advance, before those same items are used in multiple choice tests, enhances the **reliability**, **validity**, and **instructional utility** of the items themselves and the tests constructed from them (see Yan, 2007).

Better Communication

The principle is straightforward: *better communication of the subject matter results in better comprehension, learning, and connection to one's own world of experience*. When teaching and learning are more successful in this way, testing is also more reliable, valid, and useful. Reliability is improved because the better students understand the material, the more they are apt to get the same excellent results from one occasion to the next. Also, validity is improved because there is greater agreement about the subject matter and thus about why some answers to the questions are better than others. That is, there is more agreement between students, teachers, researchers, and so forth, about which answers are correct, or incorrect, and why. Better communication is just that. It is better.

Making Information Accessible

Our purpose as teacher/communicators is to make information accessible. The objective of this book and the materials that accompany it is also to make the material of the course and all the research to which it is connected as accessible as possible.

> The objective of this book and the materials that accompany it is also to make the material of the course and all the research to which it is connected as accessible as possible.

The DVD includes an *Instructor's Manual* showing how to construct a countless variety of multiple-choice tests from the items included there. It is also easy to construct essay tests from the Discussion Questions at the end of each chapter. Instructors also can expand and modify the PowerPoint summaries to suit their distinct styles and preferences. Abundant reading resources are contained in the list of references at the end of the book and these are made completely searchable on the DVD. The Discussion Questions suggest many ways to expand on material in any given chapter and on the key issues that come up along the way. The Reference List and Index of Subjects and Authors are also provided in digital format making them conveniently searchable.

Case-Based Problem-Solving

We use a case-based approach referring to real persons in actual situations for several reasons. For one, such an approach is completely consistent with what we know of language acquisition and valid learning in general. The most effective teaching is necessarily grounded in true representations of actual persons, things, events, and situations in the real world. This is the main reason that we follow the Harvard model of case-based problem-solving. The cases themselves are grounded in the real world, well documented, and referenced against the most reliable and valid and up-to-date theory and re-search (Mostaghimi et al., 2006; Tosteson, Adelstein, & Carver, 1994).

When we look to real cases of actual human beings, we stop thinking of problems in the abstract and begin seeing them as real problems that affect individuals like ourselves. This, we believe, is what the Harvard reformers meant by the phrase "care for the patient." When we see the patient, client, student as a human being, we start thinking of the problem as if it were our own. We identify with the parents of Ethan Kurtz. After seeing him at nine months as a happy bright-eyed boy, we are shocked when at 18 months he is unresponsive to his name. The symptoms of hand-flapping, social unresponsiveness, and full-blown autism are shocking. When we see the video of Ethan Kurtz where he retreats into severe autism, as if a prisoner inside his own body, we identify with his dad, Stan Kurtz (see "Children's Corner," n.d., retrieved March 20, 2009, from http://www.childrenscornerschool.com/stankurtz.htm). We share the intense desire and motivation to get Ethan back.

Like Bryan and Laurie Jepson (see Jepson & Johnson, 2007), Jon Shestack and Portia Iverson (see and hear Shestack, 2003, at the Autism Summit retrieved March 20, 2009, from http://www.tv worldwide.com/events/nimh/031119/agenda.cfm), and Jenny McCarthy (2007)—when we learn about the regression of children whose mind and personality seem to have been kidnapped leaving a "bewildered body behind," we determine to find out what we can do to help get them back. Through firsthand acquaintance with real cases we put ourselves in the shoes of the parents and others who love the individuals with disorders. When we hear the story ("The Myelin Project," 2009, retrieved March 7, 2009, from http://www .myelin.org/en/cms/?14) and when we learn what Augusto and Michaela Odone did—as recounted in the film *Lorenzo's Oil* (retrieved March 20, 2009, from http://www.myelin.org/en/c ms/?14)—to rescue their son from a fatal genetic disorder, we ourselves are motivated.

Another reason for using a case-based approach is that it shows more clearly than any other that the main goal in the study of communication disorders is to improve the quality of the lives of affected human beings. Persons affected directly or indirectly by impairments in abilities to communicate, typically want more than thick, rich, descriptive research concerning the behaviors associated with the disorder—as useful as such descriptions may be. They do not want to wait for half a century while researchers develop more of **epidemiology** and statistics. It is not enough to advocate increasing the number of caregivers, or enhancing the resources and facilities dedicated to the treatment of communication disorders, or improving the pay of persons who treat disorders. It is not enough to train

Real life cases move us to action. They give us the energy to burn the midnight oil, to spend the resources, and to do what it takes to make things better. They enable us to define and carry out the research needed to answer the critical questions about diagnosis, causation, and intervention.

professionals to provide care and treatment. It is not enough to raise public awareness about communication disorders or to inform the public and professionals about the emotional, economic, and personal costs associated with communication disorders. All these goals are desirable and may be helpful in moving toward our deeper objective, but we agree with the American Speech-Language-Hearing Association (ASHA) as noted in Chapter 12: the highest and best goal is to discover the causes of disorders in order to cure, prevent, or lessen their negative impact.

Why Study Communication Disorders?

> The obvious purpose of this book and all its accompanying resources is to introduce students to the nature and classification of communication disorders, but the best reason—perhaps the only legitimate one—for studying communication disorders is, as much as possible, to learn how to prevent them, to cure them whenever they cannot be prevented, and to make them less severe whenever they cannot be prevented or cured.

Human beings, after all, are not like rock crystals, physical phenomena, numbers, art, music, or literature that might be studied out of curiosity. Human beings with disorders are persons.

If they have one or more communication disorders that prevent them from enjoying human experience in all its dimensions, as human beings they merit our highest compassion, our complete attention, and our best efforts to help them. As fellow human beings, we must strive to enable persons with communication disorders, as much as possible, to achieve their full potential as human beings. As we will see, communication systems—including all the skills, abilities, and knowledge sources that make such systems possible—are essential to the full enjoyment of ordinary human experience. Noam A. Chomsky—an MIT linguist who happens to be the most quoted intellectual of modern times—has suggested that if we were to take away all our distinct human capacity to communicate, especially through language, our experience would be reduced to something like "an amoeboid creature," which would be "utterly impoverished and lacking the intricate special structures making possible a human existence" (1980, pp. 33–34). Does he go too far? Perhaps so, but the question is not only how much *do communication disorders limit human experience* but whether it is possible for some or all of the abilities lost to be recovered. This is the question on the minds of people who love the individual whose capacities to communicate with others or to interact with the world have been impacted by one or many communication disorders.

As we will see, communication systems—including all the skills, abilities, and knowledge sources that make such systems possible—are essential to the full enjoyment of ordinary human experience.

Disorders as Amusement

Sometimes communication difficulties, breakdowns, and disorders are regarded as subjects of amusement and "comic relief"—as blindness was regarded at a burlesque show observed by Valentin Haüy (see the account in Chapter 3). The voice and behaviors of a joke-teller may change to sound like a person who is mentally disabled, who speaks with a cleft palate, or just has a "funny" accent. The gait of a performer may change to imitate that of a person with **cerebral palsy**, or some other motor-disorder, or a person with a physical deformity such as a cleft palate or lip. Comedians may imitate stutterers for effect. In many situations, these antics may be amusing, but for the persons affected by communication disorders—and those who love them—the loss of any ability to communicate is genuine. Some may regard autism, for instance, as "quirky," "cute," or "a special gift," or "a blessing in disguise" and many have argued that there is no "autism epidemic" (Gernsbacher, Dawson, & Goldsmith, 2005). But to the contrary, see Chapter 5, Jon Shestack (2003) said, "There is nothing 'cute' or 'quirky' about autism." Shestack is the Founder of Cure Autism Now, which recently merged with Autism Speaks (retrieved March 20, 2009, from http://www.autismspeaks.org/).

> We join Jon Shestack in the hope that autism, for instance—to single out the most prominent disorder of the 21st century, one still described in medical textbooks as an "unsolved mystery"—may soon be relegated to the history books.

For all the foregoing reasons, in this course, we take the perspective of the persons most affected by communication disorders. For us, the goal of this study and all the work associated with it is restoration to the point of a cure and/or complete prevention of the disorder. That is our objective. We join Jon Shestack in the hope that autism, for instance—to single out the most prominent disorder of the 21st century, one still described in medical textbooks as an "unsolved mystery"—may soon be relegated to the history books.

For reasons that will become clearer as we go along, we believe that the current epidemic of metabolic disorders including autism (Jepson, 2007), **ADD/ADHD**, Alzheimer's, **multiple sclerosis**, and many more will require and produce a revolution in the way toxin-related disorders are treated in the future.

SUMMING UP AND LOOKING AHEAD

In the next chapter, we deal with genetic and bodily disorders that affect appearance, anatomy, and every aspect of human experience. Such disorders also may influence seeing, hearing, smelling, touching, and tasting. In obvious ways, our senses ordinarily depend on an intact, functional body. Above the senses which provide the most basic kinds of signs, the next level of signs involve movement, especially volitional movements that result from intentional actions. Yet intentional voluntary movements could not exist, much less have any social meaning, if they were not accompanied by meaningful sensations. So, meaningful movements, especially facial expressions such as smiling, gesturing, and all intentional social acts, must be aided by sensory signs. Language likewise depends on sensations and movements. Voluntary movements are crucial to speaking, writing, manual signed languages (as of the Deaf), and intentional acts in general. Even acts such as breathing, swallowing, clearing one's throat, sniffing, or blinking the eyes involve movements that can convey meanings in human interactions.

In the following chapters, we consider the integration of our anatomy with sensory, motor, and linguistic systems. In Chapter 2 we consider how bodily disorders impact communication. As we will see throughout this book, communication disorders always spill over into related domains and have cascading effects. For this reason, disorders that impact the body and its growth tend to affect how we perceive ourselves and others, and how they perceive us. As a result, communication development and all the social relations, skills, and knowledge systems that depend on communication can be affected dramatically by the disorders to which we turn in Chapter 2.

Above the senses which provide the most basic kinds of signs, the next level of signs involve movement, especially volitional movements that result from intentional actions.

STUDY AND DISCUSSION QUESTIONS

1. Why is successful communication harder to explain and to account for than breakdowns, failures to communicate, and disorders? (Consider the analogy of designing a lightbulb, an airplane, a computer, a space shuttle, and so on. Which is more difficult to account for, the many initial failures or the ultimate achievements and successes of ordinary acts of communication? Why are successes necessarily more complex than the failures that often precede them?)

2. Why do parents like Jonathan Shestack and Portia Iversen want more than just an explanation of their child's disorder — or an intensive microanalysis of his behaviors? Is what they are asking for unattainable? Is it reasonable? Should students of communication disorders be satisfied with less than a viable method of preventing or curing a particular disorder? Why so or why not? What is your personal view?

3. What are the arguments for and against claims that there is an epidemic of autism? What is your own conclusion and why do you think as you do? What evidence can you muster in favor of your own and opposing views?

4. What arguments show that the acquisition of any natural human language cannot be accomplished by the rote memorization of sentences? How can a child's memory produce a system of systems that is universal, abstract, and completely general?

5. What facts tend to support or refute the gas pain theory of smiling? What reasoning has been offered in its favor? What can we learn from that theory, if anything?

6. Why did Einstein argue that understanding sensory impressions requires reliance on the abstract relations that hold between them? Here is a problem to stimulate your thinking: How can you be sure that the classroom you are sitting in on a certain occasion, say, is the same one you were in a few minutes or a day before? How do you know it is the same room that your classmates also are in? Or, if you are working in a distance setting, how do you know you are following the same course as other students who are working through this book? Or, how do you know that a particular pencil, pair of sunglasses, or book sack, is your own?

2

Genetics to Anatomy: Craniofacial Anomalies

OBJECTIVES

In this chapter, we:

1. Overview the major classes of bodily disorders that affect communication;
2. Discuss cleft lip, cleft palate, and **spina bifida**;
3. Review and expand on their diagnosis by 4D ultrasound;
4. Consider treatment options for bodily disorders;
5. Discuss the contrast between conditions before and after treatment; and
6. Put bodily disorders in perspective relative to sensory, sensory-motor, and sensory-motor-linguistic disorders.

University of Ulster LIBRARY

KEY TERMS

Here are some key terms of this chapter. Many you may already know, but it may help to review them. These terms are explained in the text and they are defined in the Glossary at the end of the book. They appear in **bold print** on their first appearance in the text.

anosmia	dysostosis	mandibulofacial dysostosis
apraxia	embryological development	nasalized
bifida	embryologist	neurogenic disorders
branchial arch syndromes	epigenetic disorder	ossification
cesarean section	epigenetic systems	pancreas
chromosome	euthanasia movement	paranormal phenomena
cleft lip	FAE	parosmia
cleft palate	FAS	partial birth abortion
comorbidity	fetal alcohol effects	pediatric surgeons
congenital anomalies	fetal alcohol syndrome	pervasive developmental
craniofacial anomalies	fontanelles	disorders
craniosynostosis	Franceschetti syndrome	philtrum
cranium	genetic disorders	prosody
cystic fibrosis	genotoxin	prosopagnosia
diabetes mellitus	germ cells	sickle cell anemia
diagnosis	gestational period	single nucleotide
domino theory of disorders	hemoglobin	polymorphism (SNP)
Down syndrome	hydrocephalus	spina bifida
Duchenne smile	hypernasality	syllables
dysarthria	hyponasality	synostosis
dyslexia	hyposmia	teratology
dysphagias	imperforate anus	velopharyngeal insufficiency
dysosmia	late-term abortions	

All communication disorders ultimately affect bodily entities and when it comes to human communication, disorders affect bodily persons. Disease, injury, metabolic imbalance, immune system deficiencies, cumulative impact of toxins, emotional trauma, abuse, prejudice, drug addiction, and so on, affect the body in ways that interfere with, disrupt, and can lead to persistent disorders of communication. There are vastly more ways for things to go wrong than for them to go right. For this reason, great thinkers such as C. S. Peirce, Albert Einstein, Jean Piaget, and Fred Hoyle have all argued that accidental success in communication is extremely unlikely. By contrast, communication failures and breakdowns are highly probable.

There are, according to a general theory of signs developed out of the rich reservoir of theories of language and communication (see J. W. Oller, S. D. Oller, & Badon, 2006) four major classes of disorders that impact communication. They consist of (1) bodily, (2) sensory,

(3) sensory-motor, and (4) sensory-motor-linguistic disorders. This organization is simpler than its predecessors and, as we have shown elsewhere (see our review in *Discourse Processes*, 2005), it is also more comprehensive.

Theory of Signs

Only a general theory of signs—one that is deeply grounded in the sciences of abstract logic and mathematics as well as linguistics, genetics, biochemistry, psychology and sociology —can hope to cover the full scope of communication disorders from genetics to social breakdowns. It must also be kept in mind that although relying on a simpler, more consistent and more comprehensive theory does not change the facts of communication disorders, it does provide a better basis for classifying, understanding, and explaining them. Also, a better theory of what causes communication disorders and how they arise from breakdowns in normal communication processes is certain to lead to better understanding and better practice in treating them. As we will see, even in this introductory excursion as we look back over more than 300 years of history in dealing with communication disorders, understanding how communication works is a huge advantage in treating communication disorders.

There are many subclasses within each of the major divisions of communication disorders and many more combinations and interactions within and between them. Because there are more ways for things to go wrong than to go right, the existence of many different communication disorders is unsurprising. Rather, it is surprising that development often proceeds successfully and that communication is commonly possible in spite of all the things that can and sometimes do go wrong. If things go well, the genetic specifications that are available in our parents' **chromosomes** from before our conception lead to the development of a normal body. However, along the way, during the process of development and ordinary living, many factors can interfere with successful communication. Those factors include genetic errors as well as injuries owed to toxins, disease, and metabolic imbalances. In fact, toxins, as we will see, are a primary source of genetic errors along with exposure to harmful radiation. Other factors in producing bodily disorders include physical injuries, disease, and their interactions with genetics. To begin, in this chapter we focus attention especially on anomalies and disorders that directly impact the body. Then, with that discussion as a foundation, we look ahead briefly to the three other major classes of communication disorders that are discussed in succeeding chapters.

> Because there are more ways for things to go wrong than to go right, the existence of many different communication disorders is unsurprising.

BODILY DISORDERS

Many bodily disorders, even if they happen to be severe, can be corrected or alleviated by appropriate and timely treatment. Even in severe cases, normal abilities, functions, and appearance can sometimes be partially or almost completely restored by surgery. Commonly, the treatment for **craniofacial anomalies**, in particular, will involve surgery. However, even with genetically linked disorders of the gut and brain, especially those with a significant metabolic disease component that may be triggered by toxins, sometimes something as simple as a diet change, treatment with an antiviral medication, or enhanced detoxification may result in dramatic improvements in communication abilities (see Chapter 5 and the video of Ethan Kurtz in Chapter 1.)

Commonly, the treatment for **craniofacial anomalies***, in particular, will involve surgery*

Mind and Body

No matter what the treatment, it is useful to keep in mind that absolutely all disorders of human communication, with no exceptions, involve bodily systems at their basis. Also, it should be kept in mind that the body depends for its well-being on an intact genetic system enabling our normal development and thus access to higher communication abilities. The idea of a mind or personality without any body to express it is like an idea without any signs to represent it or words to say what it is. Minds and personalities depend on bodily forms to express them. This is one of the reasons we have chosen to use actual *Cases* of persons with disorders as our primary reference points throughout this course.

We also know from studies of language acquisition and learning in general that knowledge must ultimately be grounded in experience in the real world to be fully coherent. Therefore, the study of actual cases of persons with disorders in their real contexts of experience is necessary in making sense of the subject matter.

Bodies and Words

In keeping with the fact that **embryological development** unfolds over time from conception to birth, from birth to maturity, and from maturity until death, it makes sense to begin the story of disorders of communication with the kind that arise during the earliest stages of the growth and formation of the body. As we will see here and in subsequent chapters, the body is the essential residence of the mind, personality, and of all our communication abilities. If it were not for those abilities—ones situated necessarily in individual bodies of persons—there could be no communities or social groups. Communities consist of, and for their very existence absolutely depend on bodily individual persons who can communicate with each other. If it were not for our communication abilities, social, political, and historical contexts as we know them could not exist. So bodies are important.

Also, as we demonstrate throughout the course, the health and well-being of the body and of human communities depends absolutely on words. On the one hand, the body depends on the words in our genetic systems as well as nutrition, rest, and exercise. The words of the genetic system provide for the **epigenetic systems** of metabolism, immunity, and detoxification. All these higher systems engage in complex interactions that are normally provided for in our genetics. Those interactions, when all the communications are going well, provide protection from disease, injury, and chemical assaults from toxins.

On the other hand, our abilities to communicate with each other—and thus the well-being of our bodies along with our minds and personalities—depend greatly on interactions with other persons mainly through language.

The well-being and freedom of the mind, body, and personality, deeply depend on access to ordinary communication through the amazing powers of words and especially of the unique human language capacity.

Anomalies as Abnormal

Normal experience in communication is called "normal" because communication efforts usually work as intended. More often than not, communication goes right. We intend to perform certain tasks, and we are often able to do them. We intend to strike certain keys to form a particular sentence, and we succeed. We punch up a particular number and we hear the right voice on the other end of the line. We buy a ticket, order a meal, sign up for a class, or whatever, and everything works more or less as intended. The plane arrives at its destination, our meal nourishes us, the class meets and proceeds as expected, and so on and on.

It is because things normally develop according to the intended design that bodily disorders are commonly referred to as "anomalies"—abnormalities of form or function. Commonly, but not in all instances, there may be a genetic abnormality at the basis of a bodily anomaly. There is a large class of genetic disorders that can have a cascading series of effects, like the domino that knocks over another, which in turn strikes another. Of course, genetic transmission must work in a cascading fashion from parent to child, grandchild, and so on (Figure 2–1). More than 6,000 **genetic disorders** had already been catalogued by 1981 and many adjustments to the list have been made since then (Gardner & Snustadt, 1981; also see the Genetics Education Center, 2009, Web page retrieved March 20, 2009, from http://www.kumc.edu/gec/support/index.html).

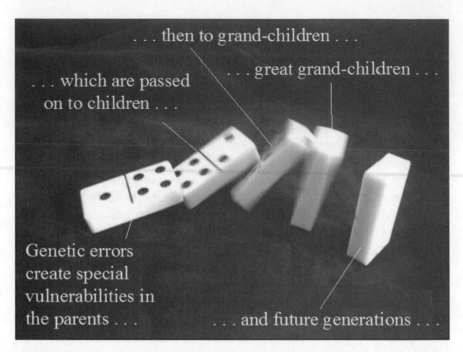

Figure 2–1. The cascading effects model of genetic errors across generations.

Genetic disorders have the potential of impacting the atoms, molecules, proteins, cells, tissues, and/or organs of the body in one way or another. However, genetic anomalies must remain silent until and unless they are put into action during development by environmental and metabolic factors.

In this chapter, and throughout this course, we are concerned with anomalies, problems, and imbalances that directly or indirectly lead to one or more communication disorders. Among the more common bodily anomalies that impact communication fairly directly are **craniofacial anomalies**. The best known of the disorders in this class consist of a *cleft lip* and/or **cleft palate**. These anomalies are similar in many respects to **spina bifida**—a kind of cleft where the spinal cord is exposed. The term *palate*, when we are speaking of the oral cavity, refers to what is commonly called the "roof of the mouth." The term *bifida* means "split" in Latin (see "Spina bifida" retrieved February 16, 2009, from http://en.wikipedia.org/wiki/Spina_bifida).

Establishing the Boundaries

The body is an amazingly differentiated system of distinct organs that are normally well integrated through communicating parts and yet are sharply distinguished by multiple layered boundaries. For instance, the fingernail emerges from beneath the skin but is a hard shell-like covering distinct from the skin and yet attached to it right out to the end of the finger. There, at the end, the fingernail separates itself from the skin completely. The distinct layers of tissue and their boundaries can be seen and felt from every angle of sight and touch.

Ordinarily, as a baby develops in its mother's womb, the seams and boundaries where growing tissues, for example, of the skin, bones, and bodily organs are normally joined are knitted together and integrated smoothly. There are, however, many more ways for embryological development to go wrong than for it to go right. In fact, **embryologists** are the first to admit that we can hardly tell what is going on in the developing embryo when things are going along normally. The process runs itself with incredible speed, efficiency, and accuracy. It is because the process usually works according to design that well-formed babies are more common than miscarriages or deformed individuals. However, many things can go wrong.

In this chapter we are especially concerned with the development of the skull, head, and the face where the main organ systems of speech and language are situated. With that in mind, consider the many **sutures** of the **cranium** (the skull) where bone tissues are joined as shown in Figure 2–2. The sutures are the joints between the distinctly colored bone plates, which are shown in Gray's diagram

> . . . boundaries where growing tissues, for example, of the skin, bones, and bodily organs are normally joined are knitted together and integrated smoothly.

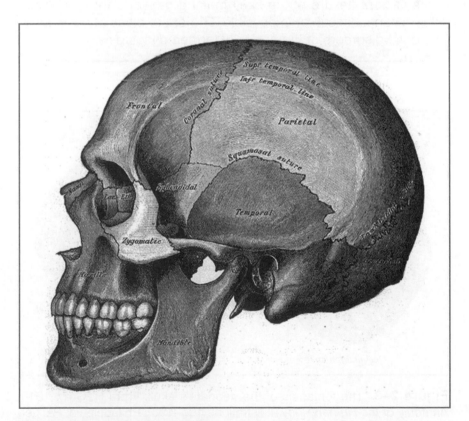

Figure 2–2. The distinct regions of the cranium. From H. Gray, 1918, *Anatomy of the Human Body* (Illustration 188). Philadelphia, PA: Lea & Febiger. Copyright © 2000 by Bartleby.com, ON-LINE ED., Inc. at http://www.bartleby.com/107/. Retrieved February 16, 2009, from http://www.bartleby.com/107/illus188.html. Reprinted with permission. All rights reserved.

as somewhat jagged lines between the pieces of bone. Each plate develops somewhat independently as soft and pliable tissue and then differentiates itself from surrounding tissues and hardens into bone—a process called **ossification**. Normally, at birth, the bones of the skull are not fully joined at the location of the "soft spots" in the baby's skull. These are technically called **fontanels**.

The major ones are the frontal and occipital fontanels at the top and back of the skull as seen in Figure 2–3 (on the left) and the sphenoidal and mastoid fontanels (at the right side of the figure). By comparing Figures 2–3 and 2–2 we can see that the major fontanels appear at the points where several bone plates of the skull come together. When either the bony or soft tissues fail to join, the result is a cleft, or **bifida**. If the bone plates close too soon, the resulting disorder is referred to as **synostosis**. When the bones of the skull join and harden too soon the outcome is **craniosynostosis**. In the latter case, some of the bone plates join too early resulting in a deformed skull with potential complications caused by insufficient room for the developing brain. There may also be insufficient flexure of the skull making passage through the birth canal difficult or impossible. The entire class of developmental disorders of the bones is termed dysostosis.

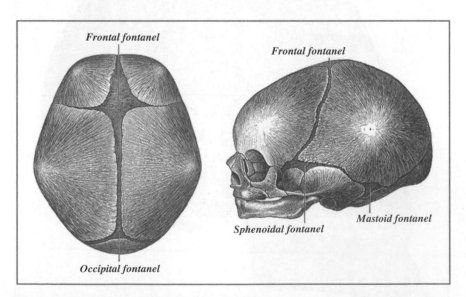

Figure 2–3. The fontanels of the neonate's skull. From H. Gray, 1918, *Anatomy of the Human Body* (Illustrations 197–198). Philadelphia, PA: Lea & Febiger. Copyright © 2000 by Bartleby.com, ON-LINE ED., Inc. at http://www.bartleby.com/107/. Retrieved February 16, 2009, from http://www.bartleby.com/107/illus198 and http://www.bartleby.com/107/illus197. Reprinted with permission. All rights reserved.

Passing On Genetic Injuries and Errors

Because genetic disorders result from damage to the genome, they lead to problems downstream—a cascading effect across generations as suggested in Figure 2–1 where the dominoes represent a succession of generations from parents to children and so on. Such cascading genetic injuries can be caused by radiation or by toxins. Some toxins have the potential to damage germ cells—that is, the chromosome carrying cells that we pass on to our children and grandchildren. Those **genotoxins**—gene damaging poisons—are a major source of errors leading to genetic deformities and diseases. Also, genetic damage may arise from some combination of factors. As suggested in Figure 2–4, genetic errors can lead to problems in the body, sometimes highly visible and audible ones, such as a cleft lip and palate, which tend to lead to additional difficulties of emotion, cognition, behavior, and communication.

   The toxins that produce or exacerbate genetic and related communication problems may come from dental fillings, medicines, vaccines, pesticides, legal or illegal drugs, industrial pollution, food preservatives, the leftover parts or byproducts of a destroyed virus or bacterium, diseased or damaged parts of our own bodies, and all kinds of environmental contaminants. The most ubiquitous genotoxin in the environment during the latter half of the 20th century and now in the 21st century that is also the most widely studied **neurotoxin**—a poison damaging nerves—is mercury in all of

Bodily malformations typically are communication problems from start to finish. The difficulty may begin with a communication problem at the level of genetics, but it may end with a host of problems at the level of social interactions.

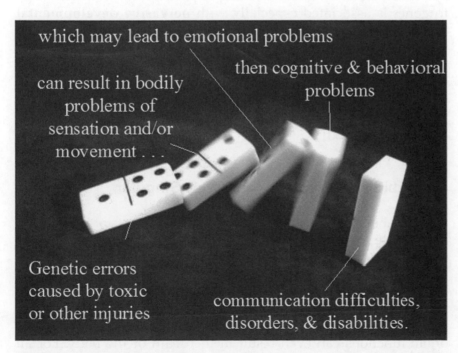

which may lead to emotional problems

then cognitive & behavioral problems

can result in bodily problems of sensation and/or movement . . .

Genetic errors caused by toxic or other injuries

communication difficulties, disorders, & disabilities.

Figure 2–4. Genetic damage can begin with toxic injuries producing a cascade leading to communication disorders.

its common forms. The largest single source of mercury in all manufactured products combined is the silverish gray metal material called **dental amalgam**. This is the material in what are called "silver fillings" because of their color, but they consist of a mixture containing more mercury than the several other metals combined. The mixture is approximately 50% mercury by weight and is known not only to be involved as a causal agent in autism (see Chapter 5) but also in essentially all the so-called **neurogenic disorders** of speech, language, hearing, and so on (Chapter 10).

As it turns out, many of those disorders are certainly *not caused by the nervous system* (as suggested by the term *neurogenic*) but are caused, in many instances, by damage as far removed from the central nervous system as the small intestine. We now know that disease of the gut can affect the production of chemicals involved in neurotransmission, which in turn can produce extreme impact on the central nervous system (Jepson & J. Johnson, 2007; also see Wakefield, 2005 retrieved February 16, 2009, from http://www.chem.cmu.edu/wakefield/). Again, the process is something like a series of falling dominoes where the most obvious impact—for example, loss of ability to speak in some cases—may be caused by an infection in the intestines. It may be initiated by a toxin such as mercury (see J. W. Oller & S. D. Oller, 2009).

For all of these reasons, some toxins are of special interest not only as agents that make communication disorders worse for the persons exposed, but because they can also affect the genes that will be passed on to future generations. Because our genes shape every system of the body, genotoxins are of particular interest. Damage to genes is associated especially with **pervasive developmental disorders** such as autism, but gene injuries can affect everything from a particular protein involved in maintaining the heart beat to molecules that enable neurons to fire correctly. To see a video showing how mercury damages the tiniest microtubules that surround neural fibrils, click on the hyperlink to How Mercury Damages Neurofibrils on the DVD (see the published report by Leong, Syed, & Lorscheider, 2001).

> Damage to genes is associated especially with **pervasive developmental** disorders such as autism, but gene injuries can affect everything from a particular protein involved in maintaining the heart beat to molecules that enable neurons to fire correctly.

Comorbidity: Disorders Are Rarely Singular

Figure 2–1 shows how the cascading series of effects of injuries can accumulate from basic chemicals expressed at the atomic level, to the macromolecules of genetic systems that control bodily structures, defenses, and transportation systems—especially those that help rid the body of toxins. Damage to these structures can result in damage to cells. An accumulation of that kind of damage can result in loss of functions of bodily organs. In their turn, loss of organ functions can even result in the death of the body. For all these reasons, the study of communication disorders can no more be separated rationally from the study of complex organismic systems than the study of aeronautical engineering can be separated from the basic sciences of physics, chemistry, and thermodynamics. When a cascading series of effects begins in, or interacts with, our genetic endowment, it is said to be epigenetic. For as long as the organism survives the developmental process, it is safe to say that all of the genetic, metabolic, and organic problems that arise in human experience must be epigenetic. They have to involve interactions between the genetic system and higher systems of proteins, metabolism, and so forth.

Behavioral manifestations impacting communication also commonly have significant genetic and epigenetic components. Some are known and many more are being uncovered as the mysteries of the human genome are being unraveled (Sanford, 2005). One thing is clear: environmental factors can impact the body and all of its related systems through epigenetic interactions.

Interdependent Systems

In addition to all of the foregoing factors, of course, there are social and linguistic factors that, if our systems are functioning correctly, enable us to transcend material limits to a very high degree in the exercise of what Nobel Laureate Roger Sperry called "free will" or what Noam Chomsky has described as "linguistic creativity." However, the will cannot be truly free if the body is severely damaged or prevented from its normal functions—for example, by being damaged, shackled, enslaved, or killed. The important fact to appreciate is that the body functions as a whole. It is a complex and dynamic system of balanced and interrelated systems. It is essential to see that a relatively intact body is crucial to the development and functioning of the senses; that valid signs produced by functional sensory systems are necessary for building up motor signs; and that motor signs in their turn are crucial to the building up of linguistic signs. Understanding the relations between these interrelated systems is essential.

With respect to disorders, because of the interdependencies of the various representational systems of the body, the actor inside it, and the mind that is also in the body, we have proposed what we call the *domino theory of disorders*. It is also known as the *cascading effects model* (see Figure 2–1 modified from J. W. Oller, S. D. Oller, & Badon, 2006, p. 377). The idea is simple and certainly not new. A disorder at any level or stage of development can have far-reaching effects on subsequent developments and on all of the systems of representation dependent on whatever may be affected by the disorder. As we will see here and in Chapters 3 through 10 especially, a disorder at any level, but particularly one that appears early in development, is apt to have a cascading series of effects on subsequent (and usually higher levels of) development.

For all the foregoing reasons, situations where more than one disorder, disease, or problem can be found in the same individual or group of individuals—a condition generally referred to as

It is essential to see that a relatively intact body is crucial to the development and functioning of the senses; that valid signs produced by functional sensory systems are necessary for building up motor signs; and that motor signs in their turn are crucial to the building up of linguistic signs.

comorbidity—is common. We must expect this because of how our bodily systems and all our systems of representation are naturally and inevitably interrelated. As a result, disorders that are popularly regarded as distinct may turn out to be the same and some that seem to be the same may turn out to be different disorders that merely have common symptoms. The expectation that the **diagnosis** of a particular disorder necessarily precludes the diagnosis of one or several related disorders is generally the result of failure to understand how intricately representational systems are interrelated. Distinct systems of representation can have multiple interactions with each other at many different levels. Because of the complexity of the representational systems that have to be understood and used, it is unremarkable that communication disorders occur and that where we find one we are apt to find others. The inevitable tendency to apply multiple terms to the same disorder or the same term to different disorders is also predictable.

The Real Material World: The Body Is Situated

Communicators are always situated in some real space-time-matter context. In Figure 1–3 we show the body as in the material world at the bottom of the picture. The body is a physical form and it appears inevitably in the material, physical world.

The bodies of human communicators are inevitably "situated" in the real world of human discourse (Ballard, Hayhoe, Pook, & Rao, 1997; Barsalou, 1999; Gibbs, 2003; M. Johnson, 1992; J. W. Oller, L. Chen, Pan, & S. D. Oller, 2005; Pylyshyn, 2002).

It is important to realize that even if we engage in the construction or interpretation of some fiction, or, say, a fantasy beyond imagination, we are still situated bodily in the world somewhere. Even if we imagine ourselves to be in a distant galaxy far removed from our solar system, in doing this we need to be situated somewhere in the real world. Where we really are may have little to do with what is going on in the fantasy, but our bodily systems are still involved in a crucial way to enable us to dream, imagine, or develop the fantasy. Imagination does not exist in a total vacuum apart from material contexts and it is not completely separated from our bodies. If we start dodging punches at the movies, for instance, because there is a fight scene on the big silver screen, any movements we actually make will be situated right where we are even if they are coordinated somewhat with actions depicted on the screen. Just ask the persons sitting next to you at the movies. Or, if you bump one of them, they may volunteer to point out the fact that your body is sitting in a seat at a theater, and that you are only involved in the scene on the big screen in a vicarious way. Still, it is true that imagination and understanding of words is not much dependent on where we happen to be at the time.

Your understanding of this paragraph, for example, does not depend (much) on whether you are at a table in the library, or on a jet at 30,000 feet. It hardly depends at all on whether you are reading a printed page or viewing the text on a liquid crystal device or a plasma screen. It does not matter whether you have the DVD in your laptop or whether you do not have it with you at all. You might think about this paragraph, or its meaning, an hour after reading it, or two years later on. No matter where or when, if you think of these words or ideas at all, you will be situated somewhere. Your body will be, must be, and is involved in any interaction just as the bodies of the authors are involved in writing, editing, and rewriting the words of this book. All of us are situated somewhere in space and time in every interaction between us.

It is important to keep in mind, as suggested in Figure 1–3, that the bodies of communicators who are interacting are invariably part of the stream of experience in the material world. Ordinary human communication always involves bodily interactions of one or many persons. So-called **paranormal phenomena**, which are outside of the scope of this course, only become "paranormal"— that is, outside of or above what is normal—by being associated in some way or other with the bodies of persons who are in the "normal" world. That is, whatever paranormal dimensions there might be, can be of interest to normal people only to the extent that those phenomena impact us—if at all—in the real (the "normal") world. Representations are creations of the representer, but only to the extent that they actually connect with the real world can they shape or change things in that world to the slightest degree.

Genetic and Epigenetic Disorders

Many disorders seem to have a primary genetic component. Among them are **sickle cell anemia**, **diabetes mellitus**, **cystic fibrosis**, **Down syndrome**, **Treacher-Collins syndrome**, and many more. In this section we consider each of those along with **fetal alcohol syndrome (FAS)** which is less likely than many others to be caused primarily by its genetic component. However, the fact that not all children exposed to alcohol toxicity while they are in their mother's womb develop FAS, there is reason to suppose that some women and their genetically linked offspring are more particularly susceptible to FAS. This is what is meant by an **epigenetic disorder**—one that arises above the genetic systems but interacting with them. All of the genetically linked disease conditions, many of which we will not discuss here, can have pervasive and far-reaching adverse consequences on communication abilities. In some instances the impact is relatively direct and in others it is indirect.

Sickle Cell Anemia

This blood disorder is a condition known to be caused by a **single nucleotide polymorphism (SNP)**—pronounced "snip"—in the gene specifying **hemoglobin**, which is the main protein ingredient in our red blood cells. Without it, blood cannot carry oxygen to the rest of our body. There are 600 nucleotides in the gene in question

So-called **paranormal phenomena**, which are outside of the scope of this course, only become "paranormal"—that is, outside of or above what is normal—by being associated in some way or other with the bodies of persons who are in the "normal" world.

and one SNP produces sickle cell anemia. As seen in Figure 2–5, in this disease, blood cells lose their round shape. Because of their deformation, the red cells—some of them sickle shaped—clog the smallest blood vessels, the capillaries, producing excruciating pain and sometimes death (see "Sickle Cell Disease," 2009, retrieved February 16, 2009, from http://en.wikipedia.org/wiki/Sickle-cell_disease). This debilitating disease can indirectly affect the entire course of development and essentially all communication processes. It is especially damaging to hearing, and because it can affect blood supply to the central nervous system may also result in mild to severe intellectual and emotional problems.

Diabetes Mellitus

This form of diabetes is a genetically linked disease affecting sugar metabolism and related systems in about 7% of the U.S. population according to the American Diabetes Association (retrieved February 16 2009, from http://www.diabetes.org/about-diabetes.jsp). Because of its pervasive impact on the body, and since it is known to be impacted by some of the same toxins that contribute to pervasive developmental communication disorders, the upsurge in diabetes in recent years is linked with a host of disorders that impact communication more directly. Although diabetes is not itself thought of as a communication disorder, it can cause complete blindness, which is an extreme sensory disorder. It can also result in general neurological deterioration especially at the extremities.

Although diabetes is not itself thought of as a communication disorder, it can cause complete blindness, which is an extreme sensory disorder.

Cystic Fibrosis

This disease is largely inherited and results commonly in chronic lung infections, consequent difficulty breathing, and digestive problems. The **pancreas** is so significantly affected in this disease that

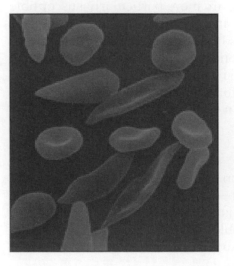

Figure 2–5. Sickle cell anemia is seen in red blood cells that become deformed into an oblong shape. Micrograph retrieved February 16, 2009, from http://en.wikipedia.org/wiki/Image:Sicklecells.jpg. U.S. Government publication by the National Institute of Diabetes and Digestive and Kidney Diseases. Image in the public domain.

it used to be called "pancreatic cystic fibrosis" or "cystic fibrosis of the pancreas" (Andersen, 1938) as it was originally designated by its discoverer Dr. Dorothy Hansine Andersen [1901–1963]. Because it affects the lungs, it is one of the diseases that is occasionally seen by speech-language pathologists in clinical settings. Because of its impact on breathing it affects voice production and the quality of speech.

Down Syndrome

Known primarily by its impact on outward appearance (Figure 2–6), Down syndrome was named for the British doctor, John Langdon Down [1828–1896], who first described it in 1866. The likelihood of occurrence of Down syndrome is a function of the age of the mother with younger mothers, before age 30, having an incidence of about 1 child in 900, while the oldest mothers, after age 49, have an incidence of 1 in 12. Between these boundaries a smooth growth curve can be plotted (National Institute of Child Health and Human Development, 2006, retrieved February 16, 2009, from http://www.nichd.nih.gov/publications/pubs/downsyndrome.cfm#The Occurrence). The disorder is caused, as determined by Jerome Lejeune (see Lejeune, 1960; Lejeune, Gauthier, & Turpin, 1959) by what is termed "triplication" (three instead of two copies) of chromosome 21 (Leshin, 2003, retrieved February 16, 2009, from http://www.ds-health.com/trisomy.htm).

The likelihood of occurrence of Down syndrome is a function of the age of the mother with younger mothers, before age 30, having an incidence of about 1 child in 900, while the oldest mothers, after age 49, have an incidence of 1 in 12.

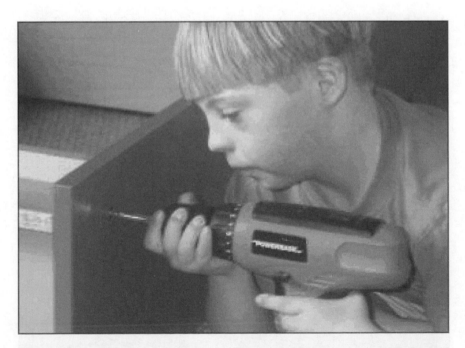

Figure 2–6. Jordan, son of EN, Excalibur with Down syndrome. Retrieved February 16, 2009, from http://en.wikipedia.org/wiki/Image:Drill.jpg. Used under the GNU Free Documentation License, Version 1.2.

Individuals with Down syndrome generally have lower than average intelligence accompanied by mild to severe learning disabilities. They often seem naive and tend toward concrete thinking. Some have severe intellectual disabilities. They are often seen by teachers of special education and by speech-language pathologists. Rarely do children with Down syndrome fail to acquire significant verbal skills, though reading and writing may present special challenges in instances accompanied by severe retardation.

Treacher-Collins Syndrome (TCS)

This disorder, illustrated in Figure 2–7, is known by various names and has been attributed to a defective gene at chromosome 5q32-133.3 (Loftus, K. Dixon, Koprivnikar, M. J. Dixon, & Wasmuth, 1996; Magalhaes, da Silveira, Moreira, & Cavalcanti, 2007; McKeown & Bronner-Fraser, 2008). TCS is also known as **mandibulofacial dysostosis** and as **Franceschetti syndrome**. It is one of what are also called **branchial arch syndromes**. The branchial arches are the tissue systems that develop into the head and neck. The problems in TCS are more severe than cleft lip and/or palate and more difficult to repair, but like the more common clefts, TCS can leave almost everything intact except for the main structures of the head, face, and neck. The impact on social interaction, articulation of speech, and thus on communication can be severe.

Fetal Alcohol Syndrome (FAS)

A multiple systems developmental disorder, FAS (Figure 2–8) is triggered in genetically susceptible individuals by the mother's

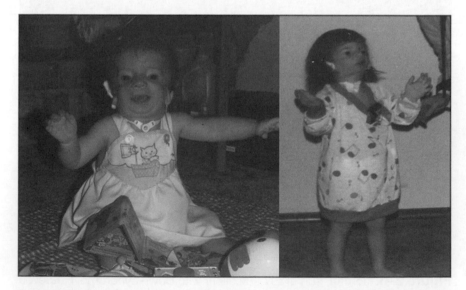

Figure 2–7. Emily as an infant and later as a toddler. Photograph used by permission. Copyright © 2009 by Plural Publishing, Inc. All rights reserved.

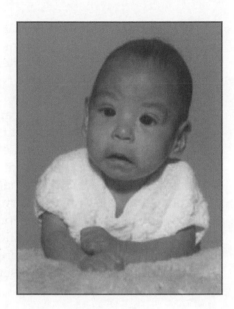

Figure 2–8. A baby with fetal alcohol syndrome. Retrieved November 5, 2007, from http://en.wikipedia.org/wiki/Image: FASbaby.jpg. Used under the GNU Free Documentation License, Version 1.2.

consumption of alcohol during or prior to her pregnancy. "It's estimated that each year in the United States, 1 in every 750 infants is born with a pattern of physical, developmental, and functional problems referred to as fetal alcohol syndrome (FAS), whereas another 40,000 are born with **fetal alcohol effects (FAE)**"(see "Fetal Alcohol Syndrome," 2009, retrieved February 16, 2009, from http://www.kidshealth.org/parent/medical/brain/fas.html). However, not all children exposed to alcohol in the womb are impacted by FAS.

An Important Study

A longitudinal study that began in 1974 with 1,529 children born to mothers who consumed varying amounts of alcohol finished up with 500 cases 25 years later each of whom was assessed for FAS symptoms on 11 occasions. The study showed a significant dose-related correlation with severity of symptoms.

Neuropsychological and neurobehavioral performance measures are correlated with prenatal alcohol dose, without substantial confounding by socio-demographic or rearing conditions, smoking, nutrition, or other drugs. Deficits in attention, arithmetic skill, spatial-visual memory, and IQ, as well as increased alcohol problems and psychiatric disorders are among offspring outcomes correlated at several ages with maternal drinking during and before pregnancy recognition. (Streissguth, 2007, p. 81)

The risks are evidently higher early in the pregnancy, or possibly just prior to and during the time of conception. While it is generally argued on the basis of evidence from humans that the consumption of alcohol by the father is unrelated to FAS, research with mice shows that alcohol consumed by the father on the day of conception results in smaller litters, more runts, more aggressive offspring, and a greater number of early deaths in the offspring (Meek, Myren, Sturm, & Burau, 2007). It is also interesting that although FAS is probably not caused by any particular arrangement of genes, it seems to impact the metabolism of the developing fetus so as to create a greater likelihood of the child becoming an alcoholic as an adult. Other symptoms at birth include facial abnormalities, low birth weight, a smaller than normal head, flattened cheekbones, an indistinct **philtrum**—the groove under the nose and just above the upper lip—poor coordination, delayed social development, reduced imagination and curiosity, and a host of learning difficulties impacting language and reasoning. Except for the facial abnormalities, FAS resembles autism in some of its key symptoms (see Chapter 5).

WHEN THINGS GO WRONG

> It is unremarkable that things sometimes go wrong in communication and that disorders occur. What is remarkable is that communication *commonly works as expected*.

It is unremarkable that things sometimes go wrong in communication and that disorders occur. What is remarkable is that communication *commonly works as expected*. If this were not so, we would not use terms such as "abnormal," "disorder," "anomaly," and so forth in cases where things go wrong.

Disorders Are Not Normal

Undeniable indirect evidence that communication commonly succeeds is that communication disorders are outside what is expected. They are not normal. The fact is that successful communication is normal—that is, common and expected. By contrast, when communication disorders arise, in one way or another, things have not gone so well. In some cases of communication disorders, things have gone terribly wrong. The study of what is known as teratology—based on the Greek root meaning marvel, prodigy, or monster—suggests the fact that anomalies can be extreme. We do not like this term because it seems to suggest, falsely, we believe, that injured human beings, for example, with craniofacial anomalies—the most common instances being cleft lip or cleft palate—are less than human.

We agree rather with Mother Teresa (Figure 2–9) who said, "If you don't want the little child, that unborn child, give him to me" (as quoted by Reagan, 1984, p. 36).

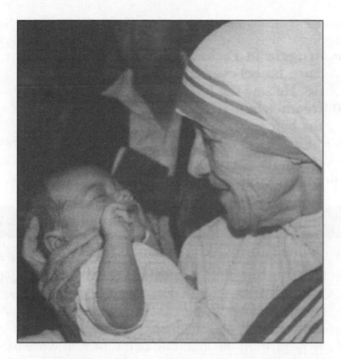

Figure 2–9. Mother Teresa at a meeting of the American Family Institute. Copyright © 1984 by the Human Life Foundation, Inc. From *Abortion and the Conscience of the Nation* (p. 37), by R. Reagan, 1984, Nashville, TN: Thomas Nelson Publishers. Copyright 1984 by the Human Life Foundation, Inc. Reprinted with permission. All rights reserved.

Teratology

When serious disorders arise in infancy, one of the great moral questions of the ages reverberates across the millennia. We hear its echoes in the 21st century. Is there such a thing as "life not worthy to be lived"? When that question comes up, all of the personal freedoms, the values, and the laws protecting them, are on the line. The problem was well put in the context of the Nuremberg War Crimes Tribunal by Dr. Leo Alexander who worked with the Chief American Counsel. He pointed out the connection between attitudes toward disabilities and beliefs about human worth. In pre-Nazi Germany there was a

> subtle shift in emphasis in the basic attitudes of physicians. It started with the acceptance of the attitude, basic in the **euthanasia movement**, that there is such a thing as life not worthy to be lived. This attitude in its early stages concerned itself merely with the severely and chronically sick. (1949, p. 45)

Among those disposed of were

> the mentally defective, psychotics (particularly schizophrenics), epileptics and patients suffering from infirmities of old

Is there such a thing as "life not worthy to be lived"?

age and from various organic neurologic disorders such as infantile paralysis, Parkinsonism, multiple sclerosis and brain tumors. (1949, p. 41)

An Immense Separation

There is an amazing division in history between those who would help the disordered, disabled, the injured, diseased, and sick among us and those who would prefer simply to dispose of them.

The Small Wedged-in Lever

The Nazi mentality tending inevitably toward the disposal route —just kill them—was not a sudden decision embraced in the full force of its meaning. It was accepted little by little as one expediency led to another until the Nazis were at war with the whole world. Dr. Alexander shows how the "just kill them" mentality grew from the idea that some people were too sick or disabled to be worth saving to the view that only the hypothetical super race consisting of Germanic Nazis were worthy of life:

> Gradually, the sphere . . . was enlarged to encompass the socially unproductive, the ideologically unwanted, the racially unwanted, and finally all non-Germans. But is it is important to realize that the infinitely small wedged-in lever from which the entire trend of mind received its impetus was the attitude towards the non-rehabilitatable sick. (1949, p. 45)

There was a common doctrine taught in German math classes well before the Nazi era that certain lives of the genetically damaged, injured, and so forth, would take up too much space, breathe too much air, and cost too much money.

Dr. Alexander reached a very different conclusion from the Nazi doctors. There was a common doctrine taught in German math classes well before the Nazi era that certain lives of the genetically damaged, injured, and so forth, would take up too much space, breathe too much air, and cost too much money. In response, Dr. Alexander (1947) wrote, "The value of even one human life is infinite" with the result that "one times infinity is just as infinite as 500 times infinity" (retrieved February 16, 2009, from the transcript at http://nuremberg.law.harvard.edu/php/pflip.php?caseid=HLSL_NMT01&docnum=2&numpages=78&startpage=1&title=Closing+argument+for+the+United+States+of+America.&color_setting=C, p. 76).

As we study the full range of genetic, developmental, and communication disorders that directly affect the body not only in its appearance but in its functioning, we discover that disorders that affect the structure of the body can also impact the senses in some cases, and/or movements, and the senses and motor systems can affect higher systems of communication. All of the cases we consider in this chapter would have been candidates for extermination under the Nazis. However, the rewarding careers of speech-language pathologists, **audiologists**, teachers of special education, and **pediatric surgeons** like C. Everett Koop (see "C. Everett Koop," 2009, retrieved February 16, 2009, from http://en.wikipedia.org/wiki/C._Everett_Koop) show that many of these disorders can not only be corrected or alleviated, but that the children can be enabled to lead productive and valued lives.

Dr. Koop (1984), for example, described the "rehabilitation of youngsters who were born with **congenital anomalies** incompatible with life but nevertheless amenable to surgical correction" (p. 43). He was referring to surgeries for everything from craniofacial deformities such as cleft lip or palate, to spina bifida, or an **imperforate anus**. He himself treated many children with the last problem—where there is no exit point for fecal body wastes. He says that no surviving person nor parent of such a patient ever came back and said, "Why did you work so hard to save the life of my child?" (pp. 43–44). In a survey of 25 families of children operated on for an imperforate anus between 15 to 25 years after the surgery "almost every family referred to the experience of raising the defective youngster as a positive one. A few were neutral. None were negative" (p. 44).

THE CASE OF SAMUEL ARMAS

The baby pictured in Figure 2–10 is Samuel Armas.[1] At the time this picture was taken little Samuel would have almost fit completely in the hand of the doctor doing the surgery to repair his spina bifida. Samuel was just past the half way mark in the normal **gestational period**. Dating his life from his conception, he was 21 weeks old at the time of his surgery, and as far as we know to this very day (February 16, 2009), he remains the youngest baby ever operated on for spina bifida.

In Figure 2–10, all we see of tiny Samuel is his small hand reaching out to grasp the finger of the surgeon, Dr. Joseph Bruner. This picture is one of a series of four shots taken in rapid succession in 1999 by Michael Clancy (2001). The four distinct photos shot at 60 frames per second can be viewed on the DVD (retrieved February 16, 2009, from http://www.michaelclancy.com/story.html). Clancy had been commissioned by *USA Today* to document the surgery at Vanderbilt University Medical Center with the permission of Dr. Joseph Bruner, the physician who performed the surgery. The procedure involves something like a **cesarean section** except in this case instead of taking the baby from the womb, the entire

In Figure 2–10, all we see of tiny Samuel is his small hand reaching out to grasp the finger of the surgeon, Dr. Joseph Bruner. This picture is one of a series of four shots taken in rapid succession in 1999 by Michael Clancy (2001).

---

[1]We are indebted to Raquelle Horton for calling Samuel's story to our attention.

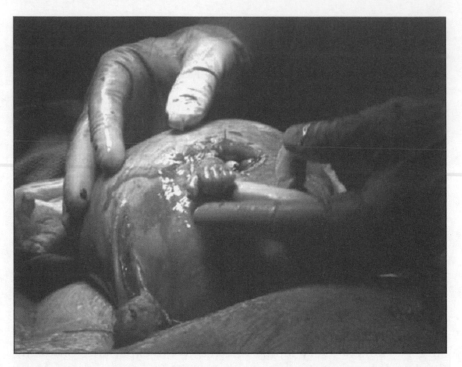

Figure 2–10. The spina bifida surgery on Samuel Armas by Dr. Joseph Bruner. Copyright © 2005 by Michael Clancy. Retrieved February 16, 2009, from http://www.michaelclancy.com/story.html. Reprinted with permission. All rights reserved.

womb is removed and a small opening is made through which the surgery to repair the spina bifida can be performed on the baby. Then the womb is replaced inside the mother until the gestational period of approximately 40 weeks is completed. Without the surgery, Samuel's life would have been a lot less normal than it is today. Figure 2–11 shows what Samuel looked like about four years after his surgery.

Samuel in Congress

On September 25, 2003, at the age of 3½, Samuel Armas went with his parents and Mr. Clancy to testify in Congress about his surgery. When asked by Senator Sam Brownback of Kansas if he knew who that baby in the picture was, he said, "Baby Samuel." When he was asked what was done to him on the day of that hand reaching out from mommy's womb, Samuel said, "They fixed my boo boo."

The photo and the story behind it inevitably was swept up in the storm of controversy that has been going on since before the time of Hippocrates over severe diseases and disorders. The question then and now is when, if ever, is a doctor justified in deliberately causing or assisting in the causation of the death of the patient or an unborn child? Senator Brownback observed during the Senate

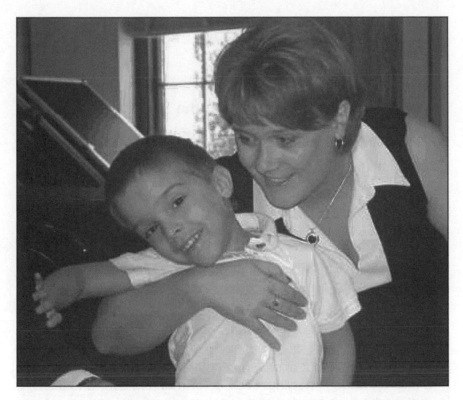

Figure 2–11. Samuel Armas at about four years. Copyright © 2003 by Jonathan Imbody. Retrieved February 16, 2009, from http://freerepublic.com/focus/f-news/1012548/posts. Reprinted by permission. All rights reserved.

hearings, "There is little debate about whether the child in utero is alive; the debate is over whether or not the child has a life worthy of protection." In testifying before the Senate Committee, both Julie and Alex Armas, Samuel's parents, noted how they were affected by the news that their baby not only had the condition known as "spina bifida" but also **hydrocephalus**—a condition popularly referred to as "water on the brain" but more accurately described as excessive cerebrospinal fluid in the cranium. Such a condition can cause not only an enlarged head but can also result in mental disabilities, including inability to acquire language. Typically it also results in the inability to control the bladder and a persistent unstable gait and posture (National Institute of Neurological Disorders and Stroke, 2009, retrieved February 16, 2009 from http://www.ninds.nih.gov/disorders/hydrocephalus/detail_hydrocephalus.htm).
    Alex Armas said,

> It's every parent's worst nightmare to learn that something is very wrong with your child. The doctor painted a grim picture for us and stopped just short of suggesting an abortion.

Alex went on to explain why, for him and Julie, "ending the pregnancy was never an option." After the surgery during the 15 weeks

It's every parent's worst nightmare to learn that something is very wrong with your child.

prior to his birth, Alex recalled, "the hydrocephalus stopped progressing and started to slowly decrease." By the time he was born, Samuel's hydrocephalus had resolved.

A Moral Quandary Emerges with the Tiny Hand

Worldwide interest followed the pictures of Samuel Armas's tiny hand reaching out to touch the doctor. It inspired one writer at *USA Today*, Robert Davis, on May 2, 2000, to title his article, "Hand of a Fetus Touched the World." But the article would dispute the following claims of Michael Clancy who describes what happened on the day of the surgery in his own words:

> ### An Intentional Connection
>
> As a doctor asked me what speed of film I was using, out of the corner of my eye I saw the uterus shake, but no one's hands were near it. It was shaking from within. Suddenly, an entire arm thrust out of the opening, then pulled back until just a little hand was showing. The doctor reached over and lifted the hand, which reacted and squeezed the doctor's finger. As if testing for strength, the doctor shook the tiny fist. Samuel held firm. I took the picture! Wow! It happened so fast that the nurse standing next to me asked, "What happened?"
> "The child reached out," I said.
> "Oh. They do that all the time," she responded (retrieved February 16, 2009, from http://www.michaelclancy.com/story.html).

The events described by Michael Clancy occurred on August 19, 1999 and were recorded in the pictures he took that day. Those pictures were first published on September 7, 1999 in separate articles in *USA Today* and in *The Tennessean Newspaper*. The article by Robert Davis appeared 9 months later on May 2, 2000. Davis's article seemed to doubt the integrity of Michael Clancy and the validity of the photos. The basis for the challenge, it seems, was a flare up of the longstanding debate between abortionists and anti-abortionists in the good old USA.

An Urban Legend?

It is interesting that the very doctor who performed the surgery described the pictures as having spawned "an urban legend." Robert Davis quoted the surgeon who reported an alleged bit of hearsay implying that the pictures of baby Samuel were fraudulent:

Worldwide interest followed the pictures of Samuel Armas's tiny hand reaching out to touch the doctor.

One person said the photo had been reviewed by a team of medical experts and they had determined that it was a hoax," Bruner says with a laugh.

Dr. Bruner's account was that certain "opponents of abortion" were responsible for the claim that the baby had reached out on its own volition. But the writer of the article in *USA Today* continues quoting Dr. Bruner:

> "Not true," Bruner says. "Samuel and his mother, Julie, were under anesthesia and could not move."

Yet, the four photos shot at 60 frames per second on Mr. Clancy's Web site show the hand of the baby moving on its own. We can also see the tiny fingers of Samuel's hand grabbing on to Dr. Burner's middle finger just covering the tip and nail of Bruner's finger and we can see the pressure in the grip of the tiny fingers which could not occur apart from movement initiated by the baby. It is true that photos can be manipulated, but the gripping fingers of baby Samuel are under no one's control but Samuel's.

A Posed Picture

Whether Samuel Armas was consciously intending to grab Dr. Bruner's finger or whether Dr. Bruner gave him his middle finger on purpose is hardly the issue. The question is whether the doctor could have produced the visible tightness of the grip. The answer is plain that only Samuel could squeeze the tip of the doctor's finger, or ball his little fingers into a small fist. The reader can compare a posed picture of an unconscious baby of 24 weeks undergoing a similar surgery by the same Dr. Joseph Bruner (n. d., retrieved December 27, 2007, from http://www.life.com/Life/eisies/eisies 2000/scienceSingle_blowup.html).

The posed picture looks different. It shows Dr. Bruner supporting the baby's limp arm so that the hand will remain on the doctor's finger. The thumb in the posed picture is not gripping the doctor's finger and the doctor is visibly pulling on and sustaining the limp arm with both hands. Contrasting with the posed picture, the four shots of Samuel Armas show his fingers contracting and holding on to the doctor's finger. It also came out that the posed picture was taken prior to the surgery on Samuel Armas and that Dr. Bruner, evidently, was looking forward to making the cover of *Life Magazine*.

The Underlying Issue

As Dr. Bruner revealed in his comments to Robert Davis at *USA Today*, the underlying motivation for the controversy was Dr. Bruner's sympathy for the abortionists' side of the argument. He did not

> The question is whether the doctor could have produced the visible tightness of the grip.

want the surgery he performed to repair Samuel's spina bifida to be used in arguments against abortion. It was probably inevitable, however, that the Armas story would be told. In fact, it would inevitably become an element in the hearings soon to take place in Congress leading up to the passing of the 2003 law banning **partial birth abortion** (see "Partial Birth Abortion," 2009, retrieved February 16, 2009, from http://en.wikipedia.org/wiki/Partial_birth_abortion and see the references included there).

In partial birth abortions—also referred to as **late-term abortions**—the baby is deliberately killed by the doctor in the process of delivery. In fact, in all abortion procedures, the baby is killed by the doctor, but with late-term abortions the baby is effectively born alive and killed while coming out. It hardly seems possible in the modern world, much less in the land of the free and home of the brave, but by 2003 approximately 300,000 such abortions were paid for under Medicaid (see the extensive discussion and cited sources at the URLs already given). The total number of abortions performed from 1973 to 2003 was about a million per year with a high of 1,429,247 in 1990 and a low of 615,831 in 1973 (Strauss et al., November 24, 2006, Table 2).

Three and a Half Years Later: Samuel Armas in Congress

Six Congressional Hearings on partial birth abortion occurred prior to the signing on November 5, 2003 of the law banning them in the United States (Gorney, 2004, retrieved February 16, 2009, from http://www.harpers.org/archive/2004/11/0080278). Interestingly, the testimony of Samuel Armas on September 25, 2003 would take place before the U. S. Senate Subcommittee on Science, Space, and Technology just a few weeks before the passage of the law (see the video record of the signing retrieved August 23, 2008, from http://www.whitehouse.gov/news/releases/2003/11/20031105-1.html#). At that time, Samuel was almost four years old.

Ostensibly the purpose of the pictures of Samuel's spina bifida surgery and his testimony was to laud advances in medicine. Among them was the use of four-dimensional real-time video of babies—4D ultrasound—in the womb about which we will have more to say in the next section. The subtext of the meeting that day, however, was the deeper moral question of whether or not the parents of Samuel Armas did the right thing in not aborting him on account of his hydrocephaly and his spina bifida. Samuel's act at 21 weeks of gestation defies theories that deny humanity to unborn babies and shows the intrinsic criminality of black marketeers who sell the organs of aborted babies. See the 20/20 exposé (Crutcher, 2007) of a doctor selling aborted human baby parts (retrieved February 16, 2009, at http://lifedynamics.com/Abortion_Information/Baby_Body_Parts/index.cfm by scrolling down and clicking on the link at the bottom that says Click Here to see Miles Jones profit clip).

The pictures taken by Michael Clancy showing the volitional movement of a tiny baby before its birth play havoc with theories that a "fetus is just a lump of tissue" and not a human being with senses, freedom of movement, and significant cognitive awareness.

There can be no doubt that Samuel Armas was a living human being when the surgery to correct his spina bifida was performed.

In personal correspondence with us on September 21, 2007, Michael Clancy wrote, "I was pro-choice [pro-abortion] when I walked into that operating room. Now, I'm a Crusader for life." He says, "You couldn't have worn my shoes and not become actively pro-life." On the evening of his message, he was en route to a meeting of a pro-life organization where he would give a plenary address the following day.

There can be no doubt that Samuel Armas was a living human being when the surgery to correct his spina bifida was performed.

The Partial Birth Abortion Act

On November 5, 2003 after extensive debate in the U.S. Congress, President Bush signed into law the **Partial Birth Abortion Ban Act of 2003**. The law made it illegal in the United States for reasons stated in the opening paragraph of the law to perform the procedure described in the following quotation:

> A moral, medical, and ethical consensus exists that the practice of performing a partial-birth abortion—an abortion in which a physician delivers an unborn child's body until only the head remains inside the womb, punctures the back of the child's skull with a sharp instrument, and sucks the child's brains out before completing delivery of the dead infant—is a gruesome and inhumane procedure that is never medically necessary and should be prohibited. (retrieved February 16, 2009, from http://news.findlaw.com/hdocs/docs/abortion/2003s3.html)

After considering the pictures of the surgery on Samuel Armas—along with a great deal of testimony including some from Michael Clancy—the U.S. Congress in 2003 made illegal a procedure that was forbidden before 380 BC by what is known as the "Hippocratic Oath" (see Chapter 12, especially Figure 12–8). In that historical compilation in the time of Hippocrates, it was already common practice for physicians to promise *not* to do two things:

Hippocratic Oath

I will neither give a deadly drug to anybody who asked for it [to enable medically assisted suicide, known now as euthanasia], nor will I make a suggestion to this effect. Similarly *I will not give to a woman an abortive remedy* [our emphasis]. (For discussion see "Hippocratic Oath," 2009, retrieved February 16, 2009, from http://en.wikipedia.org/wiki/Hippocratic_Oath.)

It seems curious that the government of the United States of America—the torch bearer of freedom in the modern world with its great Statue of Liberty in New York harbor—in the year 2003 returned just part way to the moral standards laid down by medical practitioners prior to the time of Hippocrates. The standards set in the famous "Hippocratic Oath" as recorded prior to his death in 380 BC were already higher than the current ones of the so-called "free" world.

4D ULTRASOUND: MOVING PICTURES OF THE BABY IN THE WOMB

Thanks to Dr. Stuart Campbell's pioneering work we can see the growth of the baby in the womb (S. Campbell, 2004; from http://www.createhealth.org/ visited April 11, 2009 click on "Video Life Before Birth," and also see the Baby in the Womb on the DVD).

Moving pictures looking inside the womb were critical to discovering Samuel's spina bifida and arranging for its repair. The technology involves creating multiple sequential images from the echoes of sound waves and then removing their natural distortions with the aid of software that converts them to real-time moving pictures of the baby in the womb. Such pictures are radically changing the way people view the human baby before it is born. Dr. David Chamberlain (2009) writes:

> Through many windows of observation, we can now see—for the first time in human history—what is actually happening in the womb. There is good news and bad news. We can no longer think that the placenta can protect the prenate from anything bad going on in the mother's body, or that the mother's body can protect the prenate from bad things going on in her world. Mother and baby face together the perils of air, water, and earth compromised by the toxic residues of modern chemistry and physics. Parents are perhaps the last ones to learn (and their children the first ones to suffer) these tragic realities of modern life. (retrieved February 16, 2009, from http://www.birthpsychology.com/lifebefore/)

Dr. Chamberlain might also have mentioned the perils of a surgeon's knife.

One thing that has changed dramatically is our ability to know what is going on inside the womb. We can now look inside in a relatively noninvasive way to see what is happening before the baby is born. The moving images of human life before birth have certainly changed medicine and have also helped to shape public policy concerning disabilities and disorders. As we saw in Chapter 1, the baby by its 12th week can blink its eyes, jump around, take steps, and suck its thumb. A little later in the pregnancy it can produce a perfect **Duchenne smile**. By 21 weeks, Samuel Armas could reach out and touch the world.

False Theories Refuted

Because of advancing technologies enabling us to see inside the womb, the gas theory of smiling has been exploded. Similarly, 4D ultrasound shows the falseness of the elaborate mythology promoted by Ernst Haeckel (Pennisi, 1997) about human babies going through a phase of development where they breathe through gills like a fish.

Many such false claims, though still widely circulated in high school biology texts, are immediately refuted by the evidence from actual videography of the human baby in the womb. Not only does the technology show certain claims by Haeckel, for instance, to have been fanciful fictions rather than science, but video of babies in the womb demolishes all the nonsense claiming that human babies are not fully distinct human beings until after they are born.

Just as the testimony of the Armas family and the pictures from Michael Clancy influenced the U.S. Congress, students commonly report that they have a different view of themselves and of all human babies after seeing what a human baby can do of its own free will and what it can certainly feel and know before it is born. As the resolution of such pictures improves they will inevitably have even greater diagnostic value and a growing impact on our knowledge of ourselves. As of the time of this writing accuracies of up to .03 mm (that is, 3 hundredths of a millimeter) are already attainable in representing the edges of a moving image. It is certain that the images will continue to improve as new technologies and programs become available.

Language Before and After Birth

Moving pictures of embryological development from conception forward are informative. From moving ultrasound video, we know that by 12 weeks of gestation normal infants can move their fingers, by 18 weeks they yawn and smile, and by 26 weeks they blink and cry. Mothers regularly report that their unborn babies are responsive to human voices especially during the last three months (the third trimester) of the pregnancy. The research shows that infants before birth also respond differently to their mother's language as contrasted with a foreign language. Even in the womb the baby seems to distinguish the rhythms, stress patterns, and intonations—the so-called **prosody** of its own native language. One author has suggested that the prosody of discourse is everything that cannot be included in the writing of its surface forms (see "Prosody (linguistics)," 2009, retrieved February 16, 2009, from http://en.wikipedia.org/wiki/Prosody_(linguistics)).

At birth, infants can distinguish **syllables** such as "ba" and "pa" (Dehaene-Lambertz & Pena, 2001). By their seventh month after birth human infants begin to babble in repetitive sequences, like "bababa" but at birth human infants are already able to engage in turn-taking vocal exchanges that resemble a conversation. Also, the movements of a normal human newborn tend to fall into rhythm with the sounds, syllables, words, phrases, and turn changes of adults who speak within the hearing of the infant (Condon &

Because of advancing technologies enabling us to see inside the womb, the gas theory of smiling has been exploded. Similarly, 4D ultrasound shows the falseness of the elaborate mythology promoted by Ernst Haeckel (Pennisi, 1997) about human babies going through a phase of development where they breathe through gills like a fish.

Sander, 1974). This phenomenon, known as *entrainment*, is among the milestones already achieved by normal human babies at birth or soon after.

Human Rights from Conception

. . . human babies are genetically human before their conception, after that time, during embryological development, the human baby shows special responsiveness to the human voice and to its own native language.

In addition to the fact that human babies are genetically human before their conception, after that time, during embryological development, the human baby shows special responsiveness to the human voice and to its own native language. There is no question that human babies are human beings with the unique language capacity from conception forward. Therefore, the question of whether to save a human baby with a split spine, a cleft palate, or any other defect, comes down to the one put by Senator Brownback: " . . . whether or not the child has a life worthy of protection." There was no question whether Samuel Armas was a human being or not, or whether he was alive. The question was whether someone with the sort of disability Samuel Armas had was worth saving. Interestingly, under American law at the time, and under British law, Samuel's life could have legally been terminated.

A Profound Quandary

Does an unborn person such as Samuel Armas qualify as a human being? Did Samuel receive the rights and privileges granted, according to the American Declaration of Independence and the 14th Amendment to the U.S. Constitution, to all human beings by their Creator? Or were unborn babies excluded from the statements in our Declaration of Independence, the Bill of Rights, and the 14th Amendment? (see Chapter 12.)

The connection between disorders and disabilities, especially severe birth defects, with the laws, policies, and ethical statements impacting them inevitably bring out some interesting moral issues. There was no hesitation in condemning the Nazis at the Nuremberg trials for slaughtering a quarter of a million persons with disabilities, but some of the same nations that condemned those acts have permitted a great many more late term abortions of human infants.

Under British law since 1967, the United Kingdom has provided that an abortion can occur at any time of the pregnancy provided that "two doctors agree that a woman's health or life is gravely threatened by continuing with the pregnancy or that the fetus is likely to be born with *severe physical or mental abnormalities* [our italics]" ("More on UK Abortion Law," 2007, retrieved February 16, 2009, from http://www.efc.org.uk/Foryoungpeople/Factsaboutabortion/MoreonUKabortionlaw#1).

When the Condition Is Severe

In December 2001, a test case arose in Britain when a baby at 28 weeks of gestation was aborted because it was going to be born with a cleft lip and palate. A challenge to the decision was initiated by Joanna Jepson on the ground that she herself had been born with a similar condition, a deformity of her jaw, which did not prevent her from having corrective surgery and living a productive and useful life. Figure 2–12 shows Joanna after her surgery. She argued that the baby had been killed unlawfully.

The doctors defending themselves could not deny that one of them killed the baby, but they argued that it was a lawful death and won in the British courts (see BBC, 2003, retrieved February 16, 2009, from http://news.bbc.co.uk/1/hi/health/3247916.stm for a version of the story). In effect, the court's judgment was that the baby had no rights as a human being. So we can see that the moral question of what life is worth preserving is a genuine one in the 21st century. Hear "Abortion at 24 weeks for a cleft palate" (2003; retrieved March 20, 2009, from http://web.archive.org/web/20050101061713/www.bbc.co.uk/radio4/womanshour/24_11_03/tuesday/info4.shtml).

In the next section, we deal with craniofacial disorders specifically of the kind that have provided a basis in the United Kingdom, at least since 1967, for the taking of the child's life. We also look at pictures before and after surgery showing that severe defor-

In December 2001, a test case arose in Britain when a baby at 28 weeks of gestation was aborted because it was going to be born with a cleft lip and palate.

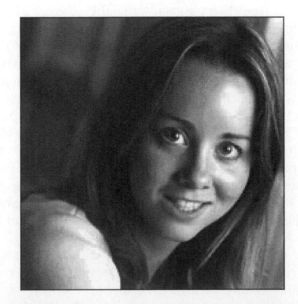

Figure 2–12. Joanna Jepson today after surgery for a congenital craniofacial anomaly. Retrieved February 16, 2009, from http://web.archive.org/web/20060115213036/www.jjepson.org/index.php. Copyright © 2007, Joanna Jepson, St. Michael's Church in Chester. Reprinted by permission. All rights reserved.

mities can be repaired. Is it worth the risk? In the year 2000 Zogby polled 1,031 Americans with the question:

> If you had a disease that was fatal, and was causing great pain and discomfort, which of the following courses of action would you prefer: Physician assisted suicide, wait and let nature take its course, or not sure?

Of the 1,031 persons polled nationwide, 63.5% would choose to live with the pain, 6.1% were undecided, and 30.4% said they would take doctor assisted death. Although there was no difference by gender, the respondents from 18 to 29 and over 65 were more likely to tough it out. Similarly, Blacks were less likely than Whites to choose euthanasia (see "Poll Shows Little Support for Assisted Suicide," 2000, retrieved February 16, 2009, from http://www.nrlc .org/euthanasia/facts/suicideassistpoll.html). The Zogby poll did not ask persons with facial deformities if they would rather have been aborted, but Dr. C. Everett Koop did survey individuals upon whom he had performed corrective surgery for an imperforate anus. None of those he surveyed, or their families, chastised him for enabling them to live.

Craniofacial Anomalies

Among the champions of individuals with cleft lip and/or palate is Stacy Keach (see "Stacy Keach Official Website," 2009, retrieved February 16, 2009, from http://www.stacykeach.com/). Stacy, who has been the Honorary Chairman of the Cleft Palate Foundation since 1994, was born with a cleft lip and partial cleft palate. At the web site of that organization, he says, "A facial birth defect doesn't get in the way of achievement. Parents need to instill a positive sense of self-esteem in their children so they can pursue their dreams" (Cleft Palate Foundation, 2006, retrieved February 16, 2009, from http://www.cleftline.org/). If we consider the success Keach has had as an actor his statement carries a lot of weight.

The standard treatment for cleft lip or palate is surgical repair. Figure 2–13 shows the results of such surgery for three different children who were treated at Rady Children's Hospital of San Diego, California. As in the cases of Joanna Jepson and Stacy Keach, surgical repair can offer the hope of a life without the stigma of an extreme facial deformity. On the contrary, as Keach reminds us, and as Joanna Jepson has argued, both based on their own experience as individuals who received surgical help—Keach as a young child and Jepson as a teenager—dreams can be fulfilled and a facial deformity does not have to get in the way of achievement.

In addition to surgical intervention, other therapy may also be desirable to enhance language and speech articulation. As we will see in Chapters 5 and 8, especially, bodily repairs can sometimes

The standard treatment for cleft lip or palate is surgical repair. Figure 2–13 shows the results of such surgery for three different children who were treated at Rady Children's Hospital of San Diego, California.

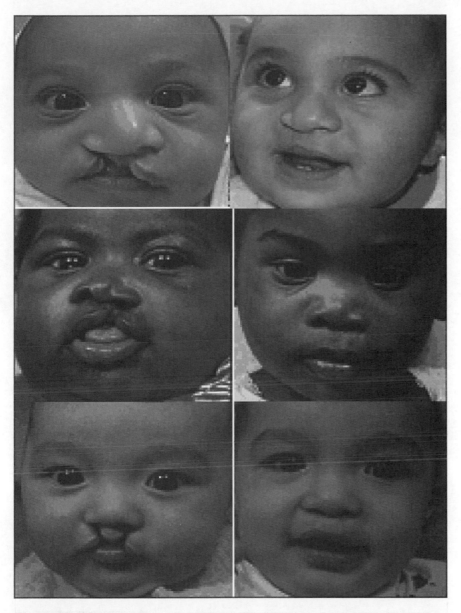

Figure 2–13. Photos on the left side represent the condition and appearance prior to surgery and on the right after surgical repair of cleft lip and/or palate. Retrieved February 16, 2009, from http://www.chsd.org/12293.cfm. Copyright © n.d. by Rady Children's Hospital of San Diego. Reprinted by permission. All rights reserved.

leave some of the nerves and muscles needing training that would not be necessary in uninjured tissues. In the case of Samuel Armas, for instance, though his body seemed to correct the life-threatening and potentially debilitating hydrocephalus, he needed braces to help manage his lower extremities. As far as we know, he did not require or receive any speech therapy. However, when surgical intervention is needed to repair a cleft lip and/or palate, therapies for voice and articulation are commonly needed to establish control over nerves and muscles that have either not formed completely or that may have been incompletely formed, incompletely repaired and/or damaged by the craniofacial surgery.

Cleft Lip and/or Palate

With clefts, the problem is that the complex tissues of organs that normally join up and merge along natural seams or borders—for example, the plates of the skull, the bones of the face, mouth, and jaw, the two sides of the upper lip that join at the middle—fall short of a smooth and complete connection. It is as if the builders of a bridge are working to connect, and fuse the structure in the middle of the gorge but never get the two sides to meet up. There are different ways that the failure to meet up can occur. Some of the most common are diagramed in Figure 2–14. In the drawings seen there, the failure to join is generally caused by underdevelopment of one or both sides. Another possibility not pictured is that one side may develop too much and the other not enough.

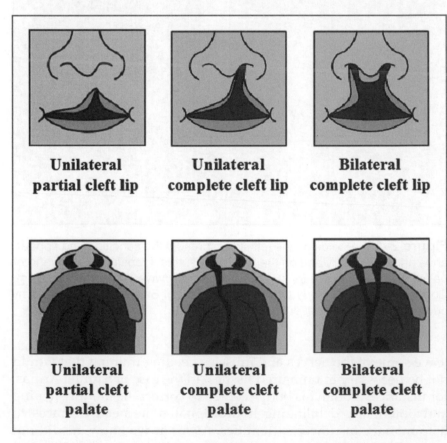

Figure 2–14. Schematic of common clefts of lip and/or palate. Retrieved February 16, 2009, from http://en.wikipedia.org/wiki/Cleft_lip_and_palate. Image in the public domain.

Disorders of this kind are estimated at about one birth per 700 ("Statistics by Country for Cleft palate," 2009, retrieved February 16, 2009, from http://www.wrongdiagnosis.com/c/cleft_palate/stats-country.htm), but they are among the ones commonly treated by speech-language pathologists. Among the articulatory problems, which we deal with in Chapter 8, are these: The sounds formed at the lips, for example, the ones we represent in writing with the letters "p," "b," and "m," for instance, may be unattainable without repair of the cleft. Also, if the palate is open into the nasal cavities on one or both sides, all speech sounds will be **nasalized** producing the condition called **hypernasality** because without repair of the palate, there is no way to close off the entry to the nasal passages when vocalizing. Since one of the causes of this condition is failure to block flow of air through the nasal passages by what is termed **velopharyngeal closure** as illustrated in Figure 2–15 the condition is often referred to as **velopharyngeal insufficiency**. To discover how the velic closure is achieved, try alternately saying the syllables "puh" or "buh" versus "muh," "tuh" or "duh" versus "nuh." Notice how the back of the velum feels in each of the indicated contrasts. Or try saying "sing" versus "sick" or "sig" and notice what is going on in the very back of your mouth and pharynx. Normally, when we are producing the non-nasalized stop consonants represented by the letters "p," "b," "t," "d," "k," and "g," the nasal passages are closed off at the back of the velum by pressing it against the wall of the pharynx. In the nasal "m," "n," and "-ng" by contrast, the connection from the pharynx into the nasal passages

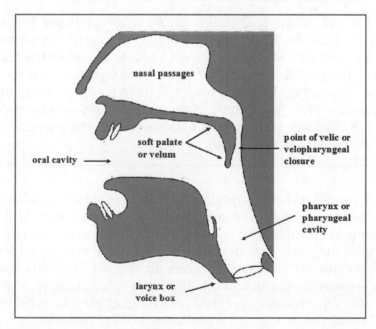

Figure 2–15. The vocal anatomy of velic or velopharyngeal closure.

is held open. In case the passage of air from the pharynx through the nasal cavities is blocked by abnormal tissue growth or, say, by mucus and swelling from a cold, nasal sounds will seem like muffled stop consonants and the entire stream of speech is said to be **hyponasal**—that is, lacking the normal nasal resonances.

The problem of insufficient velopharyngeal closure can arise from various causes. Among them are deformities of the velum itself or failure for the hard palate to close. The usual treatment in such cases is surgical repair of the malformed tissues.

Surgical Repair

In Figure 2–13, we see before and after pictures of surgical repairs of clefts of the lip and or palate. Because the muscles and nerves impacted by the cleft(s) are apt to be imperfectly formed, and also because of the trauma of the repair procedures, considerable attention may be needed to help the individual achieve normal sounding articulation of speech. The good news is, however, that not only are the physical difficulties commonly repairable, but children who undergo the surgery are usually able to learn to speak intelligibly and to live productive and normal lives.

As Stacy Keach said, a birth defect does not have to interfere with the achievement of a child's dreams, but an unrepaired craniofacial deformity can be overwhelming.

As Stacy Keach said, a birth defect does not have to interfere with the achievement of a child's dreams, but an unrepaired craniofacial deformity can be overwhelming.

Min Zhu Lei

At the home page of Operation Smile (2009, retrieved February 16, 2009, from http://www.operationsmile.org/) the picture of a three year old little girl named Min Zhu Lei bears the caption, "They point. They stare. They call me names. When will it stop? Someday." The story of Min Zhu Lin tells and shows the difference after her surgery. (Other stories can also be seen at this Web site.) It is difficult to overestimate the importance of the surgery in such cases.

Of course, it is also important to keep in mind the common fact that disorders rarely come in singular focused packages. Multiple problems are commonly comorbid. For that reason it is essential to prioritize the most serious problem first, deal with it, and then work downward to lesser priorities in the list. It would hardly make sense to treat articulation difficulties—for example, to try to remediate hypernasality—ahead of arranging for the repair of the cleft lip and palate that is the root source of the problem.

It would be better still to determine the source of the genetic or other damage that is causing the clefts in the first place to prevent them from occurring. It is for that reason that we focus as much attention as we do in this introductory course on the root causes of genetic damage caused by environmental toxins, infections, and so forth. In the following sections, we sum up the kinds of problems that can arise at higher levels of the representational systems on which our distinctly human experience depends. Along the way we keep in mind that the problems we are concerned with throughout this book and in all of its accompanying course material, occur in and affect bodily persons. For this reason, as noted in Chapter 1, we deal with cases of actual human beings.

SENSORY DISORDERS

Sensory difficulties include the loss, distortion, and/or lack of integration of one or more of the senses of sight, hearing, smelling, touching, and tasting. In Chapter 3 we deal with some interesting historical cases that have involved the loss of both sight and hearing, and cases where only sight or hearing was lost. In the most extreme case imaginable, the loss of all the senses would prevent all learning and knowledge of any kind.

The Extreme Limit of No Senses

Our bodies would not be able to make sense of experience at all, presumably, without our senses—that is, our abilities to see, hear, smell, touch, and taste. Aristotle [384–322 BC] argued that loss of any one of the senses must entail a corresponding loss of understanding and experience. In *Posterior Analytics* (ca. 350 BC), he wrote:

> . . . the loss of any one of the senses entails the loss of a corresponding portion of knowledge, and . . . since we learn either by induction [logical reasoning] or by demonstration [perception and/or action], this knowledge cannot be acquired. (Book I, Part 18, para. 1, retrieved February 16, 2009, from http://classics .mit.edu/Aristotle/posterior.1.i.html)

Logically, Aristotle's claim must be correct.

Among the most famous and difficult cases in history there are several amazing success stories about individuals who lost or failed to develop one or several senses. In Chapter 3 we deal with cases of complete loss of both sight and hearing as in the cases of Helen Keller and the less well-known case of Laura Bridgman. We also consider historically important cases of individuals who lost either sight or hearing. We give special attention to the story of Louis Braille [1809–1852] ("Louis Braille," 1852/2009, retrieved February 16, 2009, from http://en.wikipedia.org/wiki/Louis_Braille) —the inventor of Braille writing for the Blind and Alexander

If a child had no senses at all, language acquisition, knowledge of the common world, and the normal sharing of human experience would not be possible.

Graham Bell [1847–1922] ("Alexander Graham Bell," 1922/2009, retrieved February 16, 2009, from http://en.wikipedia.org/wiki/Alexander_Graham_Bell) often referred to as a champion on behalf of the Deaf. Bell himself was not deaf, but he married a woman who was deaf as was his own mother. He was sometimes referred to as the "Father of the Deaf."

Less Well-Known Sensory Losses

In addition to blindness and deafness, there are similar but less well studied, and less well understood, disorders that affect the other senses as well. Our sense of smell involves detecting certain molecules of gas in the air. Molecules of gas diffuse rapidly as the atoms themselves move around at about 1,000 miles per hour. Although they do not move in a straight line, the smell of a cigarette, for instance, can permeate an entire floor in a large hotel in a matter of seconds. The complete loss of smell is known as **anosmia** and a diminishing of smell is called **hyposmia**. Disorders of smell can involve phantom smells, **parosmia**. All of the less extreme disorders of smell, where there is less than a complete loss, are captured under the general term **dysosmia** (Costanzo & Becker, 1986; Vokshoor & McGregor, 2006). The sense of smell is susceptible to influence from conditions that affect respiration, for example, nasal congestion and allergies. Sometimes, a reduction of allergies alone can significantly improve the sense of smell.

There are similar disorders of taste. Our sense of taste also depends on molecules of the substance we taste, but mainly these are detected in a liquid rather than gaseous form. A complete loss of the sense of taste is called **ageusia** whereas the cover term for the variety of possible lesser losses are termed **dysgeusia**. Interestingly, there are many combinations of flavor to detect, but we are programmed to handle just five distinct tastes.

Five Distinct Tastes

We are programmed to handle just five distinct tastes: sweet, sour, bitter, salty, and **umami** (Chandrashekar, Hoon, Ryba, & Zuker, 2006; R. K. Palmer, 2007). The last of these is the underlying flavor of **monosodium glutamate (MSG)**—a flavor enhancer which has since been shown to be neurotoxic (G. G. Ortiz et al., 2006). Because glutamate is the most abundant excitatory neurotransmitter in the body, MSG may tend to produce **excitotoxicity** in autism (Jepson & J. Johnson, 2007, p. 251). The umami taste was described by Japanese chemist Kikunae Ikeda in 1909 ("Umami," 2009, retrieved February 16, 2009, from http://en.wikipedia.org/wiki/Umami) and subsequently, in the form of MSG, has been used in many foods to artificially make the food taste better.

Because tasting involves touching whatever is tasted, and because tasting normally requires touching with the tongue, disorders of taste involve a potential disorder of touch as well. However, the sense of touch, to the extent that it can be isolated, is referred to as **proprioception**. For one thing, this sense tells us where our body is and what it is doing. It is rare but possible for a disease or injury to single out the sense of touch. For instance, a certain Ian Waterman in 1972 at the young age of 19 suffered a viral infection that caused him to lose "all feeling below the neck" becoming "unable to tell without looking how his body is positioned" (Azar, 1998, retrieved February 16, 2009, from http://www.apa.org/monitor/jun98/touch.html). The fact that he is able to compensate for his loss shows the remarkable ability of substituting information from one sense for the loss of another. For Waterman, according to his own account, however, it has been a difficult and costly substitution.

Movement Without Sensation of Touch or Pain

Without any sensation at all a moving organism would eventually die of self-inflicted injuries resulting from bumping into objects. In fact, there is a still common disease where the sense of touch and pain are almost completely lost but without an accompanying loss of the capacity to move. The disease in question is **biblical leprosy** also known as **Hansen's disease** (Hansen, 1874; Figure 2–16; see also Sasaki, Takeshita, Okuda, & Ishii, 2001; "Leprosy," 2009, retrieved February 16, 2009, from http://en.wikipedia.org/wiki/Leprosy#_note-Heller_2003).

Without any sensation at all a moving organism would eventually die of self-inflicted injuries resulting from bumping into objects.

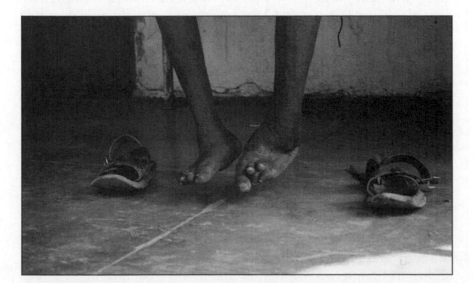

Figure 2–16. The destruction of extremities due to current day biblical leprosy. Retrieved February 16, 2009, from http://www.leprosy.ca/site/c.an KKIPNrEqG/b.2012733/k.8C01/The_Disease.htm. Reprinted with permission. Copyright © 2009 by the Leprosy Mission Canada. All rights reserved.

Persons with this disease still have significant strength and capacity for movement but are relatively unable to tell when they injure themselves. Leprosy attacks the sense of touch and more particularly reduces the affected person's capacity to sense pain. It may also produce cramping of the muscles as seen in the lower part of Figure 2–16. Partly because of this loss and the infection, injuries accumulate until body parts are destroyed. According to the Leprosy Mission of Canada there are still new cases of leprosy being detected every day. With this disease, the extremities can be completely destroyed by injuries as seen in Figure 2–17. The disease can be treated but it is still virulent according to the The Leprosy Mission Canada (see their Web site retrieved February 16, 2009, from http://www.leprosy.ca/site/).

SENSORY-MOTOR DISORDERS

Through our bodily movements, informed by our senses and our minds, as writers we cause words to appear here on this page and throughout this book. Through the reader's movements which are coordinated with ours (to some degree), our readers perceive our words and our words connect us with each other. As a result, our bodies and bodily movements are involved in this interaction however far apart we may be in space and time. Without movements of fingers on a keyboard, the words would not appear on the page (or screen). Without movements of the perceiver's eyes—or hands if the reader happens to be using a **Braille text**; see Chapter 3 for the story of Braille writing—no perception and thus no comprehension of the words can occur. Movements are actually indispensable in making sense of sensations. Have you ever had the experience in that borderland between being awake and falling asleep where you have to move to see where your arm or hand is? Movement is essential, it seems, even to the determination of our posture—whether we are sitting, standing, or lying down. Without a whole hierarchy of interrelated systems of control, neither voluntary movement, nor necessary involuntary movements would be possible. Along the way, as they say, there can be "many a slip 'twixt the cup and the lip."

Electrochemical and Autonomic Control

Sensory-motor representations are involved at multiple levels of the body and nervous system. There are many motor problems (as shown in Chapters 5 through 8) that involve balance in all senses of the word—coordination, rhythm, and the starting and stopping of muscular contractions or glandular secretions. The motor control systems at issue govern such processes as the beating of the

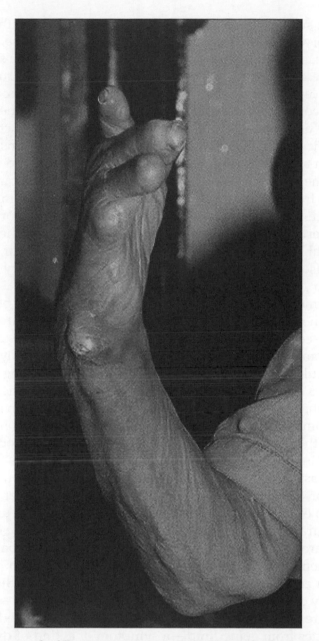

Figure 2–17. Digits lost to leprosy. The destruction of extremities due to current day biblical leprosy. Retrieved February 16, 2009, from http://www.leprosy.ca/site/c.anKKl PNrEqG/b.2012733/k.8C01/The_Disease.htm. Reprinted with permission. Copyright © 2009 by the Leprosy Mission Canada.

heart, contractions of the smooth muscles in the **gastrointestinal tract**, circulation of the blood, the functioning of the **lymphatic system**, and nervous processes at the electrochemical level.

Movements that are timed and controlled by the nervous and immune systems are termed "autonomous"—meaning self-directed or automatic and involuntary. The autonomic nervous system

Movements that are timed and controlled by the nervous and immune systems are termed "autonomous"—meaning self-directed or automatic and involuntary.

regulates such rhythms as the beating of the heart, breathing, and digestion; whenever we are not thinking about one of these, and provided we are not consciously over-riding the autonomic system—which we can do with breathing, for instance—it will run things more or less automatically all by itself. The autonomic nervous systems control all kinds of glandular secretions that need to be balanced and managed in order for our bodies to function. The autonomic systems serve in part as switching systems turning things on and off in response to communications to and from the body at the electrochemical level. **Autonomic disorders** can involve any level from the brain down to distinct atoms in very small quantities, such as **trace metals**, associated with the building or destruction of certain complex biomolecules. Movements at the level of individual cells, molecules, and atoms, are critical to our immune systems (see "Immune System," 2009, retrieved February 16, 2009, from <u>http://en.wikipedia.org/wiki/Immune_system</u>).

The movements and communications between the blood and the lymph in repairing injuries and warding off attacks are remarkable but seem to be far below the level of consciousness and even farther from volitional control. Some of the responses of bodily cells and biomolecules are almost instantaneous, like the bleeding of a cut, and others are sustained over long periods of time, like the swelling of a sprain, the scarring of the cut, or the recovery from an infection.

> Communication between cells and transportation of molecules between them and their parts are essential to repairing bodily damage from injuries and poisons, and to warding off attacks from bacteria, parasites, and viruses.

Communication between cells and transportation of molecules between them and their parts are essential to repairing bodily damage from injuries and poisons, and to warding off attacks from bacteria, parasites, and viruses. All such molecular movements remain largely or completely outside of voluntary control, yet they are crucial to our health in general not to mention enabling us to keep our postural balance when we are sitting, standing, lying down, or moving around. We do not consciously (or voluntarily) balance the electrochemical systems at the muscular level that keep our muscles from cramping—a symptom of a **spastic disorder** that can be caused by drinking too much coffee or by a disease such as **tetanus** (see Figure 6–23). The autonomic systems are also involved in keeping muscles from going limp—a symptom of a kind of **dysarthria** that can be caused by alcohol consumption or drugs that cause the muscle to relax. In disorders of the autonomic nervous system, it is not that the person affected is unwilling for the muscle systems to work properly, but many aspects of their functions are at a subconscious level outside of the control of conscious intentions. They cannot be controlled directly by our will.

On the Border

At the boundary of voluntary versus involuntary movements are movements such as swallowing that we can initiate by volition but that continue under autonomic nervous control. After we initiate the movement voluntarily, the autonomic system, if it is working correctly, takes over and does the rest for us. Breathing is something we can also control, but when we are not doing so deliberately, the autonomic system does the work. The autonomic system can also control all kinds of more or less conscious and intentional functions that we can decide on a whim to do or not to do. That is, the autonomic system can take over all kinds of process that we initiate and sustain on a voluntary basis, but that we do not normally need to attend to consciously moment by moment. These include such activities as walking, running, riding a bicycle, clapping our hands or tapping our foot to a rhythm, dancing, playing a familiar song on a musical instrument, reciting a memorized poem, and so forth. As the tasks become more difficult, at the edge of our competence, conscious effort and voluntary control are more apt to be needed. The highly articulated and planned movements that come increasingly under volitional control and cognitive supervision and planning include such things as playing a competitive game, say, of racquetball or ping pong. As the steps in a sequence of moves becomes more subject to change, as we move, say, from casual conversation to something like a formal debate, or from a chat with mom on the phone to a job interview, conscious volitional control comes more and more to play a central guiding role.

In Chapter 6 we give special attention to sensory-motor disorders traditionally associated with swallowing and indirectly associated, commonly, with speech. The reason that these are usually classed with speech and language disorders—some would say inappropriately—is because swallowing, like speech, comes under conscious control to some degree and is thus subject to possible benefit from therapeutic intervention. Swallowing disorders, called **dysphagias**, it is true, are a very different class of disorders from the disorders involved in speaking and writing. However, it is also true that both can be helped by the sort of coaching and therapies that speech-language pathologists can provide.

Motor Control of Conscious, Voluntary, Articulated Actions

As we move to the higher cortical control of the fine grained articulated movements necessary in speech, writing, and the manual signing of language, we come to the sensory-motor disorders that are commonly referred to as **apraxias** which also logically include the higher order linguistic **ataxias**. The apraxias impact the production of learned and skilled movements (see Chapter 6) and the linguistic ataxias disrupt the capacity to form and coordinate articulated

As the steps in a sequence of moves becomes more subject to change, as we move, say, from casual conversation to something like a formal debate, or from a chat with mom on the phone to a job interview, conscious volitional control comes more and more to play a central guiding role.

sequences of them. These terms, apraxia and ataxia, however, are also used for disorders at lower levels of motor control—for example, the ability to turn a crank, to insert and turn a key, or to simply stand up and take steps.

In some kinds of motor planning, where a certain element A must precede B which comes before C, and so on, but there is difficulty in coordinating or arranging the sequence—logically speaking, this sort of difficulty should be classed as a high order "ataxia." For instance, if we say, write, or sign, *The dog bit the man*, our production is in a sequence that makes sense. But if we jumble the order as in *dog the bit man the*, or if we jumble the letters as in, *gto deh mnb tia eht*, we get an idea of the sort of thing that goes wrong in theoretical high order ataxias of speech where sequencing is lost or disrupted in spite of the fact that some of the units of structure are accessible. This type of ataxia is apt to be identified as Wernicke's aphasia (discussed in Chapter 10). In Chapters 4, 8, and 10, especially, we deal with the rich and deep integration of the systems that enable the highly articulated movements of speech and/or manual signing.

The motor disorders associated with swallowing, voice, and the muscular movements and expressions that accompany speech are dealt with in Chapter 6. Such articulated and speech coordinated muscular functions cannot be strictly differentiated from the higher functions of speech which are dealt with more intensively in Chapters 7 and 8. Contrary to some oversimplified theories, the systems of speech, prosody, facial expression, and gestures, are normally richly inter-connected. As we will see in Chapters 6 through 8, the differentiation of motor disorders is an area filled with an almost unlimited multiplication of competing and overlapping terms. Distinctions are often proposed, or claimed, that cannot be made reliably and terms that supposedly should lead to distinct therapies or treatments may not do so at all. Or, in some cases where different therapies are recommended and/or applied there may be little or no evidence that the differences are at all effective—that they matter at all.

In fact, the supposed distinction between apraxias and ataxias is a notorious case in point especially when speech and language are involved. The categories of linguistic ataxias and apraxias are almost always found together and the distinctions between them, are not as precise as sometimes claimed. Even the distinctions between movement and sensation are far less precise than is commonly supposed and as we will see in Chapter 4, the integration in the case of speech and language perception is so complete that sensation is dramatically informed and in some instances shaped by what we know of movements and of higher intentional meanings. (Refer to the discussion of the McGurk effects in Chapter 4.)

Consider what you are doing while reading a text or listening to a spoken version of one. Consider the text you are presently

As we will see in Chapters 6 through 8, the differentiation of motor disorders is an area filled with an almost unlimited multiplication of competing and overlapping terms. Distinctions are often proposed, or claimed, that cannot be made reliably and terms that supposedly should lead to distinct therapies or treatments may not do so at all.

reading as an example. Are you moving your eyes as you read? Even in what are commonly thought of as passive systems of sensation and perception, movement is critically involved. In fact, highly articulated intentional movement is essential to reading comprehension. Without movement on the part of the person doing the reading, the process of reading, for instance, will bog down and stop completely. Staring at a text is not the same as reading it. We must move our eyes and we need to turn the pages or scroll from screen to screen. Similarly, in understanding speech, or manual signs, movement is critically involved. Hearing of speech involves subtle movements and adjustments within the ear itself, as we will see in Chapter 4. Also, comprehension of speech involves movements to a much greater extent.

If a reader/listener depends on an audio-playback system, the recording must involve the voice and movements of the tongue and mouth of the speaker who says and/or reads the words out loud. Even if the voice were artificially produced, it would still involve processing of the linear sequence of symbols created by the producer(s) and displaying them in a particular timed sequence to the automatic text-reader in some way or other. Also, the audio playback system has to operate in time and space on a mechanism that is controlled by the bodily actions of speakers/listeners. Someone has to load the DVD in a recorder, set up the recording, and turn on the recorder during the recording phase and someone has to load the disk in the drive, select the right directory, choose the file, set the volume controls, and issue the play command during the playback process. There is a lot of *coordinated motor activity* associated with the interpretation as well as the production of either a spoken or printed version of any text.

To a much greater extent than may be realized the movements involved in so-called "passive" language processing are intentional and volitional. In reading, we depend on intentional bodily movements much more than commonly realized. To read a given text, we must get the text where we can see it, or in the case of a Braille reader, feel it. In the case of a seeing reader, we must move our eyes across the page, or in the case of Braille reading, we must move our fingers across the raised spots on the page. Imagine how soon communication would come to a halt if the communicator were completely unable to move. If the heart stopped beating, or if we could not breathe or swallow, communication would soon cease. Bodily movements are involved in sensory impressions to the extent that congenitally blind individuals orient their eyes toward a heard sound (Garg, Schwartz, & Stevens, 2007). Also in interpreting speech Nicholls and Searle (2006) showed that lipreading is more influenced by the right visual field showing a left hemisphere dominance for perception of speech as well as motor production. The depth of the integration of movement and sensory impression is remarkable.

SENSORY-MOTOR-LINGUISTIC DISORDERS

Language Disorders

Language disorders are without contest, the most important among all those that affect human communication. It is for this reason that when language is disrupted at its basis that pervasive developmental disorders of childhood, which we discuss in Chapter 5, are so devastating. Viewing things from an individual's point of view, without sufficient language and communication, employment and social relations are impaired. From a broader perspective, without language there would be no history, science, mathematics, education, or law. There would be no literacy, musical scores, no choreographed dance, theater, movie making, opera, symphony, and no arts. The development of the language capacity is crucial because it is essential to our ability to plan intentional actions and to regulate and carry out volitional bodily acts and to enter into social relations. Even breathing and swallowing as we will see in Chapter 6 must be integrated with highly articulated actions in producing speech. Such actions as producing meaningful speech are vital to social relations between human beings and to all of the truly distinctive human aspects of experience.

The language capacity is without rival the most distinctive trait of human beings marking us as different from other creatures.

The language capacity is without rival the most distinctive trait of human beings marking us as different from other creatures. It is also the key to the life of the mind. Without it, as Einstein once observed, our lives would be mentally impoverished. Language provides the basis for social systems and our primary means of communication, thinking, and reasoning. As we will see, especially in Chapter 10, language is the essential governing communication system that enables our many related cognitive and neurological systems to make sense of experience. This unifying system enables us to understand who we are and how we fit into our families and communities. Through language we understand and produce the stories of our lives.

Sensory-motor-linguistic disorders, for all of these reasons, are very important. They encompass the full range of problems from cognitive/psychological, and/or social/interactive difficulties that are dealt with especially in Chapters 6 through 10. Chapter 7 zooms in on the special problems associated with speech articulation. Chapter 8 goes on to discuss sensory-motor-linguistic problems that impact the fluent production of speech and/or signing. Chapter 9 deals with problems of literacy and especially the large class of poorly understood disorders lumped together under the huge umbrella of **dyslexia**. Chapter 10 overviews neurological problems and especially the kinds of disorders that impact adults. Chapters 11 and 12 kick it all up a notch and zoom out to the perspective of the assessment and diagnosis of disorders and then to how they are regarded in the light of law and ethics. Throughout the whole book, the focus is on communication disorders, but, as we have already seen from the beginning, language systems of great complexity and depth are central to understanding communication disorders.

Dysfluencies

The disorders loosely classed as **dysfluencies** straddle the borderline between sensory-motor disorders that indirectly affect speech and writing, and language disorders that clearly involve the emotions and all of the cognitive systems of social interaction. A hugely important part of chronic stuttering, for example, is how the person who stutters feels about, thinks about, and reacts to how others are perceived or thought to be reacting to the stuttering. As a result, the stuttering itself is often spoken of as the **primary disorder** (or difficulty), while the emotional reactions and all that they give rise to—for example, grimacing, closing of the eyes, foot stomping, teeth grinding, and so forth—are termed **secondary behaviors**, or simply **secondaries**.

Because speech and manual sign systems invariably involve the surface forms of language, it is obvious that the articulate movements and rhythms of speech (and signing) cannot be entirely distinguished from the higher functions of language. Although some disorders involving loss of or failure to develop fluency in speech and language may fit in the "motor-speech" category, it is evident in many ways, especially in Chapter 8, that fluency disorders commonly involve higher systems of language.

Language Subsystems That Can Go Wrong

Problems that specifically impact the sounds, syllables, rhythms, intonations, and the processing of these aspects of sound systems generally fall under the scope of **phonology**. Ones that impact the specific processing of words may be termed **lexical** and ones that affect substructures of words, for example, plural marking or tense marking of words like *cat* as contrasted with *cats* and *walk* as contrasted with *walked*—can be loosely classed under the scope of **morphology** or what may be called **morphosyntax**. Usually "morphology" is associated with relations within words—such as the association of *associate* with, say, *association*, or *flammable* with *inflammable*. By contrast, changes in words that are necessary to achieve agreement with some other word or phrase—for example,

Language systems are complex and multilayered as are each of the three major classes of sign systems—sensory, motor, and linguistic. Language also is a multilayered system of systems. For evidence of this that is easy to understand, see especially Chapter 4. Language systems are layered and they involve multiple interrelated components.

we say *The dog barks* but *The dogs bark*, where the change in *bark* is associated with whether or not the subject *dog* is singular or plural—are termed "morphosyntactic." Problems in sequences of words, phrases, and higher structures are loosely classed under the scope of **syntax**, whereas problems with managing abstract meanings go to **semantics**, and problems in fitting language to social and material contexts of interaction go to **pragmatics**.

Syntax is essentially about sequencing of units whether they are words, phrases, or higher structures. Semantics is about abstract meanings, for example, classifications and qualities that are general and run across all possible cases such as being male or female, red or not red, abstract or concrete, and so on. Pragmatics is also concerned with meanings, but particular, concrete, bodily meanings rather than abstract and general ones. For instance, whether or not a certain page of this book contains the word "pragmatics" or a picture of Mother Teresa are pragmatic questions. However, the abstract qualities shared by pages, pictures, and printed words—that all of them can be referred to in words, tend to involve or be associated with flat surfaces, involve vision, and so forth—are semantic facts.

Major Classes of Language Disorders

The complexity and interdependencies of the various components of language systems make the disorders associated with language exceedingly complex. However, we can sum up major classes of language disorders involving loss or failure to develop which is generally attributed to damage to brain tissue according to the impact on particular aspects of language processing.

Aphasias are the disorders (see Chapter 10) especially associated with the governing part of the brain that is not only involved in producing speech and writing, but especially in planning, reasoning, and the main discursive (meaningful) functions of language. These disorders are almost completely and exclusively associated with the controlling half of the brain. The conceptual disorders described as **agnosias** are those that impact our ability to make sense of holistic shapes, contexts, and scenes. These functions are subordinated to the linguistic and especially semantic functions in the process that we have described above as "pragmatic mapping." We illustrate in greater detail what is meant by pragmatic mapping and how it is accomplished in Chapter 3.

The most studied type of agnosia involves a loss of or simply a congenital inability to recognize faces which is known as **prosopagnosia**.

The Linguistic Apraxias

Connecting the conceptual processes of semantically and conceptually understanding whole shapes, persons, scenes, and contexts of experience are the sensory-motor (mainly indexical) processes involved in the pragmatic mapping of a name, for instance, *Mother Teresa* onto the person in the photo of Figure 2–9. That mapping, if you think about it, clearly involves an actual or at least a mental movement that allows the association of the words, *Mother Teresa*, as printed here on this page, with the person pictured on an earlier page. That implicit connection constitutes an indexical sign and the production, by some means, of the surface form of a linguistic expression. If such a normal production, cannot be carried out, for whatever reason, the disorder would properly fit into the general class of linguistic apraxias.

The most important of those are the ones that directly affect our ability to produce intelligible linguistic forms in speech, manual sign, or writing.

Chapter 5 addresses childhood disorders, especially those of the pervasive developmental kind such as autism, while Chapters 6, 7, and 8 single out disorders involving motoric functions and, especially in Chapters 7 and 8, the articulation of fluent speech. Chapter 7 deals with what have traditionally been termed articulation disorders and Chapter 8 with fluency disorders. Chapter 9 addresses problems particularly (though not exclusively) associated with literacy, especially the class of disorders that fall loosely under the term *dyslexia*. Chapter 10 looks to adult disorders with special attention to a host of conditions that we now know are substantially impacted, if not caused, by environmental toxins. Overarching all of the foregoing disorders of language, learning, and the ability to make the connections between words and facts are the general deteriorative disorders called simply **dementias**. With all of the foregoing in mind, we take a deeper look into the many ways things can go wrong in pragmatic mapping in Chapter 10. Then in Chapter 11 we deal with the assessment and diagnosis of disorders and in Chapter 12 with systems of law and ethics pertaining to communication disorders.

SUMMING UP AND LOOKING AHEAD

In this chapter, we focused our attention first at the bottom of the representational hierarchy—the place where all communication abilities begin—in the developing body of a communicator within the physical world. We tend to take this level of representational systems for granted, but it is inevitable that communication disorders are connected both with genetic systems and with particular individual persons in bodies. Communication disorders are associated

Describing social situations may be very important, but it cannot account for the root causes of communication disorders that are profoundly genetic, congenital, or epigenetic in nature. To suggest that such disease conditions should be treated socially or behaviorally is a logical mistake of a high order.

with bodily persons. Contrary to approaches that leap immediately to the complexities of social contexts, all communication disorders involve bodily individuals, and there are many cascades of disorders beginning in the bodily makeup of an individual person.

In this chapter, however, we have also seen that behavioral, social, and even political systems do come into play in the treatment of individuals with physical deformities and disabilities. Deformities, disabilities, and debilitating diseases, have served throughout history as a watershed for public policy. The crucial question that inevitably comes to the surface in trying to determine what to do about severe deformities and disabilities is whether a life is worth whatever it may cost. Historically, we find two extremes: some, like Dr. Leo Alexander, Dr. C. Everett Koop, Mother Teresa, Joanna Jepson, Stacy Keach, Alex and Julia Armas, and so on, have cast their vote in favor of doing all that is possible to affirm that lives are of worth, irrespective of the cost.

Others have regarded human life more in terms of supply-side economics where the persons in power, the haves, decide everything for the have-nots. After adding up the numbers and doing the math, the authorities may come to the conclusion as was done in the United Kingdom in 1967—if the baby is deformed—and in the United Sates in *Roe v. Wade* (1973)—if the baby is just unwanted—that unborn babies may be killed. The Germans reached a similar conclusion much earlier, and under the Nazi rule, they narrowed the definition of "a life worth living" until it excluded all persons with deformities, diseases, disabilities, or merely different from the ideal super race consisting of—surprise, surprise—only persons like themselves, or rather their preferred ideal selves.

The deep-seated economic, legal, and ethical controversies over how to treat persons with disabilities, as we will see, have formed an important subtext throughout history. More than commonly realized, the question of what to do about chronic diseases, disabilities, and disorders, has been a defining element in the background of the major conflicts of world history. In the following chapter, we delve more deeply into disorders of the senses, especially loss of seeing and hearing, as those disorders impact communication.

STUDY AND DISCUSSION QUESTIONS

1. What is the domino theory of disorders?
2. Why is comorbidity of different disorders both common and expected?
3. What are the four major classes of communication disorders?
4. How does the sign hierarchy, and its interconnectedness, help us to differentiate and classify distinct kinds of communication disorders?

5. How do genetic and epigenetic disorders relate to bodily systems?
6. What evidence is there that the Nazi purges did *not* begin with ethnic cleansing?
7. Discuss the impact of 4D ultrasound on modern views about human development.
8. How do bodily disorders impact higher systems of sense, movement, and language? Illustrate with specific examples.

3

Auditory and Other Sensory Disorders

OBJECTIVES

In this chapter, we:

1. Relate sight, hearing, and touch to acquiring language and literacy;
2. Discuss blindness and deafness as challenges to acquiring language and literacy;
3. Review the history of writing for the Blind;
4. Learn about the distinct manual language systems of the Deaf;
5. See how language and literacy are acquired by individuals who are both blind and deaf;
6. Review highlights of the history of education for the Blind and the Deaf; and
7. Critique specific cases of language acquired by deaf-blind children.

KEY TERMS

Here are some key terms or names in this chapter that appear in **bold print** on their first appearance. They are explained or defined in the Glossary at the end of the book.

alphabetic writing
American Sign Language
    (ASL)
audible electronic text
authenticity
calligrapher
conventions
derived signed languages
digital text
eugenics
facilitated communication
gene pool
Grade 1 Braille
Grade 2 Braille
Grade 3 Braille
hard of hearing

high functioning autism
    (HFA)
interpretation
Laura Bridgman
manual babbling
manual modality
Manually Signed English
    (MSE)
native models
natural signed languages
oral babbling
phonetic code
phoneticians
plagiarism
Postmodernism
profound deafness

raised print
referring term
replication
rigid transliteration
San Diego twins
self-contradiction
sensory prejudices
Signed Exact English (SEE)
simultaneous interpretation
social Darwinism
synthesized speech
text to speech
translation
TTS
visible speech
visuocentricity

Language acquisition is the process by which we learn to associate impressions of the surface-forms of language with the sensory impressions of everything else through a complex of sign systems that we collectively call *grammar*.

In this chapter we begin to see just how deeply our language capacity is related to our nature as human beings and to our freedom to communicate with each other. Here we consider the impact of different kinds and degrees of sensory disorders. We focus especially on the most severe disorders of sight and hearing—blindness and deafness. The processing of sensory impressions, such as those involved in understanding speech or writing, requires highly abstract concepts. Those concepts can only be accessed through the scaffolding that is provided by the symbol systems of some particular language. Two very distinct kinds of sensory signs are involved in language acquisition. On the one hand there are:

1. the sensations of the surface-forms of language as it is spoken, signed, written, or read, and on the other hand, there are
2. the sensory impressions of everything else in the world, and in our thoughts.

In this chapter we see how language acquisition depends on sensory information and how disorders of the senses, especially of seeing and hearing, can interfere with or even completely obliterate our ability to learn and understand language. Without language we can hardly find out what is going on in the world. We have little freedom of body or mind.

FREEDOM OF THE BODY AND THE MIND

Communication depends on systems of representation. The highest of these is language but our senses enable our most basic representations of the world which are essential for language acquisition. We see, hear, smell, touch, and taste the world around us. Usually, our senses inform us correctly, but sometimes the senses do not work as expected. Sensory disorders come in many different combinations and degrees of severity. In the most severe cases, where all the senses are completely dysfunctional, as Aristotle [384–322 BC] noted long ago, communication and learning of any kind are impossible. More recently, Chomsky (1995) referred to experience without language as "amoeboid." He argued that without the language capacity, we would hardly be free to do anything that is distinctly human. He said:

> The scope and limits of development are logically related . . . Take language, one of the few distinctive human capacities about which much is known . . . the growth of language allows very restricted options. Is this limiting? Of course. Is it liberating? Also of course. It is these very restrictions that make it possible for a rich and intricate system of expression of thought to develop in similar ways on the basis of very rudimentary, scattered, and varied experience. (retrieved February 23, 2009, from http://www.ditext.com/chomsky/may1995.html)

Deaf and Blind: The Prison and Slavery Analogies

In 1832, at the age of 2, Laura Bridgman [1829–1889] contracted scarlet fever ("Laura Bridgman," 2009, retrieved February 23, 2009, from http://en.wikipedia.org/wiki/Laura_Bridgman) which left her alive but deaf and blind. According to the historian, Lash, her senses of smell and taste were also severely impaired (Lash, 1980, p. 16ff). It was supposed that of her five senses she had only one left that was still somewhat intact—her sense of touch.

Laura Bridgman Described by Dickens

In 1842, when she was 10 years old, she was visited by the famed British reformer and author, Charles Dickens [1812-1870], who described her in *American Notes* as

a fair young creature with every human faculty and hope and power of goodness and affection enclosed within her delicate frame and but one outward sense—the sense of touch. There she was before me, built up, as it were, in a marble cell, impervious to any ray of light or particle of sound; with her poor white

Sensory disorders come in many different combinations and degrees of severity. In the most severe cases, where all the senses are completely dysfunctional, as Aristotle [384–322 BC] noted long ago, communication and learning of any kind are impossible.

hand peeping through a chink in the wall, beckoning to some good man for help, that an immortal soul might be awakened. (as quoted by Lash, 1980, p. 18; also see Dickens, 1842, retrieved February 23, 2009, from http://en.wikipedia.org/wiki/American_Notes)

Dickens went on to tell of Dr. Samuel Gridley Howe ("Samuel Gridley Howe," 2009, retrieved February 24, 2009, from http://en.wikipedia.org/wiki/Samuel_Gridley_Howe), a medical doctor and philanthropist who had come along not only to rescue Laura Bridgman from her "marble cell" but who also set the stage for the teaching of other deaf-blind individuals including the more famous Helen Keller [1880–1968] ("Helen Keller," 1955/2009, retrieved February 24, 2009, from http://en.wikipedia.org/wiki/Helen_Keller). In fact, Lash's book is mainly about Keller.

Howe himself was also deeply involved in the American anti-slavery movement. Not only did he himself oppose slavery, but his wife, Julia Ward Howe [1819–1910], also an abolitionist, was the author of "The Battle Hymn of the Republic" in 1861. (See "Julia Ward Howe," 1910/2009, retrieved February 24, 2009, from http://womenshistory.about.com/library/bio/blbio_howe_julia_ward.htm). Many individuals may not realize that the anthem of the American Civil War was also a statement about the abolition of slavery. As described in Chapter 12, the association of communication disabilities and slavery was more than skin deep. The mind and the body are obviously connected, especially when it comes to the abstract concept that we call freedom. We cannot really have freedom of the one—the mind or the body—without freedom of the other. If the mind is enslaved by disabilities the body is not free, and likewise, if the body is enslaved, in what sense is the mind free? In Dr. Howe's thinking, in the first third of the 19th century, the freeing of the mind and the freeing of the body from any kind of enslavement were one and the same objective. In reality, the mind and body have always been connected logically and historically in politics, war, law, and education.

The struggles that have played out on the battlefields, in the courts, in the legislatures, and in our schools, in the quest for racial equality, especially in America, have inevitably been linked to the rights and freedoms of citizens with disabilities.

As we will see in Chapter 12, persons who are different from others because of communication disabilities have benefitted from recognition of the rights of persons different in color and race. Struggles for freedom of the mind and body did not begin when America was discovered, nor in the slave trade that plundered Africa and condemned the United States to our own unique Civil War. The underlying premise as Howe saw it was that deaf-blind citizens, like all human beings, should be enabled to pursue the full benefits of communication. Standing in the way of full participation and employment—often compared to the bars and walls of a prison or to the despised institution of slavery—stood disabilities such as blindness and deafness.

Language and Literacy as Essential

In the teaching of the blind and deaf, Dr. Howe saw language and literacy as the highway leading to communication and employment. With respect to deafness and blindness, to understand the extreme problem that Dr. Howe set out to solve, it is important to see just how difficult it is for a person who is both deaf and blind to acquire a language. Being cut off from language means being cut off from literacy, and without literacy, a person is cut off from access to education. Without education, and without the capacity to communicate with others, earning an income is nearly impossible. As we noted in Chapter 2, disabilities tend to have cascading effects like falling dominoes.

In addition to his concern for the "immortal souls" of human beings, Howe wanted to enable deaf-blind individuals to be employed and to have productive lives. Today, gainful employment remains one of the most pressing needs of persons with communication disorders. Temple Grandin (2005), for example, is a contemporary professor, engineer, and author with **high functioning autism (HFA)**. In her talks, she commonly makes the point that employment is among the most essential goals for persons with disabilities. At the same time, when it comes to education, training, and therapies for persons with communication disorders, the goal of gainful employment is one of the most difficult to achieve and it is often set aside as a near or complete impossibility.

Howe understood that having such disabilities as deafness and blindness together presents a far more difficult challenge to language and literacy than they do separately. Nevertheless, he believed it was just possible that a deaf-blind person could be taught language and literacy through the sense of touch. In many respects he anticipated arguments about the nature of speech and language that would require another hundred years or more to be clearly expressed by linguistic theoreticians and researchers. He believed it should be possible to acquire language and literacy primarily through the avenue of touch without any sight or hearing.

In 1832, after doctoring wounded soldiers who were fighting for Greek liberation from Turkey, Howe visited the best known school for the blind in Europe. Later that same year he returned to America to become the first Director of the new Perkins Institution for the Blind in Boston. In 1837, he met the deaf-blind Laura Bridgman and took on the task of teaching her language and literacy. On his wedding trip to Ireland in 1843, Howe wrote a few words that show how he felt about cases such as that of Laura Bridgman. While in Ireland he had met a deaf-blind adult and he wrote about why and how she might possibly be taught language:

> The whole neighborhood would rush to save this woman if she were buried alive by the caving in of some pit . . . Now if there were one who had as much patience as zeal, and who, having

With respect to deafness and blindness, to understand the extreme problem that Dr. Howe set out to solve, it is important to see just how difficult it is for a person who is both deaf and blind to acquire a language.

observed carefully how a little child learns language, would attempt to lead her gently through the same course, he might possibly awaken her to a consciousness of her immortal nature. (see Lash, 1980, p. 20)

When he had first met Laura Bridgman he had asked if the "immortal" soul—the mind, personality, and language ability—were not just as worth saving as her body. Howe evidently realized that language is crucial to literacy and that literacy unlocks the door to education and thus to employment.

Pragmatic Mapping as the Key

Howe's method of teaching language began with his own understanding of how normal language acquisition works. He observed that children associate arbitrary spoken and written signs with things, persons, and sequences of events. Howe understood correctly that language acquisition depends on the association between an arbitrary sign, such as a word, with something else.

Nowadays, this type of association is referred to as *pragmatic mapping*. This descriptive phrase has been widely adopted in work on language acquisition, theoretical linguistics, and especially in language teaching and clinical applications. The process of pragmatic mapping requires an association of an abstract word or symbol (a sign) with some concrete object or context. For instance, a symbol, say, the word *key*, as shown in Figure 3–1, is associated through the actions of sign users with its object, a KEY. Understanding this basic process, Howe used actions to demonstrate the

> In the early days of his work with Laura Bridgman, Howe concluded that language "was the key to her development, and the first step was to show Laura that words—arbitrary signs—were the means of communicating. . . . He began with a spoon and a key, upon which he pasted in **raised print** the words *key* and *spoon*" (Lash, 1980, p. 16).

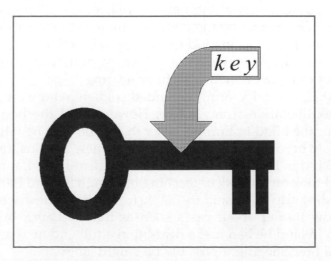

FIGURE 3–1. The pragmatic mapping of the word *key* onto an actual KEY accomplished by pasting the word in raised print onto the object—an experiment by Dr. Howe with Laura Bridgman that enabled her to make the connection.

abstract relation of the word to the object. Among the actions he used was to actually paste the printed word *key* onto an actual KEY. Then, he showed Laura by guiding her hand with his, the KEY and the distinct raised letters of the word *key* pasted onto the object. The word, *key*, by this method could come to be associated with its object. Laura Bridgman learned language through demonstrations of the pragmatic mapping relation that she could understand through her remaining sense of touch. To make the association, she still had to have the language capacity, but the first step had to involve the demonstration of the pragmatic mapping of words onto objects.

Laura Bridgman learned language through demonstrations of the pragmatic mapping relation that she could understand through her remaining sense of touch.

VALENTIN HAÜY AND LOUIS BRAILLE

Howe got the idea of using raised print from a visit in 1830 (Lash, 1980, p. 15) to the first well-known school for the blind. It was called L'Institution Royale des Jeunes Aveugles (the Royal Institution for Blind Youth; retrieved February 23, 2009, from http://en.wikipedia.org/wiki/Louis_Braille). It had been established in Paris in 1784 by Valentin Haüy [1745–1822] who became known as the "Father and Apostle of the Blind" (Knight, 2009, retrieved February 23, 2009, from http://www.newadvent.org/cathen/07152b.htm). Howe visited the school several years after Haüy's death in 1832 but he was inspired by what Haüy had done.

Dealing with Blindness Without Deafness

Haüy had intended to be a priest, but ended up as a **calligrapher** and foreign language teacher and later as an interpreter and translator for the French Ministry of Foreign Affairs. His background in the learning and teaching of languages helped him to see the importance of language and literacy to persons with sensory disabilities, especially blindness. His work as a translator and interpreter also gave him insight into the processes associated with acquiring language and literacy and their importance to education and employment. Like Temple Grandin and Samuel Howe, Haüy saw communication as a necessary basis for participation and employment in society. A significant event in shaping Haüy's future occurred in 1784, the year he started the famous school "des Jeunes Aveugles" [for blind youngsters].

According to one account, Haüy was leaving the Abbey of Saint Germain des Prés after services when he gave a coin to a 17-year-old blind boy named François Lesueur. The boy protested that Haüy was too generous by calling out the denomination of the coin. Some believe this very event enabled Haüy to realize that the Blind could learn to read by using their sense of touch instead of sight. In

When Haüy saw a burlesque show in 1771 where blind beggars were "made the object of ridicule and general merriment" he is reported to have said to himself, "I shall substitute truth for mockery, . . . I shall teach the blind to read and to write, and give them books printed by themselves" (see Kimbrough, n. d., retrieved February 23, 2009, from http://www.brailler.com/braillehx.htm).

any case, Lesueur became Haüy's first pupil (Kimbrough, n.d.) and the incident with the coin may have led Haüy to develop his system of raised print. Haüy discovered that by printing letters large and impressing them deeply on suitably stiff paper when it was wet and flexible, the raised letters when dried and hardened could be identified with training and effort by touch alone. His system of raised print foreshadowed the development of a less tedious, faster, and more efficient system for the blind that is now known simply as Braille.

Before Braille Writing

The Braille writing system was largely developed by a blind boy of 15, Louis Braille [1809–1852] while studying at Haüy's school. Braille's system was completed in 1824, just two years after Haüy's death. It had been known all along that a blind child could acquire a language more or less in the same way that a sighted child does ("Blind Children's Learning Center," 2009, retrieved February 23, 2009, from http://www.blindkids.org/speech.html), but literacy for the blind was largely unknown until after the establishment of Haüy's school. A few books were first provided in oversized raised print at the Haüy school sometime after 1784 (Knight, 2009). Today, there are approximately 2,000 titles still available using Haüy's system of raised print writing. They can be found listed in French at the *Bibliothèque gros caractères* [Big Letters Library] at the *Musée Valentin Haüy* (2009) in Paris [Valentine Haüy Museum] (retrieved February 23, 2009, from http://www.avh.asso.fr/rubriques/association/musee_avh.php.) Partly, because of the wide success and familiarity of Haüy's writing system, Braille writing would not be adopted officially at any institution in the United States until 1860 when it was finally accepted for use at the Missouri School for the Blind (Kimbrough, n.d.).

At the time of its invention in 1814 by the 15-year-old Louis Braille, widespread acceptance of Braille writing was a distant hope that would take several decades to be achieved throughout the world and across many languages. It is interesting that the acceptance of Braille writing for the blind in the United States occurred in the same year that Lincoln was elected President and just one year before the start of the American Civil War. The freedom of the Blind to read, like that of the American slaves, did not come without struggle and the cost of bloodshed. At the 2009 French Web site for the Haüy Museum, the relation between the history of blindness and all the human struggles for freedom in the world is eloquently summed up:

> La lutte pour l'autonomie de cette catégorie humaine minoritaire est exemplaire de toutes les luttes menées, entre exclusion et intégration, au nom de la liberté.

The struggle for independence by this minority category of human beings, meaning persons who are blind, is exemplary of all the struggles undertaken, between exclusion and integration, in the name of freedom.

Although it had been known since ancient times that blind children can learn to speak any language just about as easily as sighted persons, for the Blind to become able to read and write was a more difficult proposition. Even with Haüy's system of raised print—which employed ornate embossed letters impressed on stiff paper with copper wire fonts—reading by blind individuals was slow, hard work. Some of the children at Haüy's school for the Blind, for instance, could not lift the heavy books. They consisted of thick pages pasted back to back. In addition to their bulkiness, there were other obstacles for the Blind in using Haüy's system of raised print. Although blind persons could read the raised print with effort, they could not write with it at all. The process was too complex and cumbersome, and it required a lot of special equipment and processing time for heavy wet paper to dry after being impressed with the mirror images of raised letters one by one.

However, a series of events that began with Braille's own blindness would lead him to develop a system of writing by which blind persons could learn not only to read but also to write. Curiously, the instrument by which Louis Braille was blinded was also destined to be the very sort he would use in developing and perfecting the system of Braille writing. Incidentally, we should note that Braille's system consists of a pragmatic mapping of a tactile symbol in each case onto a letter of the alphabet as seen in Figure 3–2. In a more complete representation of his system, of course, some of the tactile symbols also corresponded to numbers and/or marks of punctuation that are not shown in Figure 3–2.

Although it had been known since ancient times that blind children can learn to speak any language just about as easily as sighted persons, for the Blind to become able to read and write was a more difficult proposition.

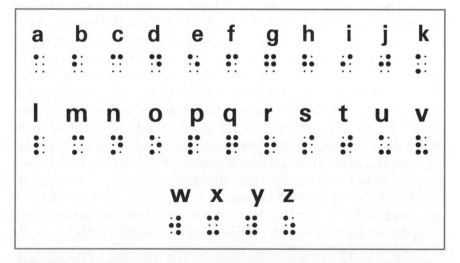

FIGURE 3–2. The Braille code as applied to the English alphabet. Copyright © 1995–2009 by the Royal National Institute of Blind People (RNIB). Retrieved February 24, 2009, from http://www.rnib.org.uk/xpedio/groups/public/documents/publicwebsite/public_braille.hcp. Reprinted with permission. All rights reserved.

In 1827, Louis Braille published a book titled *Method of Writing Words, Music, and Plain Songs by Means of Dots, for Use by the Blind and Arranged for Them.*

The Instrument of His Blindness

In 1812, at the age of 3, Louis reached up on a table where his father had been working and drug an awl, a leather-working tool, to the edge of the workbench where it fell into his left eye. According to one story (Kimbrough, n.d.), his father had been called out of the shop by a neighbor bringing news of Napoleon's invasion of Russia. The injured left eye became infected and the infection spread to the right eye, leaving Louis Braille blind at the age of four. Napoleon's wars and his eventual defeat at Waterloo in 1815 had devastating effects on Louis Braille's home town, Coupvray, France, which was a hard day's ride on horseback from Paris. However, by 1819, when Louis was 10 years old, his father was able to take him to Paris and enroll him in Haüy's school for the Blind.

At that time, there were 100 blind students and just 14 books written in Haüy's raised print for the whole school and all the students. Meantime, spurred by the fortunes of war, a military communications expert, Charles Barbier, had invented a form of secret writing in a **phonetic code** (see Chapter 7 especially Figure 7–2 showing the symbols of the International Phonetic Alphabet) that, with a certain amount of training and practice, could be read by touch at night or in the dense smoke of battle. Barbier's code was made more difficult, however, by not being based on ordinary spellings of words. To use it well, it was necessary also to understand quite a bit of the esoteric business of 19th century phonetics and linguistics. Although Barbier's code never caught on with the military, he supposed it might be of use to the blind. At any rate, when he visited Haüy's school in 1821 his secret writing code fell into the hands of 12-year-old Louis Braille who immediately began to improve it (Royal National Institute of Blind People, 2009; retrieved February 23, 2009, from http://www.rnib.org.uk/xpedio/groups/public/documents/publicwebsite/public_braille.hcsp). By redesigning the symbols so that each sign could fit under the imprint of the last joint of a single finger of an average-sized adult, Braille made Barbier's system both simpler and more readable. He also modified it to represent the letters of ordinary printed texts rather than the sounds of speech as described by **phoneticians**. He created a symbol for numbers and used it with the first 10 letters of the alphabet to represent the digits 0, 1, 2 . . . through 9. Braille not only simplified Barbier's code but also added marks of punctuation. He eliminated Barbier's dashes and figured out how to represent musical scores. As a young boy, Braille himself was an accomplished pianist and organist, so his interest in representing musical scores was as useful to his own needs as it was to other blind musicians.

In 1827, Louis Braille published a book titled *Method of Writing Words, Music, and Plain Songs by Means of Dots, for Use by the Blind and Arranged for Them.* A few years later he was one of three blind individuals who were promoted to the rank of Full Professor at the

Haüy school. In 1837 the first Braille book was published—a three-volume history of France—but it was not until seven years later at the dedication of a new building for the Haüy school that its director, a certain P. Armand Dufau, arranged for students to demonstrate the Braille writing system. For several years he had resisted the use of that system. It is interesting and informative to consider why Dufau opposed Braille writing for as long as he did, and why, in the end, he became a strong supporter of it.

The Visual Prejudice: Visuocentricity

The almost fatal objection to Braille writing was grounded in a common prejudice of sighted persons. Individuals who can see, it seems, are blind to the special needs and even the abilities of the Blind. Like the driver who frantically motions from within the vehicle for the blind person holding the stick to go ahead and cross the street in front of the car (we have actually seen this happen), the sighted persons of Braille's time also were subject to what may be termed **visuocentricity**. That is, they had a natural bias toward thinking of the world in terms that are appropriate for individuals who can see.

Like the driver motioning for the blind person to cross the street, our own inability to think of the world as it seems to a blind person does not occur to us until after the fact. The study of communication disorders, and especially of blindness, can help, if not to remove, at least to raise our awareness of visuocentricity and other **sensory prejudices**.

Visuocentricity and Braille Writing

When Braille proposed his writing system to sighted persons, it was received somewhat the way it is still viewed today by sighted individuals. We are apt to say something like, "I can't see how it works. I don't recognize any of the letters." That was the reaction in Braille's time and no doubt accounts for the preference of seeing persons for the system invented by Valentin Haüy and the continued use of Haüy's system even to this day—in spite of the fact that blind individuals almost universally prefer Braille. It was exactly as if the sighted persons to whom Braille was first introduced, ironically, were blind to the fact that Braille was invented for the Blind, not for the sighted.

It is true that Braille symbols are not transparent to sighted persons because they do not resemble the characters of the Roman alphabet. This can be appreciated by examining the Braille letters in Figure 3–2. But for the Blind, Braille writing is simple, easy to understand, and useful. Although no one has improved much on the underlying code, writers who use Braille naturally prefer

For sighted persons it is difficult even to talk about how the world must seem to a blind person. We are apt to talk about how the world "looks" or "appears" to the blind, in which case, we have already fallen into the trap of visuocentricity

The tool that Louis Braille used in creating his system was the sort of awl that had blinded him (Kimbrough, n. d.)

abbreviations and contractions that make the system work faster. They invariably simplify it and end up using fewer symbols, for instance, by expressing a whole word or phrase by using only its first letter, first syllable, or an abbreviation.

The letters and symbols of Braille writing, as can be seen from Figure 3–2, consist of raised dots as shown in darkened circles. The empty circles show places that are not raised to form the letter (or symbol) in question. With his writing system, blind individuals could use such a tool to write their own original messages and books. This was a great advantage over the raised print formerly used at the Haüy school. It is important to note that the blind students at the Haüy school understood as soon as they were introduced to Braille writing that they could also write their own thoughts in it and they immediately began to pass notes to each other in Braille. They continued to do so in spite of the fact that Braille writing was officially forbidden by the Director of the school, Mr. Dufau, for quite a few years. Evidently, being a sighted person, he preferred the Haüy system.

However, the new Braille writing system continued to be used secretly by the blind students at the Haüy school long before it was officially accepted. According to Paula Kimbrough (n.d.), its secret use lasted until February 1844. At that time, Mr. Dufau not only changed the school policy but arranged for a public demonstration of Braille writing to show how well it worked.

Demonstrating Braille Writing

The demonstration took place on the dedication of the new building for the school. Evidently, Dufau was as visuocentric as the rest of the sighted world. He had been in the group that complained they could not read printed texts in the Braille code. It took many demonstrations that Braille was a superior writing system for the Blind, for whom it was invented, in order for sighted persons like Mr. Dufau to come around. When Dufau did finally change his mind, he also realized that the invention of Braille writing would also help the school. When the new building at the Royal Institution for Blind Youth was dedicated, here is what happened according to historian Paula Kimbrough (n.d.):

> An official in the audience cried out that it was all a trick, that the child writing Braille and a second child reading it back (who had been out of the room for the dictation) must have memorized the text in advance. In reply, Dufau asked the man to find some printed material in his pocket, which turned out to be a theater ticket, and to read it to the student Braillist. The little girl reproduced the text and another child read it back flawlessly before the man even returned to his seat. The crowd, convinced, applauded wildly for a full six minutes. (retrieved February 23, 2009, from http://www.brailler.com/braillehx.htm)

Distinct Grades of Braille Writing

The basic form of Braille, now known as **Grade 1 Braille** included numbers and marks of punctuation. The system was also easily adapted to languages other than Braille's native French. For example, it has been used for writing systems as different as Arabic, Hebrew, Greek, and Chinese (see "Braille," 2009, retrieved February 23, 2009, from http://en.wikipedia.org/wiki/Braille). To save space in transcriptions a slightly more advanced form known as **Grade 2 Braille** evolved with various contractions to speed up its use. In addition, there are personalized systems with additional abbreviations and contractions that are known collectively as **Grade 3 Braille**.

Is Braille writing and reading a trick? Evidently not. But how can we be sure? Certainly there have been tricks of memorization, deliberate illusions created by sleight of hand, and even unintentional confusions that have led intelligent observers to mistake errors and deliberate lies for authentic systems of communication. How are we to tell the difference?

HOW CAN WE TEST THE AUTHENTICITY OF COMMUNICATION?

It is interesting that even the possibility of successful communication has often been doubted by skeptics. Sometimes the skepticism has ended in outright denial that genuine communication is possible at all. **Postmodernism** ends up taking this strange position. Pennycook (1994), for instance, asserted that "we cannot know ourselves or the world around us in any objective fashion" (p. 134). A skeptic like Pennycook commonly says something like, "We really never understand each other quite perfectly." Or like the man at the Braille demonstration, the postmodernist is apt to suppose that when communication seems to succeed there must be some magic trick involved, as with smoke and mirrors.

However, as we showed in Chapter 1, *ordinary communication usually succeeds*. It is for this reason that the common world—the one we know through our senses and through the agreement we achieve in communicating with others—is what we call "the real world." We suppose that world is real because we often (though not always) agree with each other about what is going on in that world. For instance, the audience at the Braille demonstration in 1844 understood the claim of the skeptic very well. They also understood, no doubt, that he might possibly be correct. They could understand his claim that perhaps the whole demonstration was a clever trick—even a deliberate deception. Maybe they had been fooled. That audience was certainly as well equipped as we are to understand the skeptic's suggestion that they had been duped, so

The very fact that breakdowns, including blindness and deafness, can be recognized for what they are shows that our senses commonly inform us correctly and validly about the world as it is.

There were three characteristics of the interactions that day showing the **authenticity** of the demonstration of the Braille system. When all three characteristics are present on the same occasion, we can be virtually certain, though perhaps not quite absolutely certain, that authentic communication has occurred.

why did they come around to accepting the demonstration as valid after the skeptic's ticket was translated into Braille and read back by a different blind student?

Characteristics of Authentic Communication

There were three characteristics of the interactions that day showing the **authenticity** of the demonstration of the Braille system. When all three characteristics are present on the same occasion, we can be virtually certain, though perhaps not quite absolutely certain, that authentic communication has occurred. Consider the three abstract qualities achieved at the Braille writing demonstration that can only be achieved when communication succeeds (as it normally does):

1. The most obvious characteristic of authentic communication is the *agreement between communicators*. In the Braille demonstration, agreement was shown in the sustained applause after the second demonstration succeeded. The audience agreed with the demonstrators that the demonstration was authentic—that is, valid and true.

2. A less obvious characteristic of authentic communication is the *intelligibility of shared meanings*. The meanings are achieved through abstract symbols of a language. The letters on the ticket were translated into Braille symbols and then back into spoken words by the Braillists. The writer and the reader of Braille understood the same meanings by those symbols as were understood by the skeptic and the whole audience that day.

3. The least obvious characteristic of authentic communication is the *creativity of the exchange*. That is, the exchange involves unrehearsed material. The Braillists could not have known what was written on the skeptic's ticket in advance. It was—assuming only that the skeptic was not himself a plant (a co-conspirator) in the audience—a piece of writing selected on a whim with no advance warning. Still the braillists were able to write in Braille what the ticket contained and to read it back without difficulty.

Let us consider each of these characteristics a little further.

With respect to *agreement between communicators*, there are three distinct levels. (a) At the most superficial level, the communicators agree on the surface forms. That is, a single raised dot in a particular position is differentiated from no raised dot, or from two raised dots, and so forth. (b) At a slightly deeper and more abstract level, the communicators agree on the **conventions** of those symbols; for instance, the conventions that associate a particular Braille symbol with a particular letter or with a mark of punctuation. In other words, the users of the Braille system all realize that a single raised dot in the upper left corner of the field of six positions represents the letter "a"; that two raised dots one above the other in the first two positions represents the letter "b"; and so on (as shown in Figure 3–2; from "Braille," 2009). And at a still higher level (c), the communicators agree on the intended meanings of the sequences of symbols; for instance, in Braille writing, the meanings consist of the words that are translated from **alphabetic writing** or from speech into Braille. The words represented were translated from the writing on the skeptic's ticket.

The second characteristic in addition to agreement between the communicators is the *intelligibility of meanings* to independent parties. This is not always so observable and testable as agreement between the communicators themselves. However, when the audience saw the second demonstration of Braille writing and reading —the writing and then the reading of the skeptic's ticket—the audience was able to verify the intelligibility of the Braille system by comparing the starting point with the end result. Because the Braille reader was able to read back the same words from the Braille transcription that were on the skeptic's ticket, the whole process was intelligible to the observing audience. The audience could verify that Braille writing was intelligible to the Braille users. The cycle of working (1) from spoken words to (2) symbol production in Braille and (3) symbol interpretation from Braille back into spoken words was completed sufficiently so that both producer and interpreter agreed on the words that were spoken at the beginning and at the end. That is, they agreed on the meanings of the Braille symbols from start to finish.

> Because the Braille reader was able to read back the same words from the Braille transcription that were on the skeptic's ticket, the whole process was intelligible to the observing audience. The audience could verify that Braille writing was intelligible to the Braille users.

A third characteristic showing the authenticity of successful communication is the *creativity of the exchange*. If the sequence of symbols that is agreed upon and which is intelligible to the Braillists and other observers involves a new sequence of symbols never encountered before, then its comprehension cannot be based on rehearsal or memory. It must be based on a real act of creative construction of an unrehearsed sequence of Braille symbols. If so, it is evident that the communicators are not relying on rote memory of past experience. In the case of the Braille writer, a new stream of surface forms in Braille had to be constructed to fit the writing on the skeptic's ticket. We suppose that the Braillists did not know that the skeptic would raise the objection he did. They could not predict that Mr. Dufau would select the man's ticket for a secondary demonstration. In the case of the reader of the Braille transcription, a stream of spoken words, not heard before, had to be produced from the string of Braille symbols taken from the skeptic's ticket.

Ruling Out Probable (Reasonable) Doubt

If all three of the foregoing characteristics are present in any successful communication, *probably*, that communicative interaction was and is authentic. But a serious skeptic might ask whether even this sort of demonstration, with all three of the characteristics of authentic communication, guarantees that a particular communication is or was successful and not a mere trick? Suppose a new skeptic comes along and says, "Yeah, but, the skeptic in the story about the demonstration of Braille could have been a plant and the whole exchange could have been set up in advance. It still might be a trick to cause the audience to believe that the Braille system works." This argument might be correct in a cleverly staged trick. However, it would require a very carefully planned series of deceptions. But suppose it was all staged.

The solution to the problem of a second, third, fourth, and any number of additional skeptics, is still the same. If the communication had not been authentic, asking for another and another and another different translation would eventually either show Braille reading and writing to be valid, or would turn up the deception. By the point that genuine communication is actually understood even once, the likelihood of a clever deception is so remote that it can be considered nil. It is not reasonable to claim doubt when in fact the reasonable basis for doubt has been effectively removed. The aphorism that "you can fool all of the people some of the time and some of the people all of the time, but you just can't fool all of the people all of the time"—commonly attributed to Abraham Lincoln—applies here. When a given result can be achieved over and over again, doubters who say that result cannot be achieved must be mistaken or themselves deceived. There comes a point after which continued doubt concerning the success of some ordinary communication becomes unreasonable.

Of course, we are convinced that the demonstration of Braille writing and reading by blind individuals really was authentic. If the **replication** of unfamiliar sequences of words or meanings can occur at all, we know that the apparent success in communicating is probably authentic. With additional replications, reasonable doubt is diminished to the point that it would be silly to continue doubting that authentic communication has occurred. However, an even more powerful and a more general refutation of any denial that authentic communication commonly occurs will be given next. It is possible, and the next section shows why this absolutely must be taken as a reasonable starting point.

> By the point that genuine communication is actually understood even once, the likelihood of a clever deception is so remote that it can be considered nil. It is not reasonable to claim doubt when in fact the reasonable basis for doubt has been effectively removed.

> If we are to suppose that overcoming communication disorders is at all possible, it is necessary to believe from the start that real, authentic, genuine communication is actually possible.

Denying Successful Communication Involves Self-Contradiction

Any intelligible denial that authentic communication is possible contains a necessary **self-contradiction**. When anyone says, "We can never really understand each other perfectly," if the statement is comprehensible at all, it refutes itself. This is obvious whether we happen to agree with the person expressing the doubt or whether we disagree. Suppose we agree. We say, "We know exactly what you mean, communication never succeeds perfectly." The agreement shows that communication has succeeded perfectly even though we have agreed with the skeptic that communication never succeeds perfectly. Communication has occurred perfectly well because we understood that the skeptic meant to say that it never occurs perfectly well. Or, on the other hand, suppose we disagree. We say, "We don't know exactly what you mean, because communication never succeeds quite perfectly." Again, communication has succeeded perfectly well in spite of the fact that we have denied the skeptic's claim that communication never succeeds perfectly. Either way (and there are no other reasonable ways to take the message) the skeptic's claim is refuted by itself. The claim contains its own contradiction.

Therefore, logically, we are obliged to suppose—or at least we *cannot reasonably deny*—that communication in some cases must succeed very well. In many cases, it succeeds perfectly well for practical purposes. That is, it succeeds exactly as perfectly as it was intended to succeed. In fact, the demonstration of the usefulness of Braille succeeded as it was intended to succeed with the whole audience in February 1844, and now it has succeeded equally well with us.

To show the relevance of refuting any general skepticism about the possibility of authentic communication we only need to point out that if successful communication were not attainable at all, the whole purpose of the study of communication disorders would be lost. But the goal of curing and/or preventing communication disorders is not lost because communication really does commonly succeed. We can rule out any extreme and general form of skepticism about authentic communication. This means that even in cases of extreme difficulty—for instance, deafness combined with blindness—there can still be a real possibility of understanding. Even deafness and blindness combined do not make communication necessarily impossible.

We can rule out any extreme and general form of skepticism about authentic communication. This means that even in cases of extreme difficulty—for instance, deafness combined with blindness—there can still be a real possibility of understanding. Even deafness and blindness combined do not make communication necessarily impossible.

Skepticism Sometimes Justified

On the other hand, we are *not* ruling out all skepticism as applied to particular cases as unreasonable. Only a completely general skepticism is ruled out. In fact, the official at the Braille demonstration did everyone a service by pressing his point until all reasonable doubt about the authenticity of the demonstration was removed. The fact is that skepticism about particular cases is often good and reasonable. It is, of course, possible for a well-rehearsed act, an error of understanding, or even a deliberate deception to be mistaken for an authentic and truthful communication. There have been important cases where claims of successful communication turned out on closer examination to be false. As a result, we should never entirely dismiss the possibility of clever deceptions or of

Sometimes we think communication has succeeded when it has not. However, the discovery of such errors and especially the discovery of deliberate deceptions absolutely demonstrates that a general (complete or extreme) skepticism is absolutely untenable.

errors in particular cases. Sometimes we think communication has succeeded when it has not. However, the discovery of such errors and especially the discovery of deliberate deceptions absolutely demonstrates that a general (complete or extreme) skepticism is absolutely untenable. If there were no genuine communications, no errors or lies could ever be discovered and shown up for what they are. If there were no authentic cases where communication succeeds, errors, lies, and even doubt itself, could not be intelligibly expressed in any case.

There are cases, nonetheless, where doubts are justified. For instance, alleged written communications about sexual abuse coming from nonverbal and illiterate children with autism merits close scrutiny (see American Academy of Pediatrics, 1998; Probst, 2005; von Tetzchner, 1997). In some cases, the individuals with autism—with the skilled assistance of a "facilitator" guiding the person's hand on a keyboard—were supposed to suddenly start communicating in writing at levels beyond anything the child had been able to do in the past. The technique has been called **facilitated communication** and has been widely advocated by certain individuals (e.g., Biklen, 1990; Crossley & Remington-Gurley, 1992).

It was sometimes claimed that a given child had supposedly become literate more or less overnight, and suddenly had begun to pour out in writing his or her own history of sexual abuse—but not without the assistance of the clinician. Upon examination, the writing that was supposed to be coming from the person with autism turned out to be coming almost exclusively from the clinician instead (Probst, 2005). In cases where the person being assisted was able to communicate independently, performance was consistently superior without the assistance of the facilitator. In cases where questions were put to the individual being assisted, to which the facilitator did not know the answer, correct answers could not be produced. By contrast, correct answers could often be obtained to questions, provided the facilitator had independent access to those answers. The claims in favor of facilitated communication have turned out not only to be generally false, absurdly so in the case of severe autism, but extremely harmful to innocent parties who were accused of wrong-doing.

Interestingly, as we will see, the test-of-authenticity offered by Mr. Dufau in response to the skeptic at the Braille demonstration in 1844 involved the same key elements as later tests of authenticity in the 20th and 21st century.

Consistency Is Critical

Because errors are possible, however, no matter how unlikely they may be, skepticism concerning particular cases should neither be lightly dismissed nor should they be casually accepted as true. The burden of proof is especially heavy when the supposed communication is potentially damaging to individuals or their families. We must carefully examine the relevant facts and apply all of the standard tests for authenticity that were used in the case of the Braille demonstration. The key to authenticity in all possible cases is always the consistency (or lack of it) between the representations of different parties and the relevant facts as known to competent observers.

Inevitable Acceptance of Braille Writing

Because of its usefulness to blind individuals, Braille writing is by far the most widely used system of literacy for the blind today. However, most users are rapidly moving to digital input methods with a standard keyboard. Blind individuals now learn to use ordinary keyboards just like the various ones used in writing this book. Only in the beginning stages of learning the layout of the standard keyboard do blind writers today rely on keyboards with raised Braille characters impressed on them. The ordinary standard keyboard with the raised dots or dashes marking the "F" and "J" keys are sufficient for blind users just as they are for sighted persons (National Federation for the Blind, 2009, retrieved February 24, 2009 from http://www.nfb.org/). Only in the beginning stages is it necessary for any skilled typist to have access to the letters printed as letters or as Braille symbols on the keys. After some skill in typing is achieved, sighted and blind typists alike only need the raised dots on the reference keys to position their hands and find the rest of the keys.

Nevertheless, in spite of the move to digital input systems, Braille remains the most commonly used display system for text in a tangible format for blind users. The device used to achieve Braille print today is "the Braille display machine, a flat box that sits under a keyboard and duplicates the screen text in Braille characters produced by plastic pegs that poke up through tiny holes. The machine can even display a flashing cursor by popping the proper pegs up and down" (National Federation for the Blind, 2009, retrieved February 24, 2009 from http://www.nfb.org/). Another modern technology that supplements and extends the usefulness of ordinary computers for the Blind are screen reader programs that convert **digital text** to intelligible **synthesized speech** which is routed to the computer's speakers. The output is **audible electronic text**. By converting digital text electronically into intelligible speech, current technologies are providing blind users of the computer an additional means of access to ordinary print.

> After some skill in typing is achieved, sighted and blind typists alike only need the raised dots on the reference keys to position their hands and find the rest of the keys.

DEAFNESS WITHOUT BLINDNESS

Individuals who are deaf from birth, or who lose their hearing at a very early age, have greater difficulty in learning to speak than blind children do. However, deaf children, provided they do not have additional severe impairments, can acquire a manually signed language, such as **American Signed Language (ASL)** or any other manual language, much in the way that hearing children acquire a spoken language ("Deafness—From Birth to Death," 2009, retrieved February 23, 2009 from http://deafness.about.com/cs/earbasics/a/birthtodeath.htm).

Babbling: Oral and Manual

Deaf infants also go through **oral babbling** by producing rhythmic syllabic utterances, such as "bababa," somewhat later than hearing children do. Hearing children reach this stage of development typically by about their 7th month after birth whereas deaf children rarely reach the stage of repetitive oral babbling before their 10th month. However, deaf children, like their hearing counterparts, do go through a stage of rhythmic **manual babbling** right on schedule by about their 7th month (Eilers & D. K. Oller, 1994; D. K. Oller & Steffens, 1994; Petitto & Marentette, 1991).

Researchers and theoreticians generally interpret these facts as showing that the underlying language capacity of deaf and hearing children is essentially the same (Petitto & Marentette, 1991; Ross & Bever, 2004). Recall Chomsky's remarks about the nature of the language capacity—without which human beings are hardly free to think, act, and communicate in the normal ways. Evidently, babbling of the repetitive kind is a timely manifestation of that universal human language capacity.

The similarity of oral and manual babble is taken as evidence that spoken and signed languages are merely different manifestations of the same underlying universal human language capacity.

Inventing Language Without Native Models

If the parents and siblings of a deaf child are not signers, children deaf from birth will commonly invent manual signs on their own (G. Morgan & Kegl, 2006; Senghas, 2003, 2005; Senghas & Coppola, 2001; Senghas, Kita, & Ozyurek, 2004; S. E. Wilcox & P. P. Wilcox, 1997).

Language Invention by Twins

Language invention has been observed in hearing twins. A well-known case of this kind involved a pair of **San Diego twins** who were at first diagnosed as "mentally retarded." It was later discovered by an intelligent and alert speech pathologist, Alexa Kratze, that the two girls had invented their own private language system. It was unintelligible to anyone other than themselves and consisted of a mixture of German and English components ("Poto and Cabengo," 2009, retrieved February 23, 2009, from http://en.wikipedia.org/wiki/Poto_and_Cabengo). There was also movie, *Poto and Cabengo 1979* about the twin girls, Grace (Poto) and Virginia (Cabengo) Kennedy, directed by Jean-Pierre Gorin (retrieved February 23, 2009 at http://vtap.com/topic/Poto+and+Cabengo/VM910480).

Similarly, it is often reported that deaf children of hearing parents tend to invent a sign system of their own when they are not exposed to a manually signed language. This situation is fairly common on account of the fact that "the overwhelming majority of deaf and **hard of hearing** students have hearing parents" (Mitchell, 2004; also see Mitchell, 2006). In fact, Mitchell's research shows that more than 90%, possibly even 95%, of deaf children are born into hearing families. **Profound deafness** at birth is relatively rare though it is more common for infants to be born hard of hearing than to be born profoundly deaf. Mitchell's research, however, showed that only about 5 to 10% of the children of deaf parents will be born deaf. Therefore, it follows that more than 90% of deaf and hard of hearing children are born to hearing parents. In all the cases where deaf children are born into hearing families, they typically are surrounded by people who are not native signers. Nevertheless, the deaf children in these situations tend to invent signs of their own. In many cases they become fluent signers in the absence of **native models** (Morford & Kegl, 2000; G. Morgan & Kegl, 2006).

Because the parents and siblings of deaf children are usually hearing persons who use a spoken language, the deaf child in a hearing family is born into a situation somewhat like a foreign country except that in this strange land, the people use a different foreign language (a spoken language that the child cannot hear)—than the language the child will invent (a manually signed language). The question is, how can a deaf child acquire a signed language when none of the family members or interlocutors in the neighborhood of the child use any signed language? How will the deaf child acquire a language to which he or she is not exposed? The situation is a lot more difficult than that of a child who must learn a foreign language under normal circumstances. It is more like the situation where a child has to invent some foreign language in a country where that language has never been used before! It is unsurprising that children typically acquire a new foreign language if they are in the country where it is used around, them, but how can a deaf child acquire or invent a manually signed language

Profound deafness at birth is relatively rare though it is more common for infants to be born hard of hearing than to be born profoundly deaf.

in a setting where little or no use of any signed language occurs? The fact that deaf children of hearing parents can learn such a language at all is strong evidence of the inborn human capacity for language acquisition.

Natural Signed Languages Versus Ones Derived from Speech

The signed languages of the world can be divided roughly into two categories: (1) there are those **natural signed languages** that are used by preference by Deaf communities, such as American Signed Language (ASL), and (2) there are **derived signed languages** which were created by reference to a spoken language by persons who either became deaf after acquiring that spoken language or who, for whatever reason, set out specifically to create a signed language based on a particular spoken language. These distinct systems tend to be intermingled to some extent, but they are even more different in some respects than English and Chinese.

Natural signed languages are, for reasons to be explained, much more like spoken languages whereas derived signed languages tend to resemble word-for-word translations that seem strange even to persons who know the original language. They are stilted, unnatural, and tedious to use. The derived signed languages are, therefore, more different from natural languages than radically distinct natural languages are different from each other. For example, signed languages derived from the surface forms of spoken languages are more different from natural spoken language systems and from natural signed languages than English is from Chinese.

ASL, a natural signed language system that is about as related to English as Chinese is, has in fact often been compared to Chinese in its underlying structure (S. E. Wilcox & P. P. Wilcox, 1997). But ASL is a natural manually signed language and is very different from the system known as **Signed Exact English** (**SEE**)—also known as **Manually Signed English** (**MSE**)—which uses signs that are directly associated with the surface forms of spoken English. Deaf individuals in America usually learn either one or the other system, that is, ASL or SEE, but rarely both. Persons born deaf, and Deaf communities, almost universally prefer natural signed languages such as ASL over systems of manual signs derived from any spoken language such as SEE. It is important to see why this preference is deeply felt and so perfectly reasonable. The reason that the Deaf prefer ASL over SEE are similar to, though more complex reasons than, those of the Blind for choosing Braille over Haüy's raised print system of writing.

To become literate in English, for instance, the language as well as the writing system must be deciphered simultaneously by the deaf person. Although literacy is commonly attained by deaf individuals who happen to have learned the signed variant of a

> Persons born deaf, and Deaf communities, almost universally prefer natural signed languages such as ASL over systems of manual signs derived from any spoken language such as SEE.

spoken language, such as MSE (see "Manually Signed English," 2009, retrieved February 23, 2009, from http://en.wikipedia.org/wiki/Signing_Exact_English), literacy in a spoken language—that is, learning to read and write in English—is less common and more difficult for persons who have been deaf from birth than for persons who became deaf later in life, after acquiring a spoken language. Persons who are born deaf do not normally use the signed variant of any particular spoken language. They use a natural manually signed language such as ASL.

Fitting Square Pegs in Round Holes Two at a Time

A common complaint against signed variants of spoken languages, such as SEE or MSE, is that they are awkward in the **manual modality**. The surface structures of spoken systems were not developed for manual signing. To produce a manual sign in SEE, for example, for every structurally functional element in spoken English (including plurals, possessives, demonstratives, and so on) requires about twice the time needed to produce the same sentence in a natural system such as ASL (Bornstein, 1973, 1979; Zak, 2005). It is tiring to use SEE when doing simultaneous translation from speech to sign and it is virtually impossible to produce all the manual signs required to show all the surface forms of spoken English at a normal conversational tempo.

The problem is about the same as trying to translate every single surface element of any natural language, one at a time, into a surface component of another language. This is not the way normal **translation** is done. Translators do not work directly from the surface forms of language A to the surface forms of language B. If they did, the result would be stilted and odd.

Rather than trying to use the surface forms of language A in language B, a more natural approach to translation or **interpretation** is to express the meanings originally expressed in A in the surface forms of B, and vice versa. Users of natural languages would find it rather strange to attempt to directly convert every surface element of language A into a new surface element of language B retaining the essential word order and structure (though not the sounds) of language A. But that is essentially what the creators of SEE set out to do. The process can be called **rigid transliteration**. It forces the surface forms of the foreign language into the surface forms of a different language. It is a little like forcing square pegs into round holes, two at a time. The interpreter/translator has to keep both surface forms in mind at the same time. This is not normal. Normally, translators—even those doing **simultaneous interpretation**, that is, producing an equivalent representation in language B almost at the same time as the representation in language A is produced by someone else—work from the meaning expressed in language A to the same meaning expressed in language B. In fact, if the speaker

To produce a manual sign in SEE, for example, for every structurally functional element in spoken English (including plurals, possessives, demonstratives, and so on) requires about twice the time needed to produce the same sentence in a natural system such as ASL (Bornstein, 1973, 1979; Zak, 2005).

being translated from language A to B, say, happens to say something in B (while the interpreter is expecting A), the interpreter (who is typically focusing on the meaning of what is said rather than its surface form) is apt to repeat in language B what was just said in language B by the speaker. Interpreters are commonly amused if and when they catch themselves doing this. Often, they are unaware of doing it.

The reader who has studied a language which is no more different from English than Spanish is, can appreciate the sort of hybrid we are talking about by transliterating a few simple Spanish sentences into an "exact" Spanish Equivalent English (the analogue of SEE) as contrasted with the same translations into ordinary English (the analogue of ASL). In Table 3–1 a few simple sentences in Spanish in the leftmost column are rigidly transliterated into an analogue in English of SEE in the middle column. In the rightmost column the Ordinary English translation of the Spanish sentences is given.

The reader can see that there are some elements in the surface forms of Spanish that do not appear at all in the surface forms of English, and vice versa. Also, it seems strange to adhere to the word order and structure of Spanish when translating into English.

Why Deaf Signers Prefer ASL Over SEE

The exact translations of the surface forms of Spanish into surface forms in English give the reader some idea of the difficulties faced by the creators and users of SEE—alias, MSE.

Table 3–1. Ordinary language forms in Spanish in the leftmost column and English in the rightmost column compared with rigid transliterations in the middle column to exemplify the oddity of SEE or MSE from the viewpoint of users of ASL

| Ordinary Language A

Example: *Ordinary Spanish (analogous to any natural language such as ASL or English)* | Rigid Transliteration from A to B

Example: *Spanish Equivalent English (analogous to the sort of system represented in SEE, MSE, or any contrived rigid transliteration from one language to another)* | Ordinary Language B

Example: *Ordinary English (analogous to any natural language such as ASL or Spanish)* |
|---|---|---|
| Hacía sol ayer. | Making-was sun yesterday. | Yesterday, it was sunny. |
| Ven acá. | Come-you-familiar here-moving. | Come here. |
| Me llamo Guillermo. | Me call-I William. | My name's William. |
| Tengo veinte cuatro años. | Have-I twenty-four years. | I'm twenty-four. |
| Son las seis y doce. | Are-they six and twelve. | It's twelve past six. |

The examples also show why SEE seems strange and awkward to Deaf signers. Ordinary English translations from Spanish seem natural and transparent while the transliteration of Spanish surface forms into English surface forms seems weird. Because of the unnaturalness of going directly from surface forms in one language to surface forms in an entirely different system, the kind of transliteration that SEE requires is stilted, strange, and artificial. It also takes about twice as long as normal translation of meanings (rather than surface forms) between natural languages, for example, from English to Chinese or vice versa, or English to ASL or vice versa. There is little wonder, then, that Deaf signers prefer natural signed languages—such as ASL over SEE, for instance. Signed languages that are based on the surface forms of a spoken language, are strange to say the least.

Why not just dispense with the artificial intermediate system altogether? This is not done in the case of Signed Exact English on account of the fact that there are persons who know spoken English prior to becoming deaf. As a result for such persons who already know spoken English and its written variants, SEE, according to its proponents, is easier for them to acquire and use than ASL. Nevertheless, any effort to create an intermediate sign for every form of the reference language results in a contrived language with strange surface forms. To sign all the spoken forms results in an unnatural and awkward sequence that is considerably slower than speech, and slower than translation into any other natural language. Interestingly, it is about as difficult to translate every aspect of a message in a manually signed language into a spoken system as it is to go in the other direction. To express in ASL the meaning of someone "helping" someone else, for example, you place your dominant hand in the shape of a fist in the palm of your other hand, and lift the dominant hand a short distance with the nondominant hand. If we translate the meaning, we get something as brief as the word "help" which takes about as much time to produce as the sign, but to express an exact translation in spoken English of every movement involved in the sign for "help" in ASL, would take much longer. Surface translations from any language to any other are awkward in both directions. They take a great deal longer to produce than is needed to translate meanings across distinct natural language systems.

> Surface translations from any language to any other are awkward in both directions. They take a great deal longer to produce than is needed to translate meanings across distinct natural language systems.

Additional Difficulties in Rigid Transliteration

Another complaint is that signed variants of spoken languages have no natural culture to back them up the way ASL and natural signed

For a free teachable, learnable, and user-friendly version of about 1200 ASL signs in a digital format—where you can see how the sign is formed and find out what it means—see "ASL Dictionary" (n.d.; retrieved February 23, 2009, from http://www.lifeprint.com/asl101/pages-layout/signs.htm).

systems do. Because SEE is not preferred by the Deaf community in America it has no "oral" literature of the sort that can be claimed for ASL. The users of SEE counter that ASL, for instance, has no commonly used writing system. Nor is there a common writing system for any of the manually signed languages of the world's Deaf communities. But some progress has been made in recent decades to provide a digital dictionary of ASL (S. E. Wilcox, Scheibman, Wood, Cokely, & Stokoe, 2009). For a free teachable, learnable, and user-friendly version of about 1200 ASL signs in a digital format—where you can see how the sign is formed and find out what it means—see "ASL Dictionary" (n.d.; retrieved February 23, 2009, from http://www.lifeprint.com/asl101/pages-layout/signs.htm).

With all the foregoing in mind, it becomes obvious that the best defense of SEE or any signed language derived from a spoken language, probably, is that it provides easier access to a vast written literature that does not exist in ASL. However, it is possible for signers who do not use SEE to learn to read English or another language with the assistance of translations provided in ASL. The fact is that learning to read and write in a particular language, as we will see in Chapter 9, is generally easier when the learner has access to the spoken language that happens to be written down. This is especially true when the writing system of the spoken language represents sounds as in our own alphabetic writing system. We will have more to say about writing systems in Chapter 9, but for now it is important to keep in mind that spoken English is a very foreign language from the viewpoint of signers who use ASL. Also, as a spoken language system, like all other spoken language systems, it is poorly suited to the direct manual representation of its surface forms.

SPOKEN LANGUAGES, MANUAL SIGNED LANGUAGES, AND LITERACY

As we have seen, children who are blind at birth or at an early age learn to speak much as hearing children do. Similarly, children who are born deaf or who become deaf at an early age commonly acquire or even invent a signed language system. Literacy is common among deaf users of SEE, and is only a little less common among deaf users of ASL. Literacy has increasingly been achieved by blind individuals since the latter part of the 18th century and especially in the 19th century after Braille came into worldwide use. Now, with computer assisted text readers, the Braille writing machine, and the increasing ease of access to automated **text to speech** (**TTS**) programs, literacy is common among the Blind.

As we also noted, for a person who was born deaf to become literate in a spoken language is more difficult than for a hearing person to acquire literacy in a second language. The deaf person must learn to decipher and comprehend the printed forms of the spoken language without ever hearing it spoken. Such a learning task is comparable to learning to decipher an ancient writing system that is no longer spoken—such as ancient Egyptian hieroglyphics, Babylonian cuneiform writing, or an ancient text from an unknown language written in Chinese characters. For a deaf user of ASL to become literate in English is more like learning to read in a language you do not know at all than learning to read in a language you already speak and understand. However, with the assistance of manually signed translations of print, persons born deaf do commonly acquire literacy. The first school in the United States which embraced the purpose of teaching literacy and of providing the benefits of education to the Deaf was established in Hartford, Connecticut in 1817 (American School for the Deaf, 2005). Shortly afterward, the Governor of Connecticut, Oliver Wolcott, called on the people of Connecticut

> to aid . . . in elevating the condition of a class of mankind, who have been heretofore considered as incapable of mental improvement, but who are now found to be susceptible of instruction in the various arts and sciences, and of extensive attainments in moral and religious truth. (retrieved February 23, 2009, from http://www.asd-1817.org/history/index.html)

Should the Deaf Speak?

Alexander Graham Bell often referred to himself more modestly as merely a "teacher of the Deaf" (Alexander Graham Bell, 2007). Among the Deaf, he is still known for his advocacy of teaching deaf individuals to produce spoken language through close observation of the articulation of speech—a method he called **visible speech**. Also, he is known to have opposed and discouraged the use of manually signed languages. Neither of these proposals was ever widely accepted by the Deaf communities of the world (S. E. Wilcox & P. P. Wilcox, 1997) anymore than the rejection of Braille writing by sighted individuals could have prevented the Blind from using Braille.

Bell's mother was deaf as was his wife, Mabel Hubbard Bell, and it was almost certainly because of Bell (see Lash, 1980, pp. 89–91, 364–377) that the most famous deaf-blind person of all time, Helen Keller, would eventually achieve the ability to speak in a manner that made her fairly intelligible to hearing persons.

Disorders and Eugenics

Strangely, Alexander Graham Bell also became deeply involved in the American **eugenics** movement. The Greek roots of the word *eugenics* mean "well-bred" or genetically gifted. The purpose of the movement in America and throughout the world was to encourage

A luminary of science through his invention of the telephone, Alexander Graham Bell [1847–1922] also shaped policies and practices so much in the education of the Deaf that he has been sometimes referred to as "the Father of the Deaf."

The eugenics movement is historically important to students of communication disorders on account of the fact that it shows again that racial discrimination generalizes to persons with disabilities as certainly as water runs downhill.

As is well documented, for instance by Gould (1981) and by Haller (1971) social Darwinism and eugenics were openly promoted and widely accepted in the United States until World War II [1939–1945].

the breeding of individuals judged to be fit and desirable and to suppress the breeding of those judged to be undesirable.

The movement has always been aimed at bettering what is loosely and misleadingly referred to as "the human **gene pool**" (Sanford, 2005). The problem with the idea of a "pool" is that it suggests that genes can be singled out for selection or elimination, but this is not the case. Only the whole genome of an individual or group can be eliminated. It is not possible by selecting whole organisms or groups of them—whether the selection is artificial or natural—to operate on single genes or gene components. The eugenics movement is historically important to students of communication disorders on account of the fact that it shows again that racial discrimination generalizes to persons with disabilities as certainly as water runs downhill.

The eugenics movement began in 1865—the year that the American Civil War ended. It came to prominence in America in the year in which slavery in the United States was abolished and Lincoln was assassinated (see "Eugenics," 2009, retrieved February 24, 2009, from http://en.wikipedia.org/wiki/Eugenics). The recognized founder of the eugenics movement was, Sir Francis Galton [1822–1911], a cousin of Charles Darwin [1809–1882]. In its least offensive forms the eugenics movement advocated improving the human gene pool through selective breeding. The movement was called **social Darwinism** on account of his prediction (Darwin, 1874, pp. 178ff) that

> the anthropomorphous apes . . . will no doubt be exterminated. The break between man and his nearest allies will then be wider, for it will intervene between man in a more civilized state, as we may hope, even than the Caucasian, and some ape as low as a baboon, instead of as now between the Negro or Australian and the gorilla. (p. 178)

Darwin, in agreement with his cousin Francis Galton (1869), claimed that some races and genetic lines of descent are intrinsically inferior to others. As is well documented, for instance by Gould (1981) and by Haller (1971) social Darwinism and eugenics were openly promoted and widely accepted in the United States until World War II [1939–1945]. For an interesting chronology paid for by the Howard Hughes Medical Institute see Cold Spring Harbor Laboratory (2003; retrieved February 24, 2009 at http://www.eugenics archive.org/eugenics/) and also see the "Chronicle [of the American Eugenics movement]" (retrieved February 24, 2009 at http://www.dnai.org/e/).

Just a year before his death, Alexander Graham Bell participated in the Second International Congress of Eugenics which took place in New York in 1921. At that meeting a resolution was unanimously adopted advocating

> the spread of popular information regarding eugenics, namely; race hygiene, race biology, the value of races, and the advan-

tages and dangers of race crossing. ("Eugenics Movement," 2006, retrieved June 15, 2006 from http://www.ferris.edu/isar/arcade/eugenics/movement.htm—a site that has since been removed)

The idea, according to B. Mehler (1988; available as of February 24, 2009 at http://www.ferris.edu/HTMLS/staff/webpages/site.cfm?LinkID=248&eventID=34) was to educate the public about the "need to prevent imbecile, abnormal, and weak-minded individuals" from multiplying themselves, and to guard against the corruption of the gene pool through cross racial breeding. Again, as we noted earlier, there was an inevitable association between theories grounded in racial prejudices and ones pertaining to disabilities.

We meet some of the present-day intellectual descendants of the eugenics movement in Chapters 7, 11, and 12. In the meantime, it is important always to keep in mind that the issues of racial freedom and the rights of persons with disabilities have been as connected throughout history as the mind is connected to the body.

FREEING THE IMPRISONED SELF

Reformer Charles Dickens compared the condition of the deaf-blind Laura Bridgman to a person enclosed within "a marble cell" and, as we saw in Chapter 1, similar metaphors have been used by articulate parents of children with severe autism. Parents have often described their child with autism as if he or she were captured inside a body unable to connect with persons in the world around them—as if the child were a prisoner in some unreachable universe—a private world of a lonely self. In fact, the term "autism" is intended to suggest this very idea. Individuals with severe autism seem to exist in a separate universe that is difficult if not impossible to reach by any means of ordinary communication. Meanwhile, the parents are trying to find the key to rescue the child who is locked inside that alien universe (see J. W. Oller & S. D. Oller, 2009).

Parents have often described their child with autism as if he or she were captured inside a body unable to connect with persons in the world around them—as if the child were a prisoner in some unreachable universe—a private world of a lonely self.

The Case of Helen Keller

When Samuel Gridley Howe learned of the eight-year-old deaf-blind Laura Bridgman in 1837 ("Laura Bridgman," 1889/2007, retrieved February 23, 2009, from http://en .wikipedia.org/wiki/Laura_Bridgman; also Lash, 1980, pp. 14–22), he set out to teach her language and literacy.

During his five-year tenure as Director of the Perkins Institution for the Blind, Samuel Gridley Howe had already established that the students should learn a manual skill, a trade making them employable, that they should engage in regular physical exercise, and that they should become "self-reliant . . . 'active' citizens of the

When Samuel Gridley Howe learned of the eight-year-old deaf-blind Laura Bridgman in 1837 ("Laura Bridgman," 1889/2007, retrieved February 23, 2009, from http://en .wikipedia.org/wiki/Laura_ Bridgman; also Lash, 1980, pp. 14–22), he set out to teach her language and literacy.

Commonwealth" (Lash, 1980, p. 16). To achieve these worthy objectives, language and literacy were indispensable.

Fifty years later, in April of 1887, when Annie Sullivan [1866–1936] (see "Annie Sullivan," 1936/2009, retrieved February 24, 2009, from http://www.lkwdpl.org/wihohio/sull-ann.htm) was hired to teach then six-year-old Helen Keller (born June 27, 1880), Annie followed the essential methods pioneered by Dr. Howe. Both of them used what is now known to be the necessary and sufficient basis for child language acquisition (see Badon, 1993; Bruner, 1975; Macnamara, 1972; J. W. Oller & Richard-Amato, 1983; J. W. Oller, 1970, 1975, 1993, 2005; J. W. Oller, S. D. Oller, & Badon, 2006). Howe had argued that we should first understand how infants solve the problem of language acquisition in order to find out how to lead persons with sensory and other communication disorders in more gentle steps over a similar path. Both Howe and Sullivan also realized that it would be necessary to exercise greater patience in leading deaf-blind individuals into language than for persons with all their senses.

The first step was to map a word onto its logical object—the process known as pragmatic mapping. Among the simpler instances of such a mapping relation is the sort between a referring term and the particular event, thing, or person in experience to which it refers. As we saw in Figure 3–1, the starting point for Laura Bridgman was guided touching of the word *key* in raised print that was pasted onto an actual KEY as contrasted with the word *spoon* similarly pasted onto a SPOON. For six-year-old Helen Keller, shown

*The first step, the one that would unlock the door of language acquisition, was to enable the deaf-blind person to discover the meaning of at least one **referring term**.*

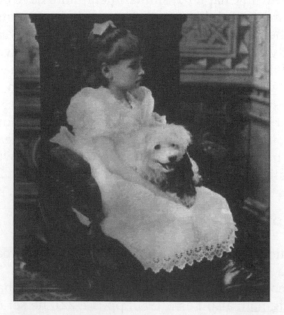

FIGURE 3–3. Helen Keller at age 7 years and two months, just five months after she met Annie Sullivan and began to acquire language. A photo in the public domain from the American Foundation for the Blind, retrieved February 24, 2009 at http://www.afb.org/Section.asp?SectionID=1&TopicID=194&SubTopicID=6&DocumetID=144.

at age seven in Figure 3–3, the salient event involved water flowing over one hand from a pump operated by her teacher, Annie Sullivan, while Annie repeatedly spelled the word *water* manually in Helen's other palm (Figure 3–4). The event became a benchmark in Helen's life to which she would often refer later on. It also provided one of the clearest illustrations in English literature of how language acquisition typically begins. In all cases, language acquisition depends on associating referring terms with their logical objects —that is, with whatever they signify (see J. W. Oller, 1975, 2005).

Helen Keller would later write in *The Story of My Life* (H. Keller, 1905) about the moment that she realized that "everything had a name" (Lash, 1980, p. 55). This was how she described the insight that opened the door to language and literacy for her. Figure 3–4 shows the scene as depicted in the 1962 movie version of the play, "The Miracle Worker," starring Ann Bancroft as Annie Sullivan and Patty Duke as Helen Keller (retrieved February 24, 2009, from http://en.wikipedia.org/wiki/The_Miracle_Worker; also see the review on the follow-up movie "The Miracle Continues," 1984, retrieved February 24, 2009, from http://movies2.nytimes.com/gst/movies/movie.html?v_id–126149).

After her teacher Annie Sullivan died, Helen Keller wrote about her memory of how her journey into the social experience of language began. For the period before she could use or understand a single word, she called herself "Phantom." This was the name she applied to the child she had been from the time of the illness at 19

In all cases, language acquisition depends on associating referring terms with their logical objects—that is, with whatever they signify (see J. W. Oller, 1975, 2005).

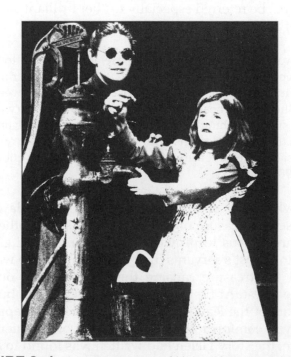

FIGURE 3–4. A re-enactment of Helen Keller acquiring her first word with the help of Annie Sullivan. From *The Miracle Worker* (p. 34), by W. Gibson, 1956, New York: Doubleday. Copyright © 1956 by Doubleday.

months that left her deaf and blind until she began to learn language again almost six years later. After April 5, 1887, when she acquired her first word, she called herself "Helen." She wrote,

> Phantom had a mug in her hand and while she held it under the spout Annie pumped WATER into it, and as it gushed over the hand that held the mug she kept spelling *w-a-t-e-r* into the other hand. Suddenly Phantom understood the meaning of the word . . . (H. Keller, 1955, p. 40)

Figure 3–3 is a picture of Helen Keller in August of 1887, just five months after she began to acquire language. Figure 3–4 is from the re-enactment of the crucial insight by Helen that words have meaning.

Was the Miracle Authentic?

Just as the authenticity of Braille's invention of writing for the blind was denied by certain skeptics long after it had been widely accepted by others, Helen Keller's so-called "miraculous" acquisition of language and literacy was also challenged.

The public inquisition in the case of Helen Keller began with an incident involving a short fictional story titled, "The Frost King."

Helen's teacher, Annie Sullivan, sent the story, as supposedly composed by Helen, to Mr. Michael Anagnos on his birthday. Anagnos was the son-in-law of Samuel Howe and had become director of the Perkins Institution for the Blind after the death of Dr. Howe. Up to the time of this particular birthday Anagnos had written a great deal about the success of Helen Keller. In one of his official reports, he referred especially to "her brilliant success in the acquirement of language" (pp. 95–96) saying:

> I am aware that my description of Helen may seem to those, who do not know her, extravagant in its praise; but her numerous friends will bear testimony most gladly to the sweetness, unselfishness and beauty of her disposition . . . Every day of her life she is teaching us gratitude and contentment; and she teaches those great lessons with such truth, patience and joyousness, that we never tire of her radiant presence. (quoted by Lash, 1980, p. 97)

The story, which was sent to Anagnos on his birthday, told how King Frost sent a treasure of rubies, emeralds, and other precious stones to Santa Claus to provide clothing and other gifts for the poor. But King Frost's servants dilly-dallied along the way and Mr. Sun melted the treasure causing the colors to run out into the leaves of the forest. At first the King was very angry, but when he saw the colors of the leaves in the autumn he was happy. He had found a way to comfort folks for the passing of summer.

Later on, the story Helen had written was found to have replicated a previously published story, "The Frost Fairies" written by Margaret T. Canby. Afterward, Anagnos would refer to Helen Keller and to her teacher, Annie Sullivan, as "a fraud and a humbug" (Lash, 1980, p. 97). Because of the "Frost King" incident, the whole idea that deaf-blind persons could acquire language and become literate came under intense critical scrutiny. Anagnos supposed that the whole "miracle" was a lie from start to finish. The emerging public reactions to the prior success of the deaf-blind children in acquiring language ranged the gamut from the claim that it was all a

1. triumph of the human spirit over adversity;
2. success, possibly exaggerated;
3. minor accomplishment owed to a remarkable memory for stories read to her by others;
4. demonstration of what Annie Sullivan could do rather than Helen Keller;
5. trumped up fraud.

The question was and remains which description best fit the facts? Let us consider each of the competing descriptions and the reasoning that fueled the doubts in the cases of alternatives 2 through 5.

When Helen Keller's successes were first reported by her teacher, Annie Sullivan, they were wholeheartedly accepted (claim 1). Michael Anagnos, for instance, the director of the Perkins Institution, was among the first to proclaim the earliest accomplishments of Helen Keller to be a triumph (Lash, 1980, p. 99). In the words of Anagnos, Helen Keller's accomplishments were hardly short of miraculous.

However, there would be some specialists in language acquisition who would point out that the Helen Keller and Laura Bridgman had both lost their sight and hearing after they had already acquired some language skills. Bridgman became deaf and blind at age 2 and Keller at 19 months. Therefore, some would caution that some of what the two deaf-blind girls learned in acquiring language, at least, if not literacy, was already known to them before their illnesses. Some would say that they merely regained what they had lost. Perhaps the claims of success were a little exaggerated (claim 2).

Others suggested that the deaf-blind success stories, like the Braille demonstration of 1844, were just extreme cases of memorization. Helen's words, letters, and other writings, by that theory, were just bits and pieces of the discourse of others that she had cobbled together without really understanding their meaning (claim 3).

Still others would argue that much of the apparent success of Helen Keller in language acquisition was owed to material directly supplied by her teacher and by others (claim 4). To support this theory it was noted that in her writings, Helen Keller would often use words and phrases describing the qualities of sights she could not see and sounds she could not hear. Therefore, some said, she had to be using the words and phrases of sighted and hearing persons. The strings of words attributed to Helen Keller could not be

Because of the "Frost King" incident, the whole idea that deaf-blind persons could acquire language and become literate came under intense critical scrutiny.

original, on this theory, so she had to be getting the words from others, in particular, from Annie Sullivan.

And finally, the most extreme critics, some of whom changed camps from wholehearted believers in Helen Keller as hardly less than a sainted genius, would go so far as to say that the apparent success of Helen Keller was not only owed to her teacher, Annie Sullivan, but that the two of them had engaged in a deliberate deception (claim 5). In this last category was Michael Anagnos, initially the strongest supporter of the success of Helen Keller. He went from the extreme of proclaiming her accomplishments to be a triumph of the human spirit, to the opposite extreme of saying privately, that "Helen Keller is a living lie" (Lash, 1980, pp. 168, 338–339).

Applying the Tests of Authenticity

A Colossal Lie?

Is it possible that the words attributed to Helen Keller were really those of Annie Sullivan? Could all the signing, reading, and writing that seemed to be coming from Helen merely have been invented by her teacher? Had Annie Sullivan, in collaboration with Helen Keller, contrived the apparent success and deceived the public? Some people would ask, how could a deaf-blind person learn to use language with so many words about light, color, and sound? Could all the words and phrases used merely be memorized passages from the writing and thought of others? There were also doubts about Laura Bridgman's success too. Could the little deaf-blind girls have merely relearned what they already knew? How much of the apparent success was real?

The most severe skeptics would say that all the linguistic output of the student was really owed to others. In the worst-case scenario, nothing of value had been accomplished: it was all a lie.

Extreme doubts about Helen Keller were triggered by the "Frost King" incident. Probably, the original story by Margaret Canby was read to Helen Keller by Annie Sullivan along with a great many other stories. However, in answer to her critics about descriptions involving sight and sound, Helen would later describe how she learned to tell the difference in colors and sounds by touch. She said she could feel the green-ness of the leaves in summer and the gradations of change as they went from soft green to crisp crunchy leaves that turned to dust in her hand. When asked how she knew there were many books in a room, she replied that she could smell their musty odor, and when she was asked how she knew there was a great crowd of people in the auditorium where she was about to speak, she said she could feel the vibrations in the floor when they stood and moved around.

Concerning the confusion of the Frost King story, she was embarrassed for her error in supposing that the story was original with herself, but she pointed out that for a person who is deaf and blind, oral readers do not always supply the full bibliography for any verbal material that they sign. The deaf-blind person receives the text, poem, or discourse in manual signs or, in her case, sometimes in fragments of raised print. It is important to realize that Braille writing was not widely available for printed material during Helen Keller's early years. Often when writing, she observed she would think of something to say simply not knowing whether she was using words she had heard from others or words that she had invented on her own.

Ruling Out Plagiarism

Oddly, one of the best known skeptics of all time, Samuel Clemens [1835–1910] who was better known by the alias Mark Twain, was among the first to defend Helen Keller concerning the accusations of **plagiarism** that were brought against her after the Frost King affair. He insisted that "all ideas are secondhand" and he never wavered from the view that her accomplishments were genuine. He wrote to her after Annie Sullivan died, saying:

> You are a most wonderful creature, the most wonderful in the world—you and your other half together, Miss Sullivan, I mean, for it took the pair of you to make a complete and perfect whole. (as quoted in Lash, 1980, p. 290)

Also, we should note that Annie Sullivan's writings—as documented in many sources but especially by the award winning author, Joseph P. Lash [1909–1987]—were often bitter and cynical, while Helen Keller's writings show her to have had a very different personality and to have been a much more optimistic person.

Whose Words Are They?

According to Lash, Annie Sullivan and Helen Keller were as different as night and day. Another point to note is that Helen Keller kept on writing long after the death of Annie Sullivan. Also, it was evidently not uncommon for Helen Keller to do and say many things over Annie Sullivan's objections. For instance, when Helen took seriously the recommendation of Alexander Graham Bell to acquire speech, according to histo-

It is important to realize that Braille writing was not widely available for printed material during Helen Keller's early years. Often when writing, she observed she would think of something to say simply not knowing whether she was using words she had heard from others or words that she had invented on her own.

When the deaf-blind Helen Keller learned to talk intelligibly at public gatherings, the naysayers, were hard-pressed to argue that it was not her own voice and her own words that they were hearing.

We thank Emily Ensminger for pointing out this link to video of Helen Keller actually speaking.

rian J. P. Lash, Annie thought it was ridiculous. According to him, Annie Sullivan doubted that it was even possible for a deaf-blind child to learn to speak intelligibly. She thought it a waste of precious time. However, a three minute film clip shows how Annie Sullivan was actually the person who taught Helen Keller to speak (see and hear it all at "Helen Keller speaks," http://www.afb.org/braillebug/hkmediaviewer.asp?frameid=29, retrieved February 24, 2009).

We also find it interesting and insightful that Helen Keller's own explanation of her first word, "water," gave a clear illustration of the nature of pragmatic mapping. It echoed the similar understanding of Dr. Samuel Gridley Howe who taught Laura Bridgman to read and write in English. Helen Keller's memory gave a living illustration of the relation between the surface form of a language act, and the external world into which language acts are mapped by intelligent sign users. When that account was written, and when it was told many times in public meetings in the words and voice of Helen Keller, the story could not have depended on the words of Annie Sullivan because Annie was long since dead and gone.

One thing that can be said for a certainty is that Helen Keller could not have memorized all the elaborate sentences she constructed in her speeches, letters, and writings.

One thing that can be said for a certainty is that Helen Keller could not have memorized all the elaborate sentences she constructed in her speeches, letters, and writings. At least since G. A. Miller (1964) published his mathematical argument about just how many sentences are possible in any language, we have had a profoundly adequate mathematical argument showing that memorizing even a fraction of a percentage of the sentences of any language is utterly impossible. This follows because no matter how good a memory anyone might have, almost all of our sentences, like the ones present in this book for the first and only time, are constructions never uttered or written before in all of human history. Most of them will never be repeated again in quite the same way, much less in the same order by the same persons in the same contexts of experience. Helen Keller's language use had all the marks of genuine and authentic communication. Her discourse throughout her education, her travels, her conversations with people, was (1) creative, (2) intelligible, and (3) led to agreement on many points with communicators in many different contexts. All this could not have been "a living lie" anymore than the demonstration of Braille writing could have been a slick trick. It has been performed on different texts many millions of times since Braille's death.

It is plainly possible to overcome great communication disorders, deficits, and disabilities.

What is even more important for our story here is that Helen Keller and those who helped and encouraged her to acquire language and literacy brought genuine hope to persons with communication disorders.

SUMMING UP AND LOOKING AHEAD

In this chapter we have seen that the senses are crucial to our learning about the world and especially to the acquisition of any language. Without any senses, any kind of learning, social relationship, or communication would be, as Aristotle noted, impossible. We reviewed two cases, however, of complete blindness accompanied by profound deafness where Laura Bridgman and Helen Keller, either learned or re-learned language and both became literate. We saw how important the process of pragmatic mapping—the linking of concrete particular objects and events in experience with the abstract symbols of language—is to the acquisition of language and literacy. Without discovering the pragmatic connections between symbols and the particular things, persons, and events in our world of experience, language itself, much less literacy, could not be acquired and would be impossible. We also saw evidence of some remarkable and very subtle prejudices against persons with disabilities and we saw how those prejudices connect persons with disabilities, historically, with individuals of diversity. In the next chapter, we consider the remarkable early integration of the senses not only with each other, but with movements—especially with the significant articulatory movements of speech—and with the deep meanings and concepts of abstract language.

> Without discovering the pragmatic connections between symbols and the particular things, persons, and events in our world of experience, language itself, much less literacy, could not be acquired and would be impossible.

STUDY AND DISCUSSION QUESTIONS

1. Why are the issues of diversity and disabilities historically linked with each other?
2. How did the process of pragmatic mapping work for Laura Bridgman and Helen Keller?
3. What improvements in particular did Braille writing offer in contrast to Haüy's system of raised print? How did visuocentricity influence the transition? What examples can you give of its influence from your own experience?
4. Why is success in communication harder to account for than its breakdowns? Or, in what ways are true representations that are correctly understood more richly developed and more complex than fictions, errors, or outright deliberate lies?
5. What is the logical difficulty of saying "it is impossible to communicate anything perfectly"?
6. If you are a skilled typist, try typing a well-known sentence on a keyboard without looking at the keys and without feeling the

raised dots or dashes that mark the reference keys for your index fingers. If you could not see, hear, or feel the keys would you (or any skilled typist) be able to type any intelligible message?

7. What evidence for or against the innateness of the human language capacity can be mustered from the cases of severe sensory impairment discussed in this chapter? Consider especially the case of deaf children born to hearing parents.

8. Consider the characteristics of authenticity as discussed with reference to the Braille writing demonstration and as applied to the question of whether or not Helen Keller actually wrote the books attributed to her. What arguments can you offer pro and con and what is your personal view of the questions at stake?

9. What major differences exist between natural manually signed languages and ones that are based on spoken language systems?

10. Discuss the prison metaphor as it relates to blindness and deafness, or to severe autism, or complete paralysis. Why do you think the metaphor is commonly applied to such cases, for example, those of Laura Bridgman and Helen Keller?

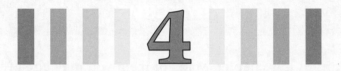

Systems Integration and Hearing Disorders

OBJECTIVES

In this chapter, we:

1. Discuss integration of the senses, especially hearing, with movements and language;

2. Review empirical evidence of early integration of senses with bodily movements;

3. Show that sensation, movement, and language are layered, ranked, and integrated;

4. Experience how movement outranks sensation and both are outranked by meaning; and

5. Explore the layered systems of hearing; and

6. Review evidence that the human hearing systems are tuned to speech.

KEY TERMS

Here are some key terms of this chapter. Many of them you may already know. It may help to review them. These terms are explained in the text and they are defined in the Glossary at the end of the book. They appear in **bold print** on their first appearance in the text.

acetylcholine
afferent nerve fibers
amniocentesis
amodal
amplitude
anxiety disorder
articulator
attention deficit disorder
audition
auditory discrimination:
auditory pattern recognition
auditory processing
auditory recognition
binaural hearing
both ends against the middle
  processing
bottom-up processing
brain stem
central auditory processes
central nervous system
cerebrum
cochlear implant
cochlear nuclei
cognitive momentum
competing acoustic signals
cortex
cortical deafness
damp
degraded acoustic signals
distributed neural networks
distributed processing
efferent nerve fibers
elicited imitation
filtering effects
formants

frequency
functional Magnetic
  Resonance Imaging (fMRI)
fundamental frequency
General American English
hand-eye coordination
hertz
homeopathic effect
hyperactivity (ADD/ADHD)
Hz
inner hair cells
integration training
kinesthetic feedback
lateralization
linear processing
linguistic expectations
lipreading
localization
masking effects
McGurk effect
McGurk interactions
median canal
multimodal
multimodal integration
neurons
organ of Corti
otoacoustic emission (OAE)
outer hair cells
parallel neural networks
parallel processing
perceptual defense
perceptual vigilance
pinna
pitch

post-traumatic stress
  syndrome
prestin
proposition
referential content
resonance
sensorineural hearing loss
sensory integration
serial neural networks
serial processing
signal detection
simple frequency theory
spectral properties
spectrogram
spectrum
sphere of reference
spinal cord
subliminal messages
synapses
temporal integration
temporal masking
temporal ordering
temporal resolution
theory of abstraction
tinnitus
top-down processing
transitive relations
triangulate
tympanic canal
vestibular canal
vestibular system
vocal folds
vocal tract
vowels

It used to be widely believed that the senses were not well integrated until months or even years after birth (Piaget, 1954). In keeping with that idea, some still hold that **integration training** can alleviate symptoms of developmental disorders such as autism or ADHD (e.g., see Auditory Integration Training, 2004; Hashemian, 2006; Silverstein, 2009). Theories of sensory integration are also closely related to ones about the development of voluntary movements. For instance, the emphasis on **hand-eye coordination** suggests that the connection between sensation and movement is learned. The research shows a close coordination between sensory-motor actions such hand-banging, babble, and extending the index finger (Masataka, 1995), all of which precede by several months the development of the child's first meaningful spoken words.

The integration of the senses (as documented in J. W. Oller, S. D. Oller, & Badon, 2006) evidently occurs well before birth and appears to be preprogramed in the genome. Babies are normally born with integrated senses of sight, hearing, smell, touch, and taste. Moving pictures of the baby in the womb, show that the integration of sensation with movement is already advanced by the twelfth week of a normal pregnancy. There are many indications of the integration of sensation, movement, and language throughout life. Also, breakdowns in systems of integration are diagnostic of disorders.

> Sensation, movement, and language are intricately associated and integrated over the whole course of normal development—even from the time in the womb which some have called "life before birth."

INTEGRATION OF THE SENSES

McGurk (1988) observed that our ideas about objects and their properties normally involve more than one of our senses. For this reason, he said, "even the simplest concepts we form are **multimodal**" (p. 3). That is, they involve more than one of our senses, more than one mode of processing. For instance, "our idea, say, of an apple includes its visible properties (color and shape); tactual qualities (shape and texture); chemical qualities (taste and smell)" (p. 6, retrieved February 25, 2009, from http://www.isca-speech.org/archive/archive_papers/avsp98/av98_003.pdf). Consider, for instance, the red apple in Figure 4–1. Imagine its taste and texture. Now compare the taste you imagined, for instance, with what you would expect of a rounder, green apple of the sort commonly used in making apple pies. How do you know the taste of the red apple that you see in Figure 4–1, as contrasted with the green apple that you only imagine? Doesn't the thought of the imagined green apple suggest a tart sour taste that almost makes your mouth pucker in anticipation?

In saying that concepts are multimodal, McGurk also made the point that the senses are integrated with respect to the concepts that we have of objects. That is, we do not have a separate and completely

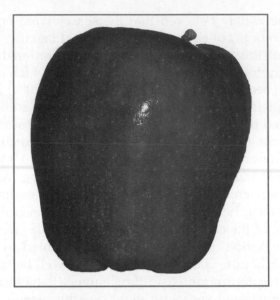

FIGURE 4–1. Image of a red delicious apple to illustrate expectations of taste and texture.

Our normal sensations of an apple produce a well-integrated and coherent concept rather than a fractured collage of different elements.

distinct concept of how an apple looks apart from how it sounds, smells, and feels to the touch when we bite into it and taste it. Our concept of any given apple seems to be unified, whole, and complete. All of the sensory properties of the apple tend to be integrated with each other and to be associated with the same unitary physical object.

We are not saying that sensory properties of a particular object cannot be abstracted and associated with other objects of similar kinds, shapes, tastes, and so on, but we are saying that sensory properties of any particular object are normally integrated in that object. They are unified right down to the history of the particular object in specific locations over space and time. Even if we eat the entire apple our concept of the apple and the experience of consuming it bite by bite remains well-integrated and coherent. Is there any doubt that we normally have integrated concepts of objects? For instance, where is your wallet or purse just now? Is your concept of it not connected to your knowledge of where you put it when you last took some money out, or a credit card? What about the driver's license and other documents that are in your wallet? Can you think of them even though you are not, say, perceiving (i.e., looking at, hearing, touching, and so on) them at the moment? Similarly, can you remember and think about your most recent meal? Are the concepts you have of these things not integrated particulars that are coherently connected with your history of experience in just the way your recollection of eating an apple is connected to your experience?

Are the Required Integrations Learned?

At the sensory level, there is a stream of research showing a close integration of sight and touch either right at birth or almost immediately afterward. Kaye and Bower (1994) studied babies within their first two days after being born. The babies were presented with one of a pair of distinctly shaped pacifiers that they had been prevented from seeing. While the baby was sucking on one of the pacifiers, a picture appeared on a computer screen of one of the pacifiers. It might be the one in the mouth or a different one never seen before. Babies preferred the visual shape that matched the one in the mouth. Considering that the visual shape on the screen was one the baby had never seen before, how was the baby able to match it with or distinguish it from the one in its mouth? See the illustration of different pacifier shapes in Figure 4–2.

Kaye and Bower (1994) concluded that the babies were relying on "abstract **amodal** or linguistic features specified by the sensory impressions" (p. 287). That is, the babies were using abstractions of some sort—intangible concepts of objects rather than the concrete objects themselves—to integrate the properties of the pacifiers across the senses of touch and vision (also see Bower, 1997). Or, we could say in McGurk's terminology that the babies were relying on

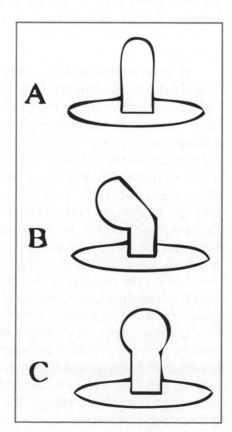

FIGURE 4–2. Redrawn images of Kaye and Bower (1994) to illustrate the pacifier experiment.

We predicted in the **theory of abstraction** that the discrimination of objects requires noticing and marking of edges (see J. W. Oller, S. D. Oller, & Badon, 2006, pp. 83, 89). This prediction is borne out by fMRI findings with adults (Macknik, 2007; Martinez-Conde & Macknik, 2007) showing that visual perception of an object is impossible without marking of the boundaries of the object noticed.

In the final analysis, it seems that the integration of the senses and the ability to abstract and generalize from touch to seeing, or hearing to seeing, must be genetically provided for before any learning takes place either in or outside the womb.

multimodal integration, or an abstraction taken from such an integration, prior to any experience that might reasonably account for that abstraction. If this is so and the experiment is understood correctly, it would seem that babies are preprogramed from before birth with multimodal integration, and or with prior knowledge of abstract concepts of certain kinds. Kaye and Bower (1994) argued that the babies were able to form highly abstract concepts of objects that enabled them to generalize across modalities.

The babies evidently are able to find the crucial boundaries of objects either by seeing or by touching. We predicted in the **theory of abstraction** that the discrimination of objects requires noticing and marking of edges (see J. W. Oller, S. D. Oller, & Badon, 2006, pp. 83, 89). This prediction is borne out by recent fMRI findings with adults (Macknik, 2007; Martinez-Conde & Macknik, 2007) showing that visual perception of an object is impossible without marking of the boundaries of the object noticed. Similarly, tiny movements of the eye referred to as **microsaccades** are also critical to illusions of motion where there is none (Troncoso, Macknik, Otero-Milian, & Martinez-Conde, 2008). The babies evidently can find the boundaries and determine the shape of the object either by touch or by vision. The question is how the translation between touch and vision is achieved by newborns. The same question arises with respect to Sai's experiment with the face and voice association (2005): how are newborns able to translate between seeing and hearing—between the visual impressions of a moving face that is producing speech and the sound of the voice that is producing the speech? We know they can do this at birth.

Human infants are born with the capacity not only to associate visual and tactile images but with integrated senses that draw inferences from vision to touch and vice versa. Can this sort of ability be learned in the womb? It has been suggested by one of our colleagues that certain experiences in the womb might help the baby to differentiate the distinct shapes of the pacifiers. For instance, a thumb has a different shape from a finger and the baby may be able to generalize the prebirth experience with thumbs, fingers, and toes to still other objects such as the distinctly shaped pacifiers that are presented for the first time after birth. However, unless the baby can see its fingers and toes in the womb, the learning of different shapes from touch, even if it does occur in the womb, does not explain the generalization of that learning to vision. To make that leap requires some abstract representation along the lines suggested by Kaye and Bower (1994).

Certainly, there is evidence of learning before birth. The question, however, is whether the learning that takes place in the womb is sufficient to explain cross-modal generalizations of the sort Kaye and Bower, also Sai, have demonstrated. If learning accounts for cross-modal generalizations, the baby must invent a means of translating between seeing, for instance, and hearing. Otherwise, if such learning cannot happen, we must suppose as Chomsky (1980;

and elsewhere) has argued, that human babies have the genetic conceptual ability to represent abstract meanings, the kind that will later be correctly called "linguistic," long before they can produce any speech, writing, or overt language of any kind.

The Senses Integrated with Voluntary Movements

Bower was also one of the pioneers in showing that sensations are tightly integrated with movements at least from birth and probably even before birth.

Bower Demonstrated Integration at Birth

In 1971 he summed up research showing that infants as young as two weeks after birth tend to perform three movements when it appears that a solid object is on a collision course with the infant's face. In the research paradigm that Bower developed, the infants were all only two weeks old or less. Each baby was placed in a situation where a virtual object seemed to be on a collision course with the baby's face. In that situation, the babies would (1) widen their eyes and open their mouths as if surprised; (2) raise their hands as if to ward off the impending collision; and (3) move their heads back as if to lessen the impact. All these actions show that the senses of sight and touch are not only integrated with each other, but that they are already integrated at the age of two weeks with the infant's capacity to produce voluntary movements.

Now here are some of the questions that researchers have considered: when did the infants learn this body-eye coordination? When and how has the infant had the opportunity to learn that visible things are commonly associated with solid and tangible objects? How often, for instance, has a visible object struck a two-week-old infant in the face? Can we suppose that the infants studied by Bower and colleagues had learned to associate touch with vision, or with the defensive movements appropriate to such experiences during their first two weeks of life? Could they have learned these associations before birth? Is vision sufficiently developed in the womb so that the observed behaviors could be acquired through the experience of the baby in moving its own hands and feet?

Other evidence of sensory-motor integration at or even before birth includes the striking of the barrel of a needle by an unborn fetus who is evidently trying to avoid the stick during an **amniocentesis** procedure (Birnholz, Stephens, & Faria, 1978). After birth, at least since Meltzoff and C. A. Moore (1979, also see Meltzoff & M. K. Moore, 1997) it has been known that human neonates can sometimes imitate gestures such as opening the mouth, sticking out the tongue, widening the eyes, and smiling. If the senses were not fairly well integrated with the infant's movements, how could the baby produce an expression on its own face that it sees on the face of another person? Presumably, the newborn baby has not commonly experienced these expressions on anyone else's face before its birth.

The baby cannot ordinarily see its own face either in or out of the womb. For this reason, we must suppose that the baby's sense of vision is already coordinated with its movements before it ever imitates anyone else's facial expressions. Sai (2005) also showed that the newborn baby's pragmatic mapping of its mother's familiar voice onto her unfamiliar face likewise requires integration of movements with sensations. The sounds that the baby can hear, for instance, are coordinated with the movements of the face, lips, and tongue of mother as she speaks. If the baby is prevented from seeing mother while she is speaking, the association of her voice with her face, Sai showed, does not occur. However, if the baby is permitted to see mother and hear her speaking at the same time, the association of voice with face (a particular instance of pragmatic mapping) occurs within the first 5 to 15 minutes after the baby's birth.

Sensory-Motor Acts Integrated with Speech and Language

> The coordination of a newborn's movements with speech rhythms suggests a deep integration of the senses not only with bodily movements, but with the particular kinds of articulated movements that are characteristic of speech and language.

The connection between mom's voice and her body is one of the earliest integrations that points toward language and that shows the normal human baby's peculiar (prior) interest in speech and language. The early connection of sensory-motor acts suggests either that (1) learning has occurred in the womb, or (2) that preprogrammed concepts exist prior to any learning, or (3) that some combination of both must be in place before birth or immediately afterward. At birth, for example, the process of entrainment, discussed in Chapter 1, consists of the observed fact that the movements of newborn infants tend to be coordinated with the articulated speech of adults that the baby overhears (Condon & Sander, 1974; Hsu & Fogel, 2003; Jaffe, Beebe, Feldstein, Crown, & Jasnow, 2001).

Interestingly, the human senses—especially seeing and hearing—have often been studied as if all the senses were separated from each other and were unrelated to bodily movements, not to mention the deeper complexities of speech and language. However, the integration of the senses with respect to the most abstract forms of representation—especially in speech, signing, writing, and meaningful linguistic discourse—is undeniable and has been demonstrated experimentally in many different ways. Logic and experience show that the senses are richly integrated with bodily movements, and, in human beings, both the senses and articulate bodily movements—as seen in speech, writing, music, dance, choreography, creative artwork, skilled athletic performances, mathematical and musical notations, and all aspects of human experience that depend on language—are far more deeply integrated and connected with each other than piecemeal studies of sight or hearing can possibly discover. Studies of isolated "pure tones" may tell us something about hearing, but they fall far short of explaining the complexities of the ordinary processes of speech perception and the comprehension of ordinary conversations and texts.

We must look to ordinary experience, and to richer and more complex experimental studies that are consistent with ordinary experience, to appreciate the integration of the hierarchical layers of representational systems within our senses, our articulate bodily movements, and our linguistic capacities. In doing so, we discover that the integration of all these representational systems—especially in the ordinary human communications that involve language— is ubiquitous. There is so much evidence of the integration that it is only amazing that it is so commonly overlooked.

The McGurk Interactions

The common phrase—"the **McGurk effect**"—is applied to many different kinds of interactions. It is misleading precisely because there are many different McGurk effects that have been demonstrated by him and by other researchers. The interactions in question involve the integration of seeing speech movements and hearing speech sounds while also processing the meanings associated with one or both. Collectively, as we will show, the McGurk interactions reveal the depth and complexity of the integration of the sensory, sensory-motor, and sensory-motor-linguistic representations that are involved in ordinary language use.

As McGurk himself explained in 1988, the interactions he discovered were stumbled upon quite by accident. He and his co-worker, John MacDonald, had no idea that the interactions they would accidentally demonstrate actually existed. If anything, the McGurk interactions are more pervasive and more revealing than McGurk himself suggested in his 1988 lecture. (see S. D. Oller, J. W. Oller, Badon, & Arehole, 2006). In setting up an experiment with infants, Harry McGurk and his graduate student, John MacDonald, found interactions across representational systems that produced some remarkable illusions. Since the development of the theory of abstraction it has become possible to explain the illusions more completely and to predict some subtle relations between them revealing a hierarchy of interactions exactly as predicted by the theory of abstraction. The illusions were discovered through mismatching of video and audio recordings. The original experimental design was described by McGurk (1988) as follows:

> Babies were to be presented with video films of talking heads in which the voice would repeat the syllables /ba - ba/ or /ga - ga/; the speakers' lips would also repeat /ba - ba/ or /ga - ga/.

A crucial line of research showing the coordination of the senses with voluntary movements and also with speech and language has developed in part from the discovery of what we prefer to call the **McGurk interactions** ("The McGurk Interactions," 1998, retrieved February 25, 2009 at http://www.isca-speech.org/archive/avsp98/av98_003.html, and Maaso, 2002, retrieved February 25, 2009 at http://www.media.uio.no/personer/arntm/McGurk_english.html; also see the McGurk syllable effects on the DVD).

> . . . By means of dubbing techniques we produced four film sequences in total. In two of them, lips and voices were coordinated in perfect synchrony, ba-voice/ba-lips, ga-voice/ga-lips. The other two comprised the mismatching combinations, ba-voice/ga-lips and vice versa. (retrieved February 25, 2009 at http://www.isca-speech.org/archive/archive_papers/avsp 98/av98_003.pdf)

As McGurk later noted,

> When we viewed our carefully dubbed films for the first time we had the shock of our lives, for we heard sounds which we had never recorded!

"The McGurk Syllable Interactions" can be experienced in a demonstration video retrieved February 25, 2009 at http://www.isca-speech.org/archive/avsp98/av98_003.html. At that site, scroll down and click on the MPEG file labeled av98_003_1.mpg (7417 KB); or go to McGurk syllable effects on the DVD.

The odd discovery was that the listener who is looking at the moving image of the face saying, /ga ga/ while the audio recording is playing /ba ba/, actually hears something strange that seems to fall somewhat in between the two articulations. The listener, provided he or she is looking at the moving video image of the face, hears something like a strange sounding /da da/, or even /ga ga/ not /ba ba/ which is what is actually on the audio portion of the recording. If the viewer looks away from the moving video image while hearing the spoken syllables, it is easy to hear /ba ba/. But if the listener looks at the recorded video image while hearing the voice, it seems that the speaker is actually saying something more like /ga ga/ or /da da/ in spite of the fact that the audio actually recorded was the syllable sequence /ba ba/. To understand the McGurk interactions, and to become convinced that they actually occur, the reader will need to experience them.

You can see and hear the syllable effects with multiple articulations on the video portion although only the syllable /ba/ is audible if you attend just to the audio portion without watching the video. The other syllables you hear when watching the video and hearing the syllable /ba/ are all the products of the interaction of your senses of vision and hearing. The McGurk interactions demonstrate just how closely those systems are integrated. On the audio portion the speaker says /ba/ repeatedly while the video goes through a series of syllables including /ba/, /va/, /ða/ as in "thar she blows," /da/, /dʒa/ as in "jar," /ga/, and /ha/ and then back through this same list in the reverse direction.

Listeners regularly report hearing at least the syllables /ba/, /va/, /ða/, /da/, and /ga/, when in fact the only syllable actually recorded on the audio portion is /ba/ (also see Rosenblum, n.d., retrieved February 25, 2009 at http://www.faculty.ucr.edu/~rosenblu/VSMcGurk.html to see a different demonstration of the same kinds of McGurk syllable effects; also Rosenblum, Schmuckler, & J. A. Johnson, 1997).

What is more, the illusions do not seem to go away with practice. They remain no matter how many times we play the moving video images while listening to the conflicting audio recording at the same time. The results were first reported by McGurk and MacDonald in a paper appearing in *Nature* in 1976. Since then, they have generated a great deal of interest and many follow up studies. A Google search for the "McGurk effect" OR "McGurk illusion" on March 23, 2009 produced 55,400 hits. The original article published in *Nature*, according to a citation search on the Web of Knowledge for "McGurk, H" in the year 1976, showed 965 articles citing the original work. You can download McGurk's 1988 lecture, for a fee, with his own explanations for the interactions (retrieved February 25, 2009 at http://www.isca-speech.org/archive/archive_papers/avsp98/av98_003.pdf).

The Interactions in Early Infancy

Initially, McGurk set out to explore the development of **sensory integration** across the life span. He himself found no evidence of visual illusions in infants to match up with the kinds observed in adults. However, Aldridge, Stillman, and Bower (2001) found that newborn babies with English speaking mothers seem to know that the vowel in French "tu" (written phonetically as /y/ and sometimes spelled "ue" or "ü")—which these babies have never heard—requires rounding of the lips. This finding suggests an integration of the type shown in the McGurk illusions but occurring in early infancy.

The fact is that the vowel /y/ does not occur at all in English. So, how do infants exposed only to English know that the production of the /y/ sound, one they have never heard or seen produced, requires rounded lips? Infants reveal their expectation by preferring to look at a face saying /y/ with lip rounding rather than a face saying the same sound with flat lips as in producing the the vowel /i/ found in "heat." This has been demonstrated in experiments with noninvasive electronic devices that measure the interest of the babies based on where they are looking and whether or not they are sucking on a pacifier that records the sucking movements. Babies show more interest in the matching video and audio —as evidenced by more attention and more sucking—than in the mismatched instances.

How do the infants born to English speaking moms know that /y/ needs to be produced with rounded lips? The key problem is how such learning could take place in babies who have never been exposed to the articulatory movements involved in the production of /y/. These results and other findings with infants suggest that a high degree of integration between the senses, the sensory-motor systems, and the sensory-motor-linguistic systems must either occur before birth, or else very soon afterward.

What Aldridge and colleagues have found in newborns appears to be a McGurk interaction in early infancy. Their results suggest that the knowledge that certain facial gestures go with certain sounds must either be innate or it must somehow be learned very early.

LAYERS AND RANKS OF SENSES AND SENSORY INTEGRATION

Setting aside the structural systems of the body itself, which we have dealt with in Chapters 1 and 2, especially as they pertain to speech and language, the three primary representational systems used in human communication are found in ranked layers where motor systems integrate and enrich our sensory capabilities of representation and language integrates and enriches both of the prior layers. The integration of the senses with motor systems, and both of these kinds of systems with linguistic systems was suggested in the diagrams of Figures 1–3 and 1–8. The ranking of the distinct systems can be thought of as shown here—where the "less-than-symbol," "<," means that whatever systems are mentioned on the left of the sign "are outranked by" the ones mentioned to the right:

(1) sensory systems < (2) sensory-motor systems <
(3) sensory-motor-linguistic systems

Both the layering and the ranking are seen in the fact that the senses provide an essential basis for the building up of motor systems, but the integration of motor systems with the senses results in a higher level of representational ability. Likewise, the motor systems together with the senses provide the necessary basis for the building up of the linguistic systems. However, the integration of language into the representations from the sensory-motor systems greatly enriches our capacity to know about the past and the future and to explore the realms of imagination. The development of each higher system also greatly influences the way we process representations of the systems lower than that given level. The interactions across the three main systems are demonstrated nicely in the McGurk interactions.

The relations between the various systems are more complex than static diagrams can easily suggest. The interactions are dynamic and take place both within and between the different major representational systems of sensation, movement, language, and the subsystems of which each of the major systems consist. For instance, the subsystems of the senses are seeing, hearing, smelling, touching, and tasting, but each of these subordinated subsystems can be further subdivided into subsubsystems, and all of them are not only thoroughly integrated, but they are also ranked as in a layered hierarchy. With respect to speech perception and processing, visual perception of speech movements, as we will see in greater detail with respect to the McGurk syllable effects below, outranks the hearing of speech sounds. Also, though the interactions of the senses of touch, taste, and smell remain to be explored, there are well-demonstrated interactions within the subsystems of hearing showing not only intensive integration of the senses, but that there are subsystems of our sense of hearing that are also layered and ranked.

First we will deal with the ranking of the integrated systems of seeing, hearing, and movement, and then we will focus more specifically on the layering and ranking of subsystems within the sense of hearing in particular.

. . . the subsystems of the senses are seeing, hearing, smelling, touching, and tasting, but each of these subordinated subsystems can be further subdivided into subsubsystems, and all of them are not only thoroughly integrated, but they are also ranked as in a layered hierarchy.

Interactions Between Seeing and Hearing Syllables Spoken

Consider the systems of seeing and hearing as they are associated with the normal processing (production and perception) of spoken syllables such as /ba/ and /ga/. We can illustrate multiple levels of processing and complex interactions across the distinct senses involved. The McGurk syllable interactions show, for example, remarkable integration of seeing, hearing, and movement in the production and perception of speech. The interactions in question clearly involve the layering and ranking of our senses of seeing and hearing, our voluntary movements, and our comprehension and knowledge of language. Let's see how this is so.

Lip-Reading Is Shared by Hearing Persons

All normal (seeing) adults rely on the visual perception of the production of speech by others to such an extent that our hearing of spoken syllables is largely dominated by what we see people saying. This is demonstrated in the McGurk syllable interactions showing that seeing outranks hearing in the cases where the articulatory movements that we see conflict with the syllables that we hear. Although **lip-reading** before the discovery of the McGurk interactions was widely regarded as a phenomenon developed to compensate for hearing loss, the fact that the various McGurk illusions are nearly universal in people who are not deaf or hard of hearing shows that normal language users are lip-readers to a much greater extent than has commonly been realized.

The fact that seeing outranks hearing is implicit in the proverbial wisdom that "seeing is believing." We do not say, "Hearing is believing." We regard a video record as carrying probative weight about a series of events, such as the events of September 11, 2001 in New York. No one who saw the video of the collapsing buildings can reasonably deny that the events of that day really occurred (see a low resolution video collage of "September 11, 2001" retrieved February 25, 2009 at http://www.metacafe.com/watch/684526/september_11/). By visiting the site where the buildings used to stand we can confirm that they are no longer there. It is because a sequence of moving pictures produced by a well-designed camera is, literally, *by design*, faithful to display images that correspond to the events recorded by the camera. For this reason the sequence of events displayed in a moving video record is usually regarded as proof that the events actually occurred. When multiple records from different vantage points exist and can be compared, the empirical

The key to authenticity and validity is the agreement that can be demonstrated across distinct modalities of representation, viewpoints, and observers.

When John Forbes Nash (2002) experienced delusional voices, he was able, according to his own testimony in a PBS interview (see a video record retrieved February 25, 2009, from http://www.pbs.org/wgbh/amex/nash/sfeature/sf_nash_07.html), to recognize them as imagined *because there was no accompanying visual part.*

The McGurk syllable interactions show why the study of isolated, discrete pure tones must be augmented with a richer and deeper theoretical understanding of the integration of hearing with seeing and how both of those senses are dynamically connected through the meaningful movements involved in the use of speech and language.

evidence is overwhelming to the point that any reasonable doubt that the events actually occurred diminishes to a vanishing point. The sensory-motor evidence provided in multiple video records of the sequence of events is validated by consistency across multiple distinct representations. By contrast, when expected agreement is not being achieved, as the McGurk interactions demonstrate, we rely on the representational system of the higher rank.

His inventions of voices were not intentional or normal and would usually be recognized as imagined fictions if everything were working correctly. When someone invents stories deliberately but does not pretend or suppose that they are real we call the resulting representations *fictions*. These are very different from lies because fictions are not usually intended to deceive, only to test ideas (as in the sciences), or to entertain (as at the movies or in a novel), or to explore (as in thinking about a future trip or vacation). But when someone tells us about a sequence of events that seems unlikely or impossible, we do not say, "Would you tell me that again so I can believe it? We are much more apt to say, "Show me." When comedian Richard Pryor was supposedly caught in a compromising position, he produced the line, "Who are you going to believe, me or your lying eyes?" J. R. Ewing (played by Larry Hagman) used the same line with his wife in an episode of the ancient TV series *Dallas*. The absurd humor of suggesting that anyone would believe a lie that is contrary to what they are seeing shows that we are more apt to believe our eyes than someone's words. Why is that? The McGurk interactions show why it is that we believe our eyes more than our ears.

The Actions We See Speak Louder Than the Words We Hear

Consider the McGurk syllable illusions. Although the recorded voice is saying /ba/ when we see the tongue move between the teeth into the position for /ða/, we hear what we see. The hearing system by itself cannot normally override the visual system. In fact, the reverse occurs. We hear what we see and, the remarkable illusion is that we perceive what we hear as if it were consistent with what we see even though it is not. We do not, however, disregard what we are seeing in order to perceive what we hear. In fact, when there is a conflict between hearing and seeing, in normal perception, we hear the sounds we are seeing the speaker produce, and not the reverse. In the case of syllable production, seeing outranks hearing. The implications of this finding for the science of the hearing systems—the study known as audiology—are important. The McGurk syllable interactions show why the study of isolated, discrete pure tones must be augmented with a richer and deeper theoretical understanding of the integration of hearing with seeing and how both of those senses are dynamically connected through the meaningful movements involved in the use of speech and language.

> ### McGurk Interactions Generalize
>
> McGurk also took the trouble to show that the interactions at the syllable level generalize to sentences (retrieved February 25, 2009, from http://www.isca-speech.org/archive/avsp98/av98_003.html; scroll down to the MPEG file labeled av98_003_2.mpg (5494 KB) or play the McGurk sentence interactions on the DVD). McGurk demonstrated that a mismatched recording where the voice of the speaker is recorded while saying, "My bab [rhyming with 'dab'] pope me pu [rhyming with 'shoe'] brive [rhyming with 'drive']," but the video recording contains a visual record of the speaker articulating the sentence "My dad taught me to drive" (both said, in the video on the DVD, in English with a Scottish accent).

What we hear plainly is the sentence, "My dad taught me to drive." As with the syllable effects, the visible articulations prevail over the actual sounds recorded. However, as we will see, once meaning comes into play, everything else is subordinated to it. If the mismatch at the level of a meaningful sentence is reversed—so that the video portion contains the articulation of "My bab pope me pu brive"—the hearer still comes up with the perception that what was said and heard was the evidently intended form, "My dad taught me to drive." Before moving on to consider the overwhelming impact of meaning in more detail, it will be useful to explain why seeing normally takes precedence over hearing in the perception of meaningless syllables.

Four Reasons for the Primacy of Sight Over Sound

There are four reasons why seeing outranks hearing in speech perception. They are (1) physical—having to do with the material world, (2) perceptual—having to do with the way our senses work, (3) motoric—having to do with how we move and the bodily constraints on our movements, and (4) linguistic—having to do with the logic and structure of language systems.

The Physical Reason

The physical fact that light moves across distances a great deal faster than sound gives an advantage to seeing over hearing. At sea level sound can travel a little less than a quarter of a mile in a second, while light travels almost a million times farther in the same second. So we can often see events at a distance, such as lightning, when we will never hear the thunder that follows it because the sound will become inaudible before it covers the great distance that

There are four reasons why seeing outranks hearing in speech perception. They are (1) physical—having to do with the material world, (2) perceptual—having to do with the way our senses work, (3) motoric—having to do with how we move and the bodily constraints on our movements, and (4) linguistic—having to do with the logic and structure of language systems.

the light travels much faster than we can snap our fingers. Even when the lightning is nearby, we can usually see it well before we hear the thunder that follows.

The Perceptual Reason

Visual processing is faster than hearing. We cannot hear the sound of the syllable /ba/ until after it is produced. The sound of the syllable must reach our ears and register an impression there before we hear it. However, we can see the movement leading up to the first segment of the syllable before any sound is audible at all. Seeing is faster than hearing. We see the tongue protruding between the teeth, leading toward the production of /ða/, for example, before we hear the consonant /b/ on the syllable /ba/ from the recorded audio. As a result, we have already anticipated the consonant sound /ð/ based on seeing its articulation before the /b/ sound arrives at our ears to be processed. The illusion that we see and hear /ða/ when the audible syllable being produced by the voice is actually /ba/ can be explained in part by the difference in the time at which the seeing takes place as contrasted with the time of the hearing. By the time the hearing of /ba/ takes place we have already processed the syllable as /ða/.

The Motoric Reason

A third reason that we rely more on the visible articulation of /ða/ than on the later auditory impression that /ba/ makes when we hear the sound is that when we produce syllables ourselves, we know that putting the tongue between the teeth is preliminary to the production of the syllable /ða/ rather than /ba/. When we do this articulatory movement, we feel the articulation. That is, we touch our upper and lower teeth by protruding our tongue to produce the /ð/ consonant. We feel the movement and the touching of the soft tissue against the hard teeth. This kind of tactile impression is called **kinesthetic feedback** because it informs our motor system that our intention to move our tongue between our teeth has been carried out.

    The action of putting our tongue between our teeth to produce /ða/, for example, is a lot more complicated than we realize because we are not normally conscious of what our tongue is doing as it carries out our intentions as speakers of a language. As Chomsky (1965, p. 59) noted long ago, much of what we do with language occurs at a level that is out of reach of conscious thought. We do not normally think about the series of movements our tongue is making as we speak. If we had to move our **articulators** consciously to produce each movement involved in the stream of speech it would take a very long time to say anything. The movements of the tongue in producing a syllable are not normally

As Chomsky (1965, p. 59) noted long ago, much of what we do with language occurs at a level that is out of reach of conscious thought. We do not normally think about the series of movements our tongue is making as we speak.

consciously controlled. The habitual acquired movements of the articulators are somewhat automatic. Also, the knowledge of how those movement are produced is deeply integrated across the various systems that are involved in speaking and in understanding speech. Before we hear the sound of a syllable, even if we are producing it ourselves, the articulatory movement can be felt. For instance, we can feel the teeth with our tongue as we are producing the syllable /ða/ before we can hear its sound. The same is true of any syllable. As a result, articulation with its tactile information takes precedence over the resulting sound that can only be heard somewhat later, after the movement is executed. Consequently, seeing a movement that we also know how to produce gives that movement precedence over what we subsequently hear. The hearing is not only subordinated to the seeing, but also to the tactile, kinesthetic, impressions that result when we speak. So, our motor experience causes us to give more weight to what we see others saying than to what we hear them saying. Again, this reason favors seeing over hearing just as the McGurk syllable effects demonstrate to be the case.

The Linguistic Reason

In addition to all of the foregoing reasons, all of our linguistic experience teaches us that certain speech sounds are produced by certain articulatory movements and not the other way around. That is, on a strictly logical basis, we know articulatory movements produce the sounds of speech, not the reverse. Speech sounds do not cause the movements that produce them. Rather, the speech sounds are caused by the articulatory movements that produce them. These facts are universal and have to do with our understanding of what are called **transitive relations**. These relations are the kind where if A has a certain relation to B and B has that relation to C, then A must also have the same relation to C. As C. S. Peirce (1897) showed, transitive relations form the essential basis for all logical thought and reasoning.

J. W. Oller and L. Chen (2007) have demonstrated that scientific measurement and our understanding of the simplest sorts of temporal relations in experience utterly depends on our ability to note the difference between a sequence such as A, B, C, as contrasted with any other arrangement of the same series. Chronological organization of events, it turns out, is essential to our being able to distinguish any pair of events. Although in noticing that A begins before B, it is not essential to mark a particular boundary between them, it is essential to be able to distinguish, say, the center of event A from the center of B. To distinguish A from B the sequence is essential and to order them into a sequence such as A, B, C—where A precedes B and B precedes C—requires the ability to take account of transitivity and to notice that A begins before B

Speech sounds do not cause the movements that produce them. Rather, the speech sounds are caused by the articulatory movements that produce them. These facts are universal and have to do with our understanding of what are called **transitive relations**.

begins, and so on. Again, as with the discrimination of objects—as predicted in the theory of abstraction and demonstrated by Machnik (2007)—with events, we must notice boundaries of some sort. From the temporal association of transitively related causes and effects, we infer causation, where the beginning of the cause must precede the beginning of the effect. For instance, first we intend to swallow, and then we initiate the swallow. We intend to say "hello" before we say it, and so forth.

Meanwhile, articulatory movements have to take logical (linguistic) precedence over the sounds they produce on account of the universal fact that in ordinary experience speech sounds are produced by articulatory movements of the vocal folds, tongue, lips, and so on, rather than the reverse. From this simple fact—that is, because articulatory movements cause speech sounds rather than the reverse—uncountably many logical and perceptual consequences follow, for example, the main syllable level McGurk interactions. What is more important still is the fact that all of our higher reasoning functions, all mathematical reasoning, all logical inferences, all probabilistic reasoning, and, in fact, all valid knowledge depends on transitive relations of the kind just described in the previous paragraph (Peirce, 1897; Tarski, 1936/1956, 1944/1949).

Affirming the impression that we have heard what we think we heard with respect to the initial consonants in the McGurk syllable illusions, the presence of the vowel /a/ encourages us to believe that the articulation that we see is the one that we are also hearing because the vowel in each syllable actually is the one in /ba/ and is the vowel we see in the articulatory movements as well. In this case, seeing is both hearing and believing.

Summing up, all of the reasons for the occurrence of the McGurk syllable illusions involve the transitive relation contained in a temporal sequence of events: If A comes before B and B before C, it follows that A comes before C. Recall the reasons one by one for the precedence of seeing over hearing in the McGurk syllable effects.

Why We Experience the McGurk Interactions

There is the *physical reason* that light is faster than sound; the *sensory reason* that seeing is faster than hearing; the *motoric reason* that speaking logically precedes the hearing of speech; and the *linguistic reason* that the impressions of speech sounds are logically subordinate to their production regardless what any competing evidence might suggest. As a result of all these logical reasons—every one of them involving transitivity—the ranking, layeredness, and integration of our various systems of representation logically require the McGurk illusions as outcomes.

Otherwise, the expectation that lips and voice will agree in the sounds produced in speech would have to be overthrown and we would have to be able to *perceive* two distinct streams of speech simultaneously. But the McGurk effects show that we cannot actually do that anymore than we can *produce* two streams of speech simultaneously.

For all the foregoing reasons—all of which are contained logically in the linguistic reason—seeing outranks hearing in all of the McGurk syllable illusions. Similarly, the production of a sequence of movements, such as putting the tongue between the teeth in saying /ða/ or putting the lips together in saying /ba/ must precede and also outranks the auditory impressions that are created by these articulatory movements. In fact, our own voluntary movements along with the tactile and other sensations that those movements produce in us, must outrank (and thus make a stronger impression) than our perception of the movements of someone else. Also, experience teaches us to expect that the sounds we produce by making certain articulatory movements will be consistent with the movements that we make. For this reason, linguistically speaking, we do not expect any mismatches of the sort that are contrived in the experiments that have led to the discovery of the McGurk syllable illusions.

So, *on account of the dynamic interactions that have to take place because of the transitivity of the actual relations between the sensations and movements involved, mismatches are compensated for in the most logical possible way by giving precedence as we have just shown to the higher ranking or prior system in every case.* Therefore, the McGurk interactions are both predicted and explained by the ranking and layering of sign systems just as is predicted and also explained by the theory of abstraction per our prior published discussions.

MEANINGFUL REPRESENTATIONS

When we reach the level of processing that involves meaningful sequences of words that have **referential content**—that is, where things, persons, and events are referred to—such meaningful representations dominate all lower systems. For instance, in sentence level structures such as, "My dad taught me to drive," a powerful **cognitive momentum** is built up as soon as we begin to comprehend the meaning. We can hardly resist the tendency when we hear the opening phrase of the sentence, "My dad . . . " to imagine the SPEAKER'S FATHER and as we hear the rest of the sentence, "taught me to drive," we can easily imagine him teaching the speaker to drive. We may also be inclined to recall or imagine our own experiences in learning to drive. We may even imagine own father teaching us to drive whether or not that was the case.

When we reach the level of processing that involves meaningful sequences of words that have **referential content**—that is, where things, persons, and events are referred to—such meaningful representations dominate all lower systems.

We also tend to supply images that are not mentioned in any of the linguistic forms. We may think of the car we drove when we were learning or we may imagine the sort of car the speaker might have been in. Similarly, we suppose that the speaker has a father and that if his statement were true, or only an example sentence pulled from the blue sky by McGurk, that the speaker is imagining or remembering actually driving a car while sitting on the driver's side behind the wheel, with dad, or perhaps someone else, coaching, and so on.

Expectancy

In processing the sentence "My dad taught me to drive" initially, when we come to the verb "taught" we are already expecting that someone will be mentioned along with whatever was taught to that someone. We are not surprised when the speaker produces the sequence "me to drive" because these words are consistent with the underlying meaning that we have already understood. Associated with that meaning are our own memories and expectations about learning to drive, and so on. We do not give much further consideration to the sounds of the syllables in the surface forms of the speech after we have settled our minds on a coherent and unified understanding of the meaning we think was intended by the speaker.

> Once the underlying meaning is conceived—the **proposition** that the speaker's father taught that individual to drive—it generates so much cognitive momentum that it carries us to other associated meanings, memories, and inferences.

Once the underlying meaning is conceived—the **proposition** that the speaker's father taught that individual to drive—it generates so much cognitive momentum that it carries us to other associated meanings, memories, and inferences. As a result of that cognitive momentum, we not only cannot believe that we are actually hearing "My bab pope me pu brive," we have significant difficulty even perceiving that sequence in the first place. Even when we look away from the video and listen closely only to the recorded voice and not the video images, once we know the underlying proposition we still hear the coherent form of the sentence rather than the syllables that have actually been recorded in the audio portion. See how many times you must play the video (the <u>McGurk sentence interactions</u> on the DVD), before you are able to hear "pu brive" rather than "to drive." Try it. You will discover that "pu brive" continues to sound like "to drive" on account of the fact that you know implicitly that this is the speaker's intention. Thus, you expect to hear "to drive" and it is exceedingly difficult to shut down that expectation enough so that you can actually hear the sounds /p/ and /b/ as the initial elements in those syllables. But "pu brive" is what is actually recorded in the voice portion. The voice recorded on the audio portion says, "My bab pope me pu brive." It is only the video that contains the visible articulations of the sentence, "My dad taught me to drive."

As soon as meaning comes into play, our minds are drawn almost irresistibly to consider images of the car, the smell of it, the feel of the steering wheel in our hands, the sound of dad's voice, the sound of the engine, the feel of the road as we accelerate, the day we took our driving test, and so on. We tend to stop thinking about the surface forms of the syllables as soon as we settle on the meaning. We see the speaker in front of us saying this and we have little difficulty imagining him behind the wheel of a car with his dad sitting next to him. In fact, for Americans, even the strange Scottish accent fades into the background as soon as we access the deeper intended meaning. When the meaning comes into play, everything is suddenly about that guy in the video and his dad teaching him how to drive a car and it is difficult for us even to notice, or care much about, the surface forms of the syllables. We do not notice, for instance, that no car is ever mentioned, but we are not apt to suppose that the speaker is talking about a tank or a golf cart. We tend to settle very early on the most likely and most coherent interpretation for what we take to be a unified and coherent assertion.

Meaningful Content Dominates

Expectations concerning movements and the sensations that they normally produce are both subordinated to **linguistic expectations** that pertain to higher levels of coherent meaning. This is well illustrated in illusions and errors that depend obviously on expectancies that are grounded in meaning.

Keeping in mind that there is a vast research literature on linguistic expectancies of different kinds (for a review and summary, see J. W. Oller, L. Chen, Pan, & S. D. Oller, 2005), consider the following examples from McGurk (1988) regarding utterances dubbed onto video or film:

> . . . if the voice for "part" is dubbed on to the lip movements for "cart" then what is normally heard, when the dub is presented alone is "part" or "cart." However, the part/cart composite is dubbed into a sentence such as "The actor played the _____," then what is heard is "part." If the spoken sentence is "The baker baked the _____," then "tart" is heard. The same composite dubbed into the sentence "The horse pulled the _____," yields a heard "cart" . . . if the voice says "My dad taught me to drive" while the lips say "My bab pope me pu brive," then "My dad taught me to drive" is heard loud and clear.

He continues to offer the explanation that

> The two streams—auditory and visual—split apart and the auditory signal, which contains the meaning, is now given priority.

Just as motor expectations outrank sensory ones, linguistic expectations outrank them both.

But we would argue that there are actually at least four distinct streams at issue. There are the two sensory streams that he mentions—seeing and hearing—plus the listener's understanding of the stream of kinesthetic movements necessary to produce the visual and auditory streams, and then there is also the stream of abstract meanings which is not exactly contained in, but which governs the other three. For this reason, as McGurk (1988) points out, when the conflict of the demonstration sentence, "My bab pope me pu brive," is reversed so that the recorded voice actually says "My dad taught me to drive," but the visible movements correspond to "My bab pope me pu brive," the meaning prevails over the visual image. Even the evident movements of the speaker's mouth are trumped by the higher level of meaning. Whereas in the perception of meaningless syllables, if the video recording shows an articulatory movement that normally results in /ða/ rather than the syllable /ba/ (recorded on the audio portion), the video will override the audio because seeing and articulatory movements outrank hearing. However, when meaning comes into play, the video, audio, and evident movements are all overwhelmed by the meaning. It is for this reason that dubbing of foreign films is fairly successful even though the articulatory movements to produce the sound tract cannot perfectly match the visually recorded syllables of the original language of the film. We can say that the deeper level of meaning outranks the more superficial streams of surface forms in all instances. It outranks the stream of movements, the visual evidence of those movements, and, in case of conflicts, the actual auditory signal.

> . . . when meaning comes into play, the video, audio, and evident movements are all overwhelmed by the meaning.

CENTRAL AUDITORY PROCESSING DISORDERS

From all the foregoing it is clear that seeing, hearing, and speaking are logically integrated in interesting and complex ways. Our systems of representation are normally layered, ranked, and integrated. The case is no different with respect to making sense of sequences of sounds through **auditory processing**. We have also noted that each of the several main systems of representation—sensation, movement, and language—consists of multiple subsystems. Furthermore, just as the main systems of representation are layered and ranked with respect to their integration, the subsystems constituting the main representational systems are also deeply layered, ranked, and integrated, so are the subsystems of each of them.

In this section, we focus on the sense of hearing in particular. More specifically, we deal with a large class of hearing disorders that are loosely categorized under the heading of central auditory processing disorder (CAPD). Our point in focusing on the sense of hearing is two-fold: first, we do so because hearing is central in the production and perception of speech, and second, because the disorders under the umbrella of CAPD help to show that the hearing system—as we noted earlier—consists of a remarkably complex layered, ranked, and integrated system of systems. Some of them are subordinated to others, but all of them appear to be deeply integrated.

Diversity of CAPDs

When it comes to CAPDs, on account of their remarkable diversity, we believe it is best to speak in the plural. However, our readers should be warned that this is not common in texts, reports, or clinical work in speech-language pathology and audiology. Nevertheless, different varieties of CAPDs are not only theoretically possible but are well-documented in the research literature as we will show in the following sections. In fact, CAPDs were being discussed for about half century before any consensus was achieved concerning whether any such phenomena existed in reality, never mind just what they might consist of, or if and how they might be manifested (see ASHA, 1996; Chermak & Musiek, 1997, pp. 6-25).

We consider this particular class of disorders here because they illustrate clearly that representational systems in general, including especially the systems involved in hearing, are both more deeply layered and more richly integrated than has been realized up till now—even by specialists in linguistics and related fields of study. Hearing, like other representational systems, is actually a complex system of systems.

> . . . representational systems in general, including especially the systems involved in hearing, are both more deeply layered and more richly integrated than has been realized up till now—even by specialists in linguistics and related fields of study.

Hearing as a Systems of Systems

As Dennis Phillips puts it in the Foreword to Chermak and Musiek (1997), hearing is not just a matter of being able to detect sounds, rather "there are whole tiers of processing levels above that of sound detection" (p. x). For instance, when we hear a sound in the middle of the night, for example, we do not merely answer the question whether or not there was a sound, but we also are usually able to tell a great deal more. We commonly are able to tell whether the sound was produced by a branch scraping against the side of the house, a bird chirping in the night, a dog barking, a creaking floorboard on the stairway, a breaking window, a voice speaking softly, or a mere whisper, and so on. Current models of our sense of hearing hold that "multiple **serial, parallel,** and **distributed neural networks**" are involved (Chermak & Musiek, 1997, p. 5). Some aspects of the hearing process seem to work in a sequence where

The grand system of communication systems of which the sense of hearing is part, as we have seen with the McGurk interactions, is dominated by language and meaning.

event A occurs first, leading on to B, which in turn leads to C, and so on. This is what is meant by **serial processing**, which may also be called **linear processing**.

However, the hearing of speech is commonly accompanied by other sensations which may include the hearing of other sounds as well as a host of other sensations going on at the same time. As we drive down the road listening to the news on the radio, we also hear the blower of the air conditioner running in the background. We hear the cars whooshing past our own vehicle and the truck that is pulling up alongside of us. We hear and see the sprinkles of raindrops hitting the windshield. We hear the noise of the road outside, and the ring of the cell phone in the side pocket of the driver's door. We hear the conversation of our spouse who is talking on a cell phone in the seat next to us and we hear another conversation between the two teenagers in the back seat, and so on. In all of these cases, the appropriate term is **parallel processing**. When serial and parallel processes are integrated across time and in different regions of the nervous system (as if on multiple computers), the appropriate term is **distributed processing**. Our sense of hearing uses all of these kinds of processing systems and to a great extent it actually enables us to do all of these kinds of processing at the same time.

Multidirectional Processing

Because the neural systems of the body are layered and ranked from the brain downward and outward to the periphery of the body, it is appropriate for this reason to speak of **top-down processing**. This is especially appropriate when we think of speech perception where the influence of meaning comes into play—as in the perception of the sentence, "My dad taught me to drive" when either the audio or the video recording says, "My bab pope me pu brive." In such cases, our expectations based on prior experience and language acquisition shape what we perceive. The influence is from the brain downward and outward to the material world, so the metaphor of top-down processing is appropriate. The actual structure of the body itself also justifies the corresponding term, **bottom-up processing**, where the physical qualities of speech sounds, or manual signs, along with their rhythms and distinct qualities are emphasized. In bottom-up processing, which human beings presumably do to a considerable extent in handling sounds that are new to us and with which we have little or no experience, for example, as in learning a new language, we must also be able to start from the periphery and work upward to higher levels. Of course, it becomes obvious, if we think about it, that the top and bottom must be connected through the middle portion of whatever processing is going on. Therefore, we have argued that in addition to top-down and bottom-up processing we must also recognize the sort of processing that consists of working "both ends against the middle" and vice versa.

If we take account of the demonstrated McGurk interactions across senses and modalities of processing—for example, influences from sight to hearing, from articulatory gestures to hearing, and from propositional meanings to hearing—it is clear that a holistic, integrated conception of hearing is required. Although the layered, ranked, and integrated system of systems that make ordinary language acquisition and use possible are mind-bogglingly complicated, they work together to virtually guarantee successful communication in the vast majority of ordinary contexts.

An Indirect Definition of Central Auditory Processes

There is sound theory and research showing that **central auditory processes** involve "multiple sources of information" that "provide constraints and corrections to guide pattern identification and interpretation" in normal hearing (Chermak Musiek, 1997, p. 5). Some of the subsystems operate very differently from others—for example, pulsing sound waves travel through air to the outer ear but in the middle ear they are transformed into pressure changes in the fluid of the inner ear. From there onward there are many additional layers connecting the ears with the higher cortex. Because each of the successively deeper systems is higher in rank than the preceding one, there is no doubt that peripheral hearing disorders differ from more central hearing problems.

It is true that central auditory processing problems have sometimes been lumped together under the singular term CAPD, but it is now clear that there are distinct levels and kinds of CAPDs. The differences also illustrate the layeredness and ranking of distinct systems involved in our sense of hearing. Although all of the hearing subsystems together seem unified and relatively simple when everything is working as expected, things can go wrong at different levels and in a great variety of ways. No class of disorders that we know of illustrates the distinct layering and ranking of its integrated subsystems better than hearing does.

ASHA (1996) has described CAPDs by referring to "behavioral phenomena" involving difficulty in "sound **localization** and **lateralization**; **auditory discrimination**; **auditory pattern recognition**; temporal aspects of **audition** (hearing) including, **temporal resolution**, **temporal masking**, **temporal integration**, and **temporal ordering**; auditory performance with competing acoustic signals; and auditory performance with **degraded acoustic signals**" (p. 41). Let us take each of these "behavioral phenomena" in the order they are mentioned in the ASHA description and then we will proceed to show just how intensively the subsystems of the hearing sense are layered, ranked, and integrated.

ASHA (1996) has described CAPDs by referring to "behavioral phenomena" involving difficulty in "sound **localization** and **lateralization**; **auditory discrimination**; **auditory pattern recognition**; temporal aspects of **audition** (hearing) including, **temporal resolution**, **temporal masking**, **temporal integration**, and **temporal ordering**; auditory performance with competing acoustic signals; and auditory performance with **degraded acoustic signals**" (p. 41).

Localization and Lateralization

Localization and lateralization together have to do with our ability to tell whether a sound is near or far from us and from which direction it is coming to us. These are things we are normally able to do on account of the fact that we have two ears and that they have some distance between them. This design feature of the system is referred to as **binaural hearing**. Mainly because of the difference in intensity of a sound that is nearer to one ear than to the other, and to a much lesser extent because of the time lapse from when a sound that has already reached one ear gets to the other ear, we can normally tell roughly from which direction it has originated.

With respect to these binaural factors in hearing, oversimplifying the problem to a two dimensional plane, each ear provides a distinct point of reference to which any sound source provides a third point, as shown in Figure 4–3. With the three points given, the angles of the triangle, and the distance at the base (between the ears) provide the means for us to **triangulate** the approximate direction to the source of the sound (as shown in Figure 4–3) and, with lesser accuracy, its approximate distance from our location (Kubo et al., 1998).

Of course, other factors enter into the determination of the direction from which sounds arrive at our ears. One of these is the shape of the ear itself, especially the **pinna** (the outer ear), and to a lesser extent, the body parts that block and thus shape the sound wave that reaches our ears. In fact, our hearing systems actually do considerably more than Figure 4–3 suggests because we can triangulate in multiple planes simultaneously. We are best at judging direction to

. . . our hearing systems actually do considerably more than Figure 4–3 suggests because we can triangulate in multiple planes simultaneously.

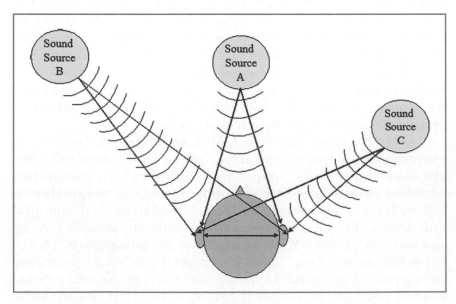

FIGURE 4–3. Localization and lateralization by triangulation of sound sources as a function of binaural hearing.

a sound in the horizontal plane, but we can also judge elevation in the vertical plane, and to a lesser extent the distance to the source of a sound within the sphere of space that the intersecting horizontal and vertical planes define.

Filters and Reflectors of Sound

In addition to the distinct **amplitude** and the timing of sounds arriving at the two ears, we also make use of the qualities of the sounds themselves as they are filtered by our own bodies and the physical shape of our ears. Soft tissues tend to absorb sounds and diminish or **damp** the sound waves by reducing their intensity. Hard tissues, such as bones and cartilage, by contrast, are fairly good transmitters and/or reflectors of sounds.

It is mainly because of **filtering effects** owed to the shape of our bodies and especially our ears that sounds emanating from a source behind us seem different to us than ones in front of us. Differences in loudness at the nearer ear as well as differences in the quality of the sound roughly enable us to tell the direction of sound sources in an unbounded sphere with the body of the hearer at its center. At any given moment the **sphere of reference** is defined relatively by whatever direction we happen to be facing and it matters very little whether we are lying down, standing, sitting, or in some other posture.

At any given moment the **sphere of reference** is defined relatively by whatever direction we happen to be facing and it matters very little whether we are lying down, standing, sitting, or in some other posture.

Auditory Discrimination and Auditory Pattern Recognition

The rattling of the small metal chain on the out-of-balance ceiling fan overhead sounds different from the clatter of the car keys that fall from the desk and strike the hardwood floor. If our hearing is functioning normally, not only will we be able to correctly tell the direction, elevation, and approximate distance of both sounds from our own bodily location, but we will also be able to distinguish the sound sources themselves to a high degree by the quality of the sounds produced. We can discriminate the sounds. We will not only notice them when they occur but we will also be able to tell them apart. This is more or less what is meant by *auditory discrimination*.

But often, we can go a step further. Without looking at the keys, just from the sound, we know what object has fallen and the kind of surface on which it has landed. The keys clattering on the floor sound very different from the small metal chain repeatedly striking the metal bell housing of the ceiling fan. When we recognize the two sounds as distinct from each other and we take the further step of correctly guessing what objects have produced the sounds in each

When sounds are associated with distinct objects in the ways described, we can say that they serve as natural symbols for distinct objects, movements, and relations in space and time. When viewed in this way, it turns out that hearing provides access to grammatical systems requiring highly complex sentences to describe only part of the information that they contain.

case, **auditory recognition** has occurred. This is the sort of process that is involved in our telling the difference between the ringing of the house phone as contrasted with the distinct ring of one of the several cell phones that may go off at any moment of the day or night. Auditory recognition may go so far as to identify the caller by a distinctive ring or melody. When sounds are associated with distinct objects in the ways described, we can say that they serve as natural symbols for distinct objects, movements, and relations in space and time. When viewed in this way, it turns out that hearing provides access to grammatical systems requiring highly complex sentences to describe only part of the information that they contain. For instance, consider the complexity of these descriptive sentences: *The keys get knocked off and fall to the left side of the desk where they clatter on the hardwood floor*, or, *The small short metal chain bouncing repeatedly against the housing of the ceiling fan becomes annoying until the person sitting at the desk gets up and turns off the ceiling fan*. These relatively simple descriptions are far less complex than the pragmatic mapping process they illustrate, and yet they serve to show that even the expression of relatively simple meanings calls into play multiple grammatical layers of sounds, words, phrases, and relations between them. Meanwhile, the relatively simple physical sounds themselves—the ones that are referred to in the complex forms of speech and language—also consist of complex fluctuating waves.

Spectral Properties of Speech Sounds

A simple sound wave can be thought of as something like the wave we see on the surface of a pond when we drop a pebble in it. The pebble causes a series of waves to emanate outward in a circle across the surface of the pond. The pebble exerts force on the water producing pressure that forces some of the water molecules downward, depending on the shape, size, and weight of the pebble as well as its velocity and the direction from which it strikes the surface of the water. Suppose the pebble is dropped more or less straight down into the middle of the pond. As it displaces some of the water molecules by its downward plunge, others are pushed upward and outward away from the source of the wave. The wave emanates outward as the molecules that have been forced upward and outward by the pebble's motion reach a limit of equilibrium between the upward momentum and the pull of gravity. When that happens, they begin to fall back toward their previous level as they continue to move outward from the point of impact of the pebble. As they fall they gain momentum, tend to overshoot their former level at the surface of the pond, and continue to fall until the momentum they gained in falling is compensated for by the upward push of the molecules seeking to fill the trough. At that point, the water begins to rise upward again, and so on. Eventually the force of friction and the loss of momentum reaches a limit of equilibrium again and the wave continues to spread outward in widening ripples. In a small pond the ripples of the wave will continue to the edge and some of them will bounce back toward the middle again until all of the energy of the wave is spent and the pond surface is still again. The energy that the falling pebble created is eventually absorbed and used up by the friction and heat of molecules bumping into and dragging on each other.

The time from the peak at which the wave reaches its greatest height to the trough where it reaches its lowest point is called the **period**, or the **frequency** of the wave. We express the number of cycles of a sound in **hertz** units, abbreviated as **Hz**. One cycle per second is one Hz unit, one thousand is a kilohertz (kHz), one million a megahertz (MHz), one billion a gigahertz (gHz), and so on.

Hertz's Unimportant Discovery

Today we measure sound waves, radio waves, and the speed of the central processors in our computers and in electronic devices, in terms of the Hz unit. The name comes from Heinrich Rudolf Hertz [1857–1894], the scientist and inventor who discovered and measured electromagnetic waves and showed that their velocity is equal to that of light. When he was asked about the importance of his discovery, he said, "Nothing, I guess . . . We just have these mysterious electromagnetic waves that we cannot see with the naked eye. But they are there" ("Heinrich Hertz," 1894/2009, retrieved February 25, 2009, from http://en.wikipedia.org/wiki/Heinrich_Hertz). He could not know at the time how important his discovery would be to the development of radar, radio, and essentially all forms of wireless communication in modern broadcasting, computing, and so on. Hertz only lived 37 years but his name is immortalized in the unit of measurement applied to wave cycles of all sorts.

Speech Production and Recognition

In speech production and recognition, much more is involved. We will have more to say about those processes, especially in Chapters 6 through 8, but here we need to note that when the sort of complex sound waves produced by the vibration of the human **vocal folds** are introduced into the cavities that consist of the throat, mouth, and nose, the qualities of the sounds that are produced are greatly affected by the shape of the cavities that the sound waves bounce around in and to some extent pass through. The shape of the cavities is dynamically affected by the movement of the articulators—especially the vocal folds, the tongue, the jaw, and the lips (see Figure 6–2 for a diagram). The sounds produced by the voice can

A speech sound is similar to a wave on a pond except that speech sounds made by the vibrations of the vocal folds are not simple waves at a single frequency.

normally be adjusted for other qualities such as loudness, openness or closure of passageways, and the **pitch** of the voice. Some of the sound waves are more or less completely filtered out as they strike soft tissues. During the production of a stream of speech, some sounds are produced by closing off the **vocal tract** completely, for example, in the production of the /p/ of *speech*. The flow of air and sound during that closure is largely or completely blocked. Other sounds, such as **vowels**, for instance, are passed through the tubes and cavities with high resonant energy—as in the vowel nucleus of the word *speech*. The reader can easily demonstrate the relative loudness of the vowel center as contrasted with the consonants at the beginning and end of the world by producing it out loud several times and listening carefully to the word while doing so.

Speech sounds consist of complexes of many waves across a broad spectrum of distinct frequencies. The strongest of those frequencies is what we hear as the pitch of the voice. It consists of the average length of time it takes for the vocal folds to close and open again. This approximated average time is called the **fundamental frequency** of the speaker's voice and is what we describe as a high or low pitched voice. Adult males, for instance, have lower pitched voices than females. In the case of speech sounds, the waves are propagated through variations in pressure caused by the vibrating vocal cords displacing molecules of air. The adult male vocal folds are typically longer and thicker and vibrate at a fundamental frequency that is typically lower than that for younger males and for females. For males, the fundamental pitch of speech is about 125 Hz whereas the female averages about 200 Hz. If our hearing is normal, we can hear sounds from about 20 Hz to 20,000 Hz. However, the range of frequencies that are prominently evident in speech, range from about 100 Hz to about 8000 Hz, and we can easily understand speech when the frequency range is chopped off below 300 Hz and above 3.4 kHz—as is still the case (at least at the time of this writing) in many currently available but antiquated phone systems (Jax & Vary, 2006). Research, however, shows that intelligibility and the naturalness of the speech transmission—as through a telephone —is improved if the range is extended from 50 Hz to 7 kHz.

The frequencies produced by both male and female voices in normal speech are smeared across a wide **spectrum** ranging from about 100 Hz to above 8000 Hz. As the complex waves within this broad spectrum pass through the throat, mouth, and nose, the waves move through the air flowing through the cavities and bounce around depending on their frequencies and the shape of the tubes and cavities the waves encounter. The energy with which a sound can continue to bounce around off the walls of a given cavity depends on the frequencies contained in the complex wave itself, the shape and dimensions of the cavity, and the relative hardness or softness of the walls of the cavities, tubes, and articulators that the wave form meets along the way. If the frequencies in the complex wave are compatible with the distance across the cavity and back, the cavity

> Speech sounds consist of complexes of many waves across a broad spectrum of distinct frequencies. The strongest of those frequencies is what we hear as the pitch of the voice.

is said to "resonate" at that frequency. By the same token, the collective reverberations of the sound within the cavity is called **resonance**. Of course, soft tissues absorb sound waves and hard ones reflect or echo them. When the length of the wave from peak to trough is an even divisor of the distance between the walls of the cavity the wave is passing through, the cavity will resonate at that frequency.

As a result, sounds of that wavelength—or an even a divisor or multiple of it—will retain their strength as they move through the vocal tract. Waves that are too long for the resonating cavity will tend to lose their energy while ones with a shorter wave length will reverberate and resonate creating the darker bands of sound energy, the formants, seen in the **spectrogram** of Figure 4–4. A spectrogram is a visual display of the **spectral properties** of a brief stream of speech. It shows how sound energy is distributed over a range of frequencies. In Figure 4–4 the range from approximately 0 kHz to 4 kHz is displayed. The word uttered is *spectrogram* as spoken by an adult user of the most common western variety of **General American English** (Ladefoged, 2001). (Click Spectrogram on the DVD to hear the recording of the word which is displayed visually in the spectrogram of Figure 4–4.)

The lighter or even blank areas in the spectrogram appear at bands of frequencies that are filtered out or silenced in the time segment displayed. The darker regions, by contrast, represent frequencies at which the cavities resonate during production of the word *spectrogram* as displayed above any given segment as indicated on the horizontal axis. Some frequencies are silenced by the shape of the cavities during the production of the sound segment.

Just as a tuning fork that produces a sound at a certain frequency (that is, wavelength) will also resonate at the same frequency if we strike another tuning fork nearby, the vocal cavities shape the sounds that come from the voice by causing some frequencies, or bands of frequencies known as **formants**, to resonate and others to be damped (weakened) or completely filtered out.

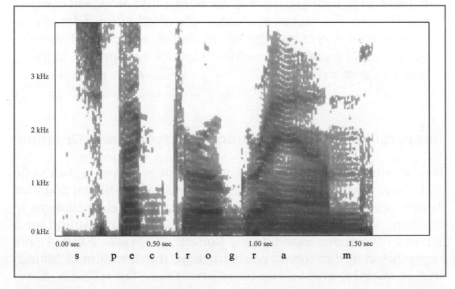

FIGURE 4–4. A spectrogram of the word spectrogram (the letters of the word appear near the center of the sound that each letter represents in the word as spoken and displayed).

Some frequencies are damped (weakened) by the soft tissues they encounter. Other frequencies resonate (bounce around repeatedly) in one or more cavities creating the dark bands of concentrated energy—the formants—that we see in the picture.

From Articulation to Hearing

Just as the tubes and cavities of the vocal tract shape the sound waves that pass through them, the sounds of speech are also shaped as they enter our ears. As we noted above in reference to Figure 4–3, because of filtering—damping and amplifying—effects, the sounds that reach our ears are differently shaped depending on which bands are affected and to what extent. A sound coming from our right side is more affected by the filtering effect of the head as it reaches the left ear than the corresponding sound that reaches the right ear without the damping effect of the head.

What We Know from the Voice
Also, just as the changing shapes of the vocal and nasal cavities cause changes in the spectral properties of speech sounds emanating from the human voice, the shape of the outer ear and the tubes leading into the middle ear change the spectral properties of the incoming sound depending in part on which direction the sound is coming from. As a result, filtering effects provide information about the relative elevation of a sound source in the vertical plane. They also supply much of our limited information about the distance to the source of a sound in addition to the nature of the vocal tract that produced it and much more. For instance, we can often tell the gender and approximate age of the speaker as well as a good deal about the general health and emotional state of the speaker at the time of utterance.

Temporal Resolution, Masking, Integration, and Ordering

Temporal resolution refers to the minimal time it takes for the auditory system to refresh itself in order to detect changes in incoming sounds, such as, the beginning or end of a sound, or a gap in a continuous sound (Gage, Roberts, & Hickok, 2006).

The "temporal" aspect of auditory processing, of course, has to do with time. *Temporal resolution* refers to the minimal time it takes for the auditory system to refresh itself in order to detect changes in incoming sounds, such as, the beginning or end of a sound, or a gap in a continuous sound (Gage, Roberts, & Hickok, 2006). Again, as predicted by the theory of abstraction, the detection of boundaries is crucial to ordinary auditory perception. The research shows that temporal resolution for a gap can be achieved by adults with normal hearing down to a rate of about two thousandths of a second. **Masking effects** with respect to hearing have to do with the way one sound, or a spectrum of sounds, can interfere with the perception of another. **Auditory integration** with respect to hearing concerns the way sounds reaching our different ears, or being processed by different subsystems within the body and brain, normally seem to produce a unified coherent sequence. The sounds are integrated and may seem to produce a coherent sequence even when bits and pieces of sound are coming from different sources and, in artificially controlled laboratory settings, are necessarily being processed independently by our two ears.

In the McGurk sentence effects, for instance, seeing and hearing seem to agree on the final interpretation of the signal, even when the visual and auditory signals are at odds with each other. We do not hear both /ba/ and /ða/ when the voice record is /ba/ and the video shows /ða/. Rather we hear only /ða/. The conflict is resolved in favor of the higher ranking system of representation in the case of the McGurk interactions. Similarly, with competing signals reaching both ears simultaneously, auditory integration often resolves them into a single coherent perception.

Discovering the Meaning

A signal that has missing parts is apt to be interpreted as if it were whole by a normally functioning auditory system. The integration at higher levels produces the illusion of wholeness even when the signal itself is not whole. This kind of integration is useful to us in noisy settings or in situations where the speech signal, for instance, is broken, intermittent, or distorted. Because of the integration performed at the higher level of meaning, we may still be able to figure out and perceive what was said.

On the other hand, if the interactions demonstrated by McGurk occurred willy nilly, without any logic, they could be detrimental. But conflicts of the sort that McGurk and experimentalists can produce in a laboratory setting are rare to nonexistent in ordinary experience. For instance, the syllable interactions demonstrated in McGurk type experiments, are logically impossible in ordinary settings. We cannot say /ba/, for instance, while actually shaping our articulators simultaneously to produce /ða/. Likewise, complex sound waves do not normally come to our separate ears in sharply differentiated bits and pieces. Therefore, the integration of our senses, and especially of our auditory systems normally enables us merely to speed up and enhance processing under conditions where noise or other competition would otherwise make comprehension difficult. Nevertheless, under experimental conditions, it is possible to demonstrate a remarkable depth and complexity of layering within the auditory systems in particular.

ABSTRACT MEANING, ANATOMY, AND PHYSIOLOGY

The sense of hearing, like our other senses, is affected by events both within and outside the body. Both kinds of events are important, but consider first the sorts of events that originate outside the body. As sound waves reach the outer ears, they begin at the periphery of the system and move toward the center. However, as we already saw with respect to the McGurk effects, what we hear is not merely a product of the surface forms of the sounds that reach our ears. Those sounds and their surface forms are important and real but do not necessarily or exclusively determine perceptual outcomes. The McGurk interactions could never be noticed at all if there were no audible difference, at the surface between, for instance, the syllables /ba/ and /ða/. But there is a difference, and that difference is accounted for by audible surface forms that make different impressions on our sense of hearing. The question is, how do they do this?

The Abstract Layer: Meaning

Interestingly, until the middle 1950s, when certain disorders in adults with CAPDs were first described in the research literature (Bocca, Calearo, & Cassinari, 1954; Bocca, Calearo, Cassinari, & Migliavacca, 1955), hearing was commonly described as if it mainly consisted of **signal detection**. That is, could the hearer/perceiver notice the presence or absence of a certain sound—say a faint tone or the dropping of a pin?

However, after Bocca and his colleagues described what Bocca himself would later refer to as **cortical deafness** in 1958, the stage was set for a series of important advances that would show unmistakably that the human hearing system seems to be directed toward abstract linguistic meanings. In instances of what Bocca called "cortical deafness," it was evident that the detection of sounds could sometimes be intact, and yet the individual could not make sense of coherent speech. After showing that CAPDs occur in adults, it took another two decades before it was confirmed that they also occur in children. The diagnosis remains controversial in part because of comorbidity with other disorders per our discussion in Chapter 1—especially neurological disorders of the type discussed especially in Chapter 10. Hearing disorders tend to be accompanied by other problems and vice versa.

It is unsurprising, therefore, that more than a little controversy centers around the extent to which CAPDs are distinct from ADHD, autism, dementias, and neurological disorders that impact the comprehension of language (W. D. Keller, 1992; Tillery, 1998). However,

On account of the interrelatedness of sensory systems, their connection and integration with motor systems, and the necessary linking of all such systems with higher cognitive functions (especially language), it is highly likely in affected individuals that CAPDs will be accompanied by other communication disorders such as, **attention deficit disorders** with or without **hyperactivity (ADD/ADHD),** not to mention any one of the many other types of disorders discussed in Chapters 5 through 10.

as Keller points out, there is no longer any reasonable doubt about the existence of CAPDs in spite of the fact that they are commonly comorbid with other conditions, some of which are not strictly auditory problems. Among the symptoms that suggest CAPDs are difficulty understanding conversation in a noisy environment, inability to process complex directions, or trouble learning or recalling new words or names. In CAPDs, there may be little or no difficulty in detecting sounds, or even recognizing isolated bits of speech in certain laboratory contexts, but in ordinary discourse situations CAPDs may significantly interfere with comprehension.

Language Acquisition and Speech Processing

Most of the sound vibrations that reach our ears, especially in speech processing, are the result of waves that travel through air in somewhat the way a wave travels in liquid. For this reason, Ray Kent (1992) suggested that auditory processing is like "words written on water" (p. 93).

Sound Transformations

A simplified view of "How the Ear Works," can be seen in a video (retrieved February 25, 2009, from http://www.youtube.com /watch?v=skXQ6Pulc4s) for persons considering a **cochlear implant**. Just how such an implant works is explained in another video, "Cochlear Implant," retrieved February 25, 2009, from http://www.youtube.com/watch?v=SmNpP2fr57A).

It involves an electronic system for stimulating the sensory nerve endings in the inner ear. It is true that the main source of information that enables us to hear speech consists of the sound waves that travel through the air outside the body and that produce vibrations in the eardrum (Figure 4–5). However, the process is considerably more complex than the simplified models suggest. We also hear our own speech especially through vibrations that are internal to our bodies and that travel to our ears mainly through our bones. The bones are better conductors than other body tissues on account of their rigidity. Because speech and language are by far the most important elements that can be affected by communication disorders, it is important to keep in mind that it is mainly the processing of speech signals that is the central concern of audiologists.

In addition to the pressure waves that move through the air and the bone conduction that we detect in our sense of hearing, speech perception is always supplemented by direct or indirect knowledge of or inferences concerning the movements of the body of the person producing the speech. This is true even when the

Because speech and language are by far the most important elements that can be affected by communication disorders, it is important to keep in mind that it is mainly the processing of speech signals that is the central concern of audiologists.

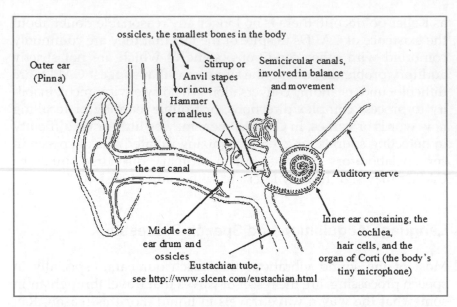

FIGURE 4–5. The peripheral hearing system leading up to the auditory nerve.

speech is only presented to the hearer in an audible recording, or on a telephone without any accompanying video, or in a foreign language. The visual and tactile elements of speech perception still come into play because anyone capable of understanding discourse relies not only on hearing but on acquired knowledge of the articulatory movements necessary to produce the stream of speech. This is still true when the listener is not producing the speech. In addition to knowledge of articulatory movements, there is a great deal more information about abstract concepts and the inferential relations between them which are accessible only through the acquisition of a particular language. All of that sort of knowledge comes into play in ordinary discourse contexts.

Articulatory Movements in Auditory Processing

When the hearer is monitoring his or her own speech while producing it, the importance of articulatory movements and their interaction with hearing is at an upper limit. However, when someone else is speaking, we refer to their body movements to a considerable extent, increasingly so in noisy conditions. All normal sighted listeners, as the McGurk interactions demonstrate, are lipreaders.

Whenever we are really able to understand a stream of speech in a particular language, we can also repeat it with a high degree of accuracy. To do this with a complex and fluent sequence of syllables, words, phrases, or sentences—ones produced at a normal conversational rate in a natural language spoken or manually signed—requires that we must also *know the language in question* (R. Yan & J. W. Oller, 2007).

The ordinary perception and comprehension of speech are deeply affected by our knowledge of how to produce the speech forms that we are perceiving and/or comprehending.

We cannot, contrary to certain claims made by T. Campbell, Dollaghan, Needleman, and Janosky (1997)—and many of their followers—repeat a fluent stream of speech in a language with which we have no experience. A person who has not acquired ASL cannot reproduce a rapid sequence of manual signs anymore than a person who does not know Russian can reproduce a substantial conversational stream of Russian speech. To do that the speaker must know the language in question—ASL or Russian. The point that ordinary perception of speech and language depends greatly on prior language acquisition has been commonly denied by the users of certain language assessment methods recommended by T. Campbell et al. (1997; but see R. Yan & J. W. Oller, 2007).

Yet, the fact that comprehending the meaning underlying fluent speech is essential to being able to reproduce it faithfully either in speech or in writing has been common knowledge in the field of language testing since the 1960s. In fact, it was noted even before 1912 by Ferdinand de Saussure [1857–1913] ("Ferdinand de Saussure" retrieved February 25, 2009, from http://en.wikipedia.org/wiki/Ferdinand_de_Saussure). De Saussure, who is regarded by many as the founder of modern linguistics, explained that speech is a continuous ribbon without distinct boundaries between its segments. To discover the boundaries between the subunits of speech it is essential to call in meanings. Saussure's claim has been tested with dictation (Valette, 1967) and with **elicited imitation** (Baratz, 1969), among other ways, and it is correct. It has been demonstrated many times over that repeating or writing bursts of fluent speech presented at a conversational rate can hardly be done at all by individuals who have not yet acquired the language in question. They can no more write it correctly or repeat it fluently than they can paraphrase it without understanding it. Language testing research has shown conclusively that no one can write intelligibly—from dictation—or repeat intelligibly—in an elicited imitation task—a sequence as brief as seven to ten words presented at a conversational rate in a language that they do not know at all. It is not just difficult to do so, it is right next to impossible. It is critical to keep this in mind when discussing the sense of hearing and its disorders.

The research shows that the ordinary perception of speech and language, through our sense of hearing, like the visual perception of manual signs, depends greatly on prior language acquisition. This point can hardly be overemphasized though it has *never, to our knowledge, been mentioned before in a text about communication disorders.*

THE DYNAMIC ANATOMY OF HEARING

At the lowest rank of the systems involved in our sense of hearing, various qualities of complex sound waves are analyzed and translated first from mechanical energy consisting of pressure fluctuations in the air into an analogous mechanical energy consisting of pressure fluctuations in the liquid that fills the inner ear.

Outer, Middle, and Inner Ear

The physical transformation from sound pressure levels to electro-chemical energy involves a series of changes between the outer, middle, and inner ear (see Figure 4–5). As the ear drum moves in response to changes in air pressure, it also moves the tiny bones of the middle ear which translate the pressure waves from air to pressure waves in the fluid contained inside the inner ear. The waves in the fluid travel through and up the spiral shaped cochlea of the inner ear.

You can see a computer simulation of this process (Givelberg & Bunn, n.d., retrieved February 25, 2009, from <u>http://pcbunn.cacr.c altech.edu/Cochlea/default.htm</u>; or to see the same demonstration click on <u>Cochlea</u> on the DVD). The analysis that subsequently takes place translates the frequency of the waves reaching the inner ear. It assesses how fast the waves are vibrating, their amplitude, how much energy or force they contain, when any given wave begins and ends, and whether at any given moment the wave is continuing or repeating.

The analysis of sounds within the cochlea involves the incredibly complex structure inside it, which is called the **organ of Corti**. It was named after the Italian Alfonso Corti [1822–1876] who was the first anatomist to stain and view some of the relevant systems under a microscope. Figure 4–6 shows what the cochlea looks like in three dimensions when it is magnified to about 60 times its

The analysis of sounds within the cochlea involves the incredibly complex structure inside it, which is called the **organ of Corti**.

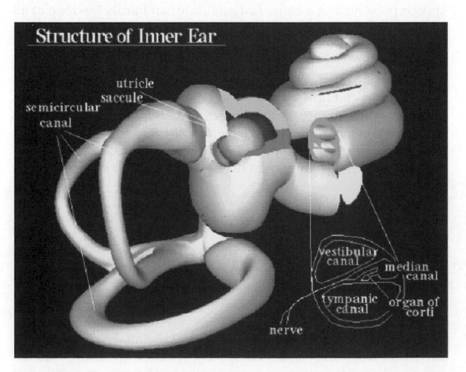

FIGURE 4–6. The semicircular canals and the cochlea of the inner ear. Retrieved February 25, 2009, from <u>http://pcbunn.cacr.caltech.edu/Cochlea/default.htm</u>. Reprinted with permission. All rights reserved.

actual volume. The figure also shows what a cross-section of the spiral coil looks like on the inside. The cochlea is connected to the semicircular canals of the **vestibular system**. They are critical to our maintaining our balance and being able to tell the orientation of our body, for instance, when we are lying down or standing up.

If we examine the cross-cut of the cochlea in the lower right corner of Figure 4–6, we discover that it is a tube containing three main smaller tubes within it. The top tube is called the **vestibular canal**, the bottom one, the **tympanic canal**, and the middle one, the **median canal**. Next to the median canal, running through the center of the cochlea, throughout its extent, is the tiny structure called the organ of Corti. It is within this tiny but richly structured tubule that much of the work of hearing is accomplished. As we have already stressed in connection with other systems of representation, the organ of Corti also is a system of systems that are tightly integrated. They are connected not only to the sense of hearing, but also to the motor system, especially balance, and to higher cognitive functions. When the fluid waves move through the cochlea, the organ of Corti is critically involved in the transformation of the energy of those waves yet again, this time, into neural (electrical) impulses.

Neural Activity and Hearing

If we magnify that tiny tubular component that is called the organ of Corti to make it about 1,000 times larger than it actually is, the cross-section can be diagramed as shown in Figure 4–7. The transformation of wave energy into neural impulses critically involves

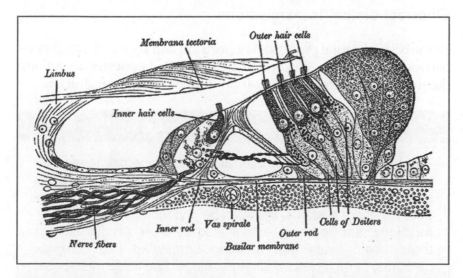

FIGURE 4–7. The remarkable structure of the organ of Corti within the cochlea. From H. Gray, 1918, *Anatomy of the Human Body* (Illustration 931). Philadelphia, PA: Lea & Febiger. Copyright © 2000 by Bartleby.com, ON-LINE ED., Inc. at http://www.bartleby.com/107/. Retrieved February 25, 2009, from http://www.bartleby.com/107/illus931.html . Reprinted with permission. All rights reserved.

Each of the outer cells function like a miniature microphone/amplifier reproducing sounds from impulses that can originate either in inner hair cells or from deeper within the brain.

the tiny "hair" cells (cilia) within the organ of Corti. There are two classes of hair cells distinguished by their positions within cochlea and by their functions. Those that fall toward the center of the cochlea are the **inner hair cells**, and those outside the midline (to the right side of Figure 4–7), the **outer hair cells**. Research shows that the outer hair cells, which are about three times more numerous than the inner ones, come under control of efferent (motor) input from the central nervous system. Evidently this efferent (motor) control within the organ of Corti is involved in making some aspects of sounds more prominent while other aspects are diminished. It is estimated that there are about 3,500 inner hair cells within the human cochlea and about 12,000 outer ones ("Hair Cells," 2009, retrieved February 25, 2009, from http://www.uni-tuebinge n.de/uni/khh/glossary.htm). Just how this process works is still under investigation (Markin & Hudspeth, 1995), but the power of sound waves that reach the organ of Corti can be greatly amplified, by as much as a factor of 100 times the strength of the sound at the periphery, by the action of the outer hair cells (Chadwick, 1998; Santos-Sacchi, 2003). It certainly appears that the sound processing that occurs in the inner ear itself is coming under the control of deeper cortical elements. We hypothesize that the capacity of the outer hair cells to amplify or diminish the level of certain sounds or aspects of them must come under the control of the language capacity. We will have more to say about that later in the discussion of sounds that the ear itself produces and which can be recorded and measured from the outer ear (see the section below entitled "Hearing Involves Motor Signals").

Electrochemical Transmissions

At the basis of neural processes are electrical and chemical interactions between cells. Nerve cells, which are also called **neurons**, are among the most basic systems of sensation, movement, and cognition.

Neurons and Synapses

The human brain is estimated to contain approximately 100 billion neurons and 100 trillion connections between them known as **synapses**. Although neurons come in a considerable variety of systems, they can be divided according to their functions, and to some extent also by their structures, into three basic kinds that function somewhat like complex switches, or multiplex switching stations. The three most basic functions, which also define the three types of neurons, are: (1) to sense stimuli either outside or inside the body and to communicate information about those stimuli to other neurons leading toward the central nervous system is the function of the *efferent* or *sensory neurons*; (2) to issue commands for movement of organs and muscles from the more central nervous system toward the periphery is the function of the *afferent* or *motor neurons*; and (3) to communicate information to and from sensory and motor neurons and with each other neurons throughout the brain and spinal column is the function of the *association* or *interneurons*.

It used to be standard doctrine that the switch inside any given neuron must be either on or off (Ramón y Cajal, 1933), but it is now known that the systems contained within single neurons are vastly more complex than this (Bullock et al., 2005) and there is no reason to suppose that we have gotten to the bottom of the systems yet. In keeping with the hierarchical model proposed in Chapter 1, it is interesting that *by far the majority of the connections within the neuronal structures of the nervous system are of type 3, that is, they consist of interneurons that integrate and connect distinct layers within the central nervous system.* It is in this third domain that the glial cells are also found. All of the distinct kinds of neurons consist of a cell body with fibers extending out from it. Ultimately the fibers at the periphery are linked either to sensors or to motor neurons but the vast majority of connective fibers in the central nervous system are interneurons linking various parts of the brain with each other and connecting both sensory and motor neurons to each other and to the spinal cord and brain.

Although neurons are known to be primary sources of electrical impulses connecting the central nervous system with the periphery, the brain also contains about 10 times as many glial cells as neurons. The glial cells, discovered in 1891 by Ramón y Cajal (see Bentivoglio, 1998, retrieved February 25, 2009, from http://nobe lprize.org/nobel_prizes/medicine/articles/cajal/index.html), help to nourish and maintain neurons and to clean up damaged and dead ones. In addition, recent research shows that glial cells are also involved in communication between cells and in their electrochemical activities in transmitting information through synapses with other nerve cells (Martineau, Baux, & Mothet, 2006). We also know that biochemical processes at the level of individual molecules are critically involved in setting up neural transmissions and in communicating information across cells.

> The exceedingly numerous glial cells are much more involved in propagating and diminishing neural transmissions than previously thought.

DISTINCT MEANING RELATED PHYSIOLOGICAL FUNCTIONS

Within the afferent nerves of the auditory system several distinct physiological functions have been identified. These functions correspond well to the kinds of information that the hearing system provides to the hearer as described above in earlier sections dealing with the descriptive phrases applied by ASHA to characterize CAPDs. Some cells start firing when a sound begins and continue as long as the sound continues. Other cells turn on and off repeatedly while the sound continues. Still others fire only at the beginning of the sound or only when it stops. Auditory nerve cells tend to fire at an increasing rate, up to a maximum limit as sound amplitude increases through the threshold above which damage to the system will occur.

Perceptual Vigilance and Defense

There is also independent evidence from research on perception of meaningful speech showing that central processing affects how well we hear at the periphery. This is particularly true when speech and language are involved.

> ### The Cortex Is Involved
>
> Two of the relevant phenomena that show involvement of the central nervous system, and especially the role of higher brain processes in perception, are **perceptual vigilance**, a tendency, for instance, to pick out your own name or that of a loved one from a conversation where perhaps nothing else is understood, and **perceptual defense**, the opposite tendency, to be *un*able to understand certain offensive words or meanings in a setting or conversation where just about everything else is easy to grasp (Borgeat, David, Saucier, & Dumont, 1994; Borgeat, Sauvageau, David, & Saucier, 1997; Erdelyi, 1974, 2004; Poloni, Riquier, Zimmermann, & Borgeat, 2003; Stip, Lecours, Chertkow, Elie, & O'Connor, 1994; York, 2005; York, Rabinowitz, Burdick, Coffey, & Tongul, 1996).

One theory that has been proposed to explain the foregoing phenomena without any necessary appeal to higher cognitive processing, or to the emotions that might amplify or diminish our response to a stimulus, and one that has not been decisively ruled out, is what may be called the **simple frequency theory**. It is the idea that words and phrases (or other stimuli) that occur more often, that is, with higher frequency, such as our own names, naturally become easier to process while ones of lower frequency, such as offensive words and meanings, are harder to process (Howes & Solomon, 1951). However, even if frequency were the only factor at work, and we do not believe that it is, it would still show that central processing—repeated experience with certain auditory patterns—results in more efficient processing at the periphery while less frequent experience makes processing more difficult. The per-

There is independent evidence from research on perception of meaningful speech showing that central processing affects how well we hear at the periphery.

ceptual vigilance for our own name, for instance, seems to be well accounted for by the simple frequency theory.

However, with perceptual defense, for example, in response to unpleasant words, or other stimuli which may be uncommon and unfamiliar to us, the simple frequency theory seems not to account for the whole story. It totally neglects the role of emotions and is not consistent with the fact that negative emotions associated with unfamiliar stimuli, for example, in cases of **anxiety disorders** and **post-traumatic stress syndrome** in combat veterans, can evidently influence the perceptual impact of unfamiliar material as much as it does unpleasant material that is familiar (Bermpohl et al., 2006; Hendler et al., 2003). Although, frequency of presentation obviously does play a significant role in perception as well as production, especially of speech material (Norris, 2006), emotional factors also must be taken into consideration to account for vigilance and defense toward verbal stimuli.

Subliminal Messages

At any rate, frequency of occurrence stimuli cannot explain the whole picture especially when it comes to abstract meanings. It is clear that high level meaning processes can augment or diminish certain aspects of peripheral processing (see Erdelyi, 1974; Maier et al., 2005). What is more, as we have seen in the McGurk interactions, perceptual effects from deep levels of meaning and processing can occur at the periphery without any conscious intention or even awareness on the part of the perceiver. With clear evidence already in hand from multiple sources and different angles of view showing that high level meanings of which we are only vaguely aware can influence peripheral processes of perception—for example, in perceptual vigilance and defense—it makes sense to wonder to what extent subconscious influences cannot also flow in the other direction. Can undetected stimuli influence our thoughts, beliefs, and actions?

In other words, is it possible for **subliminal messages**—ones that are too subtle, too quickly presented, or too faint to perceive or notice consciously—to shape our beliefs and actions? Can subliminal advertising actually work? Can it influence later perceptions, attitudes, or even beliefs and behaviors? For instance, can a message that is presented too quickly to be consciously noticed—for example, that smoking is glamorous or that drinking coca cola will make a person happier and more successful in life—cause people to smoke or drink coke?

The old controversy over subliminal messages, especially those supposedly used in advertising at movie theaters, heated up in the 1950s immediately following what was called "the Korean War." Terms like "brainwashing" and the threat that "mind-control" techniques would be abused by unscrupulous persons enhanced the widespread public fascination with subliminal messages. In

Although frequency of presentation obviously does play a significant role in perception as well as production, especially of speech material (Norris, 2006), emotional factors also must be taken into consideration to account for vigilance and defense toward verbal stimuli.

recent years the interest is still fueled by films such as *Rescue Dawn*. The story was loosely based on the true life escape of a German volunteer who flew a war plane for America but was shot down and became a prisoner of war in Laos. He escaped from there in 1966 (see the trailer of *Rescue Dawn*, retrieved February 25, 2009, from http://www.rescuedawnthetruth.com/). Before escaping, he was subjected to torture and mind control techniques by his captors.

Partly because of such war stories, and partly because of subliminal messages supposedly used in advertising, the question remains whether any such techniques can actually cause us to think or act in a certain way. The ancient controversy can be dated at least as far back as Dunlap (1900) who claimed to influence certain perceptions—sensory illusions in particular—with shadows that were too faint to consciously notice. The debate was rejuvenated a century later by Pratkanis and Aronson (1992, 2001)—who insisted that messages too faint to be consciously perceived could have no impact on the mind or actions. It is an understatement to say that there is a vast literature concerning the controversy and the basic question underlying it: do subliminal messages influence perception? The most popular example from the middle of the 20th century was the well-known, but poorly researched claim that people bought more coke and popcorn at the movies when subliminal (imperceptible) messages such as, "Buy popcorn!" or "Drink coke!" were flashed on the screen. The messages, or the images of popcorn and bubbly cola, were interspersed in the moving images of the film at rates so fast they could not consciously be noticed and perceived by viewers. Viewers were unaware that any additional messages—ads for popcorn and coke—were flashing in between the 24 to 30 frames per second of the movie they were watching.

Subliminal Influences Do Occur

The idea that subliminal messages could have any influence at all was pooh-poohed by many psychologists, advertisers, and marketing specialists, including Pratkanis and Aronson (1992) themselves. But the widespread interest of the public and certain researchers in the question did not go away. Recently, Haynes and Rees (2005) revisited the possibility of subliminal messages in a study of the visual cortex using **functional Magnetic Resonance Imaging (fMRI)**. Interestingly, when they found "feature-selective processing in [the] human cortex, even for invisible stimuli" (p. 686), the role of at least some kinds of subliminal messages seemed to be vindicated once for all.

Although Pratkanis and Aronson had reviewed more than 200 studies supposedly failing to replicate positive results concerning behavior changes related to subliminal messages, the results of

Haynes and Rees refute the strong claim that subliminal messages cannot influence perceptions. It appears to be the case that some aspects of subliminal messages—ones that cannot be consciously noticed or perceived—do register in the cortex and thus can influence subsequent perceptions. Because there is no doubt that perceptions can influence actions and vice versa, as shown in the vast literature on the McGurk interactions, the argument seems in the end seems to have gone against the skeptics. There is no doubt that there are pervasive interactions between the higher processes of expressing and interpreting meanings in speech and language and the peripheral processes of perception.

The whole discussion about subliminal messages has led to a subtle distinction between attention and awareness. Attention seems to be about what we do intentionally and willfully with our minds, while awareness involves features and connections between things over which we have no conscious control. When we notice that a sharp edge on something is similar to a straight line somewhere else, or when a certain association between meanings occurs to us, it probably has little or nothing to do with our will or conscious effort. However, when we stop listening to one conversation and turn to another, or go back to reading our book, we exercise the freedom of our will. It is interesting that this subtle difference is clearly brought out in a study by Kanai, Tsuchiya, and Verstraten (2006) in response in part to the ongoing debate about whether or not subliminal messages, invisible things that are there but not noticed, can influence our judgments.

Such messages, it seems, certainly can be registered without conscious attention or noticing, but the question still remains whether and to what extent they can influence our actions. Probably they do, but recognition of particular objects and conscious awareness of them, in keeping with our theory of abstraction (see J. W. Oller, S. D. Oller, & Badon, 2006; also Machnik, 2007), requires the noticing of edges if we are to attend to them. In simple language, attending to an icon of any object or sign requires us to find its boundaries. However, features of things we do not consciously notice, it seems, can measurably influence our thoughts, per the findings of Haynes and Rees (2005) without our noticing them consciously. Incidentally, according to the Institute for Scientific Information Web of Knowledge, as of February 25, 2009, the work of Haynes and Rees has been cited in publications by other researchers 96 times since its publication in 2005. Their findings have also persuaded other researchers and theoreticians (see Del Cul, Baillet, & Dehaene, 2007; Sarrazin, Cleeremans, & Haggard, 2008).

We do not have to attend to the icy Coke that someone else is drinking for it to influence us, presumably, to want one when the occasion arises.

Hearing and the Cortex

What all of the foregoing shows is that the sound waves of speech that begin as dynamic mechanical energy moving through air and bone are translated into electrical and chemical signals. The transformed signals move through a highly layered, ranked, and integrated system of systems leading both to *and from* the **cortex**. A great deal of what is now known about the subsystems of our sense of hearing comes from studying the actual connections between distinct structures in the brain that are known to enable us to hear as we do and to make sense of sounds. The connecting nerve fibers, and bundles of these, can be regarded somewhat as if they were highly intelligent electrical wires containing sensors and switching mechanisms of various kinds. The auditory nerve is estimated to contain about 30 to 40 thousand of these fibers (Auditory Nerve, n.d., retrieved February 25, 2009, from http://www.uni-tuebinge n.de/uni/khh/glossary.htm).

The **afferent nerve fibers** carry information from the periphery deeper into the **central nervous system** and upward to the higher processing centers of the cortex, whereas **efferent nerve fibers** carry impulses from the more central systems outward and downward from the brain to the periphery. The central nervous system consists of three parts—the brain itself, the **brain stem** contained within it, and the **spinal cord** which connects the brain stem to the rest of the body. J. Katz, Stecker, and Henderson (1992) say that central auditory processing is "*what we do* with *what we hear* [our italics]" (p. 5). So far we have only considered the first few steps, leading to the most superficial aspects of *what we hear*. It turns out that even *what we hear* at the periphery is largely subject to control from more central processes. We have already seen and explained evidence of central influence over *what we hear* in the McGurk interactions. But the control goes further.

Motor Signals in the Ear

It is surprising to discover that the hearing system is richly supplied not only with afferent (sensory) fibers leading from the periphery inward and upward, but also with efferent (motor) fibers leading outward from the cortex and connecting not only with muscles attached to the tiny bones inside the ears but also to the inner ear and from there to the entire rest of the body (Harrison & Howe, 1974).

Intelligent Active Ears

Recent research shows that the descending efferent fibers enable the central nervous system to refine and tune the responses of nerve fibers that analyze sound at the periphery (Santos-Sacchi, 2003; Suga et al., 2000; J. Yan, Q. Zhang, & Ehret, 2005). The motor processes not only amplify (by as much a 100 times; Santos-Sacchi, 2003) and filter (diminish) some signals, but sharpen the tuning to particular frequencies of some neurons. The means by which the amplification occurs has been traced down to motor activity at the molecular level through **prestin** and **acetylcholine** (Dallos, Zheng, & Cheatham, 2006; Frolenkov, 2006; Organ & Raphael, 2007; Santos-Sacchi, Song, Zheng, & Nuttall, 2006). Prestin is the motor protein that activates the outer hair cells enabling their movement and up to a 100-fold increase in the amplitude of a sound. Acetylcholine is also involved in the movements of the hair cells and is also the main neurotransmitter involved in muscle activity throughout the body.

The efferent fibers also enable the ear to reproduce the sounds that the ear hears. The manufactured "echo"—actually a reproduction—is called an **otoacoustic emission (OAE)**. Such an emission can be detected in the ear canal a few milliseconds after an external sound is presented (see Glattke, 2002; Prieve, 2002). This emission can be recorded with a miniature microphone inserted into the ear canal and is produced by motor activity in the hair cells of the cochlea. The fact that OAEs are coming from the brain to the ear rather than the reverse is demonstrated in the fact that such emissions can be produced in the absence of any external sound. We hypothesize that the activity of the inner ear in producing OAEs—whenever it involves speech in a language already acquired—must be tuned to that particular language. In theory, at least, though this idea has not yet been tested, it should be possible to detect differences in the OAEs for a known language as contrasted with a language that is not known to the hearer.

Certainly, it is known that individuals with significant hearing loss tend to produce reduced OAEs to a limit of no detectible OAEs at all (Glattke, 2002; also see Strickland, 2001). These findings show that even peripheral **sensorineural hearing loss** involves the central auditory system to the extent that OAEs are reduced or absent because of hearing loss. Again, the findings concerning OAEs and the motility of outer hair cells—especially the amplification they provide—is clear evidence that the hearing systems are both ranked and integrated. They are clearly ranked insofar as motor signals control the amplification and diminution of sensory ones—for example, motor signals outrank sensory ones. Also, if it is true that our hearing is tuned to the particular language, or languages that we acquire, it is reasonable to suppose that differences in the OAEs at the periphery should reflect changes owed to the acquisition of a certain language in contrast, say, to a very different language. That is, the quality of the OAEs produced by, say, a Japanese speaker hearing English /la/ as contrasted with /ra/ for example should be measurably different (less distinct in particular) than the OAEs

The efferent fibers also enable the ear to reproduce the sounds that the ear hears. The manufactured "echo"—actually a reproduction—is called an **otoacoustic emission (OAE)**.

of English speakers in response to the same syllables. This prediction follows from the nature of OAEs, the fact that they reflect what the inner ear is doing in processing sounds, and from the fact that Japanese speakers, unlike speakers of English, do not differentiate /la/ from /ra/ in their native language. Many other similar tests could be proposed across languages. To our knowledge no studies along this line have yet been conducted, but the hypothesis that differences in OAEs should be measurably influenced by language acquisition is reasonable and theoretically testable.

The Dynamic Motorized Cochlear Nuclei

The **cochlear nuclei** are the first major junctions of the ascending sensory auditory nerve fibers leading to the brain stem from both ears as those fibers ascend upward from the cochlea. The cochlear nuclei of the brain stem are shown in the drawing of Figure 4–8 from Gray's anatomy. This is a view of the brain stem from the back side with the cerebellum and the **cerebrum** removed from the picture. Descending from the cochlear nuclei back to the ears are motor (efferent) nerve fibers that project to the middle and inner ears. Much of the current research on central auditory processing is focused at the level of the cochlear nuclei and the tens of thousands of auditory nerve fibers ascending and descending from them.

It is interesting that the motor synapses of the hearing systems outnumber the sensory ones by a large margin, more than 10 to 1. Also, they outrank the sensory neurons as is shown in the fact that motor neurons can filter out some signals from sensory neurons and at the same time they can amplify others. It is probably because of these differences that the detection of the boundaries of syllables can be differentially refined over time by the learning of particular languages.

Interaction with Medicines

Exposure to loud noise whether owed to explosions or sustained high pressure sound can also result in the condition known as **tinnitus**—a persistent ringing in the ears that often accompanies hearing loss (Huang et al., 2006).

When the central auditory system is damaged, or even hindered by a drug as seemingly innocuous as aspirin, OAEs can be reduced or in fact stopped altogether (Huang et al., 2006). Also even temporary damage to the hearing, such as is caused by exposure to the loud noises of battle or even loud music (Nottet et al., 2006) can result in reduced OAEs.

Recent research with aspirin (salicylate) administered to guinea pigs produces tinnitus over the short term, but over the long term with repeated use, aspirin seems to "enhance active cochlear mechanics" (Huang et al., 2006, p. 2053). The researchers refer to this effect as "paradoxical" but it is reminiscent of a so-called **homeopathic effect**—according to which an agent that causes symptoms can, in smaller doses, supposedly alleviate the same symptoms (and vice

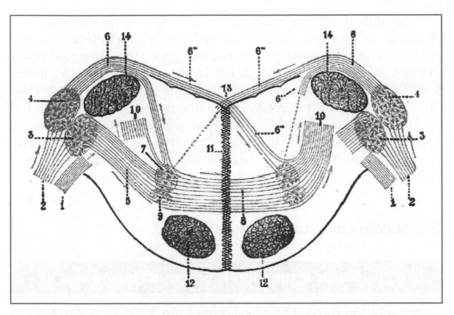

FIGURE 4–8. Terminal nuclei of the cochlear nerve, with their upper connections (Schematic). The vestibular nerve with its terminal nuclei and their efferent fibers have been suppressed. On the other hand, in order not to obscure the trapezoid body, the efferent fibers of the terminal nuclei on the right side have been resected in a considerable portion of their extent. The trapezoid body, therefore, shows only one-half of its fibers, viz., those which come from the left. 1. Vestibular nerve, divided at its entrance into the medulla oblongata. 2. Cochlear nerve. 3. Accessory nucleus of acoustic nerve. 4. Tuberculum acusticum. 5. Efferent fibers of accessory nucleus. 6. Efferent fibers of tuberculum acusticum, forming the striae medullares, with 6', their direct bundle going to the superior olivary nucleus of the same side; 6", their decussating bundles going to the superior olivary nucleus of the opposite side. 7. Superior olivary nucleus. 8. Trapezoid body. 9. Trapezoid nucleus. 10. Central acoustic tract (lateral lemniscus). 11. Raphé. 12. Cerebrospinal fasciculus. 13. Fourth ventricle. 14. Inferior peduncle. From H. Gray, 1918, *Anatomy of the Human Body* (Illustration 760). Philadelphia, PA: Lea & Febiger. Copyright © 2000 by Bartleby.com, ON-LINE ED., Inc. http://www.bartleby.com/107/. Retrieved January 10, 2008, from http://www.bartleby.com/107/illus760.html. Reprinted with permission. All rights reserved.

versa). A biochemical explanation for this well-known phenomenon has been proposed in the journal of *Homeopathy* (McGuigan, 2007). If there is a paradox in the effect of aspirin on hearing, it is that its impact seems to be homeopathy in reverse. In small doses over the short term it produces tinnitus, which is usually regarded as a bad outcome, but in longer exposures and presumably, by cumulative effects, aspirin actually reduces its own negative impact and comes to have a positive one. In the case of aspirin's effect on hearing, the short-term loss was as much as 20 to 50 dB, but with long-term administration all of the loss was recovered and the motor functions of the outer hair cells were actually improved.

In the case of aspirin's effect on hearing, the short-term loss was as much as 20 to 50 dB, but with long-term administration all of the loss was recovered and the motor functions of the outer hair cells were actually improved.

Another drug, **hydroxyurea**, which is used in the treatment of sickle cell anemia, also seems to have an impact on hearing. For unknown reasons it reduces damage to the outer hair cells that commonly occurs with that kind of anemia (Stuart, S. M. Jones, & Walker, 2006). In all these cases, the impact of these drugs on tinnitus and otoacoustic emissions demonstrate the layering and ranking of sensory and motor neurons within the hearing system. That is, all of them show that motor neurons, as we must logically expect, outrank the sensory neurons and can override or enhance their effects.

The Middle Ear (Stapedius) Reflex

> ### Motor Protection from Loud Noises
>
> Some of the descending neurons of the auditory nerve bundle connect with the middle ear enabling what is known as the **acoustic reflex** which is sometimes also called the **middle ear reflex (MER)** because it involves a rapid contraction of the main **middle ear muscle—the stapedius**. For this reason it is also called the **stapedius reflex**. This well known contraction reduces the impact of noise on the ear drum and its main function is "to protect the inner ear" from the damage that would occur if the loud noise continued at full strength" (D. J. Lee, de Venecia, Guinan, & Brown, 2006).

In normal hearing, a loud sound presented to either ear will produce the MER in both ears. Lee et al. were able to show, with surgical procedures in rats, that the interneurons enabling the MER are located in the front side, that is, the **ventral** side of the cochlear nuclei. This is the side toward the belly of the rat. It is well established that the MER reflex is dependent on interneurons within the cochlear nuclei and that the sound threshold of this reflex changes with hearing loss (Kim et al., 2006; Morata, Dunn, Kretschmer, Lemasters, & Keith, 1993). With certain kinds of hearing loss, the threshold decreases and with others it increases.

Exposure to noise can also produce what is known as a **temporary threshold shift** where the sounds the ears can detect, and which will produce the MER, must be louder than were required prior to the shift. Permanent damage to hearing is known to occur commonly with repeated or prolonged exposure to loud noise and to certain damaging chemicals and chemical mixtures. Again, all of these well-documented phenomena demonstrate a layering and ranking of the subsystems involved in hearing. The inner ear, as we are about to see, is likewise an intermediate system that is higher ranked than the middle ear but lower than, say, the cortex as we

The MER is triggered by motor neurons connected to interneurons that activate the reflex very early in the neurological process of hearing. The reflex effectively turns our middle ear off, or down, so that our inner ear (the higher ranking system) will be protected from permanent damage.

have already seen with respect to phenomena pertaining to perceptual vigilance and defense.

The sensory aspect of hearing mostly occurs through the sensory fibers of the auditory nerve connecting to the cochlea. However, as we have already noted, within the cochlea there are both afferent (sensory) fibers projecting upward from each inner hair cell in the organ of Corti toward the central nervous system and efferent (motor) fibers projecting away from the central nervous system and connecting to those outer hair cells. Each of the motor fibers in question connects to 5 to 10 outer hair cells while each sensory cell connects to only one inner hair cell. The outer hair cells by contrast are generally supplied by at least two motor connections and also by a single afferent (sensory) connector pointing back to the central nervous system. Again, within the inner ear—the cochlea and more particularly the organ of Corti—we see a layering and ranking of sensory and motor functions.

Filtering and Amplifying

It is clear that information coming from the cochlear nuclei, and certainly also from layers of the central nervous system above the cochlear nuclei—as can be inferred from the syllable and sentence level McGurk effects, for instance—must contribute to the amplification and filtering of sounds at the periphery. The motor processes that are controlled from higher up in the brain, it is believed (Drescher et al., 2006; Khan et al., 2007; Raphael & Altschuler, 2003), also enable enhanced resolution of the speech sounds that we learn to hear as we acquire one or more particular languages. Unfortunately, up to now, most of the research on the filtering and amplification of auditory signals has been done with rodents. However, noninvasive research is also possible with human participants.

Recall the hypothesis proposed above that OAEs will reveal higher resolution for the contrast between /la/ and /ra/, for instance, among English speakers than among Japanese speakers. Gray's *Anatomy of the Human Body* published in 1918 which contains 1,247 detailed diagrams that (retrieved February 25, 2009, from http://www.bartleby.com/107/) includes Figure 4–8, a diagram of some of the components and connections within the cochlear nuclei. Without going into the details, the point we want to make with this diagram is that the lowest level of central auditory processing, almost 100 years ago, had already been shown to be incredibly complex. What is more, Gray's diagram (see Figure 4–8), already suggests the kind of layering and interactions we have been talking about.

The hearing system is shown as a complex of subsystems richly interconnected within themselves, between the two ears, and with other systems of the brain and body. Presumably, it is because of the integrative processes linking the highest levels of the brain with the outer hair cells in the organ of Corti that we are able to integrate what we hear into coherent patterns in speech processing. However, the cochlear nuclei themselves is a remarkable system of interconnected systems that has long been known to involve multiple distinct layers of processing whose functions are still being worked out nearly a century after Gray's diagram was published in 1918.

CONNECTIONS ABOVE, THROUGH, AND BELOW THE COCHLEAR NUCLEI

Perhaps the most ubiquitous evidence of the connection of the ears with the rest of the body is found in the common startle response triggered by sound.

There is abundant evidence (Musiek & Lamb, 1992, p. 28) that the motor nerves of the auditory system are not only richly connected to the inner ear below them and to the cortex above—showing the ranked layers of the hearing system—but through the cochlear nuclei they extend to other vital organs and to the peripheral muscles of the body.

The Auditory (Acoustic) Startle Response

To take a well known phenomenon involving motor neurons of the auditory system, consider the **auditory startle response (ASR)** which is also known as the **acoustic startle response (ASR)**. This response is fundamentally different from the MER which occurs at a lower level. The ASR, unlike the MER, is not quite a reflex. It involves cognitive expectancy (recall the upper right corner of Figure 1–3).

The ASR is an aspect of the auditory system that is logically above the mere sensation of sound. It involves motor signals processed in the central nervous system that are projected to organs and muscles that are peripheral to the central nervous system. At this point in our developing introduction, it is no longer surprising that hearing is *not merely a matter of sensation*. The research shows that the motor nerves of the ear are connected through the central nervous system to many of our bodily organs and muscles. The ASR is commonly produced by a sound we are expecting and listening for, or by one that abruptly violates our expectation of silence or no change in, say, the sound of an airplane engine. The ASR is produced when something we were expecting (or actually expecting not to occur at all) suddenly happens. In both cases, we were expecting something different from what we hear. Either way expectancy comes into play.

Different from the MER

The auditory startle response (ASR) is different from the middle ear reflex (MER) which, as we have seen earlier in this chapter, helps to prevent damage to the cochlea from loud noises. The ASR may occur right after an MER occurs, but the ASR must have a higher point of origination on account of the fact that it involves conscious expectation. In some cases, in fact, we are anticipating or even dreading the stimulus that produces the ASR. That is not the case with the MER which is a completely uncontrollable and subconscious response of the middle ear muscles. Although both the ASR and the MER are dependent on motor signals from the central auditory system, the involvement of consciousness makes the ASR a higher level of response than the MER.

Interestingly, though the ASR is well-known and common in human beings, most of the research concerning it is being conducted with rodents. A general search on the Web of Knowledge on February 25, 2009 entering only "auditory startle response" OR "acoustic startle response" in the search yielded 1,995 hits. The vast majority of those studies, however, involve research using rodents as subjects. If we add the delimiter "human," the same search turns up 261 hits. The research shows that the ASR is common to many species. The efferent synapses of our ears are connected to our vital organs and peripheral muscles through interneurons of the higher and more central auditory system.

Those interneurons can be activated so as to inform motor neurons that are connected to the heart, the adrenal glands, and the muscles at the periphery, so that the ASR, when it occurs, produces a general bodily reaction. For instance, when waiting for the toaster to pop up, or waiting for the phone to ring—especially if we are rushed or agitated—when the sound finally occurs we often experience an ASR. It is most often caused by sounds with sharp onsets, or sudden offsets. It does not require a sound that is especially loud. The startle response, when it occurs, interferes with carrying out a planned activity such as the start of a race at the Olympics (Brown, Kenwell, Maraj, & Collins, 2008).

An ASR can be produced by a bottle crashing on a hard floor, a gun shot, an unexpected engine roaring to life, the sound of a footfall in a quiet house, or a sudden cessation of engine noise in an airplane (Björk, 1999; Thackray & Touchstone, 1970; Turpin, Schaefer, & Bousin, 1999; Wilkins, 1982).

ASR Temporarily Inhibits Processing

The ASR results in an immediate tensing of bodily muscles. We say the sound makes us "jump," though we rarely get off the floor or out of our chairs. But as **adrenaline**, also called **epinephrine**, is released in the blood, we experience a sudden increase in heart rate, we breathe faster, and our sweat glands contract (Peryer, Noyes, Pleydell-Pearce, & Lieven, 2005; Wilkins, 1982). The reaction seems instantaneous, but its peak effects last for about two seconds, inhibiting our ability to process inputs from our senses during that time. The effect then tapers off gradually in about 10 seconds (Thackray & Touchstone, 1970). The interference with perception that is caused by the ASR is an effect enabled by descending motor neurons from fairly high up in the central auditory system (Tresilian & Plooy, 2006).

Research confirms that the nerve systems involved in the ASR are above the cochlear nuclei but well beneath the level of the higher cortex in humans. We can be reasonably certain about this because of the vast amount of work done with rats and mice (L. Li &

Shao, 2003; Swerdlow, Braff, & Geyer, 2000). By many surgical interventions in rodents, whose brains are fairly similar to ours, up to and beyond the level of the cochlear nuclei, it can be shown that the ASR can be blocked by cutting nerves at the level of what is called the **inferior colliculus** in the brain stem. Although there are relatively few studies listed in the Web of Knowledge database as of March 23, 2009, on the relation between the ASR and hearing loss in humans, 23 studies were found showing a reduced ASR mainly in rodents but in a few instances also in humans with hearing loss or tinnitus. Again, the ASR shows the layering and ranking of elements within the hearing system as well as their integration.

Distinct Motor Layers Above and Below the Middle Ear

At the lowest level of the peripheral hearing system, the MER shows that there is a motor layer of processing just above the sensory system involved not only in detecting and analyzing sounds, but also in protecting the inner ear from noise damage. Motor signals are also involved in filtering and amplifying sounds to enhance hearing and to produce OAEs. The ASR shows evidence of a complex of interneuron connections at a level somewhere above the cochlear nuclei but not fully involving the cortex.

The ASR shows that motor neurons of the inner ear are connected through more central auditory systems with organs, glands, and muscles extending out to the periphery of the body. The motor nerves of the hearing system are probably involved in focusing on sounds of interest under noisy conditions, commonly referred to as *masking*. This term suggests the way noise from one or many sources tend to cover up, or drown out, the sounds we are trying to attend to, for instance, in a conversation. The research shows that persons with normal hearing and normal language functions can focus attention on a conversation of interest and largely filter out competing conversations and noise. Studies of hearing under masking noise of various sorts suggest that our ears are informed by activity in the central nervous system. We may infer that rodents can show the MER, OAEs, and ASR, but are not subject to the linguistic phenomena known as perceptual vigilance and defense. In any case, the fact that the human sense of hearing is a system of layered, ranked, and integrated subsystems is well established.

> It may be inferred that the ASR is governed by expectancies at a level beneath the cortical phenomena known as perceptual vigilance and defense. In humans, at least, the latter phenomena commonly involve knowledge of language—for example, the ability to recognize one's own name—and to subconsciously be influenced by emotional evaluations of both desirable and undesirable meanings.

SUMMING UP AND LOOKING AHEAD

In this chapter, we have reviewed evidence of the layering, ranking, and integration of sensory, motor, and linguistic systems. The integration is seen with special clarity in the McGurk interactions and, with some teasing apart of distinct functions, in problems associated with hearing and the perception and comprehension of speech, and especially in what are called CAPDs. The most basic signs involved in communication are those produced by our senses of seeing, hearing, smelling, touching, and tasting. The normal functioning of all these sensory systems, of course, presupposes an intact body. We have already seen in Chapter 2 how disorders that directly affect the body and how it appears to others can often result in communication disorders. In Chapter 3, we dealt with disorders of the senses, especially blindness and deafness. Here in Chapter 4 we have seen how deeply the systems of sensation and movement are integrated with cognition, emotions, and language. In Chapter 5 we consider disorders that range across the full scope of childhood development—the so-called "pervasive" developmental disorders such as autism. These are disorders that deeply impact the layered, ranked, and integrated systems of representation that we have introduced in Chapter 4.

STUDY AND DISCUSSION QUESTIONS

1. In broad strokes, what are some of the evidences that representational systems are layered, ranked, and integrated?
2. How can we show that a baby's senses are well integrated at birth or even before?
3. What evidence can be offered to show that an infant at less than two weeks knows that a virtual three-dimensional object that appears to be solid has mass and weight?
4. Why is it that the layering and ranking of representational processes involved in hearing, for instance, cannot be discovered by studies of pure-tone detection?
5. What evidence can be offered to show McGurk interactions, or something like them, in early infancy?
6. How can we explain the fact that the articulatory movements seen in a video tend to override a recorded voice saying a different syllable in the McGurk syllable effects?
7. If light waves/photons travel through almost empty space at great velocity what does sound travel in? How about the molecules that enable us to smell? How does it compare to touch? Which one operates faster and at greater distance? How about taste?
8. What reasons can be given for the dominance of meaning in the interpretation of ordinary conversations and discourse? Consider also the impact of perceptual vigilance and defense on the processing of emotionally charged elements of discourse.
9. What are the key features in the ASHA description of CAPDs?
10. How do the MER and the ASR show different levels of central auditory processing that are still short of the highest levels of cortical comprehension and production of language?

11. Why is the simple frequency theory of perceptual defense and vigilance necessarily incomplete? What experimental evidences does it fail to account for?

12. How does the homeopathic effect and the impact of certain medicines relate to the claim that the human hearing system is layered with respect to sensory, motor, and interneurons?

5

Childhood Disorders

OBJECTIVES

In this chapter, we:

1. Discuss why childhood disorders involve genetic factors;
2. Demonstrate that autism is the most common childhood disorder;
3. Critique theories of the accelerating increase in autism diagnoses;
4. Consider (a) diagnostic criteria, (b) public awareness, (c) monetary pressure, (d) genetic factors, (e) toxins, and (f) interactions;
5. Discuss involvement of the immune and gastrointestinal systems as well as genetics, metabolism, and the brain;
6. Review research showing similarities between autism and poisoning; and
7. Survey interventions impacting developmental disorders.

KEY TERMS

Here are some key terms of this chapter. Many of them you may already know. It may help to review them. These terms are explained in the text and they are defined in the Glossary at the end of the book. They appear in **bold print** on their first appearance in the text.

ABA
acute disseminated
   encephalomyelitis
ALS
amino acids
amyotrophic lateral sclerosis
antioxidants
applied behavior analysis
Asperger syndrome
Asperger's disorder
audiologists
autism spectrum disorders
autoimmunity
aversive stimuli
behaviorism
beta amyloids
beta-carotene
broadened criteria theory
Centers for Disease Control
CDC
cerebellar ataxia
chelation therapy
concordance rates
continuous reinforcement
delay technique
dimercaptuosuccinic acid
DMSA
dizygotic
electron
epidemic
epidemiologists
extinction
fixed-ratio schedule of
   reinforcement

free radical
gastrointestinal tract
genes plus toxins theory
genetic theory
give-me-the-money theory
glutathione
GSH
hand-flapping
HFA
high functioning autism
hyperactivity
hypotonia
infantile autism
inflammatory bowel disease
intermittent schedule of
   reinforcement
isomorphic
Kanner-type autism
Lou Gehrig's disease
macrophages
merthiolate
microglia
monozygotic
mortality
negative reinforcement
neuroAIDS
neurofibrillary tangles
neurotoxicity
operant
operant conditioning
oxidation
oxidative stress
PDD
PDD-NOS

pervasive developmental
   disorders
pervasive developmental
   disorders not otherwise
   specified
plaques
positive reinforcement
prevalence
prospective study
proton
public awareness theory
punishment
recurrence risk
redox
reduction
reinforcing stimuli
resin composite
Rett syndrome
schedule of reinforcement
senile dementia
special education
stereotyped movements
testosterone
thimerosal
toxicology
verbal behavior
vitamin C
vitamin E
xenobiotic
zone of proximal
   development
ZPD

A few decades ago, most ordinary citizens had no idea what autism was. Why is it that now nearly everyone in the world knows about autism? If you bring up the subject today, most folks will say, "Oh, I have a nephew who has it." Or, they might say, "Yeah, I know a kid who has it, and I read this book about it." Or, they may say, "Yeah, like Dustin Hoffman in *Rainman*, right?" They probably have heard about the debate concerning whether or not the worldwide autism epidemic is real or just media hype. *Why is it that almost everyone knows about autism today when just 50 years ago even specialists had hardly heard of it?* What is the explanation for the 5,030 cases in the *Omnibus Autism Proceeding* that had already been filed in the United States Court of Federal Claims by July 2006 (Edlich, et al., 2007)? Is autism just another word for the extensive and severe brain damage—**acute disseminated encephalomyelitis**—admitted in 1,322 other cases already decided since 1988 by the same court (R. F. Kennedy & Kirby, February 24, 2009)? Is the general and widespread public awareness about autism the result of a genuine increase in **prevalence**, or is there some other explanation? Is autism really becoming increasingly common or does it merely seem to be?

In this chapter we see evidence that autism and related developmental disorders are on the rise. This book is probably the first introduction in the field for speech-language pathologists and teachers of special education to take the autism epidemic seriously (also see McCarthy, 2007, Jepson & J. Johnson, 2007; and J. W. Oller & S. D. Oller, 2009). We will see that the root factors in autism are invariably involved in a plethora of relatively new childhood disorders, diseases, syndromes, and poorly understood developmental problems.

The causal factors in autism are also implicated in the causation or exacerbation of neurological diseases such as multiple sclerosis and of long-term deteriorative conditions such as Alzheimer's and Parkinson's disease.

THE STRANGE PUZZLE

How Autism Is Diagnosed

Autism is diagnosed on the basis of behavioral symptoms. For instance, there may be an almost obsessive interest in keeping things the same by repeating routines that may seem meaningless to others. The person affected may engage in **stereotyped movements**—for example, repetitive movements of the hands in front of the person's own eyes, a kind of self-stimulation called **hand-flapping**. Symptoms may also include head-banging and self-injury. We now know that many of these extreme behaviors are linked to **inflammatory bowel**

> **disease** (Jepson & J. Johnson, 2007; Bransfield, Wulfman, Harvey & Usman, 2008) and that the nonverbal children who exhibit them are commonly experiencing abdominal pain. Kanner (1943) also commented on the digestive problems of the first 11 cases that he diagnosed.

He reported symptoms such as chronic vomiting for seven of them and that or other digestive tract symptoms for nine of the 11 (see J. W. Oller & S. D. Oller, 2009). However, the key characteristics of what Kanner described as **infantile autism**, now sometimes called **Kanner-type autism**, have hardly changed. They include: failure to develop normal speech and language (or sudden loss of skills already acquired, as in the case of Dov Shestack, Ethan Kurtz, Evan McCarthy, and so on); inability (or lack of any apparent desire) to form normal social relations; and abnormal concern to maintain routines. He also described repetitive and stereotypical behaviors.

A Case in Point

About 15 years ago, Jonathan Shestack—the producer of *Father of the Bride* and *Dan in Real Life* along with other movies (see Film Scouts, 2006)—and his wife Portia Iversen had a little boy. Jon and Portia named their son, Dov (rhyming with "stove"). Jon described him as "adorable" and "cute" but about 15 months after what started out to be a normal childhood, Dov suddenly "stopped answering to his name" (Shestack, 2003, retrieved February 27, 2009, from http://www.tvworldwide.com/events/nimh/031119/agenda.cfm; just click on the Real file or one of the Windows files in the 9:30 to 10:00 AM slot on that Web page to see and hear the webcast version of his talk).

Jon tells that Dov "had a couple of dozen words. He lost them. He stopped running to greet us when we came in the door. And it really looked like he'd disappeared in front of our eyes in the space of a couple of months." When Dov was 11 years old "we were still trying get him back." Now he is 15 and they are still trying to get him back. It is true that Dov's parents are no doubt interested in whether or not there is an **epidemic** of autism—the question being addressed by **epidemiologists** such as Fombonne (2005)—but their main concern is what can be done to make him better? What can we do to get him back? How can his ability to communicate with those who love him be restored? Is there any hope of a cure? What is causing Dov's loss? How serious is it? Will his parents ever be able to reach him again? What can they do to enhance his comprehension and ability to express his needs? What can they do to once again share ordinary experiences that are commonly taken for granted?

Jon tells that Dov "had a couple of dozen words. He lost them. He stopped running to greet us when we came in the door. And it really looked like he'd disappeared in front of our eyes in the space of a couple of months."

Hearing the Diagnosis: *Autism*

At first, Jon and Portia could not get a straight answer from anyone. Some denied that Dov had any kind of problem at all. So he learned and lost a few words. It was nothing to worry about. He was just a boy. Boys develop more slowly. They got tired of hearing that "Einstein didn't speak until he was 4 years old." But finally, they talked to an individual who said the word *autism*. Jon and his wife did not know what it meant. They asked, "What can you do about *that*?" The doctor replied, "There is really nothing you can do about that. You just hold on to each other and cry and get on with your own lives." Jon described the next four days of that Memorial Day weekend as the longest days of his life. He and Portia watched videotapes of their little boy over and over asking themselves how it was that they had lost him.

What Is Causing the Increase?

In his talk before the scientists and others gathered at the National Institutes of Health for the meeting in Washington, D. C. on November 19, 2003, Shestack quoted a "sensitive and articulate" mom who described the impact of autism this way. She said, "Autism is like somebody snuck into her house when her little boy was one and a half and stole his mind and . . . his personality and left his bewildered body behind." According to the **Centers for Disease Control (CDC)**, in their *Morbidity and Mortality Weekly Report* (*MMWR*) of February 9, 2007, the rate of diagnosis based on data mainly from 1992 to 2000 is supposedly about 1 in 150 children (retrieved February 27, 2009, from http://www.cdc.gov/mmwr/PDF/ss/ss5601.pdf). We think it is higher than that rate. Sometime before 1970 the rate was less than 1 in 30,000, so the current estimate by the CDC represents an increase greater than 200-fold—20,000%. The CDC (n.d.-a) has published the following statement (retrieved February 27, 2009, from http://www.cdcfoundation.org/healththreats/autism.aspx):

> While it is clear that more children than ever before are diagnosed as having an ASD, it is unclear how much of this increase is due to changes in how we identify and diagnose ASDs, or whether this is due to a true increase in prevalence.

Could the huge change in numbers of diagnoses be owed to factors such as public awareness, better tuning of diagnostic procedures, broadening of criteria for diagnosis, or to any number of factors other than an actual increase in the incidence of the disorders? Classroom teachers are seeing the children in their schools. Caseloads of speech-language pathologists have swelled and are saturated with cases.

No one doubts that diagnoses of **autism spectrum disorders** (ASDs; see the American Psychiatric Association's *Diagnostic and Statistical Manual IV Revised*, 1994) have skyrocketed over the last couple of decades.

Many of the Cases Are Severe

Individuals with severe autism require constant care and supervision 24 hours a day and 7 days a week.

The Autism Developmental Disabilities Monitoring Network (2007), reports that between 59% and 62% of the cases examined in data from 2000 and 2002 according to their 2007 *MMWR* reports have a significant mental or cognitive impairment qualifying as "Intellectual Disability or Mental Retardation" with an IQ score equal to or less than 70 (retrieved February 27, 2009, from http://www.cdc.gov/ncbddd/autism/documents/AutismCommunityReport.pdf, p. 20). (See Chapters 11 and 12 concerning the fundamental problems associated with exclusively using English based IQ tests to determine intellectual abilities.) Many are like Dov Shestack and Ethan Kurtz. On the DVD, in the video showing Ethan's regression, notice how bright eyed and normal he was before the age of two years. For many children who are diagnosed with autism, development looks perfectly normal up to about the second year when they suddenly become unresponsive to their names, lose their former language development, become socially disconnected, and begin manifesting stereotypical repetitive behaviors.

Until recently, the mainstream prognosis was essentially hopeless, just as was told to Jon Shestack and his wife. The affected individual would never learn to talk or be able to have normal social relations with other persons. We now know that prognosis to have been mistaken for most children with autism (see Jepson & J. Johnson, 2007; McCarthy, 2007; and the Ethan Kurtz video). Although autism was, until very recently, considered irreversible and permanent—a long future without hope—we now know that it is treatable and in some cases the child that seemed to have been lost can be recovered. For instance, consider the case of Ethan Kurtz who was severely autistic at age two and remained that way until age four when a combination of factors, especially clearing his intestines of a fungal infection enabled him to advance to relative normalcy in just 21 days. On the 16 point *Scale of Autism Spectrum Disorders* (J. W. Oller & Rascón, 1999; also J. W. Oller & S. D. Oller, 2009), Ethan Kurtz advanced from Level 0, the lowest level, to above Level 15, the highest level on the scale.

Although autism was, until very recently, considered irreversible and permanent—a long future without hope—we now know that it is treatable and in some cases the child that seemed to have been lost can be recovered.

Why Has Autism Been Neglected?

Why is it that ASDs have only recently come into the public spotlight? Shestack argued that one reason is that autism does not affect rich and famous adults, except indirectly, and then only through their children. In those cases, the parents are very busy caring for the sick child. Unlike **Lou Gehrig's disease**, also known as **amyotrophic lateral sclerosis (ALS)** which eventually took the life of a world-renowned baseball player, or Alzheimer's disease that has brought down famous adults such as President Ronald Reagan, autism affects children who don't vote, don't lobby, and whose parents are so busy taking care of them that it is difficult for them to organize, raise money, or call any public attention to the problems they face. The parents of children with autism are busy being mediators between the child and the teachers, therapists, and anyone else who interacts with their child. Read Jenny McCarthy's story about her son Evan (McCarthy, 2007).

Or observe Hannah Poling in any one of multiple interviews after the government conceded that her symptoms of autism and her seizure disorder were both caused or at least made worse by vaccines. Hannah, who was 10 in December 2008, was developing normally up to her 19th month when she received with CDC mandated vaccines nine disease agents and 15 additional toxins (see J. W. Oller & S. D. Oller, 2009) all on one day. In the interview of her parents on *Larry King Live* ("The Autism Vaccine Debate," March 7, 2008, retrieved September 10, 2008 from http://www.cnn.com/video/#/video/bestoftv/2008/03/07/lkl.autism.vaccine.long.cnn?iref=videosearch). Or for a more severe case of autism, see the video of Michelle Cedillo as narrated by Sanjay Gupta (April 1, 2008) retrieved February 27, 2009, from http://www.cnn.com/2008/HEALTH/conditions/03/24/autism.vaccines/#cnnSTCVideo. Michelle Cedillo's case was decided, not in her favor, on February 12, 2009 by the U.S. Court of Federal Claims (also known as the Vaccine Injury Court; see Chapter 12), but there are still more than 5,000 other cases asserting that autism was caused by vaccines and their components (Edlich et al., 2007). Like nearly all of those children, Michelle also was developing normally until a course of mandated vaccines preceded her descent into severe autism.

As Shestack pointed out in 2003, up to then, autism was hardly mentioned in the medical textbooks. In fact, the curriculum for training speech-language pathologists, **audiologists**, or teachers of **special education** does not require any single course specifically dedicated to the study of autism. In the widely used textbook titled, *Human Communication Disorders*, a 663-page tome in its sixth edition by Shames and Anderson (2002), the terms "autism" and "autism spectrum disorders" are not even listed in the index. Clearly, more attention is needed and autism deserves a prominent place in books, courses, and curricula on communication disorders. But the study of autism spectrum disorders, or any other disorder, cannot be our final goal.

Clearly, more attention is needed and autism deserves a prominent place in books, courses, and curricula on communication disorders. But the study of autism spectrum disorders, or any other disorder, cannot be our final goal.

The Essential Goal

In his talk, Shestack went on to express his hope that in the future "autism will only be mentioned in the history books." We believe that this hope defines the essential goal for the study of communication disorders.

For this reason, Jon Shestack and Portia Iversen founded the organization, "Cure Autism Now," which recently merged with "Autism Speaks" (retrieved February 27, 2009, from http://www.autismspeaks.org/). The latter organization was founded by Bob

As important as it is to understand disorders, to describe them accurately, to understand their symptoms, to diagnose them as accurately as possible, and to minimize the loss to persons affected by them, our deeper objective must be to find their causes in order to prevent them from occurring if possible and to either cure them when they do occur or, at the very least, to reduce the severity of their impact as much as possible.

The legal and financial liabilities are high and the number of families that are being impacted by autism are staggering (see the Office of Special Masters, September 29, 2008, Docket of Omnibus Autism Proceeding, retrieved February 27, 2009 from http://www.uscfc.us courts.gov/docket-omnibus-autism-proceeding).

and Suzanne Wright whose grandson Christian was diagnosed with autism in 2004. Katie Wright, their daughter, tells the story of her son's autism in the Foreword to Jepson and J. Johnson (2007). She believes that her son Christian Hildebrand, born August 31, 2001, was vaccine injured and she explained her reasons for believing this on the basis of the history of her child in an extensive interview to David Kirby which can be viewed in four parts on YouTube (see Foundation for Autism Information and Research, April 19, 2007, retrieved February 27, 2009, from http://www.youtube.com/watch?v=IUNO25l1zFs&feature=related). Christian's first severe reaction was at two months followed six shots on one day after which he screamed for two hours. The pediatrician told her that the reaction was more severe than common, but was still normal and that Katie should continue with the vaccinations. After his fourth month and sixth month vaccinations Christian continued to go downhill. After a series of vaccinations at 37 months he descended suddenly into autism.

Is it possible that autism and many other communication disorders may be relegated in the future to the same status that is now accorded to polio and many other diseases? We believe that this is possible and that the students and teachers using this book can help in achieving that goal. To seek that outcome, it is essential, we believe, to find the causes. To the extent that vaccines are involved in producing autism, the public needs to know. The term "controversy" as applied to that question is too weak. The fact is that there is a war of ideas going on and it has divided families as well as organizations (Gross & Strom, 2007; R. F. Kennedy & Kirby, 2009). It is not difficult to see why the discussion is so intense. The stakeholders include powerful government agencies such as the CDC which has promoted the use of vaccines along with the pharmaceutical industry that is involved to the tune of billions of dollars. In addition, there are the medical professionals, organizations, hospitals, and clinics that have administered all the mandated vaccines. The legal and financial liabilities are high and the number of families that are being impacted by autism are staggering (see the Office of Special Masters, September 29, 2008, Docket of Omnibus Autism Proceeding, retrieved February 27, 2009, from http://www.uscfc.us courts.gov/docket-omnibus-autism-proceeding). The 5,000 plus cases to be heard by the Court account for only a small fraction of the number of families being affected by autism.

PERVASIVE DEVELOPMENTAL DISORDERS: AUTISM AT THE CENTER

The typically severe cognitive impairments associated with autism and its prevalence make it central to the whole class of **pervasive developmental disorders** (PDD) as described by the American

Psychiatric Association (1994). Also see the *Diagnostic and Statistical Manual of Mental Disorders, 4th edition (DSM-IV)*. It is similarly described by the World Health Organization (2007a, 2007b) in its *International Classification of Mental and Behavioral Diseases; Diagnostic Criteria for Research, 10th edition (ICD-10*, retrieved February 26, 2009, from http://www.cdc.gov/nchs/about/otheract/icd9/abticd10.htm and http://www.who.int/classifications/icd/en/).

Defining Autism

According to the popular source http://www.answers.com/autism&r=67 (retrieved February 27, 2009) autism can be defined as "a pervasive developmental disorder characterized by severe deficits in social interaction and communication, by an extremely limited range of activities and interests, and often by the presence of repetitive, stereotyped behaviors." Actually, this is an excellent summary of the standard definitions offered by experts. It closely adheres to the description of the class or pervasive developmental disorders (PDD) as described by the American Psychiatric Association (2007) and the World Health Organization (2007a, 2007b). Major changes are not expected in the forthcoming *DSM-V* which the APA is previewing at meetings coming up in May 2009 (E. A. Kuhl, February 20, 2009).

As we saw in Chapter 1, with severe autism, when parents ask for an explanation for the child's problem, a common answer is: "It's a mystery. We just don't know what is going on." Katie Wright said in her interview with David Kirby that at the time of her son's diagnosis the medical personnel consulted said, "nobody knows why . . . the word 'mystery' was used a thousand times and 'genetic.' It was 'genetic' and it was 'mysterious' and 'nobody knows' . . . " (in Part 2 of the series from about 20 seconds into the segment, retrieved February 27, 2009, from http://www.youtube.com/watch?v=_dHY5K_MP7w&feature=related). At age two, Christian descended into autism with all of the symptoms including digestive problems, diarrhea, tantrums, loss of language, social withdrawal, and so forth. As we saw in Chapter 1, the "it's a mystery" explanation does not satisfy parents. If our own child is involved, or the child of a loved one or anyone we care about, even a total stranger, we still want to know what is wrong and how it can be put right or made better. Thinking persons want to know why autism is increasingly prevalent today—why is it being diagnosed so commonly today? Why has it gone upward from the rank of an almost unknown disorder affecting fewer than 1 in 30,000 children less than five decades ago, to a diagnosis that now is affecting 1 in 150, according to the Centers for Disease Control? Just what is going on?

Needless to say, there is substantial public interest in autism today. A Google search for the term "autism" on September 16, 2006 yielded approximately 27.3 million hits. On September 10, 2008 the same search yielded 26.4 million hits while "childhood cancer"

Autism is the most common diagnosis today in childhood disorders and the symptoms of autism are the main basis for defining the rest of the disorders included among PDDs. Therefore, it makes sense to focus considerable attention on autism in the study of communication disorders. To deal effectively with the whole class of PDDs, we must ask, *What is autism? And equally important, why is it on the rise?*

yielded only 1.6 million. Another indication of the rising awareness of autism is that many parents not only know what autism is, they also know about the catch-all category called "**PDD-NOS**"—standing for "**pervasive developmental disorders not otherwise specified**." The *DSM-IV* refers to PDD-NOS (1994, p. 78) as "atypical autism" where some of the symptoms are less severe and/or there is late onset. PDD-NOS is the diagnosis for autism disorders that do not meet all the somewhat loosely defined behavioral criteria. Some argue that PDD-NOS is just milder autism. At the outside edge of PPDs we also find the so-called "personality" disorders, including **attention deficit disorder** with or without **hyperactivity**, also known as ADD/ADHD. Whether or not the latter are to be distinguished from milder manifestations of autism, and how this might be done, is uncertain.

An Autism Epidemic

It is evident that there has been an upsurge in the number of cases of autism being diagnosed (D. B. Campbell et al., 2006; Muhle, Trentacoste, & Rapin, 2004). D. B. Campbell et al. (2006) wrote "there has been a dramatic increase in the diagnosis of autism" (p. 16834). Muhle, Trentacoste, and Rapin (2004) pointed out that by 1997, the increase between 1991 and 1997 had already amounted to "an astonishing 556% reported increase in pediatric prevalence" making autism a more common childhood disorder than "spina bifida, cancer, or Down syndrome" (p. E472). Although the CDC has repeatedly questioned whether there is any real increase in the number of autism cases, their own studies (Autism Developmental Disabilities Monitoring Network, 2007; CDC, 2007) show that the rate of autism diagnosis is higher than ever before and still climbing. The latest statistics suggest that the 1 in 150 estimate, which was based on data mainly from 1992 to 2000, is too low. Evidence that this is so is seen in Figure 5–1, which shows a smooth growth curve still going upward from 1993 through 2006.

With all the foregoing in mind, we must address two questions here: (1) Why are the diagnoses still skyrocketing? And, (2) why are government agencies such as the CDC so conflicted about whether or not the increase is real?

The Data Show an Accelerating Rate

There is no doubt that the diagnosis of autism *is on the rise.* Figure 5–1 summarizes statistics gathered over 11 years under the Individuals with Disabilities Education Act (**IDEA**) and the subsequent No Child Left Behind Act (**NCLB**; see P. W. D. Wright, P. D. Wright, & Heath, 2008). Compared with all other disorders that have been tracked under IDEA and NCLB, autism spectrum disorders are

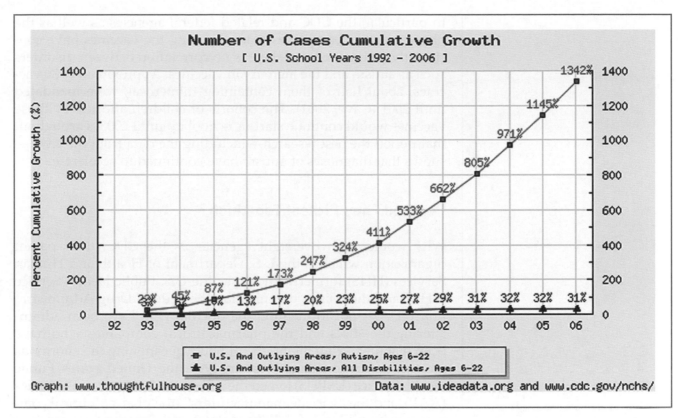

FIGURE 5–1. The accelerating diagnosis of autism in the United States of America. Retrieved February 27, 2009, from http://www.fightingautism.org/idea/autism.php? Reprinted as licensed under the rules of Creative Commons Attributions 1.0 Generic.

increasing most rapidly. Although the data in Figure 5–1 reach only to the year 2006, studies released by the CDC on February 9, 2007 showed rates continuing to rise as have studies since then.

In fact, a host of other sources could be cited showing the continuing rise in the number of diagnoses. Many of those publications, oddly, are being produced by the CDC in defense of certain vaccines that are known to produce severe injuries in some individuals with certain genetic susceptibilities—ones that are actively being sorted out as we write these words. In defending the vaccines, the CDC is both attempting to deny that there is a real epidemic of autism (e.g., see the sources cited by the CDC, August 22, 2008, retrieved February 27, 2009, from http://www.cdc.gov/nip/vacsafe/concer ns/autism/autism-mmr.htm) while at the same time insisting that the number of cases has continued to rise even when, in certain cases, the vaccines have been discontinued, or in cases where offending elements in the vaccines have been removed.

More particularly, the CDC denied any harm from the mercury containing preservative **thimerosal** that was used in multidose vaccines—including the intensive series of shots known as DTP, DTaP, HepB, and Hib—mandated for children in the United States.

It is curious that the CDC has questioned whether the rising number of diagnoses is real while at the same time insisting that the increase is not caused by CDC-mandated vaccines.

In particular, the CDC and related federal agencies as well as the pharmaceutical companies manufacturing the vaccines have consistently maintained that there is no correlation between disorders such as autism and the mercury in vaccines. Approximately 30 vaccines, about half of them containing thimerosal, were mandated until 2001 (Cave, 2001). The cohorts of children affected by those vaccines would continue starting school up until 2005. Throughout that period the best research—including the data from the CDC—shows that diagnoses of autism have continued to accelerate.

Perhaps They Protest Too Much?

Why would such oversight agencies as the CDC, their parent organization which is the U.S. Department of Health and Human Services (HHS) formerly known as the U.S. Public Health Service (PHS), and their sister organization the Federal Drug Administration (FDA)—not to mention the doctors who have been administering the shots and the pharmaceutical companies who have been manufacturing them—be publicly questioning the enormous increase in autism diagnoses? In 1999, the United States Public Health Service (USPHS) joined the American Academy of Pediatrics (AAP), and the "vaccine manufacturers" (the pharmaceutical companies with billions of dollars at stake in the mandatory vaccines that the USPHS is responsible to monitor) in an official "Joint Statement" about thimerosal.

They all claimed that there is no scientifically known injury owed to thimerosal, but they thought it was nevertheless a good idea to discontinue its use in vaccines immediately:

> . . . the U. S. Public Health Service (USPHS), the American Academy of Pediatrics (AAP), and vaccine manufacturers agree that thimerosal-containing vaccines should be removed as soon as possible. Similar conclusions were reached this year in a meeting attended by European regulatory agencies, the European vaccine manufacturers, and the U.S. FDA, which examined the use of thimerosal-containing vaccines produced or sold in European countries. The USPHS and the AAP are working collaboratively to ensure that the replacement of thimerosal-containing vaccines takes place as expeditiously as possible. (p. 1, retrieved February 27, 2009 from a carefully worded two-page statement at http://www.putchildrenfirst.org/media/1.1.pdf)

The inconsistency of saying that thimerosal should be "removed as soon as possible" combined with the claim on the same page of the same document that "there are no data or evidence of any harm caused by the level of exposure that some children may have encountered in following the existing immunization schedule" (p. 1) was hardly lost on Dr. Paul Offit (2007) who is certainly one of the most outspoken proponents of vaccines. He wrote:

Critics wondered how removing something that hadn't been found to be unsafe could make vaccines safer. But many parents, frightened by a sudden change in policy, reasoned that thimerosal was targeted because it was harmful—and their faith in the vaccine infrastructure was shaken. Doctors were also confused by the recommendation. (p. 1278)

We find it interesting that the watch-dog agencies of the governments of the United States and Europe are collaborating with the multibillion dollar pharmaceutical companies manufacturing the vaccines in the supposed effort to clean up the vaccines. But the claim that thimerosal would be removed was not actually realized very quickly. Stockpiled reserves of vaccines with thimerosal were still being used in 2005 in spite of the fact that public statements suggested that the problem had been fixed in 1999—but to the contrary see the interview with Dr. Jon Poling, father of Hannah Poling, on CNN with Dr. Sanjay Gupta (March 6, 2008, retrieved February 27, 2009, from http://www.youtube.com/watch?v=Yxfg qsZ8BV0&NR=1). In that interview, Dr. Poling points out, as we have verified (see J. W. Oller & S. D. Oller, 2009), that the last of the birth cohorts receiving thimerosal containing vaccines would not arrive in schools until the years 2009 and 2010.

Until then, claims that the rates of autism are still rising after the thimerosal has been removed from vaccines, for example, by Fombonne (2008), are misleading. Similarly, the decision on February 12, 2009 of the United States Court of Federal Claims by three of the Special Masters assigned to the *Omnibus Autism Proceeding* that the combination of thimerosal and MMR vaccination cannot cause autism is a double absurdity. First, it is contradicted by ubiquitous research demonstrating that thimerosal by itself certainly can and in many cases does cause the symptoms of autism, as we show in this chapter (also see J. W. Oller & S. D. Oller, 2009, and references cited there). Second, the idea that the MMR shot together with thimerosal cannot cause autism is contradicted by the same Court in 1,322 other cases where it concluded that the MMR vaccination all by itself can cause brain damage leading to autism (R. F. Kennedy & Kirby, 2009). What is more, in the third week of February 2009, Special Master Richard B. Abell ruled in another of the three test cases being examined by the Court under the *Omnibus Autism Proceeding* that the MMR vaccination did cause the brain damage leading to autism in the case of Bailey Banks (see Abell, n.d., retrieved February 27, 2009, from http://www.uscfc.uscourts .gov/sites/default/files/Abell.BANKS.02-0738V.pdf).

In the meantime, the CDC, FDA, the vaccine manufacturers, and the professional organizations promoting vaccines, continue to question whether or not the rising rates of autism diagnosis show a real increase. In view of all that those agencies have at stake in the on-going war of ideas, it us unsurprising that they would prefer— as all thinking persons also would prefer—for the problem of the

While denying that thimerosal had played any role in the upsurge in diagnoses of autism throughout the 1980s and 1990s, the USPHS, AAP, FDA, and vaccine manufacturers in the United States and Europe all agreed that thimerosal-containing vaccines should be discontinued immediately.

autism epidemic to turn out to be an illusion. But, evidently it is not. The increase is not only huge and still growing, but it appears to approximate a smooth, accelerating growth curve (see Figure 5–1).

THEORIES TO EXPLAIN THE INCREASING NUMBER OF DIAGNOSES

A CDC Web site (n.d.-a, retrieved September 16, 2006, from http://www.cdc.gov/od/ads/autism/autism.htm but removed sometime prior to September 10, 2008) summarized a number of theories that might explain the increasing number of autism cases:

> Several explanations are being considered for this increase in autism, including [1] administrative changes (such as evolving diagnostic criteria); [2] better awareness of the disorder; [3] changes in risk factors; childhood vaccines and their components (in particular the preservative thimerosal); increased exposure to antibiotics and food additives; and ambient environmental exposures (for example, pesticides and heavy metals).

We have added numbers in square brackets for ease of reference to the main theories to explain the "autism epidemic." In the following sections we explore and document the CDC proposals and a few others besides (for a more detailed discussion, see J. W. Oller & S. D. Oller, 2009, Chapter 2).

Give-Me-the-Money

Among the theories of "administrative changes" mentioned by the CDC, is the notion that autism is being diagnosed more and more frequently because there is more money available for a diagnosis of autism than for many other categories of disorders. This idea has been referred to as the "changed diagnosis" theory. It is an explanation proposed by Newschaffer (2006; also Shattuck, 2006; Fombonne, 2008) to explain the increase in autism cases in the U. S. We call this the **give-me-the-money theory** of the "autism epidemic." It suggests that the skyrocketing number of diagnoses is due to the fact that disorders that used to be called mental retardation, Down syndrome, and so forth, are now being called "autism." Newschaffer and others argue that it is supposedly easier to get federal funding for treatment in schools, clinics, and hospitals if you just call the disorder "autism" irrespective of whatever it actually may be.

Have parents and educators changed the diagnosis of large numbers of children because there is more money for autism than for other disorders? In fact, the diagnosis of "autism" is in many states excluded from coverage by insurance companies (Jepson & J. Johnson, 2007; Autism Speaks, 2009). The situation, however, is changing. In Louisiana HB 958, which was signed into law by Governor Bobby Jindal on July 16, 2008, provides up to almost $40,000 per year for up to a life-time maximum of $144,000 for diagnosis and treatment of autism. Even so, we must wonder it there could possibly be enough money to make parents want their own children to be nonverbal, stigmatized by stereotypical behaviors, socially withdrawn in an extreme way, cognitively impaired, and plagued by a painful bowel disorder? In fact, Autism Speaks (July 16, 2008) pointed out that Louisiana is only

> one of eight states, to date, that have ended insurance discrimination against children with autism. The law requires insurers to cover up to $36,000 a year for Applied Behavior Analysis (ABA) and other necessary treatments until age 17. (retrieved February 27, 2009, from http://www.autismspeaks.org/press/governor_signs_louisiana_insurance_law.php)

Besides, how could the give-me-the-money theory possibly explain the increasing number of diagnoses of severe autism? Those cases cannot be impacted by such a motive.

Broadened Criteria

Also in the "administrative changes" category is the idea that "evolving diagnostic criteria"—more particularly broader criteria—may have generated the illusion of an epidemic. This theory may be called the **broadened criteria theory** of the autism epidemic. As advocated and/or discussed by various authors (Fombonne, 1999, 2003, 2008; Gillberg, 1999; Gillberg, Cederlund, Lamberg, & Zeijlon, 2006; Posserud, Lundervold, & Gillberg, 2006), this theory suggests that the expanding definition of autism explains away the "autism epidemic."

It is true that the criteria for the spectrum were theoretically broadened in 1994 to officially include In 1994, with the publication of *DSM-IV*, the class of PDDs was expanded to include "Asperger syndrome" and "Rett's disorder" as subclasses along with "Autistic Disorder" and "Childhood Disintegrative Disorder." Thus, the definition of the autism spectrum was theoretically expanded, but the central category of "Autistic Disorder" was actually brought back more closely in line with the way its discoverer, Leo Kanner (1943, 1946) originally defined it. The key factors have included: social problems, speech and language delays, and repetitive stereotyped behaviors possibly including self-injury. It is true that the criteria have been broadened with reference to milder forms of "autism spectrum disorder(s)" (ASDs). For instance, **Asperger syndrome** (also known as **Asperger's disorder**) was officially included under

Compare Kanner's criteria with those of more recent authors, say, Rutter (1978) or the *DSM IV* (1994) or the Autism Society of America (retrieved February 27, 2009, from http://www.autism society.org/site/PageServer?pagename=about_whatis_characteristics), and it turns out that the same basic criteria as summarized at the beginning of this chapter have more or less prevailed across the entire history of the diagnosis of autism from 1943 forward.

Recent research based on behavioral criteria (R. A. Ritvo, et al. (2008) and R. A. Ritvo, E. R. Ritvo, Guthrie, & M. J. Ritvo, 2008) applied a scale that was 100% effective in distinguishing persons previously diagnosed with either HFA or Asperger syndrome from typical (normal) adults, but their scale could not distinguish HFA from Asperger syndrome.

the scope of ASDs along with **Rett syndrome**. It had long been debated whether Asperger syndrome should be thought of as **high functioning autism (HFA)**. It has in fact often been identified as a particularly mild, high functioning form of autism.

Regardless how the debates about HFA and Asperger syndrome may eventually be decided, the critical question is how much of the increase in the number of diagnoses of ASDs can be attributed to the broadening of the criteria that allegedly took place in 1994? If the broadened criteria of 1994 were responsible for the increase, we should see a spike after that year (as seen in the dotted line of Figure 5–2) and later leveling off. But that is not what we see. Rather, what we see is a smooth growth curve that appears to be accelerating right until the time of the latest data recorded in Figure 5–1. Say the broadened criteria accounted for somewhere between a 10% and a 60% increase sometime after 1994. Could it account for the 1300% growth in the diagnosis between 1994 and 2006? The increase that has to be explained is far greater than the proposed explanation could provide. Also, the growth curve does not fit the explanation. Why is the growth curve smooth? How come we don't see a spike in growth following 1994 and later leveling off? Why does the real picture look like Figure 5–1 instead of the expected one shown in Figure 5–2?

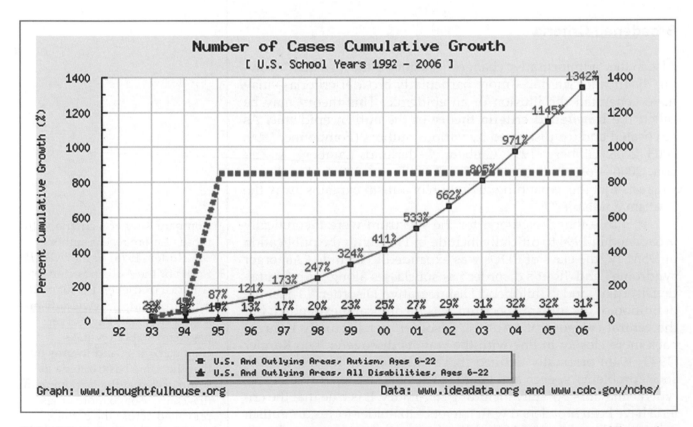

FIGURE 5–2. The dotted line shows the expected growth curve if the broadened criteria theory of the autism epidemic were correct. Retrieved February 27, 2009, from http://www.fightingautism.org/idea/autism.php? Modified and reprinted as licensed under the rules of Creative Commons Attributions 1.0 Generic.

The broadened criteria theory simply is not consistent with the data. It is also inconsistent with the more recent 2007 report from the CDC showing that the prevalence of autism continues to rise.

Public Awareness: Cause or Result?

Another possible explanation is that perhaps cases of autism spectrum disorders have always been out there in the past, at about the same level as they are today, but that they just were not noticed the way we are noticing them today. According to this theory, autism is more apt to be noticed today on account of the increase in public knowledge and awareness. This is the **public awareness theory** of the autism epidemic. It is the idea that increasing public awareness explains the explosive growth in numbers we are seeing worldwide.

It is certainly true that public awareness of autism and other PDDs has increased. The release of movies such as *Rain Man* in 1988 and other films with autism in their story line may have been partly responsible for the upsurge in the diagnosis of autism. On the other hand, such films may merely show that consumers are interested in autism because increasing numbers of children are being affected by it.

Autism as a Theme in Movies

Films featuring autism have included:

- *Backstreet Dreams* 1990 with Brooke Shields;
- *House of Cards* 1993 with Kathleen Turner and Tommy Lee Jones;
- *Forrest Gump* 1994 with Tom Hanks, Robin Wright Penn, Gary Sinise, Mykelti Williamson, and Sally Field;
- *Mercury Rising* 1998 with Bruce Willis, Alec Baldwin, Miko Hughes, and Kelley Hazen;
- *Mozart and the Whale* 2005 with Josh Hartnett and Radha Mitchell (based loosely on the lives of Jerry Newport and Mary Meinel—now Mrs. Jerry Newport); and
- *Snow Cake* 2006 with Sigourney Weaver and Alan Rickman

It may be worth noting that earlier films with autism as a thematic element did not achieve very much public interest. For instance, there was the 1969 movie *Change of Habit* starring Elvis Presley, Mary Tyler Moore, Barbara McNair, and Ed Asner. There was the French film, *L'enfant sauvage* (1969) about Victor, also known as the "The Wild Boy of Aveyron." The real child, on which the story was based, was found living in the woods near Aveyron, France in 1799 and may have been the earliest described case of autism (Lane, 1978). It is supposed that the parents of the child may have abandoned him in desperation. Interestingly, the early films on the subject did not seem to have a very great impact on public awareness whereas the more recent ones have captured a great deal of interest.

In the last several years, novels also have incorporated the theme of autism including John Dunning (2005), *The Sign of the Book*; Mark Haddon (2003), diagnosed with Asperger syndrome himself, *The Curious Case of the Dog in the Night-time*; Anne Bauer (2005), *Wild Ride Up the Cupboards* (retrieved February 27, 2009, from http://neurodiversity.com/books_fiction.html); Marty Leimbach (2006), fictional book *Daniel Isn't Talking* (see a review and comments retrieved February 27, 2009, from http://www.randomhouse .com/nanatalese/catalog/display.pperl?isbn=9780385517515); and Cammie McGovern (2006), *Eye Contact*. Someone has suggested that fictional stories written by parents of children with autism involve "autistic license" which we take to mean that some of that fictional material is true to life.

Meet Jason McElwain

When people get to know individuals dealing with autism all of them are motivated. To illustrate the point, see a high-school senior, Jason McElwain, a boy with HFA who had never been in a varsity game in his life play four minutes in the last basketball game of the season (retrieved February 27, 2009, from http://www.youtube.com/watch?v=1fw1CcxCUgg). Jason had been a team helper but not a player until March 4, 2006. His friends showed up at the game, knowing the coach intended to let him suit up and play. They came with his picture on signs they had made. Jason's coach decided it was time to let him play. The coach later said in an interview, what he was thinking when Jason first got the ball: "Oh please, Lord, just get him a basket." Jason missed a long shot, then a lay-up, and then hit one two-pointer plus six three-point shots in a row. He matched the team record for three-pointers in a single game while playing only four minutes. Jason made national news and even got to meet President Bush. Was his story part of the cause of rising public awareness about autism? Would it have made the news if people were not already especially interested in autism?

What About the Severe Cases?

The public awareness theory can, along with the other factors already considered, account for some of the increase in diagnoses of autism.

The public awareness theory can, along with the other factors already considered, account for some of the increase in diagnoses of autism. The public awareness theory is also consistent with the smoothness of the observed growth curve in Figure 5–1. That is, if it takes time to assimilate the changes in criteria for defining autism, a smooth growth curve like the one in Figure 5–1 should be expected as public awareness increases. However, all of the foregoing theories collectively run into one major problem: *How can they explain the large number of new severe cases, about 50% of the total number being diagnosed today?* The CDC estimates that about 50% of the cases diagnosed in 2000 and 2002 were also "cognitively impaired" with significant "Intellectual Disability or Mental Retardation" (retrieved February 27, 2009, from http://www.cdc.gov/ncbddd/autism/documents/AutismCommunityReport.pdf, p. 20). Also, it is worth noting that all of the *DSM* manuals from 1980—when autism was first officially recognized as a category of mental disorders—forward, all of the manuals have indicated that about two-thirds of the cases are severe. The 1994 manual describes the whole autism spectrum (alias the PDDs) as involving "severe and pervasive impairment . . . distinctly deviant relative to the individual's developmental level or mental age" (1994, p. 65). It says that only in "about one-third of cases, some degree of partial independence is possible" (1994, p. 69). *Could tens of thousands of such severe cases of autism have been overlooked in the past?*

Could doctors and teachers have failed to notice huge numbers of such cases for decades in the schools and in the clinics? Is it plausible to suppose that when Leo Kanner diagnosed the 11 cases in 1943 that there were actually hundreds, perhaps thousands more cases of children with autism who were equally or even more severely affected but who were going unnoticed by their parents and others in the world at large? If that were so, where are all those aging adults today?

Could a lack of public awareness be sufficiently deep-seated to prevent parents, teachers, pediatricians, and others from noticing thousands of nonverbal individuals incapable of maintaining social relations, dressing themselves, and who were engaging in repetitive stereotypical behaviors such as hand-flapping? The public awareness theory works fairly well with reference to mild cases of PDD with minimal impairment, but it fails as an explanation for the severe nonverbal cases of autism that constitute the majority of the cases.

Although an explosion of interest cannot cause the increase in severe cases of autism, the reverse is possible. If there are growing numbers of individuals being diagnosed correctly with autism, some of the explanations that have been proposed are wrong. If so, it is important to rule them out so that the real causes of the increasing numbers of persons being diagnosed with autism can be uncovered.

Would parents of a child who never formed social relations, never learned to talk, and who engaged in repetitive stereotyped behaviors such as high pitched shrieking, hand-flapping, and head-banging, have failed for, say, 20 years or so to notice that something was wrong?

An epidemic of autism could explain the growth of public interest in autism.

SUCH DRAMATIC CHANGE CANNOT BE UNCAUSED

Systematic (nonrandom) change does not just happen accidentally. It must have one or many real causes. In view of the inadequacies of the proposed explanations examined in the preceding sections,

One thing that can be said with confidence is that the growth in numbers seen in Figure 5–1 is *not uncaused.*

we turn next to what we believe is a more plausible possibility. It draws on evidences from genetic studies, experimental biochemistry, and a vast literature in **toxicology**—the study of environmental and other poisons.

Genetic Factors Play a Role

One indication of genetic factors in autism is that boys are about four times more likely than girls to be diagnosed. This gender bias together with studies of twins and close relatives, along with recent breakthroughs in genetics (e.g., D. B. Campbell et al., 2006) show that genetic factors are involved in autism spectrum disorders. Based on a sample of 1,231 cases of individuals diagnosed with autism, D. B. Campbell et al. (2006) found that a particular gene in the chromosome region 7q31 is involved in autism (also see State, 2006). Campbell and colleagues hypothesized that there are "environmental factors" in addition to "vulnerability genes" that "precipitate the onset of autism" (p. 16838). They refer to *epigenetic* interactions between genes and environmental factors.

Autism and neurological disorders in general tend to run in families. In identical (**monozygotic**) twins where one member has autism, the other is likely also be on the spectrum while with fraternal (**dizygotic**) twins the likelihood is about the same as with siblings—brothers and sisters who are not twins (Hu, Frank, Heine, H. H. Lee, & Quackenbush, 2006). D. B. Campbell et al. (2006) say, "Twin studies demonstrate **concordance rates** [where both twins either have autism or neither has it] of 82–92% in monozygotic twins and 1–10% concordance rate in **dizygotic twins** (Le Couteur et al., 1996). Sibling **recurrence risk** [the chance that two non-twins children in the same family will both have autism] (6–8%) is 35 times the population prevalence (Fombonne, 2003, Muhle et al., 2004), making autism among the most heritable of all neuropsy chiatric disorders" (p. 16834).

Cases Where Only One Monozygotic Twin Has Autism

For all the foregoing reasons, cases of identical twins where one has autism and the other does not are especially interesting (Gomase & Tagore, 2008; Petronis et al., 2003). They are important to study in order to find out what was different in the experience of the pair. Gomase and Tagore (2008) are especially interested in how environmental factors may have differed in such a case.

Cave (2001) reports the medical history of a pair of identical twins where Robert, who received a *thimerosal* loaded vaccine (for hepatitis B) at one month while his brother Ryan got the same shot four months later (age five months), eventually became autistic to the point of self-injurious behavior while Ryan did not become autistic. All that differed in the medical records of Robert and Ryan was the timing of the hepatitis B shot. Could it be that the shot, with its load of mercury, other toxins and disease agents, would have been less damaging after a little more maturation for Robert as it evidently was for Ryan? With identical twins, as suggested by Gomase and Tagore (2008), such a seemingly small difference in experience might provide the key to understanding the epigenetic interactions between genes and environmental toxins.

Genetics Alone as Cause of the Rise in Diagnoses?

To propose genetic factors as the whole explanation—that is, to propose a **genetic theory** of the autism epidemic—is not plausible on account of the fact that there has never been any such thing as a "genetically" caused epidemic. With respect to autism in particular, genetic factors cannot possibly change fast enough in human beings to produce the growth in Figure 5–1 or in the follow-up studies published by the CDC in 2007. Although it is agreed that genetic factors play a major role in autism, it is implausible to claim an exclusively genetic basis for autism or PDDs in general. Genetic factors cannot explain the upsurge in diagnoses. As Jon Shestack pointed out in 2003, genetic factors cannot cause the rapid increase in numbers of diagnoses that we have seen over the last several decades. No thinking researcher could propose the idea that the whole autism epidemic is just caused by genetic factors. It is easy to see that genetic factors alone can be ruled out from the evidence already in hand. Because human beings do not reproduce as fast as bacteria, fruit flies, plants, or even rabbits, a genetic theory of autism without any other interactive factors would fail to account for the growth seen in Figure 5–1.

Theoretically, damage to genes could cause an increase in diagnoses over time if we had multiple generations over the time during which the upsurge occurred, but an upsurge owing exclusively to genetics could not become evident over a handful of decades. Twenty, 30, 40, or even 60 years hardly allows time for multiple generations of human beings to turn over. Because of the slow rate of reproduction in human beings, the genetic theory by itself is powerless to explain the upsurge in the diagnoses of autism spectrum disorders as shown in Figure 5–1. Also, genetics plus the other factors already proposed cannot explain the increasing number of severe cases of autism.

There must be some other interactive factors besides whatever genetic factors there may be. For this reason, proponents of the genetic theory of the autism epidemic require additional factors to supplement their theory. Some theoreticians just add in the broadened criteria, heightened public awareness, the give-me-the-money tendency, and then assume that the rest is all about genetics. But we have already shown why those other factors come up short of offering

To propose genetic factors as the whole explanation—that is, to propose a genetic theory of the autism epidemic—is not plausible on account of the fact that there has never been any such thing as a "genetically" caused epidemic.

an explanation. Adding genetics into the mix does not escape the same basic problem: *All those theories plus genetic factors cannot account for the large number of new severe cases of autism.* For any thoughtful researcher, clinician, or parent—for example, see the remarks of Katie Wright in the interview with David Kirby cited above—it is evident that some other factors must be added to account for the increase in diagnoses. So the question is: what are those other factors?

Genetics Plus What?

Some have proposed an explanation that might be called the "genetics plus something-else theory." Previc (2007) writes:

> The incidence of autism has risen 10-fold since the early 1980s, with most of this rise not explainable by changing diagnostic criteria. The rise in autism is paradoxical in that autism is considered to be one of the most genetically determined of the major neurodevelopmental disorders and should accordingly either be stable or even declining. (p. 46)

> The rise in autism is paradoxical in that autism is considered to be one of the most genetically determined of the major neurodevelopmental disorders and should accordingly either be stable or even declining.

Previc, like many other researchers (e.g., Gomase & Tagore, 2008), is inclined to believe that there are other "epigenetic" factors, such as prenatal injuries at the level of biochemistry, that are producing the upsurge in diagnoses. In fact, the picture emerging from a rapidly growing body of research in experimental genetics and biochemistry, together with a long tradition of research in toxicology that dates back several decades, shows that some individuals, on account of their particular genetic predispositions have a harder time than others in producing or absorbing biochemicals that enable the excreting (dumping) of toxins.

The most plausible theory gaining support in the current literature (see D. B. Campbell et al, 2006; Chauhan et al., 2006; Geier & Geier, 2006a, 2006b, 2006c, 2007a, 2007b; Gomase & Tagore, 2008; Kern & A. M. Jones, 2006; MacFabe et al., 2007; Pasca et al., 2006; Previc, 2007; Rossignol & Rossignol, 2006; Yao, Walsh, McGinnis, & Pratico, 2006) involves a role for toxic injuries in combination with genetic predispositions. The injuries that set up the genetic predisposition for developmental disorders may themselves be caused by certain toxins that impact genes. Such injuries occur at the atomic and molecular levels of structure. The cumulative injuries at that level eventually show up in a cascading series of damage to cells. If the damage continues to accumulate, the injuries to cells produce damaged tissues, which result in damaged or dysfunctional organs, and eventually the whole organism is harmed. The application of such thinking as an explanation of the autism epidemic can be referred to as the **genes plus toxins theory** of the autism epidemic. As noted by various researchers, including the ones mentioned in this paragraph, this theory proposes the sort of interactive process that could produce the growth curve seen in Figure 5–1.

THE ROLE OF OXIDATIVE STRESS

The general tendency for the cumulation of atomic and molecular injuries caused by toxins is called **oxidative stress**.

How Oxidative Stress Does Harm

It is called "oxidative" because the processes of injury at the atomic and molecular levels commonly, though not always, involve oxygen. Oxidative stress damages atoms and molecules which impact, for instance, **amino acids**—the complex building blocks of proteins. As shown in Figure 5–3, the cumulative injuries have a domino effect that begins small and cascades upward to larger functional elements of the organism. In Figure 5–3, the upward cascade goes from genetics, to atoms and molecules, to living cells, tissues and organs, and eventually the whole organism. In extreme cases, oxidative stress leads to the death of the organism (see A. Chauhan, Essa, Muthaiyah, Brown, & V. Chauhan, 2008; Pabello & Lawrence, 2006; Segura-Aguilar & Kostrzewa, 2006).

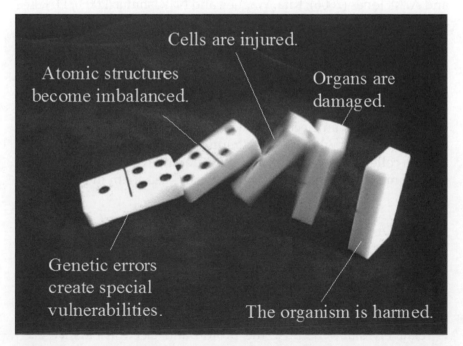

FIGURE 5–3. The domino theory (cascading effect model) applied from genetics upward through cells, organs, and interactions to the whole organism.

Although toxins can operate at much higher levels of the biochemistry, cumulative injuries can begin with an imbalance of something as small as an **electron**. An electron can be thought of as a negatively charged particle or wave. In an atomic system, an electron is attracted by the positive electrical charge of a larger particle known as a **proton**. When the negative and positive charges come into balance, the result is what is called a stable though dynamic "atomic system" (see Carpi, 1999; retrieved February 27, 2009, from http://web.jjay.cuny.edu/~acarpi/NSC/3-atoms.htm).

Oxidative Stress and the Body's Systems

Oxidative stress can cause the immune system and metabolism in general to function below par or even to go completely haywire in cases of what is called **autoimmunity**—where the body attacks its own cells, tissues, and organs.

Autism has been known, at least since 2003, to involve elevated levels of oxidative stress which also accompanies **neurotoxicity**—the sort of poisoning that impacts the whole nervous system but especially the brain. Oxidative stress also sets up a biochemical situation in which other bodily systems interacting with the nervous system get out of balance (A. Chauhan et al., 2008; Herbert et al., 2006; Jepson & J. Johnson, 2007). Autism is known to involve all of these factors and processes which are triggered by toxins.

There are a host of studies showing these connections. They include the following: A. Chauhan et al. (2006); A. Chauhan, V. Chauhan, Brown, and Cohen (2004); D. A. Geier and M. R. Geier (2008); James et al. (2004); Jernigan, Melnyk, Janak, Cutler, and James (2004); Kern, Grannemann, Trivedi, and Adams (2007); Kern and A. M. Jones (2006); Kita, Wagner, and Nakashima (2003); D. J. Lee et al. (2006); McFabe et al. (2007); Ming et al. (2005); Padhye (2003); Pasca et al. (2006); Rossignol and Rossignol (2006); Slotkin, Oliver, and Seidler (2005); Sogut et al. (2003); L. I. Sweet, Passino-Reader, Meier, and Omann (2006); Vojdani, Pangborn, Vojdani, & Cooper (2003); Yao, Walsh, McGinnis, and Pratico (2006); and Zoroglu et al. (2004).

From the biochemical point of view, oxidative stress involves either the loss of an electron which is called **oxidation**, or the gaining of an electron which is called **reduction**. These two processes are known collectively as **redox** and they are involved in essentially all normal metabolic processes. The key is to keep them in balance.

Atoms Out of Balance

To understand how out-of-balance atomic structures can do damage it is important to understand what balanced, stable atomic systems are like. The simplest stable atom is the hydrogen atom which has one proton and one electron. The hydrogen atom in that condition is relatively stable because the proton and electron balance each other with respect to their electrical charges. The negative electron is attracted to the positive proton and the two enter into a well-balanced relationship with the electron associating itself with the proton. The stable helium atom has two protons and two electrons; lithium has three protons and three electrons; and so on. Interesting complexities arise because of the fact that electrons, though attracted to protons, repel each other. However, setting those complexities to one side, in atoms (or molecules consisting of atoms) where the electrical charge becomes either positively or negatively out-of-balance, it is as if the atom gets into an active mode looking for a way to rebalance itself. An atom in that condition is said to be a **free radical**. If it seizes, and thus gains, an electron from a neighbor, the process is called reduction on the side of the former free radical, but it is called **oxidation** of the donor which loses an electron to its neighbor in order to establish its atomic balance. In the process of oxidation, the reducing agent loses electrons (gets oxidized) and the oxidizing agent gains electrons and is reduced (see "Redox," 2009; retrieved February 27, 2009, from http://en.wikipedia.org/wiki/Oxidation).

The trouble with oxidizing agents is that they become free radicals, which in the presence of certain metals can cause chemical interactions that are repeated many times over releasing more and more oxidizing agents until the cell is so damaged that it is either incapacitated or killed. As a result, the cumulative damage of oxidative stress can cascade from atoms to molecules to cells to tissues and organs and eventually to the whole organism with harmful or even lethal effects.

In the section just above this one, titled "Oxidative Stress and the Body's Systems," we already referred to many studies showing that autism and related disorders involve elevated levels of oxidative stress. In causing oxidative stress, toxins in the heavy metal category are particularly generous donors creating undesirable free radicals. Some metals are more harmful in this respect than others.

How Free Radicals Do Their Damage

The chemical reactivity of free radicals as they are seeking to establish atomic balance is something like water seeking its level. It moves, possibly with turbulence, until it achieves balance. Similarly, any given free radical will bounce around something like a loose canon until it acquires a resting place with an equal number of electrons and protons. In the meantime, until it gets tied down, it is a potential source of damage. While it is hunting for equilibrium, the free radical can combine with whatever other handy atoms or molecules offer it a landing place. It can also take electrons from its neighbors leaving them to bounce around as new free radicals.

In causing oxidative stress, toxins in the heavy metal category are particularly generous donors creating undesirable free radicals. Some metals are more harmful in this respect than others.

Standard Theory of Mortality

Unstable chemical elements, as a result of being out-of-balance, tend to be damaging to the organism within which they are bouncing around. Because such damage tends to accumulate, Denham Harman got the idea that the free radicals themselves are the primary source of aging—and thus of **mortality** (Harman, 1956)—as well as the degenerative conditions that are eventually and seemingly inevitably associated with it. For a 1998 interview with Dr. Harman, see Harris (1998, retrieved February 27, 2009, from http://www.karlloren.com/biopsy/p61.htm).

In an effort to counteract the impact of free radicals—the general descriptor for oxidizing agents—Dr. Harman began to search for **antioxidants**, chemicals and compounds that would bind the free radicals and render them harmless, thus increasing the life span of the organism. By 1969, his work began to attract the interest of other researchers and the public. When research showed that certain antioxidants such as **vitamin E** (found in wheat-germ oil see "Tocopherol," 2009, retrieved February 27, 2009, from http://en.wikipedia.org/wiki/Tocopherol), **vitamin C** (found in citrus fruits and especially kiwi, see "Vitamin C," 2009, retrieved February 27, 2009 at http://en.wikipedia.org/wiki/Vitamin_C), and **beta-carotene** (in carrots and sweet potatoes, see University of Maryland Medical Center, 2009, retrieved February 27, 2009, from http://www.umm.edu/altmed/ConsSupplements/BetaCarotenecs.html#Dietary) increase the life span of mice, rats, fruit flies, and micro-organisms, Harman's theory of free radicals—at least from the publication of Harman (1981) forward—became the dominant explanation of aging and mortality. The theory continues to be elaborated with respect to its details, but has become the dominant current theory of aging and mortality.

Kern and A. M. Jones (2006) sum up the connection of the theory of oxidative stress with autism in this way: "The increase in the rate of autism revealed by epidemiological studies and government reports implicates the importance of extrinsic or environmental factors that may be changing. They suggest that "toxicity and oxidative stress may be a cause of neuronal insult in autism" (p. 485). Toxins, of course, are introduced into our bodies from a variety of sources. Among the most surprising, controversial, and offensive sources for such toxins are medicines. We are particularly shocked to learn that medicines or other substances placed in our bodies to help us survive or to enable us to live more comfortably are actually the primary sources of oxidative stress. This is especially disappointing because we generally understand and accept the Hippocratic principle that medical practice ought to seek above all else *not to harm us* (see also the discussion of ethics in Chapter 12). However, potent chemicals, though intended to help by removing or preventing a problem, can sometimes be the source of more harm than good.

> We are particularly shocked to learn that medicines or other substances placed in our bodies to help us survive or to enable us to live more comfortably are actually the primary sources of oxidative stress.

Toxicology research shows that the mercury, still in some of the commonly used vaccines (notably flu vaccines), and the mercury in *dental amalgam* (the silver mental fillings), are among the most damaging poisons on the face of the earth. The mercury in vaccines is not the only toxin introduced in them (see Cave, 2001), but together with the mercury in dental amalgam, the mercury in vaccines and medicines is one of the main culprits known to impact nerves and genes. These and other toxins are implicated as exacerbating elements and in some noteworthy cases as primary causal agents in neurological disorders such as autism (for more research, see Chapter 10 on adult and neurogenic disorders).

In some noteworthy cases, the toxic materials are being injected or placed in our bodies by well-meaning health care professionals—notably by pediatricians administering vaccines during what are euphemistically called "wellness visits" and dentists using so-called "silver" fillings (a euphemism for mercury fillings) to repair our teeth.

Damaged Bits and Pieces

Oxidative stress accompanies many developmental and degenerative disorders. Not only autism, but essentially all of the neurological disorders affecting speech, language, and hearing are implicated. Among the ones that have been shown to be linked to stress caused by toxins, especially mercury. These include Alzheimer's (Nishida et al., 2007), Parkinson's (R. K. B. Pearce et al., 1997), multiple sclerosis (Edlich et al., 2008; Girard, 2007), rheumatoid arthritis, and many types of autoimmune and metabolic imbalances. To see what may be going on in autism it is important to consider how damaged bits and pieces of biochemicals can end up doing widespread cumulative harm.

Segura-Aguilar and Kostrzewa (2006) observe that toxins—such as mercury—interfere with important combinations of proteins and are "indigenous to Alzheimer disease, [and] Parkinson's disease" (p. 263). They go on to point out that a new variety of neurological disorders has emerged, **neuroAIDS**. In this disorder we see interaction between the **microglia**—the cells that police and clean the brain among other functions—and the **macrophages**—the main immune attack cells of the body at large. The macrophages are among the most important cells in the body's defenses against diseases.

In neuroAIDS the body's immune cells attack its own nerves creating inflammation that is "part of the neurodegenerative process" in Alzheimer's, Parkinson's, and a host of neurological disorders (discussed in greater detail in Chapter 10). As a result Segura-Aguilar and Kostrzewa conclude that we can now say that "the entire spectrum of neuroscience is within the purview of neurotoxins and neurotoxicity mechanisms" (p. 263).

A Common Problem in Autism and Alzheimer's?

It is interesting that oxidative stress and metals known to cause it are factors in autism and in Alzheimer's disease. Autoimmunity and toxic injury are both involved in these disorders. Alzheimer's disease has been known since 1906, when Alois Alzheimer [1864–1915], a German psychiatrist, published a report of a 50-year-old woman who had died with the condition just five years after he began to treat her. Her condition appeared to be an advancing **senile dementia**—a condition of deterioration associated with advancing old age. Because Alzheimer's disease commonly affects older persons it has sometimes been referred to as "old-timer's disease"—but there is no doubt any longer, if ever there was before, that Alzheimer's is impacted by toxins that damage cortical tissues.

Among the elements that are diminished in Alzheimer's is the neurotransmitter acetylcholine (see "Alzheimer's disease," 2009, retrieved February 27, 2009, from http://en.wikipedia.org/wiki/Alzheimer's_disease; also see Domingo, 2006; Ferreira, Vieira, & de Felice, 2007). The fact that abilities fluctuate within the same person in a 24-hour period, or over even shorter time spans, has led Palop, Chin, and Mucke (2006) to infer that conditions such as Alzheimer's disease cannot be exclusively caused by neuronal damage. It must involve elements of toxicity that can be intermittently overcome. Nerve cells cannot suddenly be regenerated so the changing levels must be owed to something else, perhaps ups and downs in the toxic impact of "abnormal proteins" (Palop, Chin, & Mucke, 2006, p. 768) could explain the observed ups and downs in abilities. An interesting story made into a 2004 movie, *The Notebook*, starring James Garner, Gena Rowlands, Rachel McAdams, and Ryan Gosling—from the novel by Nicholas Sparks (1996)—turned on the premise that the woman with Alzheimer's could sometimes regain lucidity and her memory for a few minutes at a time. If neurons had to be intermittently restored, the ups and downs could not be explained.

The current consensus is that certain proteins, in particular the **beta amyloids**, which are important to normal neuronal functions, literally get bent out of shape and broken in pieces by toxins, especially metals such as mercury (Leong, Syed, & Lorscheider, 2001), aluminum, lead, and so forth. Once this happens the twisted proteins end up forming the **plaques** that are characteristic of Alzheimer's disease (Ferreira, Vieira, & de Felice, 2007) as seen in Figure 5–4. There the circular formations define the offending plaques. The other hallmark of the disease consists of **neurofibrillary tangles** not seen in the figure but which can be seen in the video showing the neurotoxic impact of minute quantities of mercury provided by (Leong, Syed, & Lorscheider, 2001) on the DVD. Click on How Mercury Damages Neurofibrils. See a diagram of both plaques and tangles at "Amyloid Plaques and Neurofibrillary Tangles" (2009, retrieved February 27, 2009, from http://www.ahaf.org/alzdis/about/AmyloidPlaques.htm).

Metals such as iron, zinc, potassium, magnesium, selenium, and the like are required by the body for certain metabolic purposes. However, when metals are not properly linked to other elements for their normal constructive uses in proteins, they need to be quarantined or disposed of or else they will produce toxic stress. Some metals, in extremely small quantities, are much more damaging than others (see "Oxidative Stress," 2009, retrieved February 27, 2009, from http://en.wikipedia.org/wiki/Oxidative_stress). Of course, essentially any chemical, protein, or biological substance in sufficient quantity can produce toxic effects, but heavy metals such as mer-

Metals such as iron, zinc, potassium, magnesium, selenium, and the like are required by the body for certain metabolic purposes. However, when metals are not properly linked to other elements for their normal constructive uses in proteins, they need to be quarantined or disposed of or else they will produce toxic stress.

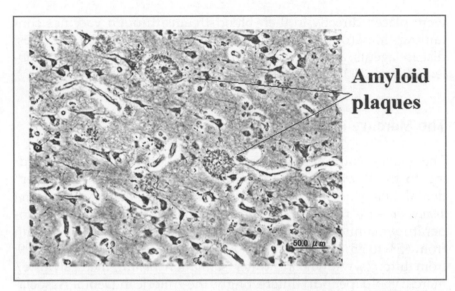

FIGURE 5–4. Amyloid plaques in the cortex of a patient with Alzheimer's disease. Retrieved February 27, 2009, from http://en.wikipedia.org/wiki/Imag e:Alzheimer_dementia_%283%29_presenile_onset.jpg . Adapted and reprinted under the terms of the GNU Free Documentation License, Version 1.2.

cury, lead, nickel, cadmium, manganese, and aluminum are toxic in relatively small quantities. Mercury is the most toxic metal naturally occurring anywhere in the world. Interestingly, mercury is the metal most clearly implicated in the case of autism spectrum disorders and it is also known to be involved in the production of the characteristic plaques and neurofibrillary tangles of Alzheimer's.

Metals are especially toxic for the same reason that they are conductors of electricity.

SEPARATING THE TOXICOLOGY OF MERCURY FROM THE POLITICS

The Environmental Protection Agency (EPA) has insisted that mercury is too dangerous to hold in your hand or to spill in our rivers and oceans. Contradicting this claim, however, both the USPHS and the EPA have argued that it is okay to put mercury in our mouths and in babies bloodstreams through vaccines. Mercury is a dangerous toxin. The primary source of mercury in medical practice is dental amalgam. For the developing human child from before birth, there has been mercury exposure mainly through the mother's body during her pregnancy. Later, however, for American children going to school, through about 2009 or 2010 (see Dr. Poling's interview with Dr. Sanjay Gupta, March 6, 2008, retrieved February 27, 2009, from http://www.youtube.com/watch?v=YxfgqsZ8BV0&NR =1), many were exposed to thimerosal in vaccines mandated by the USPHS—the CDC. For those children, multiple doses of mercury

Politically, there is "controversy" about the use of mercury in these ways, but there is none concerning the toxicology. Mercury is a dangerous toxin.

were placed directly in their bloodstreams through vaccines containing thimerosal. Also, there are other toxins in the vaccines, disease agents, and interactions between them that can cause problems (Cave, 2001; J. W. Oller & S. D. Oller, 2009).

The Mercury in Dental Amalgam

The greatest source of mercury contamination world wide according to the World Health Organization is from so-called "silver" dental fillings. Those fillings consisting of what is called *dental amalgam*—are a mixture of various metals that harden at room temperature mainly on account of the mercury in them. They contain from 45% to 55% mercury (WHO, n.d., retrieved February 27, 2009, from http://www.who.int/water_sanitation_health/medicalwaste/mercurypolpaper.pdf). Interestingly, the American Dental Association (ADA) still defends and continues to recommend dental amalgam as the preferred material for the vast majority of fillings (see ADA, 2009, retrieved February 27, 2009, from http://www.ada.org/prof/resources/topics/amalgam.asp). Their argument is that it is hard, durable, and relatively easy to work with.

Barr (2004) estimated that 55% of the world's mercury in manufactured products of any kind consisted of dental amalgam in people's mouths—an estimated 1,088 tons in the year 2004 (Barr, 2004, retrieved February 27, 2009, from http://www.epa.gov/region5/air/mercury/meetings/Nov04/barr.pdf).

As one of their arguments in behalf of its safety the ADA estimated in 2002 that approximately 70 million amalgam fillings were being placed each year in the United States alone (Bellinger et al., 2006). More recently, the ADA has raised its estimate to about 100 million amalgam fillings per year (see the ADA Web site already cited). The ADA says, if that many fillings are being placed each year, the mercury in them must be safe.

Environmental Contamination?

According to the official ADA web site (2007a) "less than one percent of the mercury released into the environment comes from amalgam" (retrieved February 27, 2009, from http://www.ada.org/prof/resources/topics/amalgam_bmp.asp). However, the World Health Organization (2003) reported that medical waste incinerators alone were accounting for about "10% of all mercury air releases" (retrieved February 27, 2009, from http://www.who.int/ipcs/publications/cicad/en/cicad50.pdf). Similarly, the Convention for the Protection of the Marine Environment of the North-East Atlantic (abbreviated OSPAR) estimated that in the United Kingdom alone 7.41 metric tons of mercury from dental amalgam are dumped in sewage, air, or on the land with an additional 11.5 metric tons being recycled or disposed of in clinical waste each year. Comparing this with the ADA estimate of 70 million amalgam fillings—which amount to approximately 12 metric tons of mercury in human mouths each year—a major source of mercury contamination worldwide is dental amalgam.

According to OSPAR, the "mercury contained in dental amalgam and in laboratory and medical devices, account for about 53% of the total mercury emissions" (WHO, 2003). The latter estimate is fairly consistent with data from Barr (2004) making the EPA and OSPAR estimates of contamination from dental amalgam about 50 times greater than the estimates of the ADA.

Body Burden

Research with human participants who have one or more amalgam fillings shows that about two thirds of the mercury in their bodies originates in the amalgam (Aposhian et al., 1992; Leong, Syed, & Lorscheider, 2001). In neonates body mercury is closely correlated with amalgam fillings either installed or removed during the pregnancy of their mothers (Counter & Buchanan, 2004; Razagui & Haswell, 2001). The research is also clear that combined toxins in medicines can produce potent interactive effects in neonates (Slotkin, Oliver, & Seidler 2005). Mercury damages the glial cells in the brains of neonates (Cedrola et al., 2003) and breaks DNA into fragments (Parran, Barker, & Ehrich, 2005). These collective findings implicate mercury as a factor in every kind of neurological disorder, in genetic damage, and especially in PDD and disorders on the autism spectrum.

Unfortunately for infants in the early stages of development, the mercury in dental amalgam is not the only source to be concerned about. As the main active ingredient in the thimerosal, which was used as a preservative in many medicines and in many childhood vaccines, mercury was introduced in substantial doses into many children. The mercury was used in thimerosal because even in small quantities it is lethal to nearly all bacteria. It was precisely because of its toxicity that Eli Lilly introduced it as a bacteriocide in the 1930s (see patents by Kharasch, 1932, 1935) for use in multidose vaccines for human beings. Since then, thimerosal (also the principle ingredient in the topical disinfectant known as **merthiolate**)—which is approximately 50% mercury by weight—has been used as a disinfectant in direct contact with bodily fluids in cataract surgery, kidney dialysis, nasal spray, contact lens disinfecting solutions, and in many other uses.

The use of thimerosal in vaccines was increasingly common through the 1980s and 1990s while the number of mandated vaccines was also increasing (Cave, 2001). As a subsidiary agency of the USPHS the CDC from 2006 has claimed that thimerosal is safe in vaccines and continues to defend its use in flu vaccines in particular (retrieved February 27, 2009, from http://www.cdc.gov/mmwr/preview/mmwrhtml/rr5510a1.htm). The Institute for Vaccine Safety provides a list—though not a comprehensive one—of vaccines and their thimerosal content updated September 9, 2008 (retrieved February 27, 2009, from http://www.vaccinesafety.edu/

Thimerosal has been used in the vitamin K shot commonly given to newborns, flu shots, eye drops (Bodaghi et al., 2005; Cave, 2001), and in medications such as Rhogam for Rh negative pregnant women. It is still present in many flu shots including FLUVIRIN and FLUARIX.

thi-table.htm). Note that quantities of thimerosal in the solutions mentioned at that site are given as a percentage of the total to be injected. In some cases, they say that certain vaccines contain "trace amounts (<0.3 mcg) of mercury left after post-production thimerosal removal" concerning which they assert that "these amounts have no biological effect" (see the footnote at the bottom of the just cited page with references to *JAMA* articles in 1999 and 2000—before much of the work showing that less than one part per billion can cause significant harm in preventing the normal functioning of critical bodily proteins (Parran, Barker, & Ehrich, 2005).

In fact, the research shows that thimerosal is not safe even in trace amounts. It has been shown to cause destruction of corneas when used in connection with eye surgeries (Bodaghi et al., 2005). It also causes neurological damage (James et al., 2005), and sometimes even death (see Rohyans, Walson, G. A. Wood, & Macdonald, 1984). Evidence that it was harmful to dogs, rodents, and other organisms, contrary to certain public denials, existed before its introduction into medicines for humans (see Kirby, 2005). It has recently been shown to cause autism-like symptoms in certain genetic strains of rodents (Hornig, Chian, & Lipkin, 2004). As a result of that study certain markers of toxicity have been identified in the urine of humans showing a link between thimerosal poisoning and autism (Geier & Geier, 2007a). Also it has been demonstrated that administration of thimerosal containing Rhogam does increase the likelihood of autism in the unborn child (Geier & Geier, 2007b). The mercury in thimerosal and in dental amalgam is cytotoxic (damaging or killing cells), genotoxic (producing harmful genetic mutations; Parran, Barker, & Ehrich, 2005), and neurotoxic (Bodaghi et al., 2005; Geier & Geier, 2006a, 2006c, 2008; D. A. Geier, Mumper, Gladfelter, Coleman, & M. R. Geier, 2008; Ghosh et al., 2007; James et al., 2005; Koch & Trapp, 2006; D. J. Lee et al., 2006; Lovely, Levin, & Klekowski, 1982; Marn-Pernat et al., 2005; Windham et al., 2006; Yole, Wickstrom, & Blakley, 2007). Concerning these facts there is no reasonable dispute.

The idea of placing mercury directly in human bloodstreams through injections or in the mouths of dental patients is—on the basis of the research in toxicology—an absurdity on its face. The only defenses that we know of for these practices are being offered by the parties with the greatest vested interests either in future profits or the potential of losses from admitting the harm done in the past. The only argument in favor of using the mercury in thimerosal in the first place was its toxicity. It is almost a universal **xenobiotic**. In very small quantities, a few parts per million, it kills or prevents cells from functioning. The argument was that the damage done to the host would be worth the cost if it prevented deadly infections. In the case of dental repairs the argument has been that elemental mercury is liquid at room temperature and forms a durable (though unstable) mixture with the other metals

The trouble was, as noted by Kharash (1935) and as demonstrated in plenty of later research studies, that the ethyl mercury in thimerosal damaged the hosts cells a great deal more than it damaged the potential infectious disease agents.

used in dental amalgam. In both cases, the dangers were weighed, to some extent, against expected benefits, and the risks of injury from short and long-term mercury poisoning were knowingly incurred not by the pharmaceutical companies or the dental associations, but by their naive patients. Now that we know more about the toxicity of mercury, it seems that the sensible thing—as independent researchers have long recommended (see the review by Mutter, Naumann, Walach, & Daschner, 2005)—is to discontinue all medical practices of intentionally putting mercury inside human beings.

THE LINKS TO AUTISM SPECTRUM AND OTHER DISORDERS RECONSIDERED

Among the most plausible reports suggesting the link between mercury poisoning and autism was a series of papers by S. Bernard (2004) and colleagues (Bernard, Enayati, Redwood, Roger, & Binstock, 2001, 2002; Bernard, Redwood, & Blaxill, 2004). They noticed that the clinical symptoms of mercury poisoning are essentially the same—indistinguishable in the way they present themselves to observers—from the symptoms of autism in its more severe forms. That is, the behavioral manifestations of mercury poisoning are nearly **isomorphic** with those of severe autism. For this reason, it is difficult to argue that there is *not* a connection between mercury poisoning and many cases of autism spectrum disorders. It is highly likely that other toxins, disease components, and injury producing events are involved as synergistic factors in addition to mercury, but there can be no reasonable doubt that mercury is a causative factor in producing the upsurge of diagnoses of autism and related neurological disorders.

> It is highly likely that other toxins, disease components, and injury producing events are involved as synergistic factors in addition to mercury, but there can be no reasonable doubt that mercury is a causative factor in producing the upsurge of diagnoses of autism and related neurological disorders.

Empirically Proving a Null Hypothesis?

On the other side of the question, those who have tried to prove that no connection exists between mercury poisoning and autism or other neurological disorders have undertaken a logically impossible task compounded by overwhelming contrary empirical evidence.

Trying to Prove a Null Empirically

To claim no impact from mercury in neurological conditions such as autism requires empirical proof of a null hypothesis. This is logically impossible because it requires ruling out all possible ways that mercury might cause neurodegenerative conditions. No number of experiments in any combination would be sufficient to do this because of a simple fact: *It is never possible to prove a null hypothesis by any number of empirical tests.* The most that can be hoped for is to disprove a null hypotheses—that is, we *can disprove the null claim* that there is no association whatever between mercury poisoning and autism, *by just one demonstration that mercury causes neurological disorders and in fact there are hundreds of such empirical disproofs of the claim that mercury has no relation to neurological problems.*

The Wright brothers disproved the universal claim that flight is impossible for humans. Edison disproved the claim that no metal could sustain a sufficient electrical current to produce an affordable lightbulb. Henry Ford empirically disproved all the general arguments against the possibility of horseless carriages. Roger Bannister showed a human could run a mile in under four minutes. It just takes one positive demonstration that mercury poisoning causes the symptoms of autism to prove that mercury is not safe in vaccines or in human teeth.

It has long been accepted that empirical science advances by empirical disproofs of general or universal claims (Platt, 1964; Popper, 1959). The Wright brothers disproved the universal claim that flight is impossible for humans. Edison disproved the claim that no metal could sustain a sufficient electrical current to produce an affordable lightbulb. Henry Ford empirically disproved all the general arguments against the possibility of horseless carriages. Roger Bannister showed a human could run a mile in under four minutes. It just takes one positive demonstration that mercury poisoning causes the symptoms of autism to prove that mercury is not safe in vaccines or in human teeth.

It is irresponsible to continue putting a toxin of such known potency inside human bodies. Only persons working on behalf of the vested interests at CDC, the American Dental Association, the American Academy of Pediatrics, and similar agencies, are claiming that additional empirical studies are required to show that mercury is harmful when injected, ingested, or implanted in teeth. The essential problem is admitted by Clarkson and Magos in their 2006 review article where they say: " . . . epidemiological studies, no matter how well conducted, can never prove the absence of risks" (p. 641). Actually, Clarkson and Magos understate the problem faced by the ADA, the CDC, and by all the professionals who have tried to defend the practice of putting mercury directly inside human bodies. For a devastating critique of their attempted defense see Herbert et al. (2006). No amount of failed research can refute a single successful study linking mercury poisoning to neurotoxicity and to communication disorders such as autism.

Once the biochemistry of the toxins had been researched and demonstrated in rats, there was no excuse for repeating the poisoning on a large scale with humans. Does it make sense to suggest that we should wait another 50 years or so for the epidemiologists to figure out how to show on a huge scale that mercury has caused vast, insidious, and long-lasting damage in human populations? We already have evidence of widespread mercury poisoning that occurred in Minamata, Japan and in Iraq as we will see next.

Correlation of Toxicity and Autism

Bernard et al. (2001) showed that the symptoms of autism and mercury poisoning are essentially similar. Cave (2001, pp. 67–69) includes a table summing up the symptoms of autism and mercury poisoning in a different order than the one which we use in this book. Here, we group the symptoms in terms of their impact on (1) the body, (2) the senses, (3) the motoric capacities, and (4) language, cognition, and social connections. However, we are still dealing with the same symptoms treated by Bernard et al., and by Cave. As is well documented, the symptoms in cases of severe autism and in actual events of mercury poisoning—some events involving substantial populations—are virtually identical.

In Minamata, a manufacturing process led to the dumping of mercury from about 1932 until 1968. Much of it ended up in the bay where it contaminated the fish and poisoned their consumers. In 1956 cases of mercury poisoning (see "Minamata Disease," 2009, retrieved February 27, 2009, from http://en.wikipedia.org/wiki/Minamata_disease) began to turn up. If those cases were being seen today, many of them would probably be diagnosed as autism, PDD, or a neurological disorder. Another instance of widespread mercury poisoning of a large population occurred in Iraq in 1971 to 1972 (Cox, Marsh, Myers, & Clarkson, 1995; also see University of Minnesota, n.d., retrieved February 27, 2009, from http://enhs.umn.edu/hazards/hazardssite/mercury/mercriskassess.html). As in Minamata, the symptoms of mercury poisoning were remarkably similar to those seen in severe autism.

We list symptoms shared by mercury poisoning and autism from the lowest to the highest affected representational systems. We begin with symptoms of damage to the autonomic systems (especially, digestion). We work upward from there through the symptoms associated with sensory, sensory-motor, and sensory-motor-linguistic systems. Each of the symptoms is well documented in scientific research cited in Bernard et al. (2001):

1. *Physical symptoms* (in the body and autonomic systems) shared by severe autism and mercury poisoning include skin rashes, inflammation of the skin, itching, tremors and loss of balance, difficulty sitting, crawling, walking, loss of normal muscle tone, for example, abnormally tense or abnormally lax muscles, unexplained grimacing and/or staring episodes, abnormal reflexes, unexplained and seemingly purposeless repetitive jerky movements, self-injurious behaviors such as head-banging, in extreme cases rendering the person unconscious, sleep disorders, problems chewing and/or swallowing, loss of control of urination or bowel movements, diarrhea, intense abdominal pain/discomfort in bowel movements, inflammation of the colon, loss of appetite, extreme narrowing of taste preferences, nausea, vomiting, lesions in the gut, and abnormal permeability of the colon.

Widespread poisoning occurred in Minamata, Japan where many people ate fish contaminated with mercury and in Iraq where hundreds of people ate seed grain intended for planting that had been treated with a mercury preservative.

2. *Sensory symptoms* shared by severe autism and mercury poisoning include sensitivity in the mouth and extremities, sensitivity to certain sounds, for example, the humming of a fluorescent light, and/or mild to profound hearing loss, sensitivity to touch possibly with extreme aversion to a gentle touch, oversensitivity to light, and/or blurred vision.

3. Shared *motor symptoms* commonly observed in severe autism as well as in mercury poisoning include circling, rocking, toe-walking, hand-flapping, head-banging, rocking or spinning motions, and unusual postures.

4. *Linguistic, social, and behavioral symptoms* common to severe autism and mercury poisoning include loss of speech production and/or comprehension, social withdrawal, mood swings, impaired face expression and/or loss of facial recognition or comprehension of ordinary emotional expressions of joy, fear, sadness, and so forth, in others, expression of irrational fears, irritability, aggression and extreme panic/anger tantrums, failure to make eye contact or lack of evidence of joint attention, apparent loss of intelligence, inability to concentrate or attend or respond normally, individuals may stop responding to their own names, regression to a babbling (echoic) repetition of surface forms without evidence of comprehension of meaning, loss of short term, verbal, and auditory memory for meaning, loss of ability to comprehend a series of events shown in actions or pictures, loss of ability to imitate or produce a series of intentional movements, loss of power to sequence, plan, or organize actions, or to comprehend complex commands, and carry them out.

Coincidence or Causality?

One of the critical factors in determining causation is the sequence of events. Which event comes first and which event comes later? We also look for correlated sequences of events.

Searching Out Causes

Researchers are a little like detectives investigating a possible crime. Like juries, they consider evidence and render a verdict. When many coincidences occur, chance can usually be ruled out as an explanation. Although it is often pointed out that correlation does not prove causation—for example, that fire trucks do not cause fires anymore than thunder causes lightning—the events in these trivial examples *are* causally related. The fires do have a role in bringing about the presence of fire tucks, and lightning does cause thunder by dispersing air molecules that come back together with a bang. Reliable correlations do not arise by chance, so they involve causation in some way or another.

When it comes to mercury poisoning and the neurological symptoms that follow from it, since the mercury is introduced prior to the poisoning, we are justified in supposing that the mercury is causing the symptoms. Mercury causes the symptoms of mercury poisoning.

But what about mercury and autism? Mutter, Naumann, Schneider, Walach, and Haley (2005), along with others, have noted that the observed increase in autism, and related neurological disorders, in the last several decades coincides with a parallel sequence of events involving increasing exposure to mercury poisoning. Since the 1950s exposure to dental amalgam has increased with the rising standard of living and the greater accessibility of dental care. Similarly, the number of vaccines required by law in the United States, and recommended worldwide by the Centers for Disease Control and the World Health Organization have risen in step with the skyrocketing incidence of autism and related communication disorders.

Is it merely a coincidence that the first cases of severe childhood autism were documented by Leo Kanner (1943) just a few years after thimerosal was introduced as a preservative in multidose diphtheria vaccine (Cave, 2001; D. A. Geier et al., 2008)? Subsequently, the number of vaccines, including those containing the mercury preservative, mandated for use in the United States, continued to rise concomitant with the rise in autism and related neurological disorders. Although the FDA, and other agencies such as the CDC and AAP (all with vested interests), deny any causal link between the rising number of children with autism and the concomitant rise in mercury dosing from mandated vaccines, there is no evidence in favor of their claim and there is a great deal of evidence disproving it.

The FDA only cites studies that have found no significant results. This is like trying to show that Roger Bannister never broke the four minute mile by referring to all the runners before and after him who failed to do so. On the FDA Web site (June 3, 2008) addressing the thimerosal issue retrieved February 27, 2009, from http://www.fda.gov/cber/vaccine/thimerosal.htm#pres), why are there no citations of the toxicology studies with rodents, sheep, pigs, dogs, monkeys, and humans that found positive results? Studies with rodents and monkeys show that the mercury in thimerosal and in dental amalgam crosses the blood-brain barrier and persists with a varying half-life depending on the type of mercury and the age of the organism poisoned by it (Burbacher et al., 2005).

Both the ethyl mercury in thimerosal and the elemental mercury in dental amalgam cross to the central nervous system. With dental amalgam the leakage into the bloodstream and vital organs occurs mainly as the liquid mercury contained within the amalgam is heated, or disturbed by pressure. For example, brushing the teeth, chewing, or drinking a cup of coffee causes liquid mercury within the amalgam to release mercury vapor (see "Smoking Teeth," 2009,

Both the ethyl mercury in thimerosal and the elemental mercury in dental amalgam cross to the central nervous system. With dental amalgam the leakage into the bloodstream and vital organs occurs mainly as the liquid mercury contained within the amalgam is heated, or disturbed by pressure.

retrieved February 27, 2009, from http://www.iaomt.org/index .asp; or click on Smoking Teeth in the DVD). Leakage to the blood also occurs when body tissues come in contact with the liquid mercury in the amalgam, for example, if the filling is at the gum line, or exposed to the tongue, cheeks, or to other tooth surfaces where the tissues come in contact with the toxin, noticeable inflammation occurs. You can see the inflammation in the tissues and in the gums it is referred to as "tattooing" (Edlich et al., 2008).

The ethyl mercury still being placed in some vaccines for children, notably the influenza vaccine produced by Aventis-Pasteur, is known to be highly neurotoxic in extremely small quantities—less than 1 part per billion. In defense of putting thimerosal in vaccines, the FDA in 2008 cited research claiming that thimerosal is safe in contact lens solutions from which it was removed by the FDA long before. Why was it removed from contact lens solutions? Because thimerosal used in surgery was shown to destroy human corneas (Bodaghi et al., 2005).

While the FDA says thimerosal is safe, its parent agency, the USPHS, the American Association of Pediatrics, and the pharmaceutical companies that manufacture vaccines recommended eight years ago that mercury containing vaccines should be discontinued or replaced as soon as possible by ones without the mercury (see the quote on p. 300).

If the mercury in vaccines is safe why is it prudent and advisable to remove it immediately? The rational conclusion is that thimerosal never was safe and that it is only politically expedient to say that it was. Interestingly, that claim is only being made by factions with huge interests at stake. The pharmaceutical companies are saying that the mercury was always safe and the watchdog agencies are saying that they were there all along looking out for the public safety. For these claims to avoid scrutiny, it is essential that the causal role of mercury in autism and a host of related disorders remain a manufactured mystery. In part 2 of her interview with David Kirby, Katie Wright expresses the dismay felt by many parents of children diagnosed with autism when pediatricians, neurologists, and many doctors keep saying: "It's a mystery. We don't know what's causing it. But we are sure it isn't vaccines." See Katie Wright's remarks at the opening of that segment (Foundation for Autism Information and Research, April 19, 2007, David Kiby, author of *Evidence of Harm*, in an interview with Katie Wright, daughter of NBC/Universal former Chairman, Bob Wright: A F. A. I. R. media production of www.AutismMedia.org, retrieved February 27, 2009, from http://www.youtube.com/watch ?v=IUNO25l1zFs&feature=related). But the "mystery" dodge is false. We do know that mercury is causally involved in a great many neurological disorders and diseases, and that it is certainly involved in either causing autism outright in many cases or in making it worse.

If there were no evidence whatever of any harm ever having been done by mercury, why would the FDA (2009) agree that removing thimerosal is "a prudent measure in support of the public health goal to reduce mercury exposure of infants and children as much as possible" (retrieved February 27, 2009, from http:// www.fda.gov/cber/vaccine/ thimerosal.htm#pres)?

TREATING THE WORST PROBLEM FIRST

The general rule in therapeutic interventions of all kinds is to treat the most severe problems first. The rule is well put by LaPointe and J. Katz (2002, p. 500). They say,

> When the lifeboat springs a leak, we do not worry about how soon it can be given a fresh coat of paint.

If a person is strangling to death and also bleeding from a superficial cut, we would generally try to clear the airways before patching up the cut. Similarly, if an illness, toxin, injury, or some combination of factors has caused an excruciating bowel disease accompanied by metabolic imbalances resulting in severe autism, wouldn't it make sense to deal with the gut condition before trying to address the resulting behavioral symptoms?

The best behavior therapy in the world cannot compete with the sort of improvement that is possible if the disease condition that is causing the inability to produce articulate language is removed. As LaPointe and Katz put it, we should seek "relief from the greatest evil" in setting priorities for therapy. This is an excellent rule to follow. We should treat the most serious need first. As rewarding as it may be to see a child progress from no words at all to an intelligible production of a single meaningful word, in dealing with debilitating disease conditions such as severe regressive autism, a very different kind of treatment may be far more effective.

The best behavior therapy in the world cannot compete with the sort of improvement that is possible if the disease condition that is causing the inability to produce articulate language is removed.

Treating the Gut

Commonly, with PDD, and especially with severe autism, parents have been encouraged to accept a future without hope—a prognosis of no progress followed by eventual institutionalization. This was the prognosis accepted by Dr. Bryan Jepson himself when his son Aaron was diagnosed with autism. He accepted the idea that it was just "another untreatable illness" (2007, p. 3). The psychiatrist that he and Laurie Jepson consulted advised them to prepare themselves "for the time when he [their son] would need to be institutionalized" (p. 2). The psychiatrist told them not to waste their money on "experimental treatments" because he had accepted the idea that the causes of autism cannot be discovered or known and that parents should be content to treat the behavioral symptoms— to reduce the hand-flapping, shrieking, head-banging, and so on, and to try to recover some of the lost verbal ground.

However, if oxidative stress, out of balance metabolism, gut disease, and toxicity are involved wouldn't it make sense to deal with those problems first? In the case of Katie Wright's son Christian, the Jepson's boy, Aaron, and many other children, treatment of problems focused in the intestines enabled huge progress. In the case of Ethan Kurtz, if it were not so well documented by his father Stan Kurtz (2009; retrieved February 27, 2009, from http://www.stan kurtz.com/; also see Ethan Kurtz's Recovery on the DVD), it would appear as either an incorrect diagnosis of a normal child or nothing short of a miracle. After two years worth of physical therapy sessions, applied behavior analysis, and severe diet restrictions, it was the clearing of fungus from Ethan's intestines that led to his remarkable recovery. Ethan went from not responding to his name, floppy child syndrome, hand-flapping and all the major symptoms of severe autism to speaking in full sentences in a period of just 21 days.

Also, his father reported that after his intestinal problems cleared up, without any chemical chelators, Ethan started dumping mercury on his own. As Jepson and J. Johnson (2007) argued, if the delicate balance of multiple systems can be restored, it seems that the bodily systems have considerable power to heal on their own. Systems that have been dysfunctional may again start functioning after a retreat from what Jepson called the "toxic tipping point" (p. 46). In fact, doing so is a logical and valid empirical test that should enable rejection of the null hypothesis that there is no relation between toxicity and autism. Next, we review evidence that removing toxins and restoring metabolic balance does, in fact, dramatically improve symptoms. Afterward, in the following section, we consider therapies that directly address the behavioral symptoms—"behavior modification approaches."

If toxins are causally involved, getting them out of the picture ought to give positive results.

Removing Dental Amalgam

In the case of dental amalgam, the mercury can be drilled out and removed, preferably in chunks, to be replaced by any one of several **resin composite** materials that do not contain mercury. For procedures that minimize the hazards to patients and health care professionals see "Safe Removal of Amalgam Fillings" (2007, retrieved February 27, 2009, from http://www.iaomt.org/articles/category_view.asp?intReleaseID=288&catid=30).

The dangers of putting mercury in human mouths and in taking it out are similar—except that it leaks into the body and brain for the whole time it is present in the mouth while it quits leaking into the body and brain after it is removed. Both processes, however, can result in inhalation of mercury vapors, swallowing of substantial quantities of mercury, and absorption of mercury into bodily tissues, the bloodstream, and the brain. If it is dangerous to take the mercury out of the mouth, it follows that it is much more dangerous to put it in and leave it there to do its damage over a long period of time.

> ## Propaganda Versus Fact on Dental Amalgam
>
> Contrary to many denials in trade magazines (for example, *JADA*, the *Journal of the American Dental Association*), paid advertisements, Web articles, and editorials published by the American Dental Association and agencies with a vested interest in defending the medical uses of mercury, there are well-designed research studies showing that the removal of dental (and other forms of) mercury improves symptoms of neurotoxicity. It is interesting that the ADA has published a lot of literature saying that it is safe to put dental mercury in human mouths (see ADA, 2009, retrieved February 27, 2009, from http://www.ada.org/public/topics/fillings.asp) but the same organization insists that it is dangerous to remove amalgam. The ADA acknowledges that the amalgam will contaminate waste water, get into fish that may be consumed by humans, and, therefore, is dangerous to remove from human mouths (see ADA, 2005, retrieved February 27, 2009, from http://www.ada.org/prof/resources/topics/topics_amalgamwaste_summary.pdf). How could the minute amounts that might end up back in someone's mouth be more dangerous than the whole amount that was there in the first place?

The research on the removal of dental mercury shows that getting it out of the body dramatically reduces symptoms of neurotoxicity (Mutter, Naumann, Walach, & Daschner, 2005; Mutter, Naumann, Schneider, & Walach, 2007; Wojcik, Godfrey, Christie, & Haley, 2006). Although evidence of the damage done by the mercury can persist long after some or most of the mercury has been removed (Mutter, Naumann, Schneider, Walach, & Haley 2005), the research shows improvements follow removal whether by drilling out amalgams or more complex **chelation** procedures.

The Chelation Alternative

Removing potent toxins such as mercury, lead, and heavy metals after they are already in the body is serious and can be dangerous if done without sufficient care. Just as consuming poisons can harm us, getting them out of the body can also produce harm. The problem is similar to rescuing an injured person by helicopter from a flood, burning building, or a cliff face. The rescue itself needs to be handled carefully.

For mercury that has been injected, inhaled, or ingested into the body in such a way that it crosses from the blood into vital organs —and especially into the brain—the removal process is complex,

Removing potent toxins such as mercury, lead, and heavy metals after they are already in the body is serious and can be dangerous if done without sufficient care. Just as consuming poisons can harm us, getting them out of the body can also produce harm. The problem is similar to rescuing an injured person by helicopter from a flood, burning building, or a cliff face. The rescue itself needs to be handled carefully.

can be unpleasant, and can also be dangerous if not done properly. The good news is that the results from well-designed studies show that symptoms of neurotoxicity are dramatically reduced by getting the mercury out of the body. To remove toxins from the blood and other body tissues after the fact, as we saw in Chapter 5, requires some form of detoxification and/or **chelation therapy**. The term "chelation" comes from the Greek root meaning "crab's claw" (see the *Oxford English Dictionary*). Its Latin cognate is *chele* which also means "claw." The word "chelation" suggests capturing the toxin as with a claw so that it can be pulled out of the protein where it is lodged and escorted out of the body (Muran, 2006; Vallant et al., 2008).

The healthy body has an important antioxidant—a detoxifier known as **glutathione** (**GSH**; Figure 5–5)—that is critical to the multistage processes by which toxins are commonly removed form the body. Children with autism and individuals with auto-immune disorders typically show significantly reduced levels of GSH (Buyske et al., 2006; Geier & Geier, 2006b; James et al., 2004, 2005; Mutter, Naumann, Schneider, Walach, & Haley, 2005; Sogut et al., 2003). Maintaining adequate levels of GSH is important to protecting DNA (Lima, Fernandes-Ferreira, & Pereira-Wilson, 2006) and in general

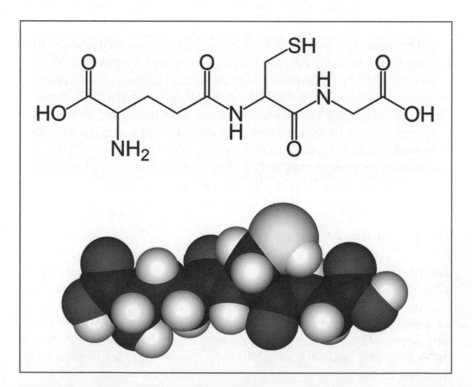

FIGURE 5–5. Glutathione (GSH). Retrieved February 27, 2009, from http://en.wikipedia.org/wiki/Image:Glutathione-skeletal.png and http://en.wikipedia.org/wiki/Image:Glutathione-3D-vdW.png. Theses images were released to the public domain by Ben Mills, Benjah-bmm27.

to guarding against damage from oxidative stress (Franco et al., 2006; Kaur, Aschner, & Syversen, 2006; D. J. Lee et al., 2006).

We include the chemical formula in Figure 5–5 and the colorful picture from Ben Mills ("Glutathione," 2009, retrieved February 27, 2009, from http://en.wikipedia.org/wiki/Glutathione) because GSH is such a crucial molecule to normal health. It is naturally manufactured by the body when things are working normally and is a critical component within the body's systems that guard against and damage at the atomic and molecular levels. The depth and complexity of the representational systems of the human body are nothing short of amazing. If the body's systems are working properly and are not overwhelmed by disease, oxidative stress, or other debilitating factors, they normally sequester and/or excrete toxins including heavy metals. Consistent with the gender bias in the diagnosis of autism, on the whole, females excrete toxins better than males. Evidently this is partly owed to the male hormone **testosterone**. It seems to reduce the male capacity to detoxify and/or may interact with certain toxins increasing their impact (M. R. Geier & D. A. Geier, 2008). Although the biochemistry remains to be worked out in detail, it appears that testosterone itself is susceptible to toxins and generates free radicals inducing oxidative stress (Prasad, Kalra, & Shukla, 2008). As a result, the demand for glutathione can be increased through the interaction of a toxin such as mercury with testosterone. The resulting impact of the toxin will thereby be increased. In some cases, additional help from a chemical that can latch on to the heavy metal and pull it out of the body may be of benefit and in some cases may be necessary for survival (for example, see Vallant, Deutsch, Muntean, & Goessler, 2008).

Large numbers of persons exposed to mercury and lead in the smoke at Ground Zero on September 11, 2001 were treated by chelation with **dimercaptosuccinic acid (DMSA)**, an FDA approved sulfur compound that attracts and captures the mercury molecules enabling the body to eliminate the mercury atoms mainly through the urine and feces (Kokayi, Altman, Callely, & Harrison, 2006). The first group evaluated for treatment were 160 uniformed service personnel—mainly police and fire—who were residents of Lower Manhattan exposed to the severely polluted air at Ground Zero for extended periods of time. Of these individuals, 85% showed "excessively high levels of lead and mercury" from inhalation of smoke and gases from materials off gassing these toxins. Most of them had eight or more of the following symptoms prior to treatment: respiratory problems, digestive problems, skin rashes, sleeplessness, anxiety, depression, weight gain, elevated blood pressure, lethargy, and recurrent headaches. After treatment for not less than three nor more than four months, 60% of the 100 individuals treated showed improvement in all of their symptoms. George et al. (2004) report studies seeking more effective chemical chelators and Olivieri, et al. (2002; also Cabrera, Barden, Wolf, & Lobner, 2007) are trying to find ways to protect cells from toxins already in the body.

Large numbers of persons exposed to mercury and lead in the smoke at Ground Zero on September 11, 2001 were treated by chelation with **dimercaptosuccinic acid (DMSA)**, an FDA approved sulfur compound that attracts and captures the mercury molecules enabling the body to eliminate the mercury atoms mainly through the urine and feces (Kokayi, Altman, Callely, & Harrison, 2006).

If removal of mercury relieves symptoms, it is reasonable to infer that it is a factor in causing them.

Meanwhile, the demonstrated effectiveness of chelation, along with the removal of dental amalgam, is prima facie evidence that mercury causes some of the symptoms of autism and related systems disorders. It may not be the only factor, but it is certainly one of those involved in producing and/or exacerbating them. The only arguments in favor of using mercury containing medicines or dental amalgam with mercury are being published by persons and organizations that have vested interests or legal responsibility for the known harm done by such practices over a very long period of time to millions of individuals. On a positive note, finding out what is causing symptoms of neurotoxicity is a crucial step toward curing them.

From Normalcy to Autism

In the case of Ethan Kurtz (see the video on the DVD), development up to about 18 months. By 20 months, however, Ethan had stopped talking, quit responding to his name, and had descended into severe infantile autism. As can be seen in the video, at nine months he was a normal, smiling, responsive child. By 20 months he stopped responding to his name or to any social interaction. He developed all the symptoms of severe autism—hand-flapping, lack of eye contact, retreat from social interaction, and loss of any apparent interest in or comprehension of language addressed to him. Ethan at 20 months was completely nonverbal.

For the next several months, there was no improvement and Ethan was diagnosed with autism in 2004 at age three. By this time he also had extreme hypotonia—a full body limpness of muscles as was noted by his physical therapist, Dr. Cheri Kay (at approximately 48 seconds into the video linked in this paragraph). When he walked his movements were uncoordinated as in **cerebellar ataxia** which is characterized by a general lack of coordination of the muscles and limbs. His speech therapist also noted that Ethan showed little interest in most play objects at the clinic except for a "Mickey Mouse thing that you pushed and it twirled around" (refer to the Ethan Kurtz video at approximately 1:37).

Severe Gastrointestinal Problems

In addition to all of the outward characteristics of autism, Ethan Kurtz also had digestive problems and there was evidence of infections in the **gastrointestinal tract** (GI). In fact, inflammation of the gut are characteristic of autism in about 70 to 80% of cases (Jepson & J. Johnson, 2007, p. 87). As Jepson notes, Kanner (1943, 1944, 1946)—the psychiatrist credited with discovering autism—commented that several of the individuals he diagnosed had abnormalities of the gut. However, he set them aside in favor of the idea that autism is a neurological and behavioral condition. In our own careful re-reading of Kanner, we found that at least seven and perhaps nine of his original 11 patients with autism also had symptoms of digestive disease or gut problems (for a detailed accounting, see J. W. Oller & S. D. Oller, 2009).

D'Souza, Fombonne, and Ward (2006) in a **prospective study** —one looking for GI disease in individuals already diagnosed with autism—found GI symptoms in 80% of the cases they examined. Similarly, Valicenti-McDermott et al. (2006) found a rate of 70% in children with autism against 28% in neurotypical controls. In Ethan's case, there was evidence of "bacterial and fungal overgrowth in his intestines" as noted by his father (approximately 15 seconds into the <u>Ethan Kurtz</u> video). Up to the age of four years, Ethan was not making significant improvement. But the more Stan Kurtz studied autism and his son's case, the more he became convinced that Ethan was experiencing conditions owed to disease.

When he was told Ethan was "too autistic to learn," Stan, quit his job as a technology executive and crisis intervention counselor, and began to work full time on the recovery of his son. Stan could not believe what he refers to as

> the resistance from doctors, specialists, family and friends. I was told by prominent doctors that I should focus my energy on fund-raising, that autism treatment was not science-based, and that parents don't change medicine (see Kurtz, 2007; retrieved February 27, 2009, from <u>http://www.stankurtz.com/</u>).

But Stan was not easily deterred. He came to believe, as we also believe, based on the research, that autism is as Jepson (Jepson & J. Johnson, 2007) puts it: "a complex metabolic disease affecting multiple organ systems" (p. 5). Stan concluded that "many types of autism and chronic illness are a combination of undiagnosed viral, fungal and/or bacterial infections that interfere with the body's ability to clear toxins" (see Kurtz, 2007).

Testing the Treatments

Readers may find it interesting that Jenny McCarthy (2007) reports also testing drugs prescribed for her son Evan on herself.

In the process, Stan discovered a great deal about autism and related disorders, and through a combination of dietary change, antifungal treatments, not only did his son's GI problems clear up, but also, within 21 days after antifungal treatment for his GI tract, Ethan made huge advances in speech and language. Ethan went from essentially a nonverbal, nonsocial, extreme form of autism, to speaking in intelligible sentences (see the <u>Ethan Kurtz</u> video from approximately 2:49).

Stan set about to address Ethan's autism, as few others have, by testing, as he put it, "on himself every drug, treatment, nutritional supplement, and alternative food source he could find."

There are still some elements in the articulation of surface form that a speech-language pathologist might focus additional attention on, but for all intents and purposes, Ethan made a full recovery from severe autism. As a result of his recovery from the disease conditions in his intestines, he also made vast gains in all aspects of language. While each individual is different and may respond to treatments differently, we come back to the essential rule as summed up by LaPointe and J. Katz: our priority as clinician/teacher/therapists is to provide "relief from the greatest evil" first and then to work our way down to the lesser problems. None of this, however, is to minimize the potential impact of physical therapy and behavioral therapy.

BEHAVIORAL INTERVENTIONS FOR DEVELOPMENTAL DISORDERS

With developmental disorders, therapies aimed at behavioral advances must be guided by knowledge of how and why development normally progresses. What makes a child advance from crawling to walking, for instance? Or why does an infant tend to move from babbling to meaningful speech? If we understand how and why these advances normally occur, then we will be in a better position to help individuals with disorders advance in spite of the disorders that stand in the way.

Understanding Where the Child/Patient Is

Recall the statement by Samuel Gridley Howe about the need to exercise patience in reducing the process of language acquisition and literacy to steps that are even more gentle and less demanding than those that are commonly followed by an infant. Howe supposed correctly that with tutoring and assistance even a person who became deaf and blind as an infant could acquire a language, become literate, eventually earn a living, and lead a productive life. As examples, we have Laura Bridgman and Helen Keller. The key, according to Dr. Howe, was to define a series of steps that an individual severely deprived of normal sensations would be able to follow. Howe's ideas and his approach were similar to what would be later recommended by Lev Vygotsky (1934/1962, 1930–1935/1978).

Working in the Zone

Vygotsky argued that a child can do things with a little help from a more advanced individual that would be impossible for that same

> The key, according to Dr. Howe, was to define a series of steps that an individual severely deprived of normal sensations would be able to follow. Howe's ideas and his approach were similar to what would be later recommended by Lev Vygotsky (1934/1962, 1930–1935/1978).

child to accomplish without assistance. He said it was as if, with the help of a more advanced person, the child could become "a head taller than himself" (1930–1935/1978, p. 102).

Vygotsky on the ZPD

He referred to the next step in the logical sequence up to the child's given level of competence as "**the zone of proximal development**" (**ZPD**). The question for any parent, therapist, or clinician dealing with any developmental disorder is just where the ZPD lies for any given individual. What, in other words, is the next step in development that the child is ready and able to make with assistance?

To discover that ZPD, and to define the series of steps involved in reaching it, or in surpassing it, requires knowledge of normal human development. In order to understand and to assist infants and children with severe communication disorders, as Dr. Howe observed, must be much more detailed with respect to the dynamics of human communications and interactions than is common knowledge. Although it is true that normal, so-called "typically developing" children, as is often noted by linguists, do not need any special tutoring beyond what they commonly receive from peers, siblings, and other interlocutors, children with disorders may need more intensive assistance and may have to advance in even smaller increments than a child without a developmental disorder would require. Typically it takes a child about a year to fifteen months to advance to the first word, but for deaf-blind children such as Laura Bridgman and Helen Keller, it took about eight to ten years. Similarly, it may require many more exemplars in much smaller steps for a child affected by a developmental disability to acquire a gesture, sign, symbol, or naming relation. A child affected by neurotoxicity, for instance, may require more time and smaller step sizes than a child who has not been injured by toxins.

The highest priority must be to address the causes of the disorder and secondary to that to we must find the ZPD for the injured child and work within it to optimize advancement. The essential question is what can the child do when functioning at his or her highest level. The level just above that is the one we must aim for and then we must adjust our goals step by step as the child advances.

Applied Behavioral Analysis

One of the most widely used and effective approaches to intervention, one that zeros in on the ZPD, is what is known as **applied behavior analysis (ABA)** therapy. It aims to break down the processes of gesturing, vocalizing, signing, speaking, reading, writing,

Although it is true that normal, so-called "typically developing" children, as is often noted by linguists, do not need any special tutoring beyond what they commonly receive from peers, siblings, and other interlocutors, children with disorders may need more intensive assistance and may have to advance in even smaller increments than a child without a developmental disorder would require.

and/or any other representational processes into exceedingly small steps. The key is to move the child in very gentle steps from whatever the child is already able to do to a more advanced level that is within reach. ABA is grounded in the theory of behavior developed by B. F. Skinner (1957). His theory is sometimes loosely referred to as **behaviorism** because he tried to explain away any need for reference to unobservable emotions and acts of thought. He emphasized observable behavior as contrasted with unobservable internal mental and emotional events.

B. F. Skinner

In Skinner's theory, an **operant** is a behavior that is, or is believed to be, subject to the consequences that follow from it or to the conditions that ordinarily follow from it.

Skinner's theory is more accurately described as **operant conditioning**. The idea is that an actor—an operator—acts on the world and experiences the consequences of those actions. For instance, Skinner's best known classic example of an operant **verbal behavior**, is shown in his claim that people learn to ask for water when they are thirsty on account of the fact that this often results in the consequence of getting a drink. The desirable result of the behavior of getting a drink of water after asking for water when thirsty increases its likelihood of reoccurring in the future. A desirable consequence of an operant behavior, therefore, is said to serve as a **positive reinforcement** for that behavior. In other words, it makes the behavior more likely in the future. At the same time, Skinner's theory predicts that **negative reinforcement**, also known as **punishment**, will result in a reduction of the operant behavior. Research shows that punishment is less effective in controlling behaviors than positive reinforcement (see Holland & Skinner, 1961, now available on line; retrieved February 27, 2009, from http://www.bfskinner.org/educational.html). The old adage that you can catch more flies with honey than with vinegar holds true in the research with operant conditioning.

Skinner's theory has been criticized as an oversimplification in the case of language, or what Skinner called "verbal" behaviors (see Chomsky, 1959; Morris, 1958), but it is agreed that Skinner's theory provides an excellent basis for many aspects of teaching, learning, and therapy for disorders. **Reinforcing stimuli** increase the likelihood of a given behavior (action) whereas **aversive stimuli** reduce its frequency or strength. Skinner observed that a rat that is fed a pellet of food each time it presses a bar, will tend to continue the bar-pressing behavior. If, however, no food is provided for bar-pressing for a sufficient number of instances, the bar-pressing will stop and the consequence for the behavior is **extinction**.

If every instance of a behavior is reinforced, the **schedule of reinforcement** is described as **continuous reinforcement**. If the reinforcement appears on every second, third, fourth, or nth occurrence of the behavior, the learner is said to be on a **fixed-ratio schedule of reinforcement**; if reinforcement appears unpredictably the learner is on an **intermittent schedule of reinforcement**, and so on.

Reinforcement Schedules

Skinner discovered that behaviors on continuous schedules of reinforcement are easier to extinguish than ones on intermittent schedules, for example, if the computer starts every time we press the start button, we expect it to do so on the next occasion. If it does not start up as expected, we may give up trying after only one or two failures. But, suppose we have an engine that is difficult to start and that requires multiple tries to get it going. In that case, we will persist and try many times before we give up. Skinner's explanation for the difference in our persistence has to do with the differences in schedules of reinforcement. An intermittent schedule of reinforcement makes the behavior more difficult to extinguish.

Dr. Vincent Carbone

One of the therapists who has achieved significant advances with children who have various developmental disorders including autism, is Dr. Vincent Carbone. Not only is Dr. Carbone able to get individuals with severe disorders to advance in communication abilities, but he is also successful in training others in the ABA methods that he uses following Skinnerian principles. The first step in ABA therapy is to observe and analyze what the child is doing in interactive contexts.

The first step in ABA therapy is to observe and analyze what the child is doing in interactive contexts.

Some of the observed behaviors may be desirable and others may be undesirable and counterproductive. For instance, the first objective may be merely to reduce certain disruptive behaviors and to encourage more cooperative ones. Screaming at a high pitch, for example, is not conducive to speech acquisition or to improved speech articulation. By contrast, looking at the parent/therapist to observe a modeled behavior is a step in the right direction. It can help move the child toward functional speech and/or signing behaviors and better socialization skills.

Also, the analysis phase of the program must ask what events cause the child to do things that are undesirable, ineffective, and perhaps even disruptive from the point of view of interlocutors as contrasted with actions of the child that are productive, acceptable, useful, cooperative, and the like. In each case, what is the child under observation/treatment trying to achieve? What causes the child to express distress, glee, calmness, or agitation? Once this analysis has been done, it is possible to put the child on a program where desirable behaviors are shaped in the direction that the therapist/parent wants the child to go, and in a way that will enable the child, step-by-step to move from less effective behaviors to more effective ones.

In his workshops on ABA, Dr. Carbone often shows video clips of real children as they progress from one therapy session to the next over a period of days, weeks, or longer. In one such clip, we see a child of five or six coming into the clinic with his mom. The little boy is agitated and pulling away. As the pair walks with the clinician from the waiting room to a play area, the little boy shrieks, pulls away from the clinician and practically has to be dragged kicking and screaming from one room to the other. Dr. Carbone stops the video and asks his audience if they would like to see that little boy a couple of sessions later. He clicks on the later session and we see the same boy as he practically gallops, without the shrieking, down the same hall with the same clinician. What has happened in the interim?

A Capsulized View of the Method

Step by step Dr. Carbone shows how during the first session, the clinician observes the boy as he calms down and begins to explore the toys on the perimeter of the room with his back to her. He shows how she discovers what interests him. As soon as she knows what the little child will regard as reinforcement, she puts him on a schedule to shape his behaviors so that the shrieking, kicking, and pulling away behaviors are diminished to the point of extinction while eye contact and desirable vocalizations are shaped and enhanced in the direction of meaningful speech and effective communication. The key with this particular child, and one that will work in much the same way with any similar child, is to provide the desired activity (reinforcement) shortly after the cessation of some undesirable behavior such as the shrieking.

The Shaping Process

As Dr. Carbone describes operant conditioning, it is a process of shaping new behaviors little by little. Say, the child shows interest in a particular toy. The clinician first observes this expression of interest. In the early going, it is essential to move away from the ineffective behaviors that prevent progress in communication. For instance, when the child is shrieking or pitching a tantrum, it is hardly possible to engage in productive communication or teaching. So, the clinician must patiently extinguish the undesirable behaviors in order to shape and develop desirable ones. While the child is behaving in an undesirable way, shrieking at the top of his lungs, she gets between him and the toy with her back to the child and waits until there is a brief silence, about two seconds. Then, she turns and produces the toy, and as Dr. Carbone says, "the circus begins."

She smiles and talks to the child facing the child while the interesting toy dances between them. This "circus" continues until the shrieking or some other undesirable behavior recurs. Then the circus ends, the clinician turns her back and waits for the child to calm down again. After two seconds of silence, the circus returns, and so forth. Within a few short sessions, the child's behavior has been shaped to a degree that the shrieking is completely extinguished and the child is interacting with, vocalizing appropriately, and moving forward on the developmental scale toward speech and effective communication.

Dr. Carbone has video clips showing children who started as completely nonverbal and after a few weeks or months of therapy were able to begin talking, or in some cases using meaningful manual signs. The key is to find out what the child is interested in, that is, what is reinforcing to the child, and then use the "circus" to shape desired behaviors bit by bit in the direction of effective socialization and communication. Examples can be given of moving from a completely nonverbal child in a first grade class to one who is effectively communicating with classmates through some verbalization and manual signing.

Appeals to All Available Modalities

One of the things that we particularly like about Dr. Carbone's adaptation and extension of Skinner's operant conditioning paradigm is that Dr. Carbone uses all the modalities of sense, movement, and language and adjusts his intervention to suit the particular strengths of the child in whatever modality will work best. He uses speech, manual signs, pictures, gestures, objects, food, tickling, hugging, bouncing on a trampoline, or whatever works to reinforce desirable socialization and to extinguish ineffective or disruptive behaviors. He finds and works within what Vygotsky called the ZPD.

One of Dr. Carbone's techniques, which relies heavily on the sort of cross-modal transfer that we dealt with in Chapter 4, involves the combination of manual signing, reinforcing action, and verbalization. For instance, the gesture for hugging with the arms crossed against the chest while rocking back and forth as if hugging a child can be combined with hugging the child so as to suggest the linking of the sign with the action. This is what we call a pragmatic mapping exemplar. The child sees the gesture and then experiences the meaning of it when his mom wraps him in her arms and hugs him. Dr. Carbone, however, takes it a step further.

The Delay Technique

If we can get the child to use the gesture to suggest that he wants mom to give him a hug, and if mom reinforces the manual sign with a hug, it is possible to connect both of these representational and highly social acts with the verbalization of the word "hug."

The trick that Dr. Carbone suggests to precipitate this sort of advance is to withhold the reinforcement for a few moments or seconds after the child has done the manual sign. He calls this the

Dr. Carbone has video clips showing children who started as completely nonverbal and after a few weeks or months of therapy were able to begin talking, or in some cases using meaningful manual signs. The key is to find out what the child is interested in, that is, what is reinforcing to the child, and then use the "circus" to shape desired behaviors bit by bit in the direction of effective socialization and communication.

Once the idea is implanted in the child's head that the manual sign means "give me a hug" and is apt to produce the desired event—the reinforcing hug—it is possible for the same child, though nonverbal up to now, to get the idea that the word "hug" will produce the same reinforcement.

delay technique. For instance, in the case of the sign for hugging with the hands across the chest, delaying the reinforcement prods the child to move up to the ZPD. It provides the learner with the incentive to move up to a spoken word. Here, with her permission, is one mom's true account of exactly how this happened with her nonverbal child the evening after she attended one of Dr. Carbone's workshops (see the whole story of the Autism07 conference retrieved February 27, 2009, from http://www.autism07.com/index.html):

> I would like people to know that I have a 5-year-old son with autism and he has never spoken. I went home and tried some of the Carbone training with my son. For the first time ever he looked at me and tried to say hug. I showed him the sign for hug several times and would give him a hug. Then he started doing the sign for hug and waiting for me to give him a hug . . . Then one of the times, he showed me the sign for hug, and I did not hug him right away [Carbone's delay technique], so he said 'ug', 'ug' several times. (Mrs. Lorine Ward, Pearl River, LA)

What ABA can do in the hands of a thoughtful, patient, and persistent interlocutor—parent, therapist, or any caregiver—is to identify the ZPD for the child and then define a series of steps that can enable advancement.

Of course, there is a long journey from the first word to mature adult level communication, but the movement from no words at all to the first meaningful word is a huge advance from the point of view of any normal child, and it is a huge step also for a nonverbal individual at any age. By linking a series of such tiny, almost infinitely small steps, it is theoretically and actually possible to accomplish a great deal and to move through major milestones of development.

SUMMING UP AND LOOKING AHEAD

In this chapter, we have considered major developmental disorders with primary focus on the rapidly increasing diagnosis known as autism. Autism is at the center of the pervasive developmental disorders that can affect any or all of the systems involved in communication. As we saw in this chapter, there has been an upsurge in the number of diagnoses of autism over the last several decades. We saw why this change cannot be explained merely by changing diagnoses to follow funding, broadened criteria for what counts as autism, increased public awareness, an exclusively genetic explanation, or any combination of these factors. Crucial test cases are the severe ones that account for about 50% of the total number. It is unlikely that persons who cannot dress themselves or engage in conversation could go unnoticed in homes, schools, and the marketplace for several decades. It appears that there has been a genuine increase in the number of cases of severe autism in the last several decades. It has gone from a prevalence of less than 1 in 30,000 to about 1 in 150. It is doubtful that the severe cases being diagnosed today have been out there all along, since say the 1930s, but unnoticed.

With that in mind we asked about causal explanations. Genetics alone cannot explain the upsurge, but if we add oxidative stress to certain genetic propensities we come upon a plausible theory. The stress can be caused by toxins from vaccines, dental amalgam, and other sources. We reviewed research in experimental biochemistry and especially in toxicology showing that major sources of oxidative stress include the thimerosal in medicines, still in some vaccines, and the mercury in dental amalgam. Experimental evidence shows that toxins such as mercury in combination with other stress factors and genetic tendencies can produce all the symptoms associated with PDDs and especially neurological disorders. We saw that the agencies and professional organizations that have promoted the use of mercury—the Federal Drug Administration, the Centers for Disease Control, the American Dental Association, the American Academy of Pediatrics, and so forth—while admitting that mercury is a potent neurotoxin, genotoxin, cytotoxin, and a general xenobiotic continue to hold that its use in medicines, vaccines, and dental amalgam has done no harm. They warn us about mercury in fish, factories, water, air, and so forth, while claiming that the estimated 1,088 tons of mercury in human mouths (55% of all the industrially produced mercury in the world) has nothing to do with the still skyrocketing increase in diagnoses of autism and other neurological disorders.

The research shows that such explanations cannot possible be correct. Mercury is one of the demonstrated causes of the elevated oxidative stress associated with neurological disorders and diseases of all sorts. The research also shows that if we get the toxins out of the mix—by removing dental amalgam, thimerosal, and mercury from poisoned smoke—we alleviate neurological and other symptoms. For this reason detoxification is the first recommended step to be accompanied or followed by behavior analysis and intervention of the sort seen in Dr. Carbone's ABA. Such sensible therapies take advantage of cross-modal integration, ranking, and layering as seen in Chapter 4. Here in this chapter, we saw how ABA can work at the threshold of the first word for a nonverbal child with autism who said the word "hug" for the first time after first demonstrating comprehension and use of the manual sign. In the following chapter we expand on motor disorders that affect both autonomic and conscious processes.

> Genetics alone cannot explain the upsurge, but if we add oxidative stress to certain genetic propensities we come upon a plausible theory.

STUDY AND DISCUSSION QUESTIONS

1. Why have thoughtful researchers in recent years generally come to the conclusion voiced by Previc (2007) that the rising incidence of autism is "not explainable by changing diagnostic criteria" (p. 46)? What arguments have been produced refuting the claim that broadened criteria, public awareness, and availability

of funding for therapies are the best explanation for the 200-fold (20,000%) increase in the diagnosis of autism since the 1930s?

2. Why are severe instances of autism of special interest as test cases? Why is it that severe cases of autism would be difficult to overlook for several decades if there had been hundreds, thousands, even millions of them at large, say, since the 1930s?

3. What do you personally think of the theory that parents and others might want to change a diagnosis from, say, ADHD to autism in order to get federal funding for therapy?

4. Discuss the increasing public awareness about autism disorders. Could public awareness be causing the illusion of an autism epidemic, or is the upsurge in autism more likely to be causing the increase in public awareness? What about the severe cases of autism? To what extent are they apt to be impacted by public awareness?

5. Supposing that D. B. Campbell et al. (2006) are correct in arguing that autism "is among the most heritable" of disorders, then, why is it that it cannot be caused entirely by genetic factors? Following the same line of thought, if autism is not caused entirely by genetic factors what about other genetically linked disorders? If autism is at the center of PDDs, what about all of them? And, for autism and related neurological disorders, what made the genes to go wrong in the first place? If the genes are changing so as to make many children more susceptible to autism than prior to the 1930s, say, what could have made the genes change?

6. How do we know for sure that genetic problems are part of but not the whole picture in autism? What about oxidative stress and toxins? How do we know that mercury is bound to make things worse for persons who have the genetic propensity for autism? By the same token, why shouldn't we take seriously the empirical studies published by the vaccine industry and the American Dental Association showing that mercury in the blood and mouths of children is perfectly safe? Does the difficulty of proving a null hypothesis ring any bells?

7. In treating developmental disorders why is it important to do appropriate analysis of behaviors to determine the zone of proximal development? How do normal milestones of development enter the picture? Why do we need to know about them?

8. In dealing with communication disorders what role is played by cross-modal integration, ranking, and layering of systems? More specifically, how can we capitalize on what we know of cross-modal integration?

6

Swallowing, Voice, and "Motor" Speech

OBJECTIVES

In this chapter, we:

1. Discuss why SLPs treat swallowing disorders along with voice and speech;

2. Examine the mouth as center for intake of food and liquid and outflow of speech;

3. Analyze the form, function, and control of breathing, swallowing, voice, and speech;

4. Consider motor systems in voice, speech, breathing, eating, drinking, and digestion;

5. Expand the descriptors of voice qualities to illustrate symptoms of disorders;

6. Discuss disorders that disrupt motor functions in swallowing, voice, and speech; and

7. Introduce some treatments and priorities for motor disorders.

KEY TERMS

Here are some key terms of this chapter. Many of them you may already know. It may help to review them. These terms are explained in the text and they are defined in the Glossary at the end of the book. They appear in **bold print** on their first appearance in the text.

abducted
acetylcholine
acid reflux
adducted
adrenaline
alien hand syndrome
aspiration pneumonia
ataxic dysarthria
atrophy
axon
basal ganglia
Bell's palsy
Bernoulli effect
Botox
Botulinum neurotoxin
botulism
bulbar palsy
bulbar region
carcinogenic qualities
clinical neurology
Clostridium botulinum
Clostridium tetani
consonant cluster
contact ulcers
contralateral
corpus callosum
corticospinal tract
cranial nerves
Crohn's disease
decussation of pyramids
dementia
dendrites
diagonistic dyspraxia
dopamine
dyspraxia
epiglottis
epinephrine
esophagus
expiratory reserve volume

extrapyramidal tract
fasciculation
flaccid dysarthrias
foreign accent syndrome
fricative sounds
functional disorders
GABA
gamma amino butyric acid
gastroesophageal reflux
   disease
gaze
geniculate fibers
genotoxic
GERD
gliotransmissions
glutamate
granulomas
Gulf War syndrome
hard glottal attack
Helicobacter pylori
HPV
human papilloma virus
Huntington's chorea
Huntington's disease
hyperfunction disorders
hypertonia
hypokinetic dysarthrias
hypotonia
inspiratory reserve volume
internal capsule
intubation
ipsilateral
lability
laryngeal webbing
larynx
lateral cerebrospinal fasciculus
lower motor neuron
LMN
medulla oblongata

mixed dysarthrias
monosyllabic word
myasthenia gravis
myoelastic aerodynamic
   theory of phonation
nuclei of the cranial nerves
Parkinson's disease
parotid salivary gland
PD
peptic ulcers
pharyngeal cavity
pharynx
phonation
polyps
positions of discourse
prognosis
progressive palsy
pseudobulbar affect
pseudobulbar palsy
pyramidal tract
residual volume
singer's nodes
solar plexus
spastic dysphonia
spastic dysarthrias
stridor
stylopharyngeus
substantia nigra
tetanospasmin
trachea
tracheostomy
trigeminal neuralgia
UMN
unilateral motor neuron
   dysarthria
upper motor neuron
vegetative movements
vital capacity
vocal hygiene

| vocal nodules | vocalic center | wavelength |
| vocal timbre | voice disorder | white noise |

In this chapter, we provide an overview of disorders that are usually grouped under the categories of swallowing, voice, and "motor" speech disorders. At first look, swallowing appears to be the "odd man out" so to speak. Why is it included with the others? In keeping with the principle of prioritizing the therapy or theory-building by taking the most difficult issue first, the puzzling question about swallowing is a good place to start this chapter.

From that question we proceed to motor dynamics of swallowing, voice in nonspeech and speech vocalizations, and the motor control of speaking itself. Along the way we discover some profound differences between the motor acts of swallowing as contrasted with the use of voice in speaking. By contrast, speech is primarily intended in its normal uses to communicate with others—so all three **positions of discourse** come into play in acts of speaking (as shown in Figure 6–1). That is, in speech we have the producer, the intended audience (consumer), and the whole rest of the world in which the vocalization takes place. Speaking obviously is intended for communication but swallowing rarely plays a role in intentional acts of communication.

In this chapter, we focus special attention on the complex switching between voluntary acts and autonomic ones—also between voiced and nonvoiced segments in syllables. It is noted that speech

What does swallowing have to do with voice, speech, and language or with communication and its disorders? Why would disorders of such diverse processes as speech and swallowing come together in any way? More particularly, why are swallowing disorders treated by speech-language pathologists? Swallowing hardly seems to be related to speech, much less to other language processes such as verbal thinking, reading, writing, or manual signing.

In swallowing, only one position of discourse is usually in view —the producer of the act—and, in most cases, only incidentally does swallowing impact other observers and interlocutors.

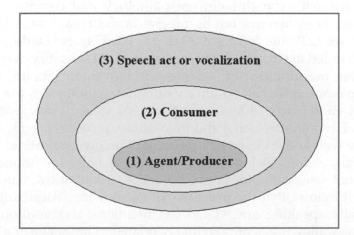

FIGURE 6–1. The inclusion of the discourse position 1 in 2 and 1 and 2 in 3—all in the same common world.

movements are carried out with much greater speed than what are commonly called **vegetative movements**—chewing, swallowing, digestion, and elimination of wastes. In introducing these processes we consider the diagnostic value of the symptoms and treatment of related motor disorders. We deal with additional motor disorders of speech in Chapter 7 on articulation and in Chapter 8 on dysfluencies. So, in this chapter, the concentration is on the interactions of motor systems involved in breathing, swallowing, voice, and speech.

SWALLOWING DISORDERS TREATED BY SPEECH-LANGUAGE PATHOLOGISTS

Our first question is the one that people usually think of when they learn that speech-pathologists are the therapists of choice to treat swallowing disorders. Why do speech-language pathologists typically end up treating swallowing disorders? It is easy to see why voice disorders would get the attention of speech-language pathologists, but why swallowing?

"Motor Speech" Processes: A Mixed Bag

It is interesting that the redundant phrase "motor speech" has commonly been used to emphasize the fact that speaking requires movement.

The phrase "motor speech" focuses attention on the underlying systems that normally enable intentional control of voice, swallowing, and speech. Of course, it isn't possible to perform any of these acts of without movement and yet not all of them involve speaking. But, as other researchers have often commented, the terminology associated with speech-language pathology and communication disorders is sometimes not as precise or systematic as might be hoped (see LaPointe & J. Katz, 2002, pp. 478-479; also Darley, 1967).

As noted in Chapter 5, movement without sensation would be senseless, meaningless, and purposeless movement. So, it is useful to keep in mind that all voluntary intentional motor acts are really sensory-motor acts unless something has gone wrong with the senses. Even unintentional and involuntary movements, for example, the well-known knee jerk reflex, still involve sensation. When voluntary actions include voice, they are usually intentional and volitional sensory-motor-linguistic actions (Bohland & Guenther, 2006). It follows that the processes of swallowing, vocalizing, and especially speaking are related by intentions and volition even though swallowing is not obviously related to language at all.

Although swallowing, voice, and speech, all come under deliberate volitional control to some extent, they are very different phenomena. The voice and speech are closely interrelated and linked to language whereas swallowing is only indirectly related to either voice or speech. Vocalization as it occurs in speech production is quite distinct from the chewing and swallowing of food or liquid. To the extent that we do actually engage in something called "speaking under our breath"—voicing may be indirectly involved in writing, and typing. Movement and volitional control are also principle features of the manual signing of the Deaf. Even intense thought tends to involve changes in facial expression, vocalizations, and spoken words in many cases. When the thinking is emotional or difficult, we sometimes do what we call "thinking out loud."

Gesturing for Our Own Benefit

We may gesture and act our way through a conversation that is happening only in our imagination. In the movies, it is popular these days for the protagonist—before going to meet with the boss, the enemy, or the potential date—to act out the anticipated conversation in front of the mirror. Several versions of the "imagined conversation" may be rehearsed before the actual conversation takes place. Sometimes, we read the instructions for some task out loud—"you hold down the control key and the shift key, and then press . . . "—and we may even repeat them aloud or under our breath while performing the actions indicated. We may say the words aloud as we type them, or repeat a number to ourselves as we punch it up on our phone, or as we are reaching or searching for the phone, and so forth. So the voice is involved even when it does not seem to be active overtly. Producing speech is essential to reading aloud, and is obviously indirectly related to producing written forms of words that can be spoken out loud, but how is any language activity related to swallowing?

As documented by Hostetter and Alibali (2004, 2008), when talking on the phone, human beings everywhere in the world are prone to gesture and point to real or imagined things or persons that the person on the other end of the phone cannot possibly perceive. The movements seem to help us in forming our own thoughts into words. Motor acts of voice and speaking are deeply and obviously involved in speech and language, but what about swallowing?

The question still remains: What does swallowing intrinsically have to do with speech-language pathology and why would swallowing disorders ever be treated by a speech-language pathologist?

Come to think of it, even swallowing—"gulp!"—can be used as an anticipatory gesture to punctuate a realization, thought, expectation, or worry.

The Clue Leading to a Three-Part Answer

The answer to this minor mystery is interesting and more complex than might be expected. It comes in three parts which have to do with the form, function, and control of swallowing, producing voice, and speaking. The three-part answer has to do with the anatomy, physiology, and neurology of swallowing, producing voice, and speaking.

To see and understand the connections and the natural association between these seemingly disparate processes, it is essential to consider them together with breathing and the whole complex of systems that enable us to function as living human beings. The solution to the puzzle begins with the anatomy of the mouth and the vocal tract. The first part of the answer has to do with form. It hinges, so to speak, on an amazing little trapdoor attached to the back of our tongues—something you probably didn't even know you had. The second part of the answer has to do with the functions involved in speech and swallowing. If that little trapdoor does not flip shut forming a slide into the throat when we swallow, life threatening choking can follow. The third part of the answer has to do with control of the motor processes making possible some overlap in the kinds of therapy that work for disorders of swallowing, voice, and speech.

Let's take the parts of the answer—anatomy, physiology, and neurology—one by one to see just why it is that speech-language pathologists are the therapists of choice for, of all things, swallowing disorders. The first part of the answer to our question has to do with the anatomy shared in part by speaking and swallowing (see A. J. Miller, 2002).

ANATOMY—FORM: THE MOUTH AS "GRAND CENTRAL STATION"

It is useful to keep in mind that the mouth—and more broadly speaking, the entire vocal tract with all of its interconnected tubes and passage ways—is the main port of entry for bodily supplies. They are brought in to be processed there and either accepted or rejected, sometimes immediately, as when we spit out some liquid or substance, or sometimes after swallowing, for example, by coughing or even vomiting. The vocal tract connects with our nose and nasal passages and provides an alternate route for breathing when demands are high, for example, when running or performing vigorous exercise.

Figure 6–2 is one of the classic drawings published in 1918 as part of the legacy of Henry Gray [1825–1861]. It is noteworthy that he only lived 34 years but he advanced the study of human anatomy so much that the 39 editions of the book he first published in 1860 still carry his name 136 years after his death (see "Henry Gray," 1861/2009, retrieved February 28, 2009, from http://www.bartleby.com/107/ and from http://en.wikipedia.org/wiki/Henry_Gray). The latest edition of what is now popularly known as *Gray's Anatomy*—a title adapted under the spelling "Grey's Anatomy" for

It is useful to keep in mind that the mouth—and more broadly speaking, the entire vocal tract with all of its interconnected tubes and passage ways—is the main port of entry for bodily supplies.

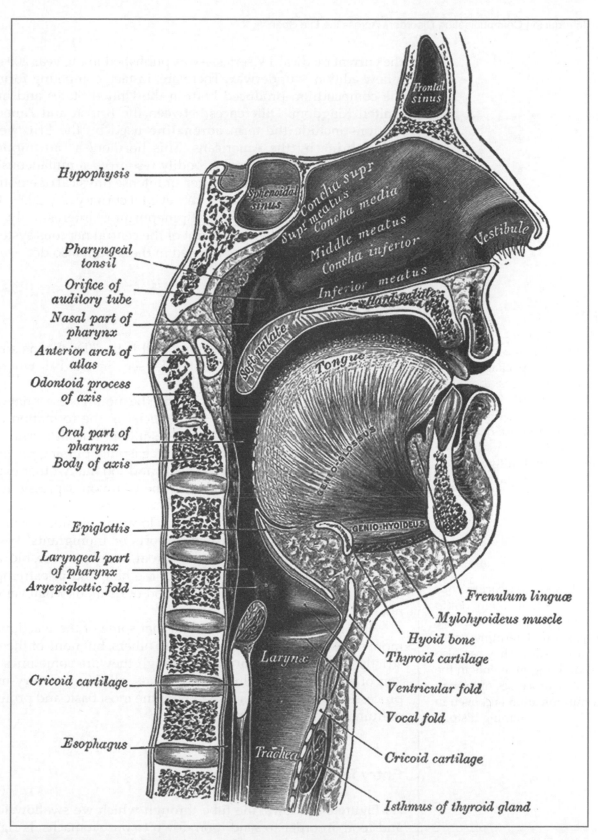

FIGURE 6–2. The anatomy of the vocal tract, sagittal view. From H. Gray, 1918, *Anatomy of the Human Body* (Illustration 994). Philadelphia: Lea & Febiger. Copyright © 2000 by Bartleby.com, ON-LINE ED., Inc. at http://www.bartleby.com/107/. Retrieved February 28, 2009, from http://www.bartleby.com/107/illus994.html. Reprinted with permission. All rights reserved.

the current medical TV series—was published in the year 2004 and a new edition is underway. There are, in fact, competing forms of the compendium produced both in the United States and in the United Kingdom. Differences between the British and American editions include the term **adrenaline** used by the Brits versus **epinephrine** by the Americans. This hormone is an important secretion that mobilizes many bodily resources simultaneously in situations that produce fear, anger, or intense physical or emotional arousal ("Epinephrine," 2009, retrieved February 28, 2009, from http://en.wikipedia.org/wiki/Epinephrine). Interestingly, this hormone comes under the control of the central nervous system—just as the speech functions focused in the mouth also do.

The Outgoing Shipping Port

The best studied facial expression of all is the "Duchenne smile," which we introduced in Chapter 1—see Figure 1–1 where an unborn baby expresses such a smile.

In addition to its speech functions, the mouth is essential to the expression of basic emotions. It is crucial in the formation of all kinds of facial expressions, not only smiling, but also grimacing, pouting, gaping in surprise, whistling, gasping, pursing the lips in thought, placing the tongue in cheek, and too many other expressions to mention. There are also all the common expressions and shapes of the mouth that precede a kiss, a curse, or a blessing.

The mouth is also the essential location of motor activities involved in expelling undesired imports or immigrants. We spit out the fly or the hair. We clear our throat, cough, sneeze, blow our nose, stick out the tongue to remove the hair, and in extreme situations we choke up, or vomit out food or drink or whatever does not sit well.

It is important to keep in mind that some of these actions are more subject to voluntary control than others, but none of them are strictly speaking "mechanical" although they are sometimes spoken of as if they were. In living persons, all these sensory-motor processes are deeply interrelated with the most basic and profound of human communication processes.

Entry for Solids and Liquids

As Figure 6–2 shows, the tube through which we swallow liquid and food, in order to send it on down to our stomachs, is right at the back of the oral cavity. It is just behind the windpipe which needs to stay clear of obstruction so we can keep on breathing. Besides, choking, getting food, or other foreign substances into the lungs

---

The mouth is the main point for shaping, packaging, and exporting our ideas, thoughts, and plans in words. The mouth is the motor center for the development and use of speech. It is also essential for the expression and differentiation of subtle emotions.

Sometimes just clearing your throat or a slight cough, not to mention a kiss or a curse, may be sufficient to determine issues of life and death. They can also be defining moments in the processes of human communication and even in shaping history.

can produce other problems such as the **aspiration pneumonias** (Shigemitsu & Afshar, 2007) and can be complicated by other digestive or breathing problems (Hunt & Gaston, 2008). To get food or liquid to the right pipe, the one that leads to the stomach rather than the lungs, what we put in our mouths has to pass right over the top of the opening of the windpipe leading into the lungs.

The anatomy of the mouth is interesting and amazing. It enables us during high energy actions such as running to open our mouths and get more air into our lungs than is possible through our nasal passages alone. Because the mouth leads directly into the windpipe, it provides an alternative method for importing air into the lungs when the demands for air are high.

The swallowing tube is the **esophagus**—at the lower left side of the drawing. Its upper opening is right at the back of what is popularly called the "Adam's apple" or "voice box." That cavity is technically termed the **larynx**. The voice box contains the vocal folds just at the upper end of the tube that carries air to and from the lungs, popularly referred to as the "windpipe"—technically called the **trachea.** The cavity behind and below the tongue, and above the larynx, is the **pharynx** or **pharyngeal cavity**. Just at the very back of the tongue and above the larynx, is a gate valve that works like a trapdoor—a lid that is hinged on one side so that it can flip downward and close off the passageway leading into the windpipe enabling food or liquid to slide down into the esophagus. That gate is called the **epiglottis**—meaning "upon the tongue." It is actually located at the back extremity of the tongue just in front of the back wall of the pharynx and directly above the larynx.

> Because the mouth leads directly into the windpipe, it provides an alternate method for importing air into the lungs when the demands for air are high.

The Little Trap Door

When it is in its relaxed position, as it is normally, it is open and allows us to breathe through our nose or mouth, or both. The epiglottis is in the open position in the diagram of Figure 6–2. In the radiographic image of Figure 6–3, it is also in the open position, and we can see its shape and position as it is poised above the larynx. When we swallow, the epiglottis flips downward to close off the passage just above the larynx and to form a slide leading down over the back of the tongue into the esophagus. So we can see from the anatomy of the tubes leading to and from the vocal tract that swallowing, breathing, and voice production are intimately related.

All of the foregoing leads us to the physiology part of the answer to the question—why are swallowing disorders treated by speech-language pathologists?

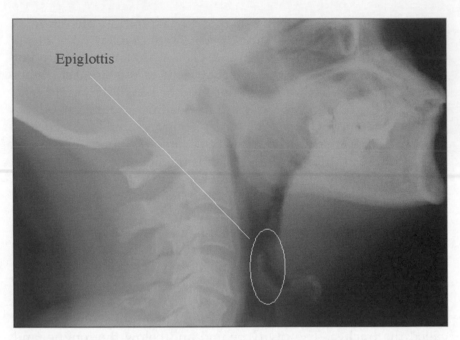

Epiglottis

FIGURE 6–3. The epiglottis as seen in a radiographic image. Retrieved February 28, 2009, from http://www.rad.msu.edu/Education/CourseInfo/ CHM_domain/ID/Morgan/default.html. Copyright © n.d. by the Department of Radiology at Michigan State University. Adapted and reprinted with permission. All rights reserved.

PHYSIOLOGY—FUNCTION: ACCIDENTS AT THE CROSSROADS

If the timing is not just right when chewing and swallowing, food, liquid, gum, a cigarette, a stray tongue or lip decoration, or any foreign substance that is small enough can enter the larynx and/or the passages beneath. This can cause choking. If coughing does not expel the foreign substance, and if the blockage is complete and lasts longer than a few minutes, of course, the result can be fatal. Or, if the food or other foreign matter passes into the lungs, infections there can lead to aspiration pneumonia or other complications.

Talking, Swallowing, and Still Breathing

It is not just because acts of swallowing occur in the same anatomical neighborhood as breathing and speech production that they have the potential to interfere with each other. The rub is not so much that it is almost impossible to talk while swallowing, but that talking while chewing and/or swallowing sets up a situation that can interfere with breathing. Between 1999 and 2000 the Centers for

Disease Control (CDC) estimated that about 3 in 10,000 recorded deaths were caused by choking. There were about 93,600 deaths by choking in the United States in 2000.

According to statistics concerning infant deaths published in 1986 by the CDC, choking on food or any object the baby puts in its mouths is the fourth most common cause of death in infants. Among the causes of injury that are recorded for infants, the only ones that pose a greater threat are car accidents, drowning, and fire (CDC, 1986, retrieved February 28, 2009, from (http://www.cdc.gov/mmwr/preview/mmwrhtml/00000741.htm). But you don't have to be a baby to choke on something. That leads us to the third part of the answer to the question about why swallowing disorders are commonly treated by speech-language pathologists.

Breathing Is Crucial

Everyone has the experience not only of biting the tongue or cheek while chewing, talking, or swallowing, but everyone occasionally chokes on food or drink. This is especially likely when trying to coordinate the complex movements involved breathing, talking, chewing, and swallowing all at the same time. That is one of the good reasons, other than manners, for not talking with our mouths full. Mom was right about that even if we may not have fully understood all the reasons why at the time.

Due to the closeness of the tracts that enable us to breathe air and swallow food and liquids, perhaps it should not surprise us that the treatment of speech disorders and swallowing disorders historically has been linked. When the motor disorders that can affect both speech and swallowing are added to the mix, plain old ordinary swallowing—without any juggling of words around the food or drink—can be a life-threatening activity.

So, it is no wonder that swallowing disorders are a matter of high priority when certain motor problems come into play. Those motor problems come under the control of different neurological systems, which leads us to the third part of the answer to the question why speech-language pathologists commonly treat swallowing disorders.

NEUROLOGY—CONTROL: VOLUNTARY AND INVOLUNTARY SYSTEMS

We discover that, after we intentionally initiate an act of swallowing, the process normally completes itself as if on automatic pilot. Also, as soon as the initial phase of the swallow is completed, we can immediately resume breathing, or speaking, but not both.

Choking is the fifth most common reason for a trip to the emergency room and poses the most serious threat for small children (see "Statistics about Accidental death," 2009, retrieved February 27, 2009, from http://www.wrongdiagnosis.com/a/accidental_death/stats.htm).

If we think about how acts of swallowing, breathing, and speaking are neurologically controlled, we discover the interesting boundary between autonomic and volitional acts.

Incompatible Aspects

We cannot breathe and swallow at the same time and we can hardly breathe in and speak at the same time. You can try it if you like. Try reading this sentence aloud while breathing in. It is possible to do so—that is, to speak while breathing in rather than out—but it is difficult, unnatural, and no community of language users in the world uses that method of producing speech (Ladefoged, 2001). Speaking normally involves an outflow of air from the lungs and it is necessary to pause the speaking intermittently in order to take a breath. When the control of swallowing, breathing, and speaking are not well coordinated, the results are unpleasant to say the least and can be life threatening.

Dominant Hemisphere Control of Volitional Movements

The initiation of swallowing, like speaking, manual signing (see J. B. Palmer et al., 2007), chewing, taking a step, scratching an itch, or taking a deep breath, involves volition. Unsurprisingly, there is clear empirical evidence from many sources showing that the dominant hemisphere of the brain—which in right handers is almost always the left hemisphere (Butler, 1997)—normally retains control of the volitional aspect of all these functions.

Volitional swallowing, both motor and sensory functions, as demonstrated by Dziewas et al. (2005) are lateralized to the dominant hemisphere—usually the left hemisphere. Figure 6-4 shows the corpus callosum that connects the two hemispheres. For a moving three dimensional view, on the DVD click this link: http://en.wikipedia.org/wiki/File:Structural.gif. Voluntary exhalation and speech production are also lateralized to the dominant hemisphere (Loucks et al., 2007).

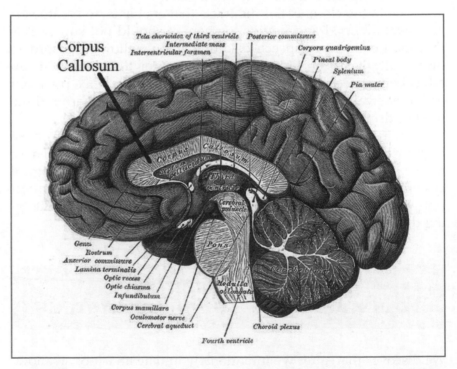

FIGURE 6–4. The corpus callosum connects the two hemispheres. Image retrieved April 17, 2009 from http://en.wikipedia.org/wiki/File:Gray 720.png in the public domain because of expired copyright.

As we discuss in greater detail in Chapter10, both hemispheres are essentially capable of performing all of the neurological functions of the body. This is known from the fact that removal of an entire hemisphere—or deliberately making one hemisphere nonfunctional, provided it is done early in development—does not necessarily result in major loss of brain functions.

Although we really have two, more or less complete brains, the two hemispheres do not normally function in competition with each other, but rather in collaboration. The dominant hemisphere provides essential control over attention, volition, verbal thought, planning, and execution of movements—especially the ones involved in speech production and in writing (Shuster & Lemieux, 2005). For manual signing, the main regions of the dominant hemisphere are still involved as in speech production but with greater participation of the parietal lobes (Emmorey, Mehta, & Grabowski, 2007). In fact, Hagler, Riecke, and Sereno (2007) showed that even pointing with the index finger activates significant regions in the parietal lobes (Figure 6–5). However, in the tasks they devised, verbal instructions are required. They draw some comparisons with monkeys but do not seem to take account of the fact that monkeys would have no hope of following the sort of instructions required to define the desired actions that human participants are able to perform in their experiments (see the discussion of their methods in below in this chapter).

> The dominant hemisphere provides essential control over attention, volition, verbal thought, planning, and execution of movements—especially the ones involved in speech production and in writing (Shuster & Lemieux, 2005).

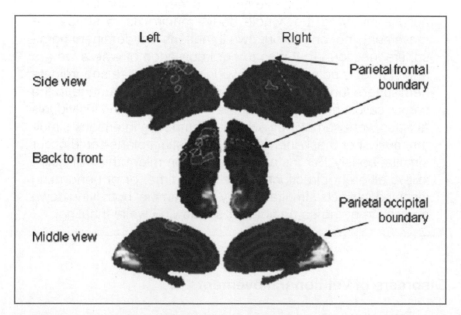

FIGURE 6–5. Regions of brain activity during pointing in contrast to eye movement. From "Parietal and Superior Frontal Visuospatial Maps Activated by Pointing and Saccades," by D. J. Hagler, Jr., L. Riecke, and M. L. Sereno, 2007, *Neuroimage, 35*(4), p. 1566. Copyright © 2007 Elsevier Inc. Adapted and reprinted with permission from Elsevier. All rights reserved.

Communication Between the Hemispheres

Connecting the two hemispheres is the bundle of fibers known as the **corpus callosum** (as shown in Figure 6–4). That large bundle of connections enables control and coordination of communication between the hemispheres. This is an oversimplification, no doubt, because there are other connections and interactions—many of them not yet well understood but some of which we will encounter later in this chapter. The corpus callosum connections in particular, however, are discussed in greater detail in Chapter 10, and it is known that damage to that bundle of nerve fibers, can produce competition between the two hemispheres in planning and carrying out certain processes especially voluntary movements. For instance, Nishikawa et al. (2001) showed that damage to the backward half of the corpus callosum creates a situation where competing intentions to carry out complex actions occur simultaneously—as if the left hemisphere had one idea and the right had another.

If the normally dominant hemisphere loses control over the normally subordinate hemisphere, the question of just who is in charge and what the body will do goes up for grabs.

The Crucial Control Issue

Nishikawa, et al. (2001) described cases of **dyspraxia** or apraxia both used as umbrella terms for disorders of learned purposeful (volitional) movements. As they explained, normally, actions involving the "whole body" require us to shape our movements not only to our own intentions—a dominant hemisphere function—but also to our knowledge of where we are and of what is going on in the world around us—a subordinate hemisphere function. In the particular cases of damage to the corpus callosum, which Nishikawa, et al. studied, the individuals affected were sometimes aware of competing intentions simultaneously. For these individuals, two distinct plans could occur simultaneously. For instance, the person might think of going in two different directions at the same time, or of performing incompatible acts simultaneously, for example, both lying down and sitting at the same time, or swallowing while inhaling.

Disorders of Volitional Movements

In certain volitional movement disorders damage to the corpus callosum, and possibly to additional brain areas, produces a condition known as **diagonistic dyspraxia** (Barbeau, Joubert, & Poncet, 2004)—a condition where the contralateral side of the body, for instance, the left hand performs involuntary movements, while the other side, say, the right hand, is performing a voluntary movement. There are many different varieties and combinations of symptoms of dyspraxia or apraxia, however, and there is no standard terminology for differentiating all the varieties that have been described or that are supposed to exist. Technically, the term "apraxia" should be reserved for a complete loss of control but this rule hardly applies if any movement whatever is possible—as is virtually always the case in the disorders described as apraxias or dyspraxias.

With respect to the diagonistic type of dyspraxia associated with damage to the corpus callosum, an intriguing set of rare cases involve what is known as **alien hand syndrome**—here the non-dominant hand seems to carry out a sequence of habitual actions all by itself, for example, as in picking lint off a garment, striking a match, or adjusting a pair of glasses on the nose (Biran, Giovannetti, Buxbaum, & Chatterjee, 2006; Giummarra, Gibson, Georgiou-Karistianis, & Bradshaw, 2008; Kikkert, Ribbers, & Koudstaal, 2006; Obhi, Matkovich, & Gilbert, 2009).

The Alien Hand

In one case of damage focused on the corpus callosum, an elderly lady's subordinate (left hand) would seemingly of its own accord start moving dishes while she was eating with the right hand and would seem to rise up and float in the air while she was walking (Kasahara, Toyokura, Shimoda, & Ishida, 2005). In another case described by Verstichel et al. (1994), a patient who was left hemisphere dominant for speaking, when asked to initiate certain gestures—tasks normally carried out by the right hemisphere—would unintentionally (involuntarily) respond with speech or writing.

Someone Needs to Be in Charge

Having just one hemisphere in control makes sense when coordinating the deliberate (volitional) movements involved in swallowing, breathing, and talking. It is good to have one hemisphere in charge because confusions of swallowing with breathing—and/or talking—can potentially be injurious or even fatal. We can easily tell from our own actions that we have volitional control over initiating acts of swallowing. We can choose to swallow a mouthful of liquid, a pill, or some food, or to spit it out. We can also choose to say a word, phrase, or sentence, or not. But the degree of volitional control of speaking is much greater than in breathing or swallowing. Except in certain kinds of habitual sudden exclamations or in disorders of motor speech—speaking does not normally occur without intention and volition although breathing and the continuation

It is good to have one hemisphere in charge because confusions of swallowing with breathing—and/or talking—can potentially be injurious or even fatal.

of swallowing can operate when we are not specifically thinking about them.

We even have volitional control over habitual verbal routines such as "Hi. How are you?" or "Thank you, thank you. Thank you very much." Reciting a memorized bit of discourse or a habitual exclamation, for example, as in saying "Ouch! Now, what did I go and do that for! __#$%#$#!!!!" and so on when you mash your finger, is not initiated in the autonomic nervous system. To a large extent, these exclamatory utterances still are under volitional control. Even the most routine verbal habits do not begin as routines. They begin under conscious control, and only later do they become rote habits (or common rituals), presumably, to reduce processing burden. Additionally, the results of various kinds of brain damage and surgeries (see Chapter 10) show that the dominant hemisphere normally controls the motor functions of speech and writing quite exclusively. If the dominant hemisphere is damaged or removed after maturity has been achieved, the subordinate hemisphere cannot produce voluntary speech or writing at all.

Even in visual aspects of speech perception, volitional control of attention—where we look and how well we listen and observe someone else who is speaking—appear to be controlled by the dominant hemisphere. The control of movements associated with speech, even carries over to intentional *visual perception* of the visual signals involved in lip shapes. Therefore, so-called "lip reading"—recall the McGurk effects discussed and demonstrated in Chapter 4; Nicholls & Searle, 2006—is an activity managed by the dominant hemisphere. Because speaking, breathing, and swallowing, share the volitional element and come under deliberate conscious control to the extent that they do, some of the therapies that work with motor problems involved in speaking, can also work, in theory at least, with swallowing.

In a study of motor control of pointing with the index finger or moving the eyes to look towards a new location—in what are called **saccades**—Hagler, Riecke, and Sereno (2007) showed that control of eye-movements and pointing are largely distinct processes. The pointing movements of their right-handed participants appeared to be controlled mainly by the dominant hemisphere while eye movements (saccades) seemed to involve both hemispheres. In fact, Jarrett and Barnes (2005) claim that **smooth pursuit** eye movements—where we track a moving object—are outside of voluntary control. However, when an object has changed directions one or two times at a certain location on a repeated path of motion, we can anticipate the change and the saccades that may be needed to continue to track the object seem to fall on the border between voluntary and nonvoluntary control. Smooth pursuit, without change of direction, by contrast, or a visual fixation where we focus on and hold a given icon in view, seems to be largely a function of the subordinate hemisphere. All of these actions tend to be referred to as "eye **gaze**" by speech-language pathologists in spite of the fact that

> If the dominant hemisphere is damaged or removed after maturity has been achieved, the subordinate hemisphere cannot produce voluntary speech or writing at all.

they are evidently quite different in critical respects and tend to be controlled by distinct neurological processes.

In the data summarized in Figure 6–5, Hagler, Riecke, and Sereno (2007) asked their adult participants either to point to a target on a screen or to look where the target had briefly appeared after a plus sign "+" in the middle of the screen changed colors. In the pointing or looking part of the task, participants could not see their pointing hand or finger and the target was no longer present. Although the pointing movements, for their participants—all of whom were right handed—clearly came under the control of the occipital lobes and the dominant (left) hemisphere, the eye movements were more or less distributed over both hemispheres. In the figure, the blue areas correspond to activity during eye movements while the red areas correspond to areas of activity during finger pointing. In personal communication, Dr. Hagler speculated that if the participants had been left handed, the right hemisphere probably would have been dominant for pointing.

What is clear from the data, by our reading, is that their right-handed subjects were relying mainly on their left hemisphere to control their pointing gestures and—we infer on the basis of a wealth of other experimental studies (especially the split brain studies of Chapter 10)—they were also relying on their left hemisphere mainly to understand the verbal instructions that were necessary to perform the tasks required by Hagler, Riecke, and Sereno (2007). It is noteworthy that Dr. Hagler and colleagues do not take special notice of what we see as the essential and crucial role of the verbal instructions that must be kept in mind in order for the human participants to perform the tasks in the study. As a result, the comparisons with macaque monkeys performing saccades or pointing may be only superficially similar to what the human participants are doing. Certainly, the macaques referred to cannot understand and keep in mind written verbal instructions about what they are supposed to do. Although the research is clear in showing that humans rely mainly on the dominant hemisphere for linguistic comprehension, and especially for the motor production of speech, it is true, as Dr. Hagler suggests, that handedness probably is a factor in the experiments. However, even left-handed individuals tend in the majority of cases, about 60% or more, to be left-brain dominant for language tasks (Squire et al., 2003, p. 1345). Therefore, we doubt the prediction that left-handed individuals will necessarily rely on their right hemispheres for verbally controlled pointing as Dr. Hagler supposes.

Seeing, Pointing, and Referring

The data from Hagler, Riecke, and Sereno (2007) offer several indications that there is a subtle tendency for pointing to be associated more with the linguistically dominant hemisphere while visual saccades show some preference for control by the subordinate hemisphere. When we take the functions of linguistic reference and pragmatic mapping into consideration (in keeping with all of the preceding chapters of this book and the references cited in relation to these processes) it is reasonable to suppose that deliberate intentional pointing should, to a significant extent, come under the control of the linguistically dominant hemisphere, just as it appears from Figure 6–5 that it does. However, the theory of pragmatic mapping suggests that visual concepts and icons, as known through smooth pursuit or enduring eye fixations, are more likely to be the province of the subordinate hemisphere.

. . . it seems that the dominant hemisphere controls intentional movements that involve the sorts of plans that we commonly express in words (symbols) while the subordinate hemisphere specializes in processing relatively enduring holistic images of sensory and conceptual icons.

We return to hemisphere dominance and differentiation of hemispheric functions in Chapter 10, but for the moment it is useful to keep in mind that the evidence from Hagler, Riecke, and Sereno (2007) does show subtle differences in the motor control of eye movements and movements of the pointing finger. The dominant hemisphere seems to specialize in abstract symbols and sequences of them that involve the greater language community while the subordinate hemisphere specializes in the construction of holistic icons that represent the external world as it is perceived by the individual.

In between, the two hemispheres are connected by the corpus callosum, which is largely responsible for communicating intentional actions that require coordination of both hemispheres. The intentional analytical constructions that we put in words are intrinsically volitional. So they usually require one of the hemispheres to be in charge—which we believe will include intentional pointing (indexes) controlled by verbal instructions. The hemisphere controlling such pointing should be the dominant one, and is expected to be the left hemisphere even in the majority of left-handed individuals who, like right-handed individuals, tend to be left-brain dominant. By contrast, saccades as suggested by Jarrett and Barnes (2005) probably fall near the border and should be distributed to both hemispheres while smooth pursuit or iconic representation should tend to go more to the subordinate (usually the right) hemisphere. Communication between the hemispheres in both directions, as we will show in greater detail in Chapter 10, greatly depends on the corpus callosum. Probably, for all these reasons we should speak of the verbally dominant hemisphere, because the subordinate hemisphere apparently excels at and even controls some nonvolitional motor tasks involving icons—for example, smooth pursuit and nonvolitional saccades in eye movements.

From Autonomous to Volitional Control of Breathing

When we are not thinking about it, breathing will normally take care of itself, but when we are speaking or swallowing, to a very great extent we bring breathing under volitional control. There is abundant evidence that the dominant hemisphere controls the volitional part of swallowing (Daniels et al., 2006; Dziewas et al., 2003; Martin et al., 2007). Also, the fact that swallowing can be done on command (J. B. Palmer, Hiiemae, Matsuo, & Haishima, 2007) shows it to be volitional and controlled by the dominant hemisphere. In the processing of speech, the control of the dominant hemisphere is dramatic. It appears to be complete in the case of motor production of speech and also of writing (see Chapter 10).

Autonomic and Habitual Aspects of Complex Movements

As we saw in Chapter 1, there are distinct nervous systems that regulate involuntary movements—for example, of the intestines and glands—as opposed to voluntary movements of muscles that in most cases are attached to our bones. Although the initiation of a swallow is a voluntary act, the completion of the process comes under the control of the autonomic nervous system. Speech also involves voluntary action not only to plan and initiate a motor sequence but to sustain it, monitor the output, and bring the act of speaking to completion. Both speaking and swallowing share the logical requirement that they need to be closely coordinated with breathing.

Breathing is more limited during swallowing than while speaking.

Both speaking and swallowing share the logical requirement that they need to be closely coordinated with breathing.

Logical Limitations

It is not normally possible to breathe in or out while initiating a swallow, though we can resume breathing just as soon as the autonomic nervous system takes over and continues the swallow. With speaking, we need to bring breathing under conscious control, and we normally speak only during controlled exhalation. We cannot speak and initiate a swallow at the same time and we do not normally breathe in air at the same time as we are speaking. These are logical limitations—breathing while at the same time initiating a swallow is like trying to get two solid objects to occupy the same space at the same time, or to get the same object to occupy two different spaces at the same time. Neither can be done without smashing or pulling apart the object. Similarly, we risk injury in trying to breathe and initiate a swallow at the same time.

The logical conflicts that incompatible actions set up are contrary to the physical systems and physiological functions of the body. In breathing in or out, we are limited by the capacity of our lungs and also by our posture—lying down, sitting, or standing—and the muscles at our disposal. We can speak or swallow at will but only within our physical and physiological limitations. For instance, as Redstone (2005) confirmed comparing normal controls with persons injured by cerebral palsy, no one can produce an extremely long sequence of syllables on one breath, and persons with physical injuries or disease have more severe limitations. A person with cerebral palsy cannot breathe in as much air as a matched person without the disorder and, as Redstone, showed, both normal controls and persons with cerebral palsy can take in more air when sitting up than when lying down.

Similarly, there are limits on how much and how fast we can swallow. However, postural change—from sitting up to reclining at 30 degrees, 60 degrees, and 90 degrees (lying flat)—does not seem to affect the completion of an act of swallowing in normal subjects (Inagaki et al., 2007). In fact, with swallowing, the autonomic system evidently exerts more pressure during the swallow to compensate for the loss of gravitational pull as the body moves from an upright posture to lying down. But it is, on account of gravity, more difficult to swallow food or drink when lying down.

Timing and Shifting Control

There is a profound difference in, say, reading out loud, and initiating an act of swallowing. With the speech act, we can choose to stop almost anywhere along the way. Try it. You can stop with the first word, in the middle of a word, or even in the middle of a syllable or at the beginning, middle, or end of a single segment such as the sound /s/ at the beginning, say, of the word *say*. But with the swallowing act, things are different. Once you initiate it, if things are functioning as they should, the swallow will complete itself.

A Matter of Timing

Normal swallowing involves a smooth slow wave-like contraction of muscles in the larynx and in the throat encircling the esophagus. It takes about three seconds to complete a swallow. Speech production is faster and involves many very quick and highly articulated, though not fully conscious, movements. If the language systems are working properly, the speech (or manual sign) movements seem to complete themselves while we think of the meanings we want to express.

Speech Production, as in Reading Aloud, Involves Many Movements

If you time yourself, and hustle a little, you can read the entire previous (italicized) sentence in just about three seconds. It contains 14 distinct syllables in General American English and it consists of 42 distinct sound segments. However, each segment can be broken down into multiple articulatory components each of which involves movements and the control of distinct coordinated muscle systems. Articulated movements are essential to go from the **consonant cluster** /sp/ at the beginning of the **monosyllabic word** *speech* to its **vocalic center**, /i/, and then to transition to the closing consonant sequence of /t/ followed by /ʃ/.

Speech Movements Much Faster Than Swallowing

The speech act in question involves of a complex of contrasts produced by the major articulators—the tongue, lips, and jaw—while at the same time breathing out mainly through the mouth, sometimes through the nose, and rapidly turning the voice on and off. In the process of producing distinct speech sounds, there are contrasts in voicing as in /z/ or no voicing as in /s/; tongue movement as in going from /k/ to /t/; whether the air continues to flow or is stopped as in /s/ versus /t/; whether the air is escaping through the mouth as in vowels such as /i/ and /a/; or through both the mouth and nose as in the vocalic center of the syllable -*ments*; or through just the nose as in the segments /m/ and /n/.

If we suppose that on the average there are at least three movements per segment—if more are required the conclusion will be even stronger—in three seconds of speaking we can complete about 150 times as many articulatory movements as are possible in one act of swallowing. This is confirmed in measurement studies. Speech movements (see C. A. Moore & Ruark, 1996; Ruark & C. A. Moore, 1997) occur at a much faster rate than chewing and swallowing. The dramatic difference in timing and speed of movements is already evident by the tender age of two years (Ruark & C. A. Moore, 1997). Also, unsurprisingly, the control of breathing at rest, which is an autonomic process, is very different from breathing while talking, which comes largely under voluntary control.

While completing a single swallow, it is possible to carry out many articulatory speech movements.

The motor dynamics are also distinct showing that the breathing associated with vocalization and speech is not a so-called vegetative (autonomic) function at any stage of development (Connaghan, C. A. Moore, & Higashakawa, 2004).

VOICE FROM THE PRODUCER'S POSITION

Have you ever used the writing gesture to borrow a pen because your voice was not working? Almost without exception everyone has suffered from trauma or infection that resulted in the loss of voice for a short time, but usually we recover our voice within a day or two. The majority of these losses are the result of a bronchial infection, too much yelling at the ball game the night before, or some temporary ailment. A **voice disorder**, by contrast, is a chronic abnormality.

A Genuine Loss of Voice

It may have been caused by an injury, disease, or deterioration, but it is not the transitory kind of condition that sometimes accompanies a cold or the flu. We hardly realize how important normal functioning of the voice is until it is gone. For most of us that condition will be only a temporary one, but even a brief time without our voice shows us just how important it is to normal speech communication. On the DVD see Chrissy's Story for a case of someone having to rethink who she was after losing her voice.

Systems Within Systems

Three major systems are involved in normal voice production: the respiratory system, the larynx, and the neural pathways that enervate the muscles that enable us to breathe and to vocalize. The potential difficulties created by voice disorders are intensified by the fact that we depend greatly on our voice for producing intelligible speech. Of course, it is important to keep in mind that the voice, as essential as it is, is not critical to the production of intelligible speech. We can achieve intelligible speech by whispering—where the voice is replaced by mere breathing either in or out. Usually we whisper while breathing out, but whispering is also possible while breathing in. Try it.

The systems involved in voice production and in speaking (as shown in Figure 6–6) include the lungs and especially the diaphragm muscles that allow us to voluntarily inhale or exhale, the trachea, the larynx, the nasopharynx, and the mouth. The nasal and/or oral pathways are the ones through which air travels first from the atmosphere into the lungs where it is stripped of some of its oxygen and then it is breathed back out again. Sometimes we take control of the breathing process to produce speech as we exhale.

Several key features of the respiratory system are involved in speech production. We can also exhale more air than we breathed in on the previous inhalation. Imagine a bucket two-thirds full of water. A cup or two of water is added and then immediately taken away, but there is always water in the bucket. The lungs operate in a similar way. Even though we are constantly inhaling and exhaling, there is normally more air in the lungs than we take in

We can normally inhale (breathe in) more air than we need. That is, our body needs a certain volume of air containing oxygen to function properly. However, it is possible, and when speaking almost a necessity, to inspire more than the required volume of air. This excess volume that we can bring in is called the **inspiratory reserve volume**.

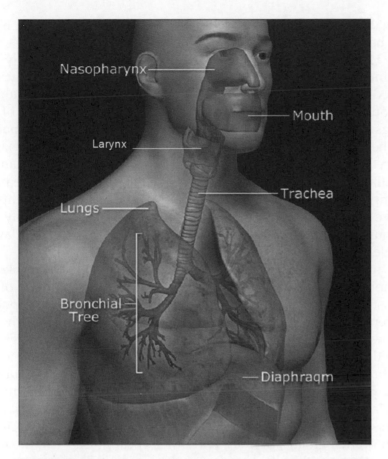

FIGURE 6–6. The respiratory system underlying voice. Retrieved February 28, 2009, from http://en.wikipedia.org/wiki/Image:3DScience_respiratory_labeled.jpg and adapted and reprinted under the GNU Free Documentation License, Version 1.2.

or breathe out. The reservoir of excess air that can be drawn on to exhale more air than we just breathed in is called the **expiratory reserve volume**.

Some Air Is Still in There

Try as you might, you can never exhale all the air that is in your lungs. Even the sensation of having the wind knocked out of you does not completely deflate the lungs. It just feels like it does. The most extreme way for this to happen is from a sharp blow affecting the **solar plexus**—that little indentation just below the rib cage centered on the diaphragm (see the pointer in Figure 6–6 for the "diaphragm"). Even when the wind is knocked out of us, we do not expel all the air in our lungs. It feels like we did because the blow can temporarily paralyze the diaphragm making it impossible (usually only temporarily) to breathe. In severe cases such a blow can be fatal.

However, there is still a volume of air that is invariably left behind even when we feel like we have exhausted our supply. It is called the **residual volume**. The measurements of air in the lungs, of course, are dependent on age, physical health, and the size of the lungs. Kent (1997) gives formulas for estimating the **vital capacity** of the lungs—if one were to maximally inhale and then exhale even the residual volume. The fact is that we have more air than we require for vital functions. The excess volume above what we need is important in reference to speech and voice because our ability to move excess air in and out of the lungs is just about exactly the amount we need to produce a full spoken sentence of about average length.

Just as sentences seem to contain thought-sized chunks of meaning in manageable package sizes, our residual volume of air is just about the perfect amount to allow us to produce a spoken sentence of average length on a single breath. Or, perhaps, we should say, without overtaxing our residual volume of air. It is interesting that the physical capacity to produce a string of syllables on a single breath seems to be approximately the same as the amount of time needed to put a well-formed thought into words. Sometimes specialists seeking to distinguish between the voicing associated with speech sounds as contrasted with the vocalizations associated with grunts, groans, belches, and other vocal noises, use the term **phonation** specifically to refer to the production of voice as in speaking, reading aloud, pretending to speak, babbling, producing nonsense syllables, or when producing speech-like hesitation forms such as *uh, ummm,* and the like. The key element that turns on and off during such phonations is the voice.

> It is interesting that the physical capacity to produce a string of syllables on a single breath seems to be approximately the same as the amount of time needed to put a well-formed thought into words.

The Larynx

The larynx, as seen in Figure 6–2 from the side view and in Figure 6–7 from back to front, is the locus of the systems where voicing is physically produced. When we view the larynx from the top, looking down with an endoscopic camera as in Figure 6–8, there are two folds that come together in an upside down V-shape. This is the upper surface of the vocal folds. These folds serve as a gate separating the lungs from the oral and nasal passages. The open or **abducted** position as seen in Figure 6–8 is normal and necessary for breathing. The closed, approximated, or **adducted** position is necessary to produce voice. It also comes in handy when evacuating the lower gastrointestinal tract, or, for the better half of the human race (according to some) when giving birth. The remarkable similarity of the opposite terms—"abducted" meaning open or pulled apart and "adducted" meaning alongside or together are just accidentally too similar to enable any easy distinction between them in

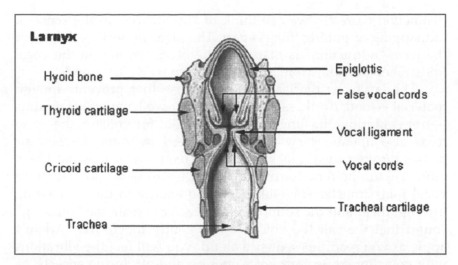

FIGURE 6–7. The larynx split down the middle and viewed from the back of the body looking toward the front. Retrieved February 28, 2009, from http://training.seer.cancer.gov/module_anatomy/unit1_1_body_structure.html. Image from the U.S. National Cancer Institute in the public domain.

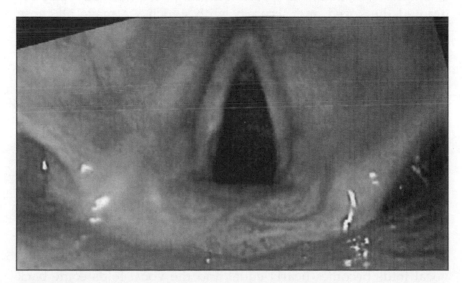

FIGURE 6–8. The vocal folds viewed with an endoscope top down, individual pictured with face upward on his back. Retrieved February 28, 2009, from http://en.wikipedia.org/wiki/Image:Larynx_endo_2.jpg. Reprinted under the GNU Free Documentation License, Version 1.2.

thought or speech. Is it purely coincidental that such terms would have been chosen in a field that studies speech disorders? Probably, but, again we are reminded of the comment by Lapointe and J. Katz about the tendency to choose terms that do not sharply distinguish their meanings and that sometimes fall wide of their semantic targets. In this case, the surface forms are so similar that they encourage students to confuse the meanings as well. To make the distinction correctly, we can think of "abduction" in the sense of kidnapping or pulling things apart. The idea supporting the use of the term "adduction" is that it too involves tension on the vocal folds. They are not in a relaxed state when we voice sounds.

The larynx is the last line of defense that prevents foreign material—food, drink, saliva, or whatever we have in our mouths —from entering our lungs. When adducted for voicing, the vocal folds also operate very much like a reed instrument when air passes through them quickly. Like the reed—or somewhat like a vibrating tuning fork, horn, or stringed instrument—the vibrating vocal folds transfer wave-like pressure energy to the air passing through them and the sound pressure waves create the "buzzing" sound that we call the voice. If you gently touch your Adam's apple as you read this sentence aloud, you will feel the vibrations with your fingers as your voice goes on and off during speech. As the sound pressure waves created by the voice pass through the variously shaped cavities above the larynx—and as we move our articulators changing the shape of the cavities, restricting, closing, and/or opening them in the production of speech—the result is the diverse stream of speech. Although we normally take for granted the speed and accuracy with which we make all those speech movements, as we will see in Chapters 7 and 8, when things go wrong in articulation, or in fluency, speech can become more difficult to understand and to produce.

> If you gently touch your Adam's apple as you read this sentence aloud, you will feel the vibrations with your fingers as your voice goes on and off during speech.

The Voicing Cycle

Van den Berg (1958) proposed what is known as the **myoelastic aerodynamic theory of phonation** to explain the production of voice. His theory takes account of the fact that voicing begins as the vocal folds are adducted—brought together—by the muscles of the larynx. Meanwhile, air is pushed out of the lungs, forcing the adducted vocal folds apart. As the vocal folds are pushed open by the air passing through them, the pressure below and above the vocal folds becomes nearly equal and the vocal folds come back together again. The pressure below builds again until the vocal folds are forced apart again and the cycle repeats.

The phenomenon of the changing pressure and movement of the air as it is forced out through the vocal folds involves what is known as the **Bernoulli effect**.

The Bernouilli Effect and Voice

The term comes from Daniel Bernouilli [1700–1782], the Dutch born mathematician, medical researcher, physicist and theoretician. He showed that the pressure of a free-flowing (nonviscous) fluid in a tube—which air approximates as we exhale air through the trachea—is about equal throughout. However, if an obstruction is introduced—for example, by closing the tube, say, by bringing the vocal folds at the larynx together—the velocity of the flow over the obstacle will be reduced as the pressure below the flow builds and the pressure above the flow is decreased. Bernoulli's principle expresses in an abstract mathematical form the relation between pressure and velocity in such a dynamic flow.

Why Is the Male Voice Deeper?

The average difference in male and female voices is owed to the size of the larynx, and the thickness and tension on the vocal folds. If the tension and thickness of the vocal folds were kept the same, a larger larynx would, on the average, produce a "deeper" voice. More tension and less thickness will also produce a "higher" voice. As we noted in Chapter 3, the fundamental frequency of the voice—that is, the pitch or underlying note that we hear in a syllable center, or a vowel, is prolonged as we speak in a relaxed and natural way—depends on the number of cycles of opening and closing that the vocal folds complete as the syllable is being produced. The number of times the cycle repeats per second (or per any other unit of time) is the fundamental frequency of the voice. We can also think of this frequency as a **wavelength**. A sound pressure change of higher frequency, one that occurs more rapidly, must also have a shorter wavelength. That is, it will occur more often over a given period of time.

Harmony and Noise

The buzzing sound produced at the level of the larynx is not much like the sound that comes out through the mouth and nose. This is because the starting "buzz" is shaped by the tubes and cavities it passes through—the larynx itself, the pharynx, and the oral and nasal cavities above. We talked about resonation in Chapter 3. It is what happens as the sound waves—that is, the changes in pressure levels—travel through the tubes and cavities of the vocal system bouncing around inside the cavities. Hard surfaces inside the cavities tend to reflect sounds just as an echo of your voice will bounce back to you from a rock wall inside a canyon. Soft surfaces, by contrast, absorb the energy of the sound waves rather than reflecting it. They are said to have a damping effect—kind of like a wet blanket at a party or like the collision of a hard ceramic cup with a soft paper towel as contrasted with the collision of the same cup with a hard desk surface. The sound of the collision is damped by the soft towel but reflected as a clunk on the hard surface.

Hard surfaces inside the cavities tend to reflect sounds just as an echo of your voice will bounce back to you from a rock wall inside a canyon. Soft surfaces, by contrast, absorb the energy of the sound waves rather than reflecting it.

You may have noticed how the body of a musical instrument, say, a flute, clarinet, sax, or trumpet, sounds in contrast to the sound produced if you only use the mouthpiece of the instrument without the rest of the shaped tube. In musical instruments, of which the human vocal system is no doubt the most amazing and versatile of all, the sound produced by the voice is partly owed to the shape and quality of the material the instrument is made of and also it is owed in part to the dimensions and surfaces inside the tube(s) through which the sound pressure waves travel. Resonance is the quality of sounds that just happen to be of the right wavelength to bounce off the walls of a given cavity so that the bouncing wave coincides (agrees with and enhances) the other waves passing through the same cavity as well as its own echoes. Waves of the same length will resonate just as striking a tuning fork will cause another tuning fork of the same frequency to vibrate. The waves coming from the one are at the right frequency to cause the other to resonate.

Waves that are even divisors of the distance across the cavity will resonate resulting in what are called *harmonics*. Resonance of this kind is what produces the pleasing quality of musical notes, for example, as sung by two or more voices, or as played on multiple instruments that harmonize. The harmony is complex and rich when the voices and instruments have different fundamental frequencies and other shaping qualities—hence, the esthetic appeal of duets, trios, quartets, and multipart choral, instrumental, and symphonic harmonies. Sounds can also blend in ways that are not harmonic but dissonant as in the clashing of cymbals, drums, and electronic sounds in a rhythmically produced cacophony of sounds that may or may not be regarded as musical, lyrical, or whatever.

Noise Versus Harmony

In the extreme case where the sounds meet more or less randomly without any harmonics we apply the term "noise." Technically speaking, noise is just a somewhat chaotic and random assortment of changes in sound pressure levels that do not harmonize. This is the sort of result we get when we produce what are called **fricative sounds** such as the /h/ of words such as *hat*, *heat*, or the /s/ of *sit* and the shushing noise of *shhhh*! If the noise is spread across the wide range of frequencies to which our ears are sensitive, we call it **white noise**.

By the dynamic production of distinct arrangements of resonance, noise, and silence in a sequence of articulatory movements made while turning the voice on and off intermittently, the remarkable spectrum of distinct qualities of speech can be attained.

Fricative noise and resonance contrast not only with each other but also with silence. By the dynamic production of distinct arrangements of resonance, noise, and silence in a sequence of articulatory movements made while turning the voice on and off intermittently, the remarkable spectrum of distinct qualities of speech can be attained.

DIAGNOSTIC VOICE AND SPEECH QUALITIES

When it comes to disorders of the voice, a great deal can be learned from observable qualities of the voice in speech production. As we have already noted, the air pressure from the diaphragm as well as the tension on the vocal folds along with the volume, shape, and quality of the vocal folds themselves affects the amplitude (power, loudness, volume), pitch (frequency), and **vocal timbre** of sounds produced by the voice. The timbre of a sound consists of all its collective qualities other than pitch and volume. Timbre is what that distinguishes one sound segment from another. Disorders of voice can affect any and all of these qualities of speech sounds and their dynamic interactions. Such qualities are subjective in the sense that we must use judgment in looking for and noticing them, but they can also be recorded, measured, and assessed by observers. The degree of agreement between different observers can then be examined statistically for reliability and validity. When we examine the voice as clinical observers, certain questions are common as discussed in the following sections.

Vocal Hygiene: Less Effort Is Better

Is the voice production difficult or effortful? Is the sound being produced easily? It is a common cliche these days to say that "less is more." In voicing, it is evidently true that less effortful speech is generally better. Effortful voicing during speech may be indicative of problems in one or more of the vocal systems and it is usually not good for the long-term health of the voice. With respect to voice, as in many other cases, the cliché is true. It is true that extremely effortful speaking, singing, or other uses of the voice, can damage the delicate tissues of the larynx, especially the vocal folds. Less effort for this reason can help keep the voice healthy and functional across the whole life span.

Related to the question about the effortfulness of speaking are a host of other issues that pertain to what is called **vocal hygiene**—the care and maintenance of the voice and related systems. Many of the recommendations concerning vocal hygiene apply across the board to the health of all our body's systems. It is recommended that all speakers, but especially ones who use their voices a lot, should take in plenty of water to keep the vocal folds from drying out. Dehydration all by itself sets up a situation for injury just from ordinary speaking. To avoid dehydration, an average sized person should apply the rule of 88—that is, to drink an eight ounce glass of water at least eight times each day. This is good for our health in general as well as the voice. It helps digestion, blood circulation, removal of toxins, uptake of nutrients, and so forth. Smoking or

A common recommendation for health of the voice is adequate hydration—that is, drink enough water.

use of tobacco products or working in contexts where noxious gases from gasoline, oil-based paints, or other known toxins are apt to be breathed or ingested is not recommended.

Tobacco and Other Toxins

Although tobacco companies denied for many years that smoking, chewing, dipping, or otherwise using tobacco products was causing cancers, all along the research was consistently confirming a causal link.

Junk Science

The term "junk science" has often been applied to deny valid research findings. In fact, the junk science has generally been produced by corporate entities with vested interests and with huge legal and financial liabilities in harm they have already done to consumers. In fact, the propaganda science produced by tobacco companies in defense of their harmful products is an excellent historical analog for the junk science propaganda produced in defense of thimerosal and other toxins in vaccines (cf. R. F. Kennedy, Jr., June 22, 2005, concerning "tobacco science and the thimerosal scandal," retrieved February 28, 2009, from http://www.robertfkennedyjr.com/docs/ThimerosalScandalFINAL.PDF).

With long-term habitual tobacco use, one of the first places the damage shows up is in ordinary breathing. The wheezy smoker's voice often is accompanied by a smoker's hack. Both the wheezy voice and the habitual hack are caused by smoke-damaged tissues. More recent research shows that the **carcinogenic qualities** of tobacco affect persons exposed indirectly as well as their offspring —tobacco smoke is also **genotoxic** (Yauk et al. 2007)—that is, it damages the genome as it is passed from one generation to the next. The male sperm cells in particular are susceptible to damage from tobacco use. Yauk et al. showed that smoking by the father causes genetic damage passed through sperm cells to subsequent generations. They did not study female lines, but the suspicion that the genetic damage can affect egg cells as well as sperm cells is a reasonable inference and well supported by other research showing damage to the unborn baby of mother's who smoke (Baler, Volkow, Fowler, & Benveniste, 2008). Interest in and concern for voice disorders is increased by the fact that they may be diagnostic of certain types of cancer or other serious disease conditions such as *emphysema* as seen in Figure 6–9.

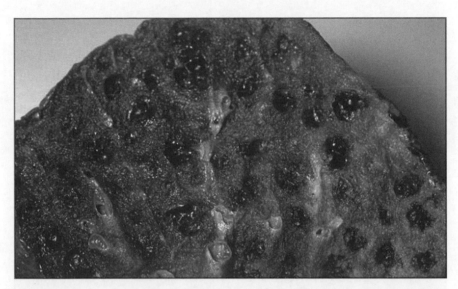

FIGURE 6–9. A sample of a smoker's lung (about 10 cm wide) with carbon deposits showing emphysema from smoking (photo by Dr. Edwin P. Ewing, Jr., 1973). From the Centers for Disease Control and Prevention; the image is in the public domain.

In addition to avoiding poisons and staying hydrated, we should also avoid unnecessary shouting, and also singing or speaking outside our comfortable pitch range (see "Vocal Hygiene," 2004, retrieved February 28, 2009, from http://pvcrp.com/vocal_hygiene .php). Straining the voice, especially when it is dehydrated, can cause damage to the voice.

Hyperfunction Disorders

The most common type of voice disorders are those caused by overuse or abuse. These are called **hyperfunction disorders** or sometimes just **functional disorders**. It is easier than we might expect to overuse or abuse the voice. Alcohol, smoking, and, of course, drug abuse and some medicines exacerbate abuse conditions because of the interactive effects of toxins and also by contributing to dehydration. Symptoms of a developing voice disorder often include pitch breaks (dropping into a lower register or "squeaking"), phonation breaks where the voice just seems to come and go producing gaps of silence. Shortness of breath and noticeable changes in the timbre of sounds can also be diagnostic of voice disorders. Changes in timbre are often described as hoarseness, breathiness, or harshness (examples of each of these are provided on the DVD). Other possible causes of such symptoms are damage from disease and/or toxins, but hyperfunction disorders are surprisingly common.

The most common type of voice disorders are those caused by overuse or abuse. These are called **hyperfunction disorders** or sometimes just **functional disorders**.

A raspy voice is also commonly associated with **vocal nodules** as shown in Figure 6–10. These are tumorous growths on or around the vocal folds or in the nearby tissues. They are anatomical anomalies that may be noticed as a persistent breathiness. The pathological growths are also called **singer's nodes**. They are somewhat like calluses that form on your hands and feet. But unlike ordinary calluses, which prevent damage to skin and bone, the hard nonpliable tissue formations in the vocal folds prevent them from operating normally. To vibrate in the normal way, the vocal folds must come together, or adduct.

> ## Vocal Nodules
>
> Vocal nodules can prevent complete closure of the vocal folds leaving spaces between them where air escapes producing the raspy sound. When air passes through the abnormal spaces, the vocal folds vibrate less than normally, and in extreme cases, not at all. To better understand why this is so, try blowing a raspberry sound with your lips. Next, hold a pen between your lips and try to make the raspberry sound again.

If you can do it at all, it will nevertheless be obvious that it is more difficult with the hard object in the way. Vocal nodules have a sim-

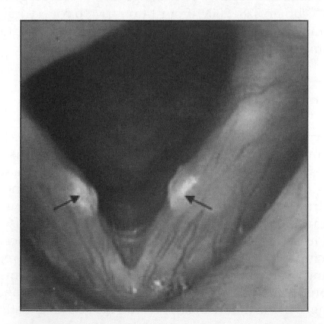

FIGURE 6–10. Contact ulcers on the vocal folds. Retrieved February 28, 2009, from http://www.gbmc.org/voice/disorders.cfm. Copyright © 1999 by The Milton J. Dance, Jr. Head & Neck Rehabilitation Center. Reprinted with permission. All rights reserved.

ilar effect. They prevent the folds from closing fully and vibrating normally, and usually cause the voice to sound breathy (check the DVD for an example of a <u>Breathy Voice</u>).

Hard Glottal Attack

To compensate for breathiness, the affected individual may push air through the larynx with more force using what is called a **hard glottal attack**. Although not recommended, this can be done by tightening the neck muscles and producing voice while at the same time pretending to lift a heavy object. What results is a combination of harsh and breathy voice, or what we often refer to as hoarseness. In an extreme variant of this procedure, a nearly complete obstruction of the larynx can result in a noise called **stridor**—a high-pitched croaky sound resembling the loud crowing of a rooster.

In emergency situations, stridor may be the precursor to complete strangulation, or, in some cases, the prevention of it. In extreme instances of blockage, it may be necessary to perform **intubation**—that is, to insert a tube into the windpipe to enable breathing. In situations where that is not possible, it may be necessary to perform a **tracheostomy**—where a hole is cut in the throat and the breathing tube is inserted directly into the trachea. Intubation itself, or endoscopic procedures that involve putting a tube into the windpipe, can damage the delicate tissues of the larynx. Such procedures are among the most common causes of the kind of contact ulcers displayed in Figure 6–11.

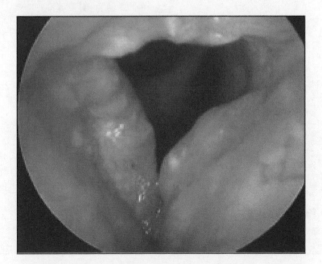

FIGURE 6–11. Singer's nodes. Retrieved February 28, 2009, from <u>http://www.med.nyu.edu/vo icescenter/conditions/voice/vocal_nodules.html</u> . Copyright © 2005 NYU Voice Center. Reprinted with permission. All rights reserved.

Acid Reflux

Another common source of damage to the voice, in addition to overexertion, is **acid reflux**—a condition better known as "heartburn." The most common treatment for acid reflux is an over the counter antacid such as the one pictured in Figure 6–12.

If the reflux is chronic it may be diagnosed as **gastroesophageal reflux disease** (**GERD**). When reflux occurs, acids that are normally contained safely in your stomach are pushed up through the esophagus into the pharyngeal cavity. Some of the acid, then, may leach into the larynx and damage the sensitive vocal folds and surrounding tissues. Vomiting can also produce acid reflux conditions, but because it occurs rarely for most people, the damage is usually temporary. By contrast, chronic abuse or chronic acid reflux, GERD, over time, can also lead to **contact ulcers** (see Figure 6–11) or vocal nodules (see Figure 6–10), or **granulomas**. Technically, a granuloma is a group of surface immune cells that engulf disease agents or dead tissue surrounded by a lymph cells forming a nodule. Granulomas are common to many diseases including **Crohn's disease**, tuberculosis, leprosy, and syphilis.

Among the supposed, although controversial, causes of chronic heartburn, the kind that does not respond to standard **antacid** treatments—for example, "Take a couple of Rolaids or Tums or a spoonful of Maalox and see if that doesn't fix it" (Figure 6–12)—is infection of the stomach by *Helicobacter pylori*. This bacterium, as seen in Figure 6–13, is associated with **peptic ulcers** of the stomach and is also found in association with more serious conditions, for example, cancers of the stomach and gastrointestinal tract ("Helicobacter Pylori," 2009, retrieved February 28, 2009, from http://en.wikipedia.org/wiki/Helicobacter_pylori; also Konturek, 2003).

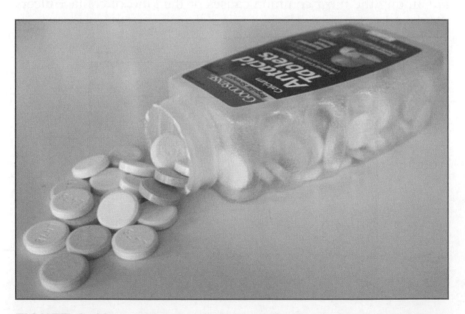

FIGURE 6–12. A bottle of generic antacid pills—a common treatment for voice disorders owed to acid reflux. Retrieved February 28, 2009, from http://en.wikipedia.org/wiki/Image:Antacid-L478.jpg. Reprinted under the terms of the GNU Free Documentation License, Version 1.2.

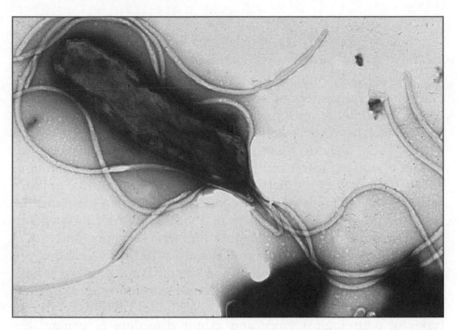

FIGURE 6–13. Electron micrograph of *Helicobacter pylori*. Retrieved February 28, 2009, from http://info.fujita-hu.ac.jp/~tsutsumi/photo/photo002-6.htm. Contributed with full permission from: Yutaka Tsutsumi, M.D. Professor Department of Pathology Fujita Health University School of Medicine.

Anatomical Anomalies

Although vocal hyperfunction can cause anatomic anomalies, there are other causes as well. Some are genetic, but most are the result of disease or trauma. In addition to granulomas, other common anomalies are **polyps**—tumors projecting from a mucous membrane. Another anomaly is **laryngeal webbing**—where tissue connections develop between the vocal folds—and there can also be wart-like growths caused by the **human papilloma virus (HPV)**. The HPV virus comes in 16 different known varieties 2 of which are involved in mouth and genital warts that can become cancerous (Brunotto et al., 2003). The tumorous growth usually is at the surface and can interfere with the normal function of the vocal folds, by preventing them from completely closing in the same way that vocal nodules or polyps do. Whereas vocal nodules usually are bilateral, affecting both folds (see Figure 6–10), anatomical anomalies, with the exception of webbing, are usually unilateral. In the cases of tumors, additional weight will be added to the vocal folds, either preventing them from vibrating, or causing them to vibrate at a lower frequency. Unfortunately, because these anatomical anomalies affect voice production, individuals will often compensate for the difference with hyperfunction behaviors, which in turn can cause further damage to the vocal folds.

DIFFERENTIATING THE DYSARTHRIAS

Neurological disorders of swallowing, voice, and speech can be compared to faulty wiring although the problems can arise at any level of the nervous system from the brain down to the body's atoms. There also are molecular interactions between toxins, for instance, with neurotransmitters and their receptors. The anatomical systems may be in the right places and the cognitive abilities may be intact (usually), but the connections between them may be deficient. Neurological disorders may not only cause problems in voice production, but they may interfere with sensation and movement in general. The neurological disorders of the voice, however, are usually classified in terms of the site of damage or the behaviors affected. Commonly both the site and symptoms are taken into consideration in differentiating the conditions. The most common types of neurological voice and motor disorders in general are dysarthria, apraxia, and ataxia.

The term dysarthria is based on the Greek root -arthria meaning joint or segment. So, dysarthria literally means *disjointed*. In fact, paralysis or weakness are the defining symptoms of dysarthrias as the term is presently used by clinicians. Most dysarthrias share some lack of coordination, and in dysarthrias of speaking, they are characterized by slow, effortful speech, distortions and substitutions, as well as resonance and volume regulation problems. It is not just the speech articulators that can be affected. The respiratory system, the voice, and swallowing are also commonly affected. Five kinds of dysarthria were distinguished by Darley, Aronson, and Brown (1975). These categories are still used today (Duffy, 2005; also see Ludlow, et al., 2008). We will discuss all five of them explaining some of the commonly affected systems along the way.

The dysarthrias are neuromuscular disorders that affect movements, coordination, and muscle tone. The specific symptoms and systems affected by the dysarthrias usually tell something about where and how things have gone wrong.

Flaccid Dysarthrias

Flaccid dysarthrias are often caused by damage in the **lower motor neuron (LMN)** system. This is the system of efferent neurons that actually connect with the muscles of the body controlling their movements. See the lower portion of Figure 6–14. It receives its commands from the **upper motor neuron (UMN)** system as shown in the top part of Figure 6–14.

The UMN System

The UMN system actually consists of two systems that interact. The one that is especially important with respect to volitional move-

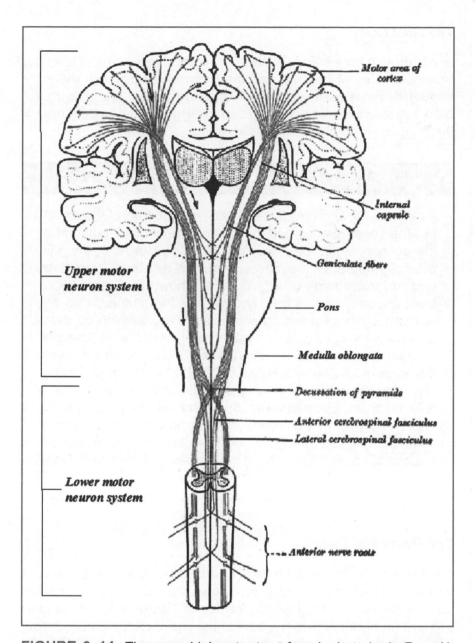

FIGURE 6–14. The pyramidal motor tract from brain to body. From H. Gray, 1918, Anatomy *of the Human Body* (Illustration 764). Philadelphia, PA: Lea & Febiger. Copyright © 2000 by Bartleby.com, ON-LINE ED., Inc. Retrieved February 28, 2009, from http://www.bartleby.com/107/illus764 .html. Reprinted with permission. All rights reserved.

ments, is the **pyramidal tract**—also known as the **corticospinal tract** because in connects the efferent neurons of the brain with each other and with those in the spine. The other UMN system, called the **extrapyramidal tract**, which is not pictured in Figure 6–14, performs a great many functions that are interrelated with the autonomic nervous system as well as with the pyramidal tract.

The Glial Cells

In addition to the neuronal cells of the cortex, consisting of afferent, (sensory), efferent (motor), and interneurons—of which there are known to be at least a hundred different types; see "Neurons," 2009, retrieved February 28, 2009, from http://en.wikipedia.org/wiki/Neurons)—there are also *glial cells*.

Gliotransmissions

As we saw in Chapter 3, the motor neurons greatly outnumber the sensory ones and the interneurons vastly outnumber the sensory and motor neurons together. However, the glial cells outnumber all the others combined by about 10 to 1. An electron micrograph of a glial cell is shown as Figure 6–15. Most importantly, it is now known, that the glial cells do not just perform housekeeping chores such as cleaning up damaged or dead nerve cells as was formerly supposed. The glial cells are also involved in transmissions within the central nervous system (Y. Zhang & Hayden, 2005; Halassa et al., 2007). The signals originating in glial cells are currently being referred to as **gliotransmissions**. The role being played by these exceedingly numerous cells is only just beginning to come to light. It is suspected that they are involved in recruiting and shepherding neurological functions that involve many distinct pyramidal cells and interneurons.

The Pyramidal Tract

Meanwhile, the *pyramidal tract* is known to consist mainly of cells that have a body that roughly resembles the shape of a pyramid as seen in the dark triangle at the center of Figure 6–16. These cells account for about 80% of the cells in the entire cortex (not counting the glial cells) and for about that same proportion in the motor neurons involved in swallowing, voice, and speech production. Each of these pyramidal cells receives input on its **dendrites**—the smaller branches from the cell body in Figure 6–16—and it also projects a larger and longer efferent **axon**. See the dark line extending upward from the pyramid (at the center of Figure 6–16) whose main excitatory neurotransmitter is **glutamate**.

As shown in Figure 6–14, the motor neurons (shown as pink lines) descend mainly from the motor cortex (also see the discussion of Figures 1–6, 1–7, and 1–8 in Chapter 1). The pyramidal system and the extrapyramidal system connect with each other and with the LMN system that reaches all the way out to the peripheral muscles.

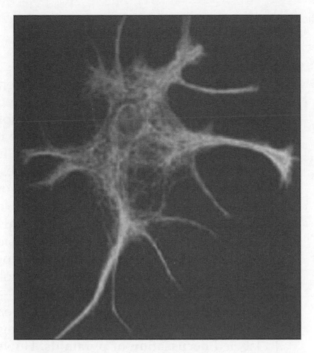

FIGURE 6–15. An astrocyte, glial cell. Retrieved February 28, 2009, from http://www.sfn.org/index .cfm?pagename=brainBriefings_astrocytes. Photo by Vladimir Parpura, M.D., Ph.D., Iowa State University and University of California at Riverside. Copyright © 2000. Reprinted with permission. All rights reserved.

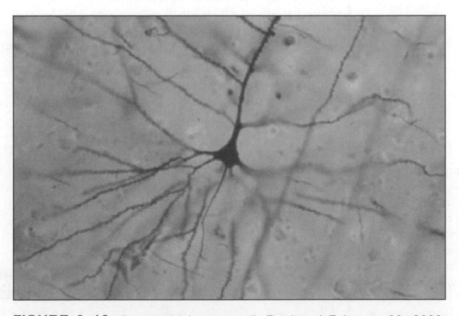

FIGURE 6–16. A pyramidal nerve cell. Retrieved February 28, 2009, from http://en.wikipedia.org/wiki/Image:GolgiStainedPyramidalCell.jpg. Reprinted under the terms of the GNU Free Documentation License, Version 1.2.

The Divisions of Efferent Fibers

There are two major groups of descending efferent fibers from the pyramidal system. The **geniculate fibers** connect with nerves descending from the opposite hemisphere at the cranial nuclei while the main bundle of fibers in the **internal capsule** continues its descent through the cerebellum and into the **medulla oblongata** where the descending capsule branches. Most of the fibers, in the **lateral cerebrospinal fasciculus** cross over to the opposite side of the body—the ones that do not cross over provide motor signals to the same side of the body that the hemisphere is located on. These are called **ipsilateral**—literally, "same side"—connections and they provide back-up motor signals preventing paralysis of one side even if the hemisphere or neurons enabling voluntary control of the opposite side—the **contralateral** connections—are damaged or shut down completely. This largest crossing of fibers appears as an "X" about two-thirds of the way down in the diagram of Figure 6–14 and is labeled **decussation of pyramids**. However, the descending efferent neurons are also crossed at most of the **nuclei of the cranial nerves** (as shown later in Figure 6–18).

Neurons that extend on to the LMN system are involved in controlling how quickly and how many muscle fibers we are able to contract voluntarily and intentionally at the periphery, for example, as in moving a hand or foot, bending over, standing up, and so forth. Damage to the LMN system can result in what is called **fasciculation**—muscle twitching—or it may result in general weakness, paralysis, and **atrophy** of muscles—shrinking and weakness owed to disuse. For all these reasons, the term *flaccid dysarthria* is appropriate because it suggests floppy, inactive, weak muscles. In the worst case scenarios, lesions occurring in the UMN system in the nuclei of the cranial nerves—the points where the cranial nerves from both sides meet and communicate with each other—can cause paralysis to large systems of muscles on both sides of the body.

The Cranial Nerves and Their Nuclei

The **cranial nerves** consist of large bundles of neuronal fibers connecting the brain with sensory and sensory-motor systems as summed up in Figure 6–17. Their nuclei are neural system hubs or transit points for electrochemical signals that connect the two sides of the central nervous system.

Among the many mnemonics to help us remember how the 12 cranial nerves are distributed with reference to their functions is the sentence, "OLd OPie OCcasionally TRies TRIGonometry And Feels VEry GLOomy, VAGUe, And HYPOactive" where the first letters in caps indicate the main functions of the cranial nerves in order.

What the Cranial Nerves Control

  I. Olfactory—sense of smell;
 II. Optical—sense of sight;
III. Oculomotor—movement of the eye;
IV. Trochlear—movement of the eye inward toward the nose;

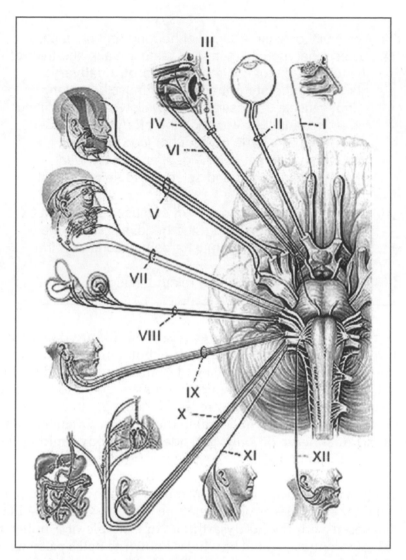

FIGURE 6–17. A schematic of the main afferent and efferent cranial nerves associated with sensory and motor systems. Retrieved February 28, 2009, from http://www.neurophys.com/ EMG/Cranial_Nerves/CranialNerves.jpg. Copyright © 1997–2003 by Neurophys.com. Reprinted with permission. All rights reserved.

V. Trigeminal—sense of facial expressions and movement of jaw in chewing;

VI. Abducens—movement of the eye outward (away from the nose);

VII. Facial—(a) movement of the face; (b) movement of the stapedius muscle involved in the middle ear reflex (see Chapter 3); (c) sense of taste from the front two-thirds of the tongue; (d) motor activation of all but one of the salivary glands, and (e) motor control of the tear gland;

VIII. Vestibulocochlear—sense of hearing and balance;
IX. Glossopharyngeal—sense of taste in back one-third of the tongue, motor control of the **parotid salivary gland**, and the **stylopharyngeus** muscle—a long skinny muscle that assists the swallowing act by lifting the larynx and thus widening the pharynx to enable swallowing of a large mouthful of food or liquid;
X. Vagus—movement of laryngeal and pharyngeal muscles; diaphragm, and spleen; and sense of taste at the epiglottis;
XI. Accessory spinal—movement of muscles in the neck enabling us to lift and turn the head, also to lift the shoulders (as in a shrug); shares functions with the vagus nerve;
XII. Hypoglossal—tongue and related muscles.

If the nuclei of the cranial nerves (Figure 6–18) are damaged or destroyed, their loss can cause dysfunctions in multiple muscle groups. The loss tends to be bilateral—affecting both sides of the body because the nuclei are typically crossed, going to both sides of the body. Peripheral lesions are less damaging, but still harmful although they tend to be unilateral in their effects. Often they damage the cranial nerve on only one side of the body limiting their impact on affected muscles.

As can be expected from the above description, patients who exhibit (fasciculations), who demonstrate weak movement or paralysis, and/or abnormal atrophying of the muscle would most likely be diagnosed with flaccid dysarthria. An example of a unilateral disorder, by contrast, would be what is known as **Bell's palsy** where one side of the face appears flat, and lacking in tone and expression by contrast with the other side of the face. See the example in Figure 6–19. Notice the left-sidedness of the smile while the right side seems less expressive. The right side reduction in range of motion associated with the facial expression suggests that cranial nerve VII is directly or indirectly restricted, possibly damaged in some way, in the left hemisphere.

In a more generalized **progressive palsy**, the disease of the UMN system together with the brainstem tends to affect some or all of the muscles controlled by the cranial nerves of the brainstem. Typically it impacts the cranial nerves IX, X, and XII, which are involved in swallowing, voice, and speech movements.

Sometimes Mistaken for Pseudobulbar Palsy

The flaccid dysarthrias resemble a distinct disorder that is called (somewhat misleadingly) **pseudobulbar palsy** ("Pseudobulbar palsy," 2009, retrieved February 28, 2009, from http://health.enotes

*An example of a unilateral disorder, by contrast, would be what is known as **Bell's palsy** where one side of the face appears flat, and lacking in tone and expression by contrast with the other side of the face. See the example in Figure 6–19.*

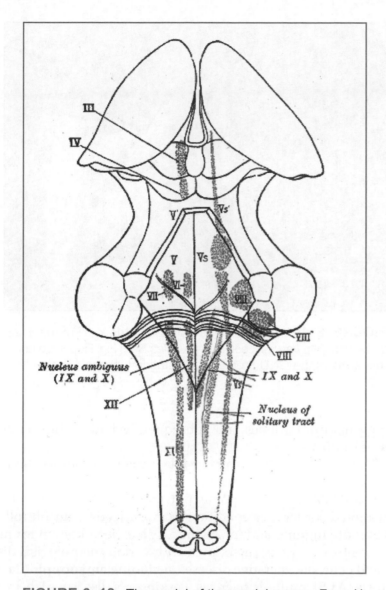

FIGURE 6–18. The nuclei of the cranial nerves. From H. Gray, 1918, *Anatomy of the Human Body* (Illustration 696). Philadelphia, PA: Lea & Febiger. Copyright © 2000 by Bartleby.com, ON-LINE ED., Inc. Retrieved February 28, 2009, from http://www.bartleby.com/107/illus696.html. Reprinted with permission. All rights reserved.

.com/neurological-disorders-encyclopedia/pseudobulbar-palsy; Kuroda, 2007). The hallmark symptoms of pseudobulbar palsy are dysarthria, limited tongue movement, and drooling (Kim et al., 2006). Another symptom commonly mentioned for pseudobulbar palsy is **lability**—proneness to unpredictable emotional outbursts. However, we hardly need to mention that this symptom—being labile—can also be associated with many other neurological disorders and with many different types of brain damage. For instance, Phineas Gage, a case discussed in Chapter 10, had a steel rod driven

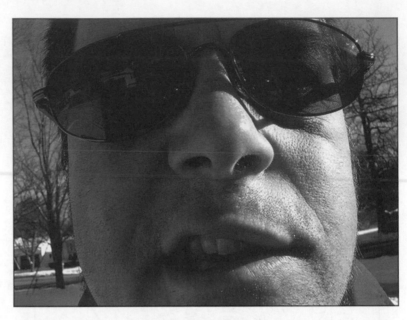

FIGURE 6–19. Left side Bell's palsy. Retrieved February 28, 2009, from http://en.wikipedia.org/wiki/Files:Bells.jpg. Reprinted under the terms of the GNU Free Documentation License, Version 1.2.

Emotional extremes are common to a host of neurological disease conditions (for example, schizophrenia and/or bipolar disorder as argued by Correll et al., 2007), hormonal imbalances in many disease conditions (for example, Lou Gehrig's disease as shown by Zimmerman et al., 2007; also see R. G. Miller et al., 2009; M. J. Strong, 2008), and toxic injuries (for example, from medications for ADHD as shown by Kratochvil et al., 2007).

through his frontal lobes and subsequently had a fairly extreme form of lability.

To see just how uninformative it is to make the observation that pseudobulbar palsy is associated with lability, consider the remarks by Duda (2007) where he points out that "involuntary emotional expression disorder . . . a condition characterized by uncontrollable episodes of laughing and/or crying. . . . has been known for more than a century . . . [to be] associated with various neurological disorders and neurodegenerative diseases, including **amyotrophic lateral sclerosis [ALS]**, multiple sclerosis, Parkinson's disease, Alzheimer's disease and other dementias, and neurological injuries such as stroke and traumatic brain injury" (p. 6). The emotional lability in question is commonly referred to as **pseudobulbar affect** (R. G. Miller, et al., 2009; M. J. Strong, 2008).

To tell for sure what region of the brain is damaged, advanced imaging techniques (see Chapter 10) may be helpful, but may not be definitive. For example, the best imaging techniques currently available cannot show the generalized impact of toxins that act at the atomic and molecular levels. Yet such toxins—for example, mercury, antidepressant medications, pesticides, or interactions among these kinds of toxic agents—can cause generalized neurological dysfunctions including lability and/or severe mood swings that do not involve a particular area of the brain anymore than destruction of the entire body does.

The so-called **bulbar region** of the brain was called that because anatomists thought the medulla, roughly at the center of the brainstem, looked like the bulb of a plant root. What is more properly called **bulbar palsy** is caused by damage to the brainstem in particular. "Pseudobulbar" palsy, by contrast, is caused by damage to the UMN system. Both can affect swallowing, voice, and speech functions, but theoretically, at least, they involve damage to distinct regions of the nervous system. In fact, it is often difficult if not impossible to pin down the exact site of damage, or the precise source, of these hypothetically distinct disorders. However, radiography and magnetic resonance imaging can sometimes identify particular lesions, and the symptoms associated with a particular case may also *sometimes* be diagnostic.

Hyperkinetic Dysarthrias

Hyperkinetic dysarthrias usually result from damage to the **basal ganglia**—a collection of nuclei deep inside both hemispheres within the temporal lobes as shown in Figure 6–20. The basal ganglia—see the positions of the sections and the expanded view in the lower right corner of Figure 6–20—are contained beneath and within the distorted horseshoe shape of the corpus callosum (see Figure 6–3). This collection of nuclei is involved in the coordination of voluntary movements. It functions in collaboration with the upper motor neuron system (UMN) of the cerebrum and also with the cerebellum.

Figure 6–21 is a diagram showing an oversimplified theory of the role of the basal ganglia in the regulation of voluntary movement. According to current understanding, the basal ganglia are involved in controlling voluntary movements by a kind of braking

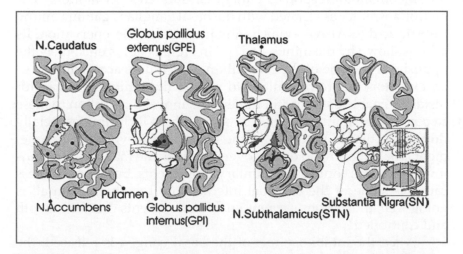

FIGURE 6–20. Four slices of the basal ganglia in the left hemisphere from front to back—see location of slices in the key (lower right side). Retrieved February 28, 2009, from http://en.wikipedia.org/wiki/Image:Anatomie-Ba salganglien-A.jpg#filehistory Public domain. Image placed in the public domain by its anonymous creator July 18, 2006.

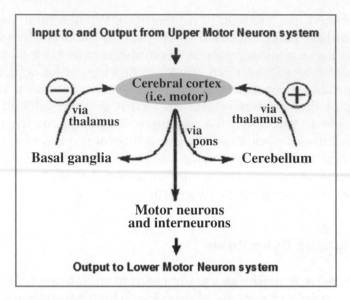

FIGURE 6–21. The interactions of UMN with LMN as mediated by the cerebellum and the basal ganglia (also known as the extrapyramidal tract). Retrieved September 12, 2008, from http://thalamus.wustl.edu/course/cerebell.html. Created by Diana Weedman Molavi, Ph.D., at the Washington University School of Medicine, Department of Anatomy and Neurobiology. Copyright © 1997 by the Washington University Program in Neuroscience http://neuroscience.wustl.edu. Adapted with permission. All rights reserved.

action inhibiting the firing of some motor neurons and thus ensuring smooth motor responses rather than sudden jerky motions. The neurotransmitter associated with the basal ganglia is **gamma amino butyric acid (GABA)**—which inhibits muscle fiber enervation. Its role, as shown by the minus sign "−" in Figure 6–21 is effectively the opposite of the role of the cerebellum, which uses **acetylcholine**—an excitatory neurotransmitter to release the inhibitions that, for instance, enable us to sit still rather than move. In addition to these two neurotransmitters, there are many others including especially **dopamine** that is involved in the regulation of voluntary movement. The diagram, no doubt, oversimplifies the many interactions involved in the control of voluntary movements, but it nonetheless captures some of the essential interactions. Together, when all is going well, the various systems enable movements that are smooth and controlled.

When the inhibitory role of the basal ganglia is released, the sort of wild, uncontrolled, dance-like movements characteristic of **Huntington's disease (HD)**, formerly called **Huntington's chorea**, are apt to occur. This condition was first accurately described by George Huntington [1850–1916] and was described by him in 1872. He used the word *chorea*—from the Greek word meaning "dancing"—to describe it because of the sweeping hyperkinetic move-

When damage occurs to the basal ganglia, movements may (1) seem sudden and out of control—a hyperkinetic effect, or (2) slow, tremulous, and effortful—which may also be a hyperkinetic effect.

ments of the limbs that are characteristic of the condition. A person affected by HD may start to take a step or move a hand when suddenly the whole leg may rise up above the level of the knee and the arm on the same or opposite side of the body may rise above the head. Or, a person sitting down may give the appearance of not being able to sit still. The arms and legs may seem to just leap into motion of their own free will. The symptoms are clear even if the exact causes are somewhat obscure.

In the contrasting case of slow, tremulous, effortful movements, the lack of inhibition may result in contraction of opposing muscle groups simultaneously where the muscles operate in dynamic tension against each other. When this occurs, it can still be hyperkinetic activity (at least in theory) that results in a spastic paralysis of the sort seen in cerebral palsy. Such a spastic hyperkinetic condition can occur at many different levels in the body—for example, it can occur in a single group of muscle fibers such as the calf in a swimmer's cramp—but if it is caused by damage to the basal ganglia, it is apt to affect the whole body. In later stages of HD, for instance, the disorder tends to affect the facial muscles along with speech and swallowing.

Hypokinetic Dysarthrias

Hypokinetic dysarthrias usually result from damage to the **substantia nigra**—see the rightmost slice of the brain pictured in Figure 6–20. This dark-colored tissue deep within the basal ganglia is involved in the production of the neurotransmitter known as *dopamine*. If dopamine production is reduced or lost because of damage to this region, the result is typically some form of **Parkinson's disease (PD)**. Dr. James Parkinson [1755–1828] first described the disease that now bears his name in 1817. He called it the shaking palsy.

Damage to the substantia nigra has also been definitively linked to increased levels of toxins such as mercury (Barlow, Cory-Slechta, Richfield, & Thiruchelvam, 2007; Blotcky, Claassen, Fung, Meade, & Rack, 1995; Carvey, Punati, & Newman, 2006; Hatcher et al., 2007; Kanthasamy, Kitazawa, Kanthasamy, & Anantharam, 2005; R. K. B. Pearce, Owen, Daniel, Jenner, & Marsden, 1997; Petersen et al., 2008; Rybicki, C. C. Johnson, Uman, & Gorell, 1993).

Spastic Dysarthrias

Spastic dysarthrias are caused by damage to the upper motor neuron (UMN) system, also known as the pyramidal tract. Damage to the UMN affects the ability to make fine motor adjustments. The affected individual may appear to be uncoordinated and to be doing more than what is needed. Movement appears to be extremely effortful. In the case of the spastic dysarthria of the voice, the condition is referred to as **spastic dysphonia**—where the vocal folds

Along with Alzheimer's disease, PD is among the most common forms of **dementia** (also see Chapter 10). PD is also commonly comorbid with Alzheimer's. The main symptoms of PD are decreased range of motion in affected systems, rigidity in the muscles, and tremors.

are too tight during speech production. Commonly, damage to the UMN affects the entire body and may result in either spasticity or flaccidity.

Another category of dysarthrias is what has been called **unilateral motor neuron dysarthria**. Just as the name implies, damage has occurred to one of the UMN or peripheral tracts in the LMN system so that only one side of the body is affected.

Ataxic Dysarthrias

Ataxic dysarthrias have generally been associated with damage to the cerebellum and/or pathways emanating from it. As with the UMN system, the LMN system, and the basal ganglia, the cerebellum is generally involved in the control of movement. Exactly how the control is exercised is not well understood but it is becoming clear that the cerebellum is involved in brain functions more generally and at higher levels of cognition than formerly thought (Mohler, 2007). Nonetheless, it is uncontroversial that the cerebellum is involved in controlling the timing and force of movements (for one explanation, see Figure 6–21).

With that in mind, an obvious symptom of ataxic dysarthrias of speech should include distorted rhythms, stress patterns, and pitch patterns in the control of speech—that is, distortions of the collection of such features which make up what linguists call prosody. Current research has demonstrated a role of the cerebellum in the control of prosody in particular and in the coordination of the rapid sequence of articulatory movements required in speech production (Spencer & Slocomb, 2007). Also Perez-Martinez et al. (2007) have proposed that the right hemisphere of the cerebrum (not the cerebellum) is also critically involved in the production of normal prosody. As a consequence, it is unsurprising that prosody can also be affected in situations where the damage is far removed from the cerebellum. In fact, Terao et al. (2007) describe three cases of individuals who developed serious problems in prosody—and in what we believe others would describe as ataxic dysarthria— without significant involvement of the cerebellum. Nevertheless, clinicians commonly assume that "ataxic dysarthria" is diagnostic of cerebellar damage.

But, it may not be. Additionally, substitutions, distortions, and what is loosely called "imprecise articulation"—a term that is about as imprecise as could be imagined to describe an articulation problem—are all descriptors commonly ascribed to ataxic dysarthrias. They cannot possibly be definitive, however, because of the fact that they apply equally well to a huge class of motor disorders that are associated with other diagnostic categories and a vastly diverse sort of damage. The damage can range from what is called **Gulf War syndrome**—ostensibly caused by exposure to toxins (Kurt, 1998) —to the peculiar manifestations of what is called **foreign accent**

syndrome. The latter is described by Blumstein and Kurowski (2006) as "an apraxia of speech, a dysarthria, and an aphasic speech output disorder" (p. 346), which they specifically refer to as "a deficit in linguistic prosody" (p. 346). The only reasonable conclusion to reach from the published research is that researchers are still far from understanding very well how prosody is controlled.

Perhaps it was inevitable, then, for Darley and colleagues to propose a sixth category of dysarthrias to pick up the slack, so-to-speak, as they might have said with a loose jaw and a floppy tongue in cheek.

Mixed Dysarthrias

Mixed dysarthrias comprise the sixth category Darley and colleagues proposed.

The Miscellaneous Category

Because of the high probability of comorbid conditions in the kinds of brain damage that cause dysarthrias, the term "mixed dysarthrias" has much to recommend it. It not only serves as a catch-all for cases where symptoms are not limited to any single one of the foregoing categories, but it is appropriate because dysarthrias tend to be diffuse and mixed in their impact. They commonly affect not just articulation, but also respiration, phonation, and the so-called "vegetative movements" associated with digestion, such as chewing, swallowing, and the mobility of food and liquid all the way through the digestive tract to the elimination of waste.

They are also commonly associated with the type of disorders that typically involve volitional complex movements which generally are classed as "apraxias"—for example, consider the "foreign accent syndrome" that Blumstein and Kurowski referred to as an apraxia specifically affecting prosody, which others assign to some sort of ataxia. In fact, the ataxias and apraxias are not as sharply distinguished as might be expected by the difference in the terms. Of course, as we noted at the outset, comorbidity is expected and is also common.

It is highly probable that an individual diagnosed with any extreme form of dysarthria will also manifest voice disorders, along with breathing and swallowing disorders. Precisely because the most common causes of damage to the nervous system are traumatic accidents, they are largely unpredictable in terms of place or effect. Much the same can also be said for the diffuse damage that can be caused by disease, toxins, genetic disorders, medical procedures, or

Although "ataxia" seems to suggest a breakdown in sequencing and order, and "apraxia" suggests inability to perform complex movements, they are both loosely associated with the same kinds of movement disorders in many instances.

some combination of these. As a consequence, higher order cognition and the emotions are commonly impacted along with the motor systems. This is especially true in the motor disorders that impact voice and speech. Typically, the motor disorders of speech are distinguished by the fact that they distinctly involve volitional control. However, volition is also involved in swallowing and breathing in spite of the fact that they are sometimes considered "vegetative movements."

TREATMENT OF MOTOR DISORDERS

The **apraxias** are different from the dysarthrias mainly because the apraxias involve impairment of voluntary movements. The affected individual has trouble completing voluntary/purposeful movements. For example, repeating a verbal routine or habitual phrase might be no problem for a person with apraxia, but the same person may be unable to repeat an unfamiliar clause or to imitate a complex novel sequence of movements. As readers will easily understand, the difficulties just described clearly fit the description of ataxias about as well as apraxias. Setting that aside, however, it is useful to keep in mind that the apraxias are perhaps best defined by difficulties with voluntary movements but in the absence of paralysis or weakness, which are the defining traits of dysarthrias.

With linguistic apraxias the therapy should generally facilitate access to and comprehension of the pragmatic mapping of increasingly complex linguistic forms onto their appropriate pragmatic contexts. Generally the therapy should begin at the highest level of linguistic performance the individual can still perform and then seek to build from there to more complex or higher functions (cf. S. D. Oller, 2005).

As with dysarthria, apraxia is often the result of a neurological injury of some type usually involving the central nervous system —especially the brain. Injuries that cause apraxia usually involve the UMN and especially the motor strip and associated areas of the frontal cortex. It is generally claimed that clinicians should distinguish the apraxias and dysarthrias because the recommended treatments differ. Because dysarthrias are generally the result of some form of paralysis and/or weakness, emphasis is placed on compensating for weakened muscles by strengthening or using others. By contrast with the apraxias, except where they are accompanied by one or more dysarthrias, successful therapeutic approaches are more likely to concentrate on the gradual restoration of skills. This is likely to involve the gradual building up of successful sequences of movements. It may require mapping of the functional contexts in which the complex movement sequences are appropriate, for example, re-learning bit by bit the processes of standing up and taking steps, or of getting some food on a spoon and bringing it to the mouth. These approaches to treating motor disorders owed to paralysis and/or flaccidity, say, by any standard are radically different from the therapies most likely to succeed in restoring linguistic skills, say, that have been lost in a language based apraxia or ataxia.

The Dysphagias

Throughout this chapter we have dealt mainly with the second most basic kinds of signs—namely, movements assisted by sensations. The movements of greatest interest to the study of human communication disorders, without any competition, are the language disorders and those related disorders that involve volitional movements resulting from intentional actions.

Volition Is Central to Meaningful Movements

We have seen that movements cannot have any social meaning at all unless they are accompanied by valid sensory representations. So, meaningful movements, especially facial expressions such as smiling, pointing, and all other intentional social acts, must be aided by sensory signs. Language too depends on sensations and movements. Voluntary movements are crucial to speaking, writing, Deaf signing, and intentional acts in general. Even acts such as breathing in or out, swallowing, clearing one's throat, sniffing, or blinking involve movements that commonly can and often do convey important meanings in human interactions. The movements of speech and language obviously depend on the higher symbol systems peculiar to language.

The dysphagias are distinct from speech and language disorders as such because swallowing does not necessarily involve anything more than an intentional movement. Difficulties in swallowing, the "dysphagias," range from problems in initiating the swallow—a voluntary intentional action—to successfully completing the swallow, which is a function performed by the autonomic system. The latter part of the swallow falls under the autonomic system, which also controls glandular functions, essential digestive processes, and so forth without our conscious or volitional involvement. However, dysphagias are an extremely important class of disorders because of their potential to interfere with breathing. They connect with the production of voice and speech on that account.

Because of that close association, as we saw above, speech-language pathologists are generally, if not universally, the therapists of choice for the treatment of dysphagias. For instance, it is estimated that approximately one-half of individuals who experience an acute stroke will also experience some degree of dysphagia (Manna, Hankeya, & Cameron, 2000). For severe brain injuries from auto accidents or other head injuries, the likelihood of an accompanying difficulty in swallowing is also very high. Approximately, 20 to 40% of individuals with a traumatic brain injury will experience some dysphagia (Winstein, 1981; Terre & Mearin, 2007).

In the tetanus disease, the neurotoxin produced by the bacterium is rapidly transferred from the point of infection along neural pathways all the way from the efferent connections at the periphery, as diagramed in Figure 6–22, to the brain.

Because the **prognosis**—that is, the course that disorders will probably follow over time and especially the prospects for self-repair or response to treatment—often differs depending on the cause of the problem, and the level at which the communication systems of the body and nervous system may be affected, it is useful, to consider the broad range of voice problems that can occur in terms of their etiology and the other systems they involve.

Similarly, degenerative diseases of the central nervous system such as Alzheimer's and Parkinsonism, are also commonly associated with dysphagia (Easterling, & Mobbins, 2008).

Voice Problems in Particular

A problem in any one of the systems involved in motor production of speech or its related bodily and neurological systems can directly or indirectly result in a voice disorder. Often, those disorders are caused by problems in more than one of the systems on which voice directly or indirectly depends. Because the voice is deeply connected with speech, and through speech with the highest levels of neurological control of language, voice disorders may be symptomatic of higher cognitive and neurological difficulties. More commonly, voice disorders are associated with problems in the bodily systems associated with breathing, swallowing, and digestion—the LMN system rather than the UMN system. However, we have seen that UMN problems can also be the direct cause of LMN difficulties. Also, because voice disorders are intrinsically related to the higher cortical functions of speech on the one hand and the essential processes of breathing, swallowing, and digestion on the other, voice disorders are of special interest and reasonable concern on the part of clinicians.

Depending on the level of the neurological involvements, voice disorders may be associated with generalized disease conditions that impact the muscles, the gastrointestinal tract, the glandular systems, or with neurological disorders that affect everything from the muscles up to the highest levels of cortical control of speech production and intentional articulate movements.

As we will see in Chapters 8 and 10, the articulate movements of speech are associated with cortical systems that are also involved in other highly skilled movements such as playing a musical instrument, dancing, and essentially all activities that involve the sorts of volitional movements and control systems involved in pointing, reaching, and grasping. Sports such as boxing, wrestling, fencing, tennis, baseball, and the like are sufficiently complex that they too involve motor control systems similar in gross respects to the muscle control involved in speech, writing, and manual signing of language. For all these reasons, the diagnostic value of voice disorders may be highly significant. Sometimes, for reasons we gave above, because of the association of voice disorders with various cancers, a correct early diagnosis of a voice disorder could be a matter of life or death.

Voice Disorders as Diagnostic

We saw above that voice disorders can be caused by anatomical anomalies, digestive difficulties, disease, and/or by excessive vocal exertion, and by neurological problems. Voice disorders can also be the result of a traumatic injury to the larynx—for example, from a blow to the throat—or to any of the related systems on which the normal functioning of the voice depends. Similarly, cumulative or traumatic neurologic damage or disease can produce a voice disorder. Rarely, an emotionally traumatic event can apparently trigger a voice disorder even in the absence of any other physical injury or disease factor (Baker, 2003). However, the most common traumatic causes of voice disorders are physical injuries to the throat, chest, mouth, or head. The most common causes of such traumatic injuries are automobile accidents but sports injuries can also damage the voice and related systems. In any case, it is important to determine just what factors are causing the problem when voice disorders are either detected or just suspected.

Muscle Tone and Levels of Control

Hypotonia

There are many motor conditions affecting the muscles and/or nervous systems of the body that can affect the voice and related system of swallowing, breathing, and speech motor control in a negative way. Some of these can affect the muscles in general and are not necessarily a direct consequence of damage to the brain or nervous system as such. For instance, **hypotonia** is the condition where the muscles lose their tone and become limp, flaccid, or floppy.

One type of hypotonia, **myasthenia gravis** (Conti-Fine, Milani, & Kaminski, 2006)—where *mya-* refers to the muscle and *-sthenia* means weakness and *gravis* means severe—is caused by an autoimmune disease that blocks the normal use of the neurotransmitter acetylcholine, which is involved in excitatory motor signals in general. This blockage prevents normal muscular recovery after use.

Figure 6–22 shows the level of the connection between the neuron and the muscle at which the neurotransmitter acetylcholine normally works to allow the muscle fiber to recover after firing. The most characteristic symptom of myasthenia gravis is muscle weakness, for example, drooping eyelids after an eye-blink, followed by gradual recovery after prolonged inactivity. Muscles that can be affected include not only those involved in blinking, eye movement, facial expressions, chewing, swallowing, breathing, head movements, but, in fact all of the muscles of the body. This includes those involved in voice production and the articulators involved in speech.

One of the noteworthy facts about this particular disorder is that, although it affects many bodily systems it is caused by neurotoxic

Figure 6–22 shows the level of the connection between the neuron and the muscle at which the neurotransmitter acetylcholine normally works to allow the muscle fiber to recover after firing.

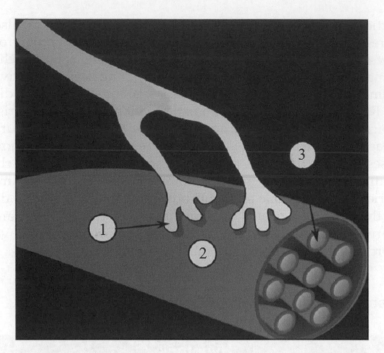

FIGURE 6–22. A diagram of the efferent nerve terminals (1) that cause a muscle fiber (2) to contract by signaling the fibrils (3) inside the bundle. Retrieved February 28, 2009, from http://en.wikipedia.org/wiki/Image:Synapse_diag3.png. Adapted and reprinted under the terms of the GNU Free Documentation License, Version 1.2.

impact on the immune system at the molecular level. When the function of acetylcholine is blocked, the resulting muscle weakness and excessive fatigue can affect swallowing and breathing. It is a serious condition.

The opposite condition, **hypertonia**, is where the muscles become rigid and cramp in a spastic condition. For instance, a general condition of spastic hypertonia where the skeletal muscles contract in an almost complete body cramp can be caused by the tetanus bacterium—*Clostridium tetani* ("Tetanus," 2009, retrieved February 28, 2009, from http://en.wikipedia.org/wiki/Tetanus). The commonly lethal results of the neurotoxin released by that bacterium are depicted in Figure 6–23. The painting shown there was created by Sir Charles Bell [1774–1842], the surgeon that many regard as the founder of **clinical neurology**. The generalized spasm of the muscles is caused by **tetanospasmin**—a neurotoxin that interferes with neurotransmitters that normally inhibit muscle contractions. In the tetanus disease, the neurotoxin produced by the bacterium is rapidly transferred from the point of infection along neural pathways all the way from the efferent connections at the periphery, as diagramed in Figure 6–22, to the brain. We have already considered many other causes of hypotonia and hypertonia. Many of these can cause swallowing to stall right from the

In the tetanus disease, the neurotoxin produced by the bacterium is rapidly transferred from the point of infection along neural pathways all the way from the efferent connections at the periphery, as diagramed in Figure 6–22, to the brain.

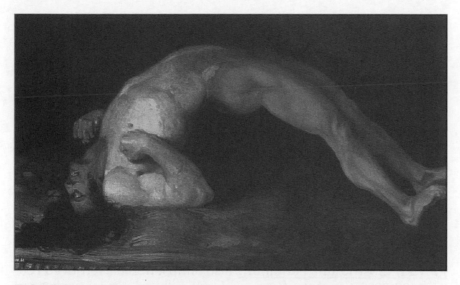

FIGURE 6–23. The impact of the neurotoxin tetanospasmin—released by Clostridium tetani—drawing by Sir Charles Bell, 1809. Retrieved February 28, 2009, from http://en.wikipedia.org/wiki/Tetanus. This image is in the public domain because its copyright has expired.

start. The epiglottis may not close off the route into the trachea and life-threatening choking can occur. The conditions in question can also interrupt a swallow with potentially fatal results.

There is another neurotoxin that is commonly extracted for medicinal and cosmetic uses including the treatment of certain disorders of the voice and of swallowing. Like the bacterium that produces tetanospasmin, *Clostridium botulinum* ("Clostridium botulinum," 2009, retrieved February 28, 2009, from http://en.wikipedia.org/wiki/Clostridium_botulinum; also see Ryan & Ray, 2004) also produces a paralyzing toxin. It is extracted and used selectively in certain medical procedures to deliberately paralyze, or render inactive, certain muscles. It is applied cosmetically to prevent "laugh wrinkles" and has other medical uses in the treatment, for instance, of cerebral palsy. It has also been applied in treating the extreme facial pain caused by **trigeminal neuralgia** or to reduce the effects of muscle spasms in the voice, or other parts of the body. The bacterium in question produces the poison that causes **botulism**.

There are several types of the botulin toxin and among them is the one used in **Botox**—a neurotoxin used in cosmetic and other medical procedures.

Botulin Toxin in Cosmetic Treatments

At the commercial site for Botox (2009, retrieved February 28, 2009, from http://www.botoxcosmetic.com/) we also find some interesting comments about possible side effects when it is deliberately injected into body tissues. They may include:

Serious heart problems and serious allergic reactions . . . difficulty swallowing, speaking or breathing, . . . The most common side effects following injection include temporary eyelid droop and nausea. Localized pain, infection, inflammation, tenderness, swelling, redness, and/or bleeding/bruising may be associated with the injection. . . .

According to one authority, less than "500 grams of it would be enough to kill the entire human population" ("*Clostridium botulinum*," 2009, retrieved February 28, 2009, from http://en.wikipedia.org/wiki/Clostridium_botulinum; also Simpson, 2000, retrieved February 28, 2009, from http://www.ncbi.nlm.nih.gov/sites/entrez?cmd=Retrieve&db=PubMed&list_uids=11086224&dopt=AbstractPlus).

Botulinum neurotoxin is sometimes used in the treatment of various kinds of palsy and other spastic muscle conditions. However, research shows that this toxin can have serious deleterious effects even in highly controlled applications. K. Howell, Selber, Graham, and Reddihough (2007) report a case of a child with cerebral palsy who was treated with botulinum toxin and subsequently developed severe swallowing and breathing problems. Similarly, C. S. Chen and N. R. Miller (2007) report a case of a person who developed a particular form of palsy associated with lateral eye movement (cranial nerve VI) after an injection. There is also controversy over whether or not botulinum toxin helps at all in cases of palsy (see Weigl, Arbel, K. Katz, Becker, & Bar-On, 2007). On the other hand, there are studies claiming improvement after injections. For instance, Russo et al. (2007) claimed that botulinum neurotoxin produced significant improvements in "body structure" for the 21 children with palsy receiving treatment as contrasted with 22 controls who did not receive the botulinum toxin in their study.

Cases where patient/client reports can be reasonably rejected are very rare indeed. Ordinarily, the final authority concerning how a person feels is that person.

However, the results of Russo et al. and similar studies have been challenged by Redman, Finn, Bremner, and Valentine (2008) on the basis of firsthand reports from the patients treated. For reasons discussed in Chapter 11, logically speaking, the studies showing verified positive effects must be given great weight, but they cannot over-ride direct firsthand reports from patients. Of course, all claims need to be critically examined and verified. At the same time, it must be kept in mind that no one has precedence concerning how a person feels over that person.

Guiding Principles for Treatment

As we noted earlier, perhaps the best rule in the treatment of any disorder is to address the most serious problem first; then, to work downward to the less serious ones until the difficulties, if possible, are resolved and/or the affected individual is enabled to control the difficulties rather than be controlled by them. The first step in successful therapy is to diagnose the problems as accurately as possible and to determine causes wherever possible. Commonly part of the solution is to educate the other persons who interact with the individual affected by the disorder, but of course, that can be done only to the extent that the problems at issue are understood by the therapist/clinician. Thorough assessment and correct diagnosis, for these reasons, are crucial. Also, there are many cases where the client/patient understands his or her own conditions and what works best in coping with them better than the doctor or therapist is able to do. The client/patient may have hours, weeks, months, and even years of experience in coping with multiple problems that the doctor/clinician/therapist only deals with intermittently for a few minutes or an hour at a time. Although it should not be the case, too often the doctor may have prescribed a long-term medication without consulting the patient or without spending an adequate amount of time in doing so. A great deal depends on the amount of time invested in diagnosis, prescription, and treatment.

> The first step in successful therapy is to diagnose the problems as accurately as possible and to determine causes wherever possible.

Applying the Rule of Three to Therapy

As Jon Shestack noted in his talk about autism, there is a rule in Hollywood for film production called the "rule of three." It says that you cannot produce a movie that is fast, good, and cheap. You can pick any two, but you can't get all three. For the treatment of disorders, he concluded, we need to aim for fast and good. It won't, however, be cheap. To get the diagnosis right and to set the priorities for treatment correctly and to do it fast—so that successful treatment can begin in time—we have to invest a lot of time, effort, and resources in advance. That is why, we must take the trouble to understand the sign systems involved in communication from top to bottom. The problems are complex. The systems are vast and the research is difficult and expensive. However, the risks and rewards are worth the effort. The goal of therapy cannot be anything less than to understand the disorders so we can prevent them, cure them if possible, or control them and reduce the losses as much as possible.

Medical Options

For many of the disorders we have met in this chapter, the recommended approach is an early surgery—for example, in the case of certain cancers, recurrent vocal nodules, and the like. In other cases, intervention may involve medication—for example, something as simple as an antacid, or possibly a course of antibiotics, or possibly an injection of Botox. Before accepting any of these recommendations, patient/clients need to be thoroughly informed. Similarly, doctors and therapists need to be fully up-to-date and current on their own understanding of the relevant research.

When they are well balanced, those systems protect the body from harm. However, one of the ways that the body's built-in protections can get out of balance is through medical procedures such as the use of dental amalgam, vaccination, or medicines containing toxins. As we saw in the case of the use of botulinum toxin, there is significant risk of disabling vital muscle systems involved in breathing and swallowing. In many cases, the recommended therapy may involve close observation and interaction with a speech-language pathologist who specializes, for instance, in swallowing or voice therapy. Gradual restoration of functions is commonly sought on a step by step basis with close observation and monitoring to avoid injury from, for example, aspiration (breathing rather than swallowing) of food or liquid. Although behavioral therapy may help, in some cases, medical intervention through diet control and/or chelation therapy (as discussed in Chapter 5) may be needed.

SUMMING UP AND LOOKING AHEAD

In this chapter, we considered movement problems in the category referred to as "motor-speech" disorders. We discussed how that large class of disparate disorders are associated through the need to coordinate breathing with swallowing and also with voice and speech production. It also came out that swallowing, and all of the so-called "vegetative" movements that can be brought under voluntary control, are often recruited for use in communication. A key question that comes up when complex actions must be coordinated, especially ones that come under voluntary control, is who is in charge? Normally, as we saw in this chapter, one of the hemispheres of the brain is dominant and the corpus callosum plays a key role in communication between the two hemispheres. Volitional articulated sequences of movements, as in speech, and in the control of coordinating multiple processes simultaneously—say, breathing while having dinner and a conversation at the same time —require a great deal of coordination between distinct systems.

When the control functions break down, movement disorders can follow, some more serious than others. Swallowing, for instance, can interfere with breathing so disorders that affect swallowing are often critical. We also contrasted the movements involved in swallowing with those in speech and showed that speech movements are many times faster. We saw that the voice as it is used in speech entails all three of the positions of discourse because of the communication of meaning. In voice disorders, we saw how symptoms can be diagnostic and we discussed the amazingly complex systems that control the voluntary and autonomic aspects of movements from the brain to the synapses of nerves at the molecular level.

With respect to therapies, we noted the guiding rule that the most severe conditions should be treated first followed by less severe ones until the disorders are resolved or brought under control as much as is possible for the benefit of the affected person. Concerning the ethics and laws governing treatments, we will have more to say in Chapter 12. In the immediately following chapter, we focus attention on the movement disorders that have to do specifically with the production of speech sounds. Traditionally, these are called "articulation disorders." They are commonly seen in early childhood and may be part of a more complex diagnosis involving additional problems. Articulation problems are also the ones that used to be the most commonly treated by speech-language pathologists—prior to what has been called "the autism epidemic" (Edlich et al., 2007; Jepson & Johnson, 2007; J. W. Oller & S. D. Oller, 2009).

STUDY AND DISCUSSION QUESTIONS

1. Why is intentional movement without any sensory input (no seeing, hearing, smelling, touching, or tasting) a logical impossibility?

2. Consider the role of gestures in communication. Do you gesture to yourself? For instance, do you ever find yourself flexing your fingers, opening and closing your fists rapidly, and shaking out your hands, as if it would help to get the thoughts flowing when you are about to write something down? Do you ever rub your hands together, as if brushing off dust or drying your palms, in anticipation of starting a task? How about shaking your head and stretching as if to shake off the sleep? Do you gesture when you are talking on the phone? Why do you or people you know do these things?

3. What crucial functions of the epiglottis did you learn about in this chapter (or perhaps already know about)? For instance, what cranial nerve is it associated with and how is it related to taste?

4. Why is communication between the hemispheres, not to mention the rest of the body and its neurosystems, so crucial in the control of voluntary behaviors such as initiating a swallow or taking a breath of air to speak?

5. Discuss the relation between the movements of swallowing and the movements of speech. Which are faster and by how much? Over which movements do we have more intentional control?

6. Explain the principles of voice harmonics. In that context, why are some voices more resonant while others tend toward raspiness, breathiness, harshness, and less harmonic qualities?

7. What are a few of the long-lasting advantages of, say, choosing to be a smoker and/or a heavy drinker? For instance, what effects can be expected in terms of impact on other conditions such as acid reflux? Vocal nodules?

8. Discuss the role of neurotransmitters in flaccid and spastic dysarthrias.

9. What are some of the competing theories about the neurologic control of prosody?

10. Why is the percentage of persons who experience dysphagia so high in the case of acute stroke or traumatic brain injury?

11. How can hypertonia (or hypotonia) produce a life-threatening condition when no brain injury is evident? How can these conditions impact a particular muscle or group of muscles, say, the ones involved in swallowing or breathing?

12. Why is it reasonable to suppose that in the future many additional systems will be elucidated at the molecular and atomic levels that are critical to the normal functioning of the body?

7

Articulation Disorders

OBJECTIVES

In this chapter, we:

1. Discuss the distinctness of surface forms of signs and why *they must be articulated*;

2. Differentiate articulation in terms of producer, consumer, and discourse in general;

3. Consider the layeredness of the mapping of intentions into surface forms;

4. Distinguish motor disorders owed to peripheral versus central neurological problems;

5. Revisit the interaction between production and perception; and

6. Discuss approaches to therapy for different articulation problems.

KEY TERMS

Here are some key terms of this chapter. Many you may already know, but it may help to review them. These terms are explained in the text and they are defined in the Glossary at the end of the book. They appear in **bold print** on their first appearance in the text.

acoustic phonetics	glottal stop	rounded
alphabetic principle	ideographic writing	sandhi
alveolar	instructional dyslexia	segmental sounds
alveolar ridge	International Phonetic	semiconsonants
articulatory phonetics	Alphabet	semivowels
aspirated	kinesics	Sequoia
aspiration	liquids	sibilant
assimilation	logographic writing	situation based
auditory phonetics	manner of articulation	slow speech
bilabial	metathesis	Smith-Magenis syndrome
bimoraic	minimal pair	spondee
breath groups	monomoraic	stress
Broca's aphasia	mora	stress pattern
cluster reduction	mora timed	stress timed language
coarticulation	motor phonetics	structural linguistics
consonants	nasal	suprasegmental
conversation analysis	normal speech	suprasegmental elements
diacritic	otitis media	syllabaries
diadochokinesis	paralinguistic devices	syllabic writing
dissimilation	parallel universes	syllable timed
duration	parsing	tip of the tongue
elision	phoneme	transcribe
ellipsis	phonemic segments	trimoraic
embodiment	phonetic features	trochee
epenthesis	phonetic segments	unrounded
extralinguistic elements	phonotactics	unvoiced
fast speech	place of articulation	velar
floppy child syndrome	plosive	voiced
fricatives	point of articulation	voiceless
glides	possible worlds	voicing
glottal plosive	prosodic	

The articulation of the signs used in communication can be defined as the motor differentiation of their surface forms. It is interesting and noteworthy that the differentiation not to mention the production of signs, any signs whatever, can only take place logically and practically at the motor level.

Motor Phonetics

For this reason Raymond Herbert Stetson [1872–1950]—the founder of **motor phonetics** and the mentor and teacher of Nobel Laureate, Roger W. Sperry (see Chapter 10)—insisted that "phonetics must be motor phonetics: the mere shuffling of symbols on a line is not enough" (1951, p. 174). To the extent that Stetson was correct, phonetics must be studied first and foremost from the vantage point of the producer of articulate language (Stetson, 1945, 1951; also see "Raymond Herbert Stetson," 1950/2009, retrieved March 3, 2009, from http://fr .wikipedia.org/wiki/Raymond_Herbert_Stetson).

Interestingly, the producer of a stream of articulated signs normally has volitional control over that stream to a greater extent than almost any other actions that human beings are capable of performing.

WHAT IS THE ARTICULATION OF SURFACE FORMS?

In terms of a general theory of signs (see J. W. Oller, L. Chen, S. D. Oller, & Pan, 2005), the process of articulation is essentially indexical and is the central element in *pragmatic mapping*. Any such mapping relies on indexes (movements) that link abstract symbolic meanings to noticeable acts that are represented in moving icons—the bodies of persons doing the articulation. Figure 7–1 suggests the general outlines of the process with respect to the surface forms of speech, manual signing, or any form of writing. A critical fact to take into account is that articulation involves movement by someone who is the articulator.

For this reason, if the surface forms of articulate language are to be recorded, they are best displayed in a moving film or video with sound. Certainly, we can capture the words of such articulated mapping relations in print, but as has been commonly noted, print cannot actually display the prosody of speech or sign. In fact, perhaps the best definition of prosody is to say that it consists of all those aspects of discourse that best express how a person feels about what he or she is saying or talking about, but that cannot be written down with the surface forms.

Prosody includes the tone of voice, rate of speech, the accompanying gestures, and the changes in pitch and volume that are difficult if not impossible to represent in printed forms on a sheet of paper, or in any static display.

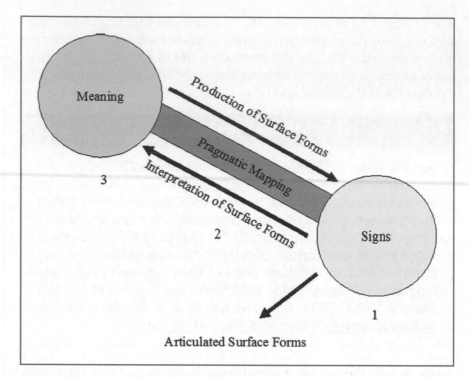

FIGURE 7–1. Articulation of signs.

ARTICULATION AND THE POSITIONS OF DISCOURSE

Ordinarily we think of articulation from the point of view of the actor who produces articulated signs as in speaking, signing, or writing. This is the producer's position, or the first position of discourse. In something as complex as a book with multiple authors, the first position is shared by multiple persons, and the articulation of elements in the book needs to be sufficient so that people reading the book can make sense of it. In the articles that appear in the Wikipedia, to take another example, the first position may be shared by many writer/editors besides the original contributor. An article in that context consists of a discourse produced by potentially many different contributors and reviewed by many more.

The second position of discourse—that of the consumer—typically involves at least two persons. There is the person addressed by the producer who perceives the stream of speech or signs and there is the person doing the production. Because the producer of discourse, provided it is intelligible, is usually also able to perceive and comprehend what is produced, the consumer's position is always at least potentially occupied by a plurality of persons. There is usually the consumer and there must also be the producer who monitors his or her own articulations. Even if the consumer is also the producer—as when we practice a presentation in front of a mirror, imagine a conversation, or re-read something we have just written to check how it sounds—the consumer's position is regarded as if it were occupied by more than just the producer. By contrast the producer's position is typically occupied by just one person at a time. Even if two individuals are talking at the same time, any given listener has difficulty attending to more than one.

Beyond the first two positions of discourse, there is also the logical third position which is occupied by all the rest of the space-time continuum and all that it may contain. The third position of discourse may contain uncountably many potential observers. So we see that the three positions logically go from one producer at the first position to more than one potential consumer in the second position to an uncountable multitude of possible observers in the third position. It turns out that the study of the articulation of discourse, and especially of speech, can be divided up into three distinct types precisely on the basis of the three positions of discourse. There is the articulation of speech or signs from the first person point of view; the auditory impression created by articulated signs on a second person; and there is the acoustic or other physical imprint (as in writing or film) that acts of articulated discourse may leave behind for all the world to observe from the third person position. Any of these three positions can be focused on, but clinician/teachers (Ball & Müller, 2005; Gough & C. H. Lee, 2007) as well as researcher/theoreticians alike (Chomsky & Halle, 1968; de Jong, Lim, & Nagao 2004; Ladefoged, 2001; Nagao & de Jong, 2007; Pike, 1947; Stetson, 1945, 1951) must logically begin with the first position of discourse—the position of the producer of articulated signs.

Distinct Domains of the Study of Articulation

The first position of discourse—the place where active articulation is occurring—is typically occupied by only one person at a time. As one of our own mentors once observed, "It is difficult for two people to hold a pencil at the same time." Similarly, it is difficult for more than one person to type on the same keyboard, or to hold the same microphone, or to occupy the position of the talking head, or the manual signing head, in a visual frame. The position of the producer of articulated signs is intrinsically singular.

At the same time, the second logical position of discourse—that of the consumer—logically takes account of at least two logically different positions which are usually occupied by two or more persons. There must be, logically at least in the second place, the position of the producer and that of the consumer. And, as we saw in Chapter 4, there are the critical McGurk interactions between the production and perception of speech forms. Manual signs have been studied less than speech, but it must be supposed that similar

More than one person can speak at the same time, but it is difficult for an audience to comprehend more than one stream of speech or manual signing, or to read and comprehend two or three emails at the same time, and no one can effectively produce two or more distinct streams of discourse simultaneously.

McGurk interactions must exist between production and perception in the manual modality as well. To recall McGurk interactions in speech and hearing, part of our perception of the syllable /va/, as produced by someone else, for instance, is in our perception of the producer's articulatory movements. We know what it feels like kinesthetically to produce that sequence ourselves. As a result, even if the syllable produced (and recorded) is not /va/ but, say, /ba/, if we see the articulatory position for /va/, it is virtually impossible for us to inhibit the auditory perception of /va/ even if the recorded syllable (as in the syllable-level McGurk interactions) happens to be /ba/.

As if this were not enough, researchers have shown even more subtle interactions between production and perception that are owed to timing.

The Dynamic Syllable

As predicted by Stetson (1945, 1951) and as demonstrated recently by de Jong and colleagues (de Jong, Lim, & Nagao 2004; Nagao & de Jong, 2007), something as simple as speeding up the production of a sequence of syllables can dramatically affect the segments perceived and even their perceived order—for example, try saying /ab/ repeatedly and speeding up the production. It begins sounding like /ab/ then transforms with more rapid production to /bab/ and then to /ba/ where the segments within the starting syllable seem to have been completely reversed.

As a result of such demonstrations, it is evident that the actual sounds of discourse, or the manual signs of ASL, for instance, must occur at a rate that is compatible first and foremost with production and secondarily with perception. Otherwise, the surface forms of discourse will degenerate into a stream of undecipherable nonsense. From such observations, it becomes clear that the articulated signs of discourse depend on our capacity to produce and to perceive them. Also, as Stetson argued and demonstrated with reference to deaf and deaf-blind individuals (also see the more recent work of de Jong and colleagues), articulatory rhythms are critical to the distinctness of the surface forms of spoken and also of manually signed discourse.

The Branches of Phonetics

When phonetics—the study of sounds—focuses on the movements of the speaker, the resulting discipline is referred to as **articulatory phonetics**. On the other hand, before a person can acquire the articulatory movements associated with a particular language—whether it is spoken, signed, or written—that individual must either have some samples of it to work from or must invent new surface forms. When the surface forms of speech are examined from the vantage point of a consumer rather than a producer, the result is **auditory phonetics**. Although there is no widely accepted term for the visual processing of the surface forms of manual signed languages, the term **visual phonetics**—a seeming oxymoron combining seeing with hearing where in manual signs there is no real need for sounds— has been used (Armstrong, Stokoe, & S. E. Wilcox, 1995, p. 107; Marschark, Siple, Lillo-Martin, & Everhart, 1997, p. 85). The focus of auditory/visual phonetics is on the sensory impressions made by the surface forms of speech and/or of manual signs. In addition, there is also the possibility of considering the surface forms themselves as physical events. When this is done, the resulting discipline is known as **acoustic phonetics**.

Thoughtful readers will notice that all of these distinctions in the study of phonetics—in terms of the first, second, and third positions of discourse (see Figure 6–1) are based on the assumption that the primary surface form of language is speech and that the primary modality of perception of speech is hearing. Hence, all of the disciplines refer to *phonetics*—articulatory, auditory, and acoustic—suggesting that they involve the sounds of speech as heard by hearing persons. There are, however, as we have noted, other manifest forms of language besides speech. There are distinct forms of manual signing, writing, computer speech synthesized from text or some digital code or other medium, and combinations of these. Also, hearing is not the only modality of sense that is involved in any of these.

As we saw in Chapter 6 (see Figure 6–1), the third logical position of discourse not only includes positions one and two but also the whole rest of the material world. It is from the third position of discourse that it is possible to record the surface forms of speech in order to replay them both in terms of their acoustic characteristics, but also in terms of the accompanying gestures, and so forth, that can be perceived kinesthetically and visually. The record may be made on magnetic tape or on a film with a sound track or some other device. It may even be a written record on a sheet of paper that can be read aloud so as to produce another stream of speech, or possibly other signs, similar to the ones that provided the basis for the written record.

As we saw with the McGurk interactions in Chapter 4, seeing, hearing, and movement are all deeply involved in the processing of the surface forms of speech and language.

Representations from Logically Different Positions

It is useful to recognize that the three positions of discourse are really logically distinct and that the three resulting ways of looking at and representing the surface forms of speech—or in some cases manual signed language—are also distinct. Each one is real in its own right to the extent that the language forms in question are actually articulated. The volitional act of articulation is attributable quite exclusively to the person producing a stream of speech or manual signs—the first person. The process of perceiving a stream of speech only indirectly involves the consumer as the second person. However, acts of interpretation may follow in which the interpreter chooses to attend to, believe, and act on what someone else said. So, any willing consumer is more than an innocent bystander who may overhear a conversation. The second person (which may be a plurality of persons in a classroom, say) in any act of communication takes on an active role as a willing participant by attending to a conversation and possibly participating in whatever may come of it. The logically third position of discourse may involve innocent bystanders, but as soon as they interpret the discourse, they become more than mere bystanders by joining the community of persons involved in that particular discourse. They are involved through intentional and volitional acts of interpretation.

As for the real-world impact of a stream of speech on a recording machine, computer, or an innocent bystander that pays no attention to the surface forms—hearing or seeing but not bothering to attend to them—volitional involvement drops off to approximately zero. However, cameras and recording devices do not set themselves up accidentally, so the producers and consumers of recorded materials are inevitably implicated as participants in such productions. As a result, volitional activity is involved implicitly even in overhearing or recording a conversation.

Parsing and Classifying the Sounds of Speech

Ferdinand de Saussure (1912) insisted that speech does not present itself with ready-made boundaries between its subunits. The same is true of manual signed languages (Armstrong, Stokoe, & S. E. Wilcox, 1995). De Saussure argued that to divide the surface forms of discourse into its component parts "we must call in meanings" (p. 103). He wrote:

de Saussure on the Sound Chain

. . . we know that the main characteristic of the sound chain is that it is linear . . . Considered by itself, it is only a line, a continuous ribbon along which the ear perceives no self-sufficient and clear-cut division; to divide the chain, we must call in meanings. When we hear an unfamiliar language, we are at a loss to say how the succession of sounds should be analyzed, for analysis is impossible if only the phonic [or visual] side of the linguistic phenomenon is considered. But when we know the meaning and function that must be attributed to each part of the chain, we see the parts detach themselves from each other and the shapeless ribbon break into segments. Yet there is nothing material in the analysis (pp. 103–104).

In fact, there is still imperfect agreement today among linguists about just what elements of the surface forms of speech should be represented in a thorough phonetic analysis or transcription. It is generally accepted that the smallest pronounceable unit of speech is the syllable, but there is no solid agreement on just what a syllable is (but for a definition, see the section labeled "Syllables" later in this chapter). When it comes to the **parsing**—that is, the dividing up—of the parts of syllables, not to mention of higher units, there is, if anything, even less agreement. Probably, this failure to agree is more because of the nature of the object of study than it is because of any lack of diligence on the part of the folks doing the study. As de Saussure noted, it is difficult to know where and how to cut the ribbon. As we have demonstrated empirically (J. W. Oller, S. D. Oller, & Badon, 2006; S. D. Oller, 2005) and in logicomathematical proofs (J. W. Oller, 2005), without bringing meaning into the picture, parsing of the surface forms of speech, as in child language acquisition, is not merely difficult, it is impossible. It is necessary to bring meaning into play. In particular it is impossible to find the essential boundaries of the surface forms of a language without appeal to meanings. To find the boundaries of speech segments, it is essential to find the boundaries of persons, things, and events in experience that are referred to and talked about in the language. The pragmatic mapping of surface forms of language onto their referents and meanings in the world of experience is crucial to language comprehension, acquisition, meaningful production, and all combinations of these uses of language.

> To find the boundaries of speech segments, it is essential to find the boundaries of persons, things and events in experience that are referred to and talked about in the language.

Language Is Deeper Than Speech or Any Particular Surface Forms

Having noted the fundamental problem of parsing the surface forms of speech, signing, or written representations, nevertheless, there have been many attempts in the past, and there are many ineffective (unreliable, not valid, and impractical) teaching and testing approaches (some of which are still being applied today with a very high failure rate), that seek to analyze language with no reference—or with as little reference as possible—to meaning. The fact is that approaches to language teaching, therapy, or any kind of linguistic analysis can only succeed to the extent that they implicitly or explicitly take the pragmatic functions of language seriously.

In the end, we know on the basis of strict logic that all approaches that limit attention to surface forms of speech, sign, or writing—or any combination of such surface forms—are bound to come up short. On that account, and because such approaches are widely used and recommended, it is all the more necessary in an introductory course about communication disorders, to take account of how approaches based on surface form analysis work as far as they do, and why they cannot get all the way home. They cannot possibly arrive at a full understanding of how languages work any more than a parrot, chimp, or gorilla can hope to engage in a meaningful conversation about history, ethics, law, philosophy, or any truly abstract subject. Keeping all this in mind, it is useful to understand how different approaches to the study of speech sounds have proceeded historically and how far they have progressed up to now. In the background, anyone studying, teaching, or seeking to modify the surface forms of speech in a clinical or educational setting ought always to bear in mind the other manifestations of language—manual signs, writing, conceptual thought, and combinations of all of them. Also, to optimize results in shaping the understanding and use of the surface forms of speech or sign systems, as we will see, access to meaning is not only advantageous: it is essential.

Deeper Than Speech

We must keep in mind the fact that language is always deeper than speech. Language is deeper, richer, and more comprehensive than any of its manifest forms. Phonetics is just about the surface forms of speech and it can never tell the whole story of language. It is true that speech is the primary form taken by articulated form of language in our early experience, but the manual signed languages of the Deaf, and the written symbols of all cultures are also highly articulated for just one reason—to enable distinctions between referents and meanings. Except for the intention to express and communicate distinct meanings, there is no advantage of an articulated stream of speech over an indistinct vocalization.

As individuals and cultures interact more and more at an adult level, we see an ever increasing dependence on written representations and, since the advent of the information age, we depend more and more on multi-media recordings and representations of interactions that go way beyond mere speech and writing.

But articulated speech is essential to the human experience, especially from before birth through childhood. As individuals and cultures interact more and more at an adult level, we see an ever increasing dependence on written representations and, since the advent of the information age, we depend more and more on multi-media recordings and re-presentations of interactions that go way beyond mere speech and writing. Now, we often have access to a vast amount of nonverbal information as represented in gestures, moving images, sounds, and combinations of all these with multiple layers of commentary in various linguistic forms—speech, signing, writing, and so forth. All these are articulated to the extent that they are at all comprehensible.

Articulation Across Modalities

With reference to speech, the main articulators are the movable parts of the mouth, especially, the tongue, the lips, and the jaw. The vocal folds are also involved in the production of voice as are the lungs and all of the muscles that control breathing. In fact, every movable part of the vocal tract, it seems, can be involved in speech articulation in one way or another. Certainly the resonating cavities of the nose and mouth are also involved. There are, without question, articulatory movements involved in manual signing and in writing, but articulatory phonetics is generally focused on the sounds of speech.

In the study of the phonetics of speech forms, it is possible to emphasize the way speech sounds are articulated (the first position of discourse), the way they are perceived (the second position), or their physical properties (the third position). Or, in some systems of phonetics, all three may be used together. However, in the study of the phonetics of speech, or the surface forms of manual signing, the articulatory production logically and actually occupies the first position and tends to receive the most emphasis. The term "articulate" itself suggests the movement of the articulators in producing the surface forms of language.

Syllables

The smallest unit of sound that can be produced as a distinct surface form in speaking is a *syllable*. For instance, the word *the* contains only one syllable whereas the words *involve* and *muscle* each contain two syllables and the word *syllable* itself contains three. Syllables not only are the smallest surface forms that can be produced as separate units bounded by silence before and after, but syllables are also the units of surface form that can carry prosodic elements such as voice qualities including *pitch* (whether the voice is high, low, rising, falling, or some combination of these), *amplitude* (loudness relative to other sounds), and **duration** (length relative to other surface forms). Many other voice qualities can be distinguished in the surface forms of speech and may be used to identify different speakers and to differentiate subtle aspects of meaning. However, pitch, amplitude, and duration are the main voice features associated with syllables.

A syllable is the sort of unit which receives a beat—a distinct pulse of energy—in speaking or in signing though the term "syllable" is usually associated with speech.

Stress Patterns

When two or more syllables appear in a sequence, as in the production of a word or phrase that has more than one syllable, all three of these features—that is, pitch, amplitude, and duration—are commonly involved in the differentiation of what is technically termed **stress**. The word *muscle*, for instance, has stress on its first syllable. For this reason it is termed a **trochee** (rhyming with "croaky" and where the syllable "-*chee*" is pronounced as *key*). You will notice that the first syllable of *trochee* (also in *croaky*) is stressed. Words such as *crazy*, *happy*, *higher*, *second*, and so on are trochees. That is, in all these two syllable words the first syllable is typically produced with higher pitch, greater amplitude, and longer duration than the second syllable of the same word. The opposite arrangement of the trochee **stress pattern** is seen in the word *involve* where the stress goes to the second syllable. The technical term for this arrangement of stress is **spondee** (rhyming with "Ron Dee" and having the stress pattern of "I see!"). When it comes to words and phrases of three or more syllables, many other arrangements are possible.

Rhythm and Timing

There appears to be a unit of structure that is abstracted from syllabic rhythms and that is deeper than the syllable itself. This unit may be called a **mora** (Sato, 1993). It is more abstract and distinct from the syllable level.

In English, stress patterns provide the main basis for the timing of our speech rhythms. For this reason, English is termed a **stress timed language**. Stressed syllables in such a language tend to be longer, higher pitched, and louder than other syllables. In many other languages, the rhythm of syllabic speech may be controlled by the syllables themselves. Those languages, including Spanish and Italian, for instance, are referred to as **syllable timed** languages. In addition, there are languages whose rhythms seem to be controlled by some combination of syllabic timing along with the underlying **phonotactics**—that is, the way syllables are structured and regarded by speakers in general or by speakers of a given language.

A given syllable may have, evidently, one, two, or three of these deeper units within it. For instance, in a word like *croaky* the second syllable is a good deal shorter than the first. That syllable is also shorter than the first syllable of *spondee*. Because there is only one stressed syllable in each of these words, why is it that the unstressed syllable (*-ky* in *croaky* and *spon-* in *spondee*) is not the same length in both? But it is easy to tell that the syllable *spon-* in *spondee* is longer by quite a bit than the syllable *-ky* in *croaky*. From such comparisons as this, it can be argued that some syllables are intrinsically longer than others because some of them involve more moras. Some are **monomoraic**, for example, the *-ky* of *croaky*, which appears to have only one mora; whereas others are **bimoraic**, that is, having two moras, as in the *spon-* of *spondee*; whereas still others, such as the word *voice* in *she raised her voice*, may be **trimoraic**—having up to three moras. That is, assuming that all else can be held equal, the word *voice* in the example sentence may be up to three times the length of, say, *-ky* in *croaky* and about one-third longer than the *spon-* of *spondee*. Taking the theoretical mora unit into consideration, researchers have discovered that there appear to be **mora timed** languages, such as Japanese (Sato, 1993) and Luganda (Hyman & Katamba, 1993). In those language, a mora is any segment given its own separate time segment at the surface. In such languages, it seems that there is a timing system made up of mora units that operates in tandem with the systems of syllable units and their distinct sound segments. Does this seem abstract? Well, it is abstract and it shows why it is difficult and rare for speech-language pathologists and audiologists to get enough training in linguistic theory to be able to appreciate fully the complexity of the communication disorders with which they are confronted.

Interestingly, the distinct rhythms that are possible in different languages seem to be used by human babies, before and immediately after birth, to distinguish and recognize their own native language Nazzi, Bertoncini, & Mehler (1998; also see J. W. Oller, S. D. Oller, & Badon, 2006).

GETTING DOWN TO THE DISTINCT SEGMENTS (PHONEMES) OF SPEECH

It is important to keep in mind in this whole chapter, but especially in this section, that we are thinking in terms of the sounds themselves—the elements that make up the surface forms of speech as contrasted with the letters or symbols that might be used to represent those sounds in writing. A letter is just a written symbol that is distinct from other written symbols by its conventional use to represent a sound—for example, take the letter "p" used to represent the first sound segment in "pitch." Theoretically, any symbol whatever could be used to represent that sound, and, as we will see, there are several distinct approaches to writing that focus on units of speech and language at levels higher than its distinct sound segments. For instance, there are writing systems that represent syllables instead of their segments, or words instead of their sound segments or syllables, or concepts underlying words instead of their surface forms. That is, in some writing systems, for example, classical Chinese writing, the system more or less neglects sound segments, syllables, and even words, and goes directly to a representation of abstract concepts.

The speech sounds that constitute syllables are generally divisible into two categories with somewhat fuzzy boundaries. There are the **consonants** on the one hand and the **vowels** on the other.

Different Classes of Sounds

With all the foregoing in mind we must still consider the phonetics of speech segments below the level of the syllable. Consonants can be defined as sound segments of a syllable that consist of a movement that blocks or hinders the flow of air from the lungs through the oral and nasal cavities. For instance, the sounds that are commonly represented alphabetically by the letters "p," "b," "s," and "h" are consonants by this definition.

In English at least, and in most languages, vowels by definition constitute the part of a syllable that can be sung. Vowels involve voicing. We may say that the vowel is the portion of the syllable that can be extended indefinitely (in producing it) until we run out of breath. Typically, vowels include the sounds that are commonly represented by the letters "i," "a," "u" and so on.

In addition to the consonants and vowels, there are certain sounds that seem to be switch-hitters and can go either way. They can fit both the vowel and the consonant categories.

The Liquids

The sounds commonly represented by the letters "l" and "r" fall into this class. They are called the **liquids**. This term seems appropriate because it suggests that these sounds in particular are fluid, changing, and hard to hold onto. Perhaps because of this, in English, for instance, we find them functioning both as consonants as in the words *red* and *led* also in *tell* and *tare*, and we also find them functioning as vowels as in *bird* and *table*.

Besides the consonants, vowels, and liquids, there is still another class of sounds that falls into the borderland between the consonants and the vowels. Although the liquids fit in both categories, this next class known as the **glides** (also known as the **semivowels** or **semiconsonants**) includes the sounds represented more or less by the letters "y" and "w" in English spelling. The segments represented by these letters—as in the words, *word, how, yet, soy, kayak,* and *awake*—do not readily fit in either the consonant or vowel categories. In view of their tendency to always to appear phonotactically on what appears to be the front or back edge of a syllable, the term *semiconsonant* seems to fit them fairly well. At the same time, they always serve as a kind of wind up or wind down for a vowel segment so the term *semivowel* is also appropriate.

Classifying Segments by Articulatory and Other Features

Classification of the segments of speech is primarily, as we have noted, grounded in articulatory rather than in auditory or acoustic (physical) features. The key features are traditionally differentiated by **place of articulation**, the **manner of articulation**, and whether or not the segment in question is accompanied by **voicing**.

Looking to the distinctions made in the **International Phonetic Alphabet** (2009; retrieved March 3, 2009, from http://en.wikipedia.org/wiki/International_Phonetic_Alphabet) as summarized in Figure 7–2 in the chart at the top reading across the top row first we have the distinctions in place of articulation and down the left-hand side we have the distinctions in manner. Within each cell, the intersection of the columns and rows of the chart, the symbol to the

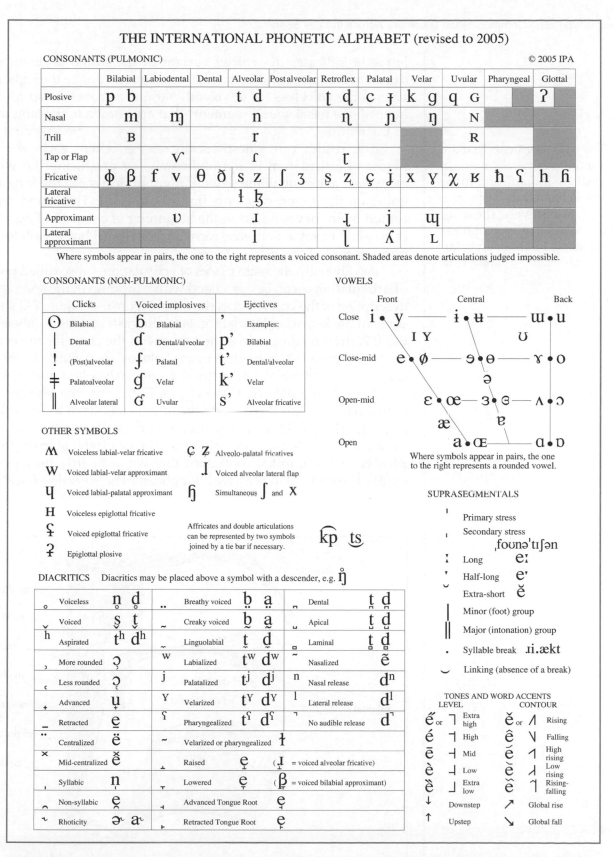

FIGURE 7–2. The international Phonetic Alphabet in 2005. Retrieved March 3, 2009, from http://en.wikipedia.org/wiki/Image:IPA_chart_2005.png#file. Reprinted under the terms of the GNU Free Documentation License, Version 1.2.

The nasal segments that are common to General American English are [m], [n], and [ŋ] as seen in the words, *mom*, *non*, and *song*, respectively. The place of articulation of each of these segments is **bilabial**, **alveolar**, and **velar**.

left side indicates the **voiced** variant of the sound segment produced at that place and in that manner and the one to the right represents the **voiceless** (or **unvoiced**) variant. Across the top row we have all the **nasal** sound segments that are known to the languages of the world.

The reader can kinesthetically assess where each of these places of articulation is, approximately, by producing the words *mom*, *non*, and *song* while paying attention to where the tongue is going on the sound segments [m], [n], and [ŋ]. The sound represented by [ŋ] never occurs at the beginning of a word in English. It is possible to say a nonsense form such as [ŋoŋ] but it violates the phonotactics of English to do so.

Additionally, the main places of articulation—also called **points of articulation**—can be associated with a location in the anatomical description of the vocal tract as shown in Figure 6–1. Figure 7–3 shows some of the key articulatory targets for English sounds as labeled in the IPA chart reading across the top row in the chart for the consonants of Figure 7–2. In English major "places" or "points of articulation" include "Bilabial, Labiodental, Dental, Alveolar," and so forth.

Next, in the IPA chart (see Figure 7–2), come the **plosive** segments which in English include the ones symbolized as [p], [b], [t], [d], [k], [g], and [ʔ]. The only unfamiliar one in this list (for non-phoneticians) is the last one which is called a **glottal stop** or **glottal plosive**. It is the initial consonant that we ordinarily hear prominently if we say "Uh oh!" with emphasis. The so-called **fricatives**

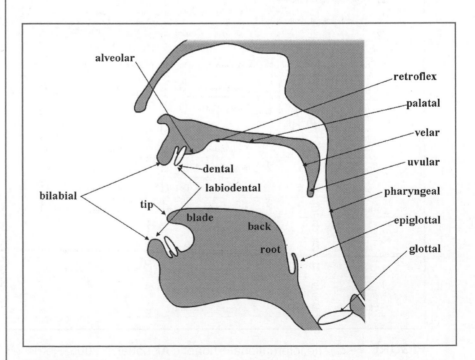

FIGURE 7–3. Places (targets) of articulation and the main parts of the tongue used in articulation.

and sounds that are produced by creating friction at the targeted point of constriction. For instance, most speakers of English produce the initial segment of the main words in *sitting on a stump sipping cider* with the **tip of the tongue** almost contacting the **alveolar ridge** just behind the upper teeth. However, one of our students recently demonstrated that she can produce that segment by producing the friction against the lower teeth. By backing the main articulator, the tongue a little farther away from the alveolar ridge, we get the General American English variant of the first segment of the words *run rat run* which is designated in the IPA system as [ɹ].

The vowel sounds differentiated in the IPA system are shown in the middle left of Figure 7–2. There are actually three dimensions to the vowel chart. It differentiates vowels by the position of the tongue relative to the front or back of the mouth and from top to bottom by the relative openness of the mouth and by whether or not the lips are rounded or flat in producing the vowel in question. For instance, [i] as in the word *see*, involves an almost closed mouth whereas [a] as in *hot* is maximally open. Also, vowels are distinguished by the relative position of the main body of the tongue. It can be shifted to the front, as is the [i] in the word *he* or to the back as it is in [u] in the word *who*. Additionally, the chart distinguishes vowels by whether or not the lips are **rounded** as in [u] or **unrounded** as in [i].

Over and above the many distinctions that the IPA enables us to represent between different consonants and vowels, it enables us also to **transcribe**—that is, to represent in the IPA form of symbolic writing—various **suprasegmental** (or **prosodic**) **elements** of speech. Symbols are included to distinguish stress, length, intonation, and tone. Besides all these marks many more subtle distinctions can be indicated thanks to the rich system of **diacritics** which are illustrated in the bottom of Figure 7–2. Theoretically, an indefinitely large number of distinctions can be represented.

However, for reasons that we are about to present, the successfulness of the IPA as a means of fully representing the surface forms of any language can easily be overrated. In fact, no matter how objective the system aims to be, because of the active interplay between the multilayered systems of language that connect its surface forms to meanings and vice versa (as suggested in Figure 7–1) and as we discussed especially in Chapter 4 earlier, all static systems of transcription come up short of fully representing the dynamics of natural languages.

In the final analysis complete observer objectivity in representing the dynamics of language is unattainable. To verify any given proposed transcription of actual discourse, meanings and intentions must be brought into play, and it will be necessary to appeal to intelligent judgments that involve inferences going well beyond the details of surface forms. This logically must be the case irrespective of how detailed the phonetic description of surface forms may aim to be.

Phonetics as Subordinate

In the final analysis, judgments about surface forms depend more on meaning and intentions than the inferences about meanings and intentions do on the shapes of the surface forms. For example, if a speaker intends to refer to one political candidate but inadvertently mentions the opponent of that person, no amount of phonetic detail will be sufficient to correct the error at that level of discourse. It will be essential to appeal to intentions and to the pragmatic level of the discourse. The phonetic level, therefore, is subordinate.

If the meanings are disregarded, or if a phonetician, say, or ethnographer, chooses to focus attention exclusively on surface forms, the view of language is dehumanized, impoverished, and destined to be less effective as we will see in Chapter 9 especially when dealing with certain failed approaches to clinical therapies, literacy, foreign language instruction, and the so-called "language arts" in general.

Keeping the Other Person in Mind

Each of the positions from which the study of the phonetics of speech, or of the articulated surface forms of manual signs or writing, can be conducted is different. The differences are as great as treating others as we would want to be treated—see the remarks of Stephen J. Cannell in Chapter 12—and treating them as we might treat a laboratory animal. If the researcher or clinician regards the surface forms of speech as connected to meanings, intentions, and the persons who are involved in producing and understanding them in ordinary discourse, we realize the most useful, humane, and rational view of language.

A Limit of Objectivity

All of the codes of ethics in medicine, speech language pathology, psychology, and so forth, as we will see in Chapter 12, acknowledge that the underlying objective is always to protect and further the legitimate interests of the patient/client/student. In fact, it has been observed by one ethnographer working with abused women that it is impossible morally to maintain observer objectivity (Guimaraes, 2007). In the case of Guimaraes, who started out with the intention of remaining objective and aloof, she says she increasingly "felt a moral responsibility . . . to intervene if I thought I could help" (p. 149). If the interests of the patient/client/students undergoing study/treatment/teaching are not known, or if the doctor/clinician/teacher or researcher claims to have no regard for those interests and concerns, the person being studied is not being treated as a human being at all, and the most fundamental of all ethical values is being violated from the outset.

To the extent that universally accepted ethical codes are valid, it is unacceptable to treat a person as if he or she were merely an object of study (T. Strong, 2005). It is for this reason that spies, private investigators, gossips, and even the most innocent seeming researchers who treat their interlocutors as mere objects of study tend to be regarded with a jaundiced eye. Individuals who claim to be able to understand the surface forms of communication with no reference to the intentions, meanings, and the underlying objectives of the interlocutors are not only mistaken from a theoretical point of view but they are taking an unethical point of view of their patient/client/students.

In Chapter 9, we show how such an agenda leads to superficial and incomplete theories of literacy and how it has produced many cases of what we have called **instructional dyslexia**. Briefly put, that form of dyslexia is produced by forcing too much attention to surface forms and away from meaning. Such misguided efforts to achieve objectivity on the part of research or theory also leads to approaches to therapy and intervention that tend to emphasize surface behaviors rather than causes and cures. Consequently, such approaches often end up treating problems of low priority ahead of more pressing needs. Logically, such approaches do not and cannot fully take account of the interests and needs of the patient/client/student.

From Extreme Objectivity to Atrocity

An interesting problem arises with respect to supposed participant observers who may claim to be aloof, indifferent, or at least completely objective toward the purposes of a conversational interaction—as in a support group, say, where parents and concerned parties are discussing shared problems such as coping with one or more communication disorders. Supposing the observation and the analysis to which it will lead has an undisclosed purpose, for example, one that is not known to the other participants involved in the conversation, should the other participants be asked to overlook this detail?

We do not think so. That sort of reasoning without regard for the other persons as human beings is what led to the Nazi atrocities that we mentioned in Chapter 1 and to which we return in Chapter 12. The only acceptable reason for research, study, and interventions in communication disorders in the final analysis is to find their causes in order to prevent them from occurring if possible and either to seek at least to cure them when they do occur, or, at the very least, to seek to reduce the severity of their impact as much as possible.

When clinical research involves human beings, the first question to be asked is how can the proposed study or intervention help the person with the disorder, or others who have similar problems, and the second question is how can we be certain that the risks and costs, whatever they may be, are worth it all. It is for this reason that universities and other research institutions have Institutional

The only acceptable reason for research, study, and interventions in communication disorders in the final analysis is to find their causes in order to prevent them from occurring if possible and either to seek at least to cure them when they do occur, or, at the very least, to seek to reduce the severity of their impact as much as possible.

Review Boards to protect the individuals who participate in research studies. Human beings are not lab animals that perhaps by necessity, may be unknowingly sacrificed for the purposes of research.

In the next section, we will see additional evidence showing that even our ability to parse the syllables, segments, words, phrases, and higher units of the surface forms of the stream of speech, writing, or signed language requires access to the meanings, intentions, and purposes of discourse.

Meaning and Participant Observers

Without access to meaning, in ordinary conversation, it is impossible to parse the surface forms of speech or sign. Therefore, participant observers are either privy to and obliged by ethical considerations to respect and in some cases to share the reasonable objectives of the persons under study/observation, or they are not full participants and have an inadequate basis for drawing inferences about what is going on in the discourse.

Conversation Analysis

The reason for the supplementation of written forms with audio and video recordings is that the full representation of movement requires movement.

Modern approaches to **conversation analysis** have made great strides in capturing the essence of turn-taking, overlapping utterances, and some of the nuances of speech acts on paper (Sacks, Schegloff, & Jefferson, 1974), but the written forms are always subordinated to the actions of the interlocutors (Richardson, Dale, & Kirkham, 2007).

If we want our readers to know what Stephen J. Cannell or John Forbes Nash or any other person sounds like in real life, we need more than written forms can provide. We need an actual recording that captures the articulate movements in real time as on tape or film. Fortunately, with modern technology we have such recordings and analysis often incorporates actual recordings of conversations in progress. For instance, in Goodwin's (2007) analysis of a father helping his daughter with a homework assignment, Goodwin suggests that it is necessary to see the participants as "social and moral actors in the midst of the mundane activities that constitute daily family life" (p. 53).

He, and other researchers using the conversational analysis paradigm, refer to the actions of interlocutors as "constitutional"—that is, as bringing into existence the conversational interaction. We agree that action is essential for the constitution of a conversation. However, we think theoreticians go too far when they say or imply that the interlocutors "constitute themselves" through conversation. This is going too far because the people exist without the conversation and they do not lose their status in the family, for instance, to use

Goodwin's example of the homework activity, if the conversation does not take place at all—much less do they lose their status if an ethnographer or outside "participant observer" is not present. Therefore, in order for participant observation, conversation analysis, and any transcription or analysis based on such methods to have validity—it must involve full participation with access to the intentions and meanings of the discourse. It cannot be based on surface forms alone and it cannot be fully captured in any kind of a static display—no matter how elaborate the transcription might be.

A musical score represents an abstraction of its music, but it is not the meaning itself. To get the meaning of a melody, or of a particularly rich harmony, or an interesting complex rhythm, the music must be performed. Try as we might—no matter how many lines are added to a written conversational analysis, no matter how many layers of overlapping parts are portrayed on different lines, no matter how delicately the overlaps are indicated in the transcription—the dynamics of the action require enactment through movement to fully express the meanings and intentions of the discourse. The meaning is contained in the rhythms, the changes, the dynamics, and the action of the music. In ordinary discourse, the speech, the manual signing, the gestures, and interactions that involve articulated signs are dynamic, intentional, and meaningful.

Articulation ultimately is in the action itself. No one has fully succeeded in getting a sequence of linear phonetic symbols to capture all the details of the actions involved in articulation. The rub lies mainly in trying to display in a static and discrete series of forms—letters, symbols, spaces, and marks of punctuation (no matter how deeply layered they may be)—a process that is inherently dynamic, moving, flowing, and changing over time.

> Real bodily movements cannot actually be accomplished with a display that is static anymore than a musical score constitutes the actual musical performance.

Speech Articulation Consists of Movement

As R. H. Stetson noted, the articulation of speech involves multilayered and highly structured movements that cannot fully be represented in a static display of any kind. A printed text cannot capture the dynamics of articulated movements. Much less can the text itself—even if it is spread over multiple layers—show all the prosodic meanings, intentions, purposes, feelings, and so forth of speakers. Stetson also argued that it is, in practice, "impossible to determine the phonetic signals of a language without reference to meaning" (1945, p. 21). Although a parrot that does not understand a word of English can imitate brief stretches in a manner that captures the surface form of a brief string of syllables, a parrot that can participate in a rich and meaningful conversation in any natural language has never been found except in fantastic fictions and in performances by parrots that are simultaneously interpreted and supplemented by human trainers. For example, when the Alex the parrot seems to comment on the corn on the cob he is eating to the trainer Irene

> . . . a parrot that can participate in a rich and meaningful conversation in any natural language has never been found except in fantastic fictions and in performances by parrots that are simultaneously interpreted and supplemented by human trainers.

Pepperberg, her commentary certainly makes the exchange look like a conversation. But careful analysis of that and other exchanges does not rule out the claim that the apparent comprehension by the parrot is an illusion created by the trainer.

Meet Alex the African Grey

As much as Dr. Pepperberg might like for Alex to show comprehension of abstract ideas and language, the phrases learned by Alex over a 30 year period of intensive training, leave him short of being able to say what he had for breakfast, much less why 2 is greater than 1. However, for an amazing demonstration of his linguistic skills, see "Goodbye to Alex, a Gifted Parrot" (retrieved March 4, 2009, from http://www.youtube.com/watch?v=sYk-wE18BTo).

The movie titled *Paulie* (1998) starring Tony Shalhoub, Gena Rowlands, and others, tells the tale of a talking bird who lives the life of a wandering human soul with feathers (retrieved March 3, 2009, from http://en.wikipedia.org/wiki/Paulie). Though it is a charming and entertaining fiction, it reminds us that mere articulation of the surface forms of speech does not constitute language, conversation, or human understanding. Also, it shows that in addition to movement, the ordinary articulation of meaningful discourse requires more than the mere copying of a surface form. Not only does the adequate representation of articulate movement logically require movement, but it requires a great deal of cognitive work that we cannot see at the surface, and yet, that is necessary if the surface forms are to constitute ordinary meaningful discourse. Nevertheless, it is important, as R. H. Stetson insisted, to incorporate movement into an adequate representation of articulatory phonetics and there is a strict logical reason for this.

Representing Movement Requires Movement

C. S. Peirce noted that it is impossible to represent movements without a moving sign—an index. Complex movements require complexes of indexes. Both theory and research show that the acquisition of a particular language critically involves a coordination of movements between the learner and the community of users who regularly employ the language being acquired (Condon & Sander, 1974; J. W. Oller, S. D. Oller, & Badon, 2006). If that coordination is disrupted, as in autism, for example, language will be dramatically impacted (Deth, Muratore, Benzecry, Power-Charnitsky, & Waly, 2008).

There is a vast amount of research bearing out this claim. One of the relevant early studies of human infancy was the demonstration by Condon and Sander (1974) that a neonate's movements are coordinated with the speech of adults within the baby's hearing. Synchronization of movements, making one set of movements match another, is the very essence of language acquisition and the noticing and coordination of movements is known to be essential to that process (Cutler, 1994; Ejiri, 1998; Sai, 2005). Without such synchronization of movements the idea of writing could never occur to anyone because there would be no meaningful speech or language to represent in writing. It is true that a new particular language system can seemingly be invented without native models, but no language system whatever can be invented or used entirely without movement.

The San Diego twins, Poto and Cabengo, evidently invented a new language ("Poto and Cabengo," 2009, retrieved March 3, 2009, from http://en.wikipedia.org/wiki/Poto_and_Cabengo) and other examples have been documented for whole groups of people in Hawaii, and elsewhere by Bickerton (1981). Similarly, Jill Morford (2006) along with other colleagues (see Morford, Singleton, & Goldin-Meadow, 1995) showed that signed languages can be invented in difficult situations over relative short time spans without native models to follow. However, there are no such inventions without movement.

As empirical proof that movement is the defining characteristic of speech, Stetson offered the fact that a deaf-blind individual such as Helen Keller could learn to produce speech by feeling the articulatory movements of other persons such as Mark Twain, Alexander Graham Bell, and a very small group of her interlocutors. She certainly could not rely on the audible production of syllables because she was completely deaf. It is not so unexpected that many deaf individuals would be able to learn to speak, but Helen Keller's case is unique inasmuch as she was also completely blind. Stetson noted that in cases of deaf persons who can see learning to speak depends mainly on visual observation of movements of someone else which are translated into articulate movements by the deaf person. In Helen Keller's case, as he noted, her success in learning to speak depended on literally feeling the speech movements with her hands.

> As empirical proof that movement is the defining characteristic of speech, Stetson offered the fact that a deaf-blind individual such as Helen Keller could learn to produce speech by feeling the articulatory movements of other persons such as Mark Twain, Alexander Graham Bell, and a very small group of her interlocutors.

All this evidence demonstrates unmistakably that movement is the main thing in defining the articulation of speech (1945, p. 21). Stetson went further to argue that there is a hierarchical structure of movements much as we have already demonstrated in Chapter 4 mainly through the McGurk interactions that were referred to there. Also, we continue to remind our readers that the hierarchy not only places visible articulated sign movements above the level of the auditory impressions they make, but it also places intentions and meanings at a still higher remove as we saw in the McGurk interactions at the sentence level in Chapter 4. With that in mind, it is also useful to see that there appears to be a hierarchy of layers within the level of essentially all truly skilled and highly articulated movements.

THE HIERARCHICAL STRUCTURE OF SKILLED MOVEMENTS

The hierarchical structure of skilled movements, which is manifested most obviously in speech and manual signed language, extends to other skilled movements as well. Stetson (1951) wrote:

> In all skilled movements the elements of the movements are included in larger units. A movement must be started and a movement must be stopped. In piano playing a series of small movements, the finger strokes, are united and included in the arm movement for the figure and the phrase, and the arm is supported by the trunk posture. (p. 155)

The movements involved in producing syllables, words, phrases, and higher units of discourse necessarily include the kinds of units normally represented by distinct symbols for segments at the phonetic level, for example, [p], [t], [k], . . . [a], [i], [u], and so on. An interesting fact demonstrated experimentally by Stetson, McGurk, de Jong, and colleagues, is that the actual resolution of syllabic sequences into particular *syllables*; **breath groups**—defined as utterances between pauses; contrastive sound segments usually designated as **phonemes**; lexical units, phrases, and higher units of discourse cannot be achieved without recourse to meaning.

Slow, Normal, and Fast Movements

Our dependence on meaning becomes obvious when we are dealing with ambiguous sequences that can be divided and grouped in more than one way. For instance, consider the sequences in the following list and see what happens when you speed up the rhythm of speech. First try saying each sequence repetitively in slow and deliberate speech at a rate of about three syllables per second—**slow speech**. Then speed up to a rate of about twice that—**normal speech**. After you have tried the normal speech rate, try the repetitions as fast as you can produce them—really **fast speech**—and see what happens:

- *at at at at* . . .(and repeat);
- *will earn, we learn, we'll learn* . . .;
- *mares eat oats and goats eat oats and little lambs eat ivy*

As Stetson noted in 1951, it turns out that the subtle points of transition between what we know are distinct phonemes, syllables, words, phrases, and higher units of structure is literally and utterly (no kidding) dependent on how fast the utterances are produced. Speech-language pathologists and diagnosticians commonly use a task where client/patients are asked to repeat rapidly the nonsense sequence *puh, tuh, kuh* as a test of what is termed **diadochokinesis**. This nine dollar word actually means the ability to perform rapidly alternating muscular movements, such as flexion and extension. The word itself is a fairly good test of a person's ability to achieve diadochokinesis in speech movements. In speech-language pathology, especially with respect to articulation, diadochokinesis refers to rapid movements of the tongue between distinct points of articulation. In English the maximal distance between points of articulation, for the tongue at least (see Figure 7–3) is between the bilabial and velar points of articulation.

When we speed up the production of a sequence such as *up up up* or *at at at* there comes a point where the syllable we seem to be saying is not the word *up* or even *pup*, though we can hear both of these in the sequence as we gradually increase our rate to the fastest rate we can maintain. In saying *at at at* at an increasingly faster rhythm, what we seem to be saying is the sequence *tat tat* and then at a still faster rate, *ta, ta, ta . . .* and so on. Why is this?

Rhythm as a Defining Feature

Stetson's results with speeding up or slowing down the rhythm required for producing surface forms have been examined in great detail more recently by de Jong and colleagues at the University of Indiana (de Jong, Lim, & Nagao, 2004; Nagao & de Jong, 2007; Silbert & de Jong, 2008). You will also notice if you slow the rate of production gradually back to a normal conversational speech rate and then all the way back to very slow, deliberate speech, the distorted sequence *ta ta ta* seems to returns to the distinct, *at at at . . .*

We can also produce similar changes in sequences such as *will earn, we learn, we'll learn* by producing them at varying rates. Even the transitions of a sequence such as *mares eat oats and goats eat oats and little lambs eat ivy* can be articulated so that all of the word boundaries are as plain as day. Or, we can speed up the production and cause the word boundaries to fade into meaningless syllabic nonsense. Why is this?

From such evidence, Stetson insisted that the real basis for phonemic distinctions, word boundaries, and phonetic disambiguation in general is strictly constituted in the motor production of speech. He argued that the rhythm of the production of syllable units in particular has special importance. His claim finds support in research with infants by Ramus and Mehler (1999) showing that the timing of syllable units is the basis by which young infants are able to distinguish English (or Dutch) from Spanish (or Japanese). Additional work along this line shows that not only are distinct languages differentiated by their rhythms in early infancy (see, for

At a nice slow rate of speech, each of the elements in the sequences *will earn, we learn, we'll learn* can be differentiated. However, at a faster rate, and especially at our fastest rate, they all sound alike.

instance, Hespos, 2007; Lewkowicz & Marcovitch, 2006; Nazzi & Ramus, 2003), but:

- toddlers use rhythms to distinguish fluent from disfluent speech (Soderstrom & J. L. Morgan, 2007);
- infants and adults alike use rhythms in particular and prosody in general to distinguish foreign accents (Kinzler, Dupoux, & Spelke, 2007);
- and even dialect differences within a given language, such as Arabic, are evidently detectable in large part from differences in rhythm (Jaffe, Beebe, Feldstein, Crown, & Jasnow, 2001; Rouas, 2007).

Adjustable Boundaries Between Segments

In written phonetic representations of language, the attempt is made to represent surface forms of speech as if the segments were discrete beads on a string. However, if we examine the way speech is produced in ordinary experience, and the way the surface forms of language change over time, we discover many different ways that the "sounds" represented in phonetic symbols tend to influence each other dynamically over time. In rapid speech many changes occur in the production of surface forms. For instance, when we ordinarily produce a surface form such as *an apple, an egg, and an orange,* we notice that the final phrase *and an orange* is apt to involve the reduction of *and* to [ən] where the sequence [nd] is reduced so that the [d] is lost. This common phenomenon, called **cluster reduction**, occurs in ordinary speech and may also occur in instances of articulation disorders and/or normal child language acquisition. The key to telling the difference is whether or not the cluster reduction occurs only in rapid speech or in slow speech as well. Does it occur regularly on certain consonant clusters?

In cases where a whole word is reduced to the point that it does not appear at all in the surface form, various terms have been applied including **ellipsis**, *deletion*, and so forth. A general term for the omission of a single segment or a whole word in rapid speech is **elision**. For instance, in rapid production of the sequence *an egg and an orange,* to take this handy example, the words *and* and *an*, especially just in front of *orange*, may be completely joined so that they appear at the surface as just one segment [nɛgnɔɹ əndʒ]. In this case the melding of two words comes out in a single [n] segment at the surface. However, they are not understood as the same word in the phrase in question even if it is articulated at as fast as possible.

We can argue that the two words are produced in **coarticulation**. As noted in the charts and symbols of the IPA (see Figure 7–2) it is possible to produce some articulations simultaneously. For instance, there may be some languages where the palatal fricative [ʃ] occurs simultaneously with the velar [x]. Of course, [ʃ] occurs abundantly in English, for example, as the final segment in the word *English*, and [x] occurs in Spanish and Arabic. Does a double articulation of both at the same time occur in any of the world's 6,912 languages? The proposed symbol for this disputed coarticulation is [ɧ]. The symbol is not commonly used because some phoneticians doubt the existence of this coarticulation. However, it is certainly possible to produce both articulations simultaneously.

Mutual Influences Across Boundaries

In ordinary speech the sounds tend to melt together in many different ways for all the reasons that de Saussure noted in his comment that speech is a ribbon with no clear cut divisions. When the segments that are clearly distinct sounds in slow speech come together in rapid conversational exchanges, they commonly become more like each other in a process unsurprisingly called **assimilation**—as in the word *income* where the [n] is apt to become [ŋ], that is, to move from an alveolar place of articulation to a velar one, in anticipation of the [k] that follows it. The [k] has a velar point of articulation so the [n] tends to assimilate to it as well. Or, the proximity of sound segments in speech can produce exactly the opposite effect which, again, unsurprisingly, is called **dissimilation**. For instance, in the word *etcetera* which is usually pronounced as [ɛtsɛtɪə], the [t] and following [s] between the first and second syllables of the word have the same alveolar point of articulation. However, some speakers of English commonly convert this word to [ɛksɛtɪə] (as if it were spelled "eksetera") where the [t] is converted to [k] with a velar point of articulation which maximizes its articulatory distance from [t].

Added Segments

Another common change that occurs when segments collide in rapid speech is the insertion of a new segment at the surface. For example, in the phonotactic system of English we find it difficult—motorically inconvenient at least—to make the transition from a voiced nasal, for instance, in *Chomsky*, *Nancy*, *fence*, and so forth, to a **sibilant** such as [s] or [ʃ] without inserting a plosive stop consonant in between the nasal and the sibilant. That is, we tend to say such words as if they contained either a /p/ or /t/ segment at the point of transition from the nasal consonant to the sibilant: for example, as if the words really should be spelled as *Chompsky*, *Nantsy, and fents*. Or to take another example, when we add the morpheme *-tion* which changes the verb *assume* to the noun *assumption*, we add a [p] in between these two sequences. Instead of saying [əsəmʃɪn] we say, [əsəmpʃɪn]. The process of adding the plosive to the string is called **epenthesis**. Similarly, we insert the same [p] in

In ordinary speech the sounds tend to melt together in many different ways for all the reasons that de Saussure noted in his comment that speech is a ribbon with no clear cut divisions.

Chomsky, and an epenthetic [t] in *Nancy* and *fence*. Assimilation, dissimilation, and epenthesis are all more or less subsumed under the broader term **sandhi** which is applied to the phonological and morphological changes that tend to occur at the boundaries of morphemes within words (see "Sandhi," 2009, retrieved March 3, 2009, from http://en.wikipedia.org/wiki/Sandhi). There are very many phenomena of this kind showing that the articulation of surface forms is influenced by deeper and more abstract systems of speech and language.

Changed Order

Still another change that commonly occurs in rapid speech is the sort of reversal of segments that occurs for instance when we speed up the production of *up, up, up*, for instance, until it seems to become *puh, puh, puh*. This sort of reversal of order, where an earlier segment exchanges places with a later one is called **metathesis**. This is what occurs sometimes in a word such as *irrelevant*, which may be rendered at the surface as *irrevelant*, where the [l] and [v] exchange places. Historically this kind of process is known to have occurred many times in well-documented languages. For instance, in Latin the underlying word for *miracle* was *miraculum* but in modern Spanish it has become *milagro* where the [l] and the [r] have neatly exchanged places. However, in French, the original Latin sequence was retained in the word *miracle*—which was also borrowed into English without the metathesis that occurred in Spanish.

THE ARTICULATION OF SURFACE FORMS

The process of articulation as diagramed above in Figure 7–1 has three essential parts. There is the conceptualization of the meaning (based on intentions), the mapping of that meaning into surface forms, and the construction and differentiation of the surface forms themselves.

A Three-Part Whole

At the top of the rank, there is the meaning which is associated with the surface forms. We saw in Chapter 4 why that meaning is by all accounts the top rank. It is highest in generality, abstractness, and function.

Second, in between the meaning and the surface form that can be perceived by ourselves or by someone else, there is the pragmatic mapping process by which the meaning is expressed in surface form. That mapping is bidirectional. As the diagram shows, we may suppose that the motor productions of articulate symbols —whether spoken, signed, or written—map articulate speech forms onto the holistic (iconic) contexts of experience. Meanwhile, the iconic representations of the facts of contexts of experience are conveyed to the symbolic and conceptual domain so that the entities which are referred to are indexed to their referring symbols. Third, in the world of experience the articulate surface forms appear as physically distinct elements—for example, in a stream of speech, manuals signs, or written symbols just as this articulate text appears on this page as it is typed on one or several keyboards. The reader will also notice that the meanings do not jump off the page all by themselves.

Reading Requires Action

Reading demands action on the part of the reader—eye movements, inferences, and thought. It is those actions by the reader that distinguish really fast expert readers with extremely high levels of comprehension as well as speed of access, from slow plodders, and, in some cases, from persons struggling to decipher one letter at a time and who we would diagnose with instructional dyslexia—see Chapter 9 and the entire system of Evelyn Wood's "Reading Dynamics" based on her master's thesis (see E. Wood, 2007, retrieved March 3, 2009 at http://www.evelynwood.com.au/). Even efficient average readers can comprehend written discourse at a rate that considerably exceeds the fastest attainable rates of speech (or reading aloud), and fast readers, such as former President John F. Kennedy, can read with excellent comprehension at rates that are about 100 times faster than they can talk.

When we work from the surface form to the meaning—from 1 to 2 to 3 (per Figure 7–1)—we are acting, for the most part, as a consumer/interpreter of those surface forms. When we work from the meaning toward the surface form—from 3 to 2 to 1, generally, we are in the process of constructing a surface form in order to represent a particular meaning. Extremely fast readers, it seems, can by-pass the motoric process of constructing surface forms of speech and are able to move along at the level of meanings as fast as they can conceptualize those meanings—that is, as E. Wood (2007) argued, at the speed of thought. Articulate speech or signing, by contrast, is more effortful because of the motoric involvement of the articulators. To produce speech at an intelligible rate not only requires more work, but it also requires movement at a rate that enables comprehension on the part of listeners—or else the intentional purposes of the speaking/signing would be lost.

Extremely fast readers, it seems, can by-pass the motoric process of constructing surface forms of speech and are able to move along at the level of meanings as fast as they can conceptualize those meanings—that is, as E. Wood (2007) argued, at the speed of thought.

In addition to planning what to say in a kind of look ahead mode, the producer of a stream of signs is also normally engaged in looking back to check the results as they emerge in the stream of signs. The question is whether the surface forms that are emerging express the intended meaning.

The Feedback Loop

There is a feedback loop from the surface form to meaning, and from the meaning to the form. Because of this loop the relation between intended or understood meaning and surface form can be checked for consistency. In addition to planning what to say in a kind of look ahead mode, the producer of a stream of signs is also normally engaged in looking back to check the results as they emerge in the stream of signs. The question is whether the surface forms that are emerging express the intended meaning.

Likewise, the consumer is checking the forms that emerge over time for consistency with the interpretations already constructed and also is looking ahead by anticipating where the discourse is going. When unexpected elements come up in the discourse, the listener is apt to pose a question to clarify a referring term, for example, "Who is George? I don't remember your mentioning him before," or "You said 'the teacher.' What teacher?" Occasionally the speaker or signer will insert a correction, for example, "Did I say 'George'? Actually, I meant 'Bill'." All this is suggested in the pragmatic mapping diagram (see Figure 3–3) as elaborated in Figure 7–1.

Articulation is the process by which the surface forms in any sequence of signs is differentiated from some other arrangement. For instance, "The dog bit the child," means something quite different from "The child bit the dog," but the same sequence of words in a scrambled order does not necessarily mean anything in particular at all—for example, "bit child dog the the." If the same sound segments themselves, or the letters in this case, are scrambled, the resulting hash is can look like this: "tbci id lhee hcg hohd." The latter hash is not pronounceable in English in spite of the fact that it contains all the same letters of the surface forms that could be arranged into the intelligible and meaningful sentences: "The dog bit the child," and "The child bit the dog."

Clearly, the intelligibility of the surface forms of speech, sign, or writing is largely dependent on articulation. Even more certainly, though this fact is not always brought out in books on phonetics, linguistics, or communication disorders, the meaningful articulation of a sequence of movements resulting in even a small segment of ordinary discourse is evidently utterly and completely dependent on the sort of intelligence that is contained in the unique human language capacity. If parrots, chimps, dolphins, or gorillas seem to be able to acquire some of the articulated gestures of speech or manual signing, closer examination will show that they had a great deal of help from human trainers in order to do so.

If parrots, chimps, dolphins, or gorillas seem to be able to acquire some of the articulated gestures of speech or manual signing, closer examination will show that they had a great deal of help from human trainers in order to do so.

The Mapping Involves Skilled Movements

In order for the differentiation of the surface forms of discourse to be accomplished, meanings have to be systematically mapped into a sequence of highly articulated movements—vocal, manual, or in some combination of them. The sequence must not only be possible to produce, but it must also conform to the requirements of the grammar of the particular language in which the forms are being articulated. Such articulation involves every aspect of the grammatical structure of language. It involves semantics, pragmatics, the lexicon, syntax, morphology, phonology, and some manifest surface form or other—spoken, signed, written, or some combination of these.

When speech is involved, the term *phonetics* is appropriate to the description of the processes of producing the speech sounds. In writing, the nature of the articulate movements depend on the kind of writing system involved, as we will see in the next major section titled "Different Writing Systems." We will see in that section that many different writing systems have been invented to express the surface forms of speech. They can be classed into several different kinds. Systems have also been invented to express meanings more or less directly without reference to the surface forms of speech. However, all these writing systems involve skilled movements to produce a distinct series of surface forms. This is just as true of writing with a keyboard or speaking into an automated dictation system that converts speech to text as it is of speaking or signing.

One of the things that is peculiar about the articulated surface forms of writing that makes them distinct from the surface forms of speech is that writing must be captured in a two-dimensional space whereas the articulation of spoken discourse, together with all its gestural and contextual accompaniments (referents, demonstrative actions, etc.), is multidimensional. This is most obvious with respect to body movements that are incorporated into speech acts, for example, smiling, grimacing, raising the eyebrows, pointing, moving the head, trunk, gesturing with the hands, or even the whole body, and so on.

> When manual signing is used, the articulatory equivalent of the *phonetic systems* of speech—sometimes referred to as *visual phonetics*—consists of hand shapes and movements (see Armstrong, Stokoe, & S. E. Wilcox, 1995).

The Distinct Dynamics of Speech and Manual Sign

Interestingly, the words and sounds of spoken discourse are typically articulated in groups by movements of the diaphragm, larynx, pharynx, velum, mouth, tongue, lips, and jaw. At the same time there are accompanying movements of the eyes, face, hands, head, and body of both the speaker and the listener that happen to be coordinated with syntactic, semantic, and pragmatic elements in the stream of speech. It is generally supposed that the stream of speech itself carries the main burden of conveying information whereas the accompanying movements of the speaker and listener, who may exchange roles many times in the same conversation, express feelings and reactions.

With manual signing of the Deaf (in American Signed Language for instance), almost the reverse is the case. Movements of the hands

As we noted in Chapter 3, manual systems that are derived from spoken languages are not only stilted, but also require about twice as much time to produce. A sentence in English, for example, can be signed twice as fast in American Signed Language as in Signed Exact English.

and body of the sign producer constitute the main acts of linguistic articulation while the movements of the eyes, voice, lips, tongue, and jaw of producer and interpreter generally express feelings (Monikowski, 1994; Valli, Lucas, & Mulrooney, 2005). Toddlers are able to associate referring terms as well as particular expressions of emotions—for example, approval or disapproval toward those referents—as early as 12 to 18 months of age (Moses, Baldwin, Rosicky, & Tidball, 2001). This shows that the articulation of speech from the vantage point of the toddler includes the gestures, line of regard (smooth pursuit and saccades), facial expression, tone of voice, and so forth, along with the surface forms of speech.

Gestures in particular help interpreters of speech to know what is being referred to and what the speaker means to say and how the speaker feels about the referents of discourse (Ozyurek & Kelly, 2007; Willems & Hagoort, 2007; Wu & Coulson, 2007). Manual signed languages derived from spoken systems, such as Exact Signed English, on the other hand, do not contrast so much with speech (see "Manually Coded English," 2009, retrieved March 3, 2009, from http://en.wikipedia.org/wiki/Manually_Coded_English). For manual systems derived from spoken languages, it is even possible to speak and sign at the same time. In that case, the signing is apt to be accompanied by some of the same facial expressions, and so forth, as speech, and the gestures accompanying the manual signs derived from speech will show a narrower range of emotions and ancillary meanings than are common to signing without simultaneous speech.

In all cases, dynamic articulation, as we have defined it, is essential. Dynamic articulation (skilled movement) is the means of producing speech, manual signing, writing, reading, or even drawing a picture, snapping a photograph, playing a musical instrument, singing a song, or shooting a segment of video or a moving picture (see Boorstin, 1990; Branigan, 1992; Gombrich, 1970, 1972; J. W. Oller & Giardetti, 1999; Stetson, 1945, 1951). Unless the signs created and used in such processes are articulated in such a way as to make them distinct from each other, it will be impossible to say what the signs are signs of.

Discrete, Distinct, and Replicable

At some level and at a slow rate of production, the surface forms of discourse (in any form) must be articulated so that they are discrete, distinct, and replicable. To be discrete, surface forms must be bounded in some way by beginnings and endings. To be distinct they must contrast with each other, and to be replicable the movements required to produce the surface form must be discriminable, recognizable, and reproducible. Without such differentiation, signs cannot function as signs of anything.

A sign that is not distinct from other signs cannot be the sign of any particular thing, event, relation, or meaning. So, articulation is not optional. It is a logical requirement. Signs not only must have some noticeable surface form, but the forms of different signs must seem different at the surface. The difference must be sufficient to enable a particular sign to be distinguished from others. A sign that has no distinct surface form cannot function as a sign distinct from other signs. It is also essential for signs to have definite beginnings and ends. Signs that do not begin cannot be produced and signs that do not end would require too much time to produce to serve the purpose of communication. For these reasons, discrete articulations that have beginnings and ends are essential.

Articulation: Required for Icons, as Well as Indexes, and Symbols

A photo, or segment of moving film, that displays no boundaries—by being out of focus say or having no contrast between light, dark, and color—cannot reasonably be said to be a photo or film of anything. A picture is not of a person, event, or sequence of events in particular unless it can be made out to have boundaries that are articulated within it (Macknik, 2007; Martinez-Conde & Macknik, 2007).

Boundaries and Edges

To be a picture or a diagram of something, it is necessary for the surface forms to involve distinct elements, edges, and identifiably bounded things, events, relations, and so on that can be discerned by an intelligent interpreter. Such discernment also necessarily involves movement of the observer, for example, especially of the eyes, body, and so forth, to connect indexically with the icons at hand, and to discriminate their boundaries and so forth.

Articulation in the sense defined is critical not only to the production of signs but also to their perception and, as a result, to their very existence as signs. Boundaries are also required for speech forms, manual signs, and written symbols. If a sequence of syllables, manual, or written signs is to be identified as a particular sequence of words, phrases, and higher linguistic units, its surface forms must be articulated sufficiently so that they can be distinguished from the other surface forms that they resemble but are not the same as, "will earn" must be distinguished from "we learn," as well as "we'll earn" and "we'll learn." Indexes similarly must be bounded by distinct icons. A pointing gesture, for instance, needs a

A sign that is not distinct from other signs cannot be the sign of any particular thing, event, relation, or meaning. So, articulation is not optional. It is a logical requirement.

beginning and an end. It must have a point of origin and a terminus or it is an incomplete and imperfect index. Pointing in all directions is like an entry in an index to a book that lists every single page. Pointing nowhere at all is like an indexical entry in a book that points to no page at all.

We conclude by strict logic that in any form of communication the articulation of the surface forms of signs, so as to make them discrete, distinct from each other, and reproducible is essential. To the extent that these requirements are met, there is hope that the sequence of signs will be intelligible. To the extent that the articulation requirements are not met, the intelligibility of the surface forms will necessarily be diminished. If it is lost altogether, the value of any icon, index, or symbol will vanish all the way to nothing.

DIFFERENT WRITING SYSTEMS

To see why it is not possible to express fully the dynamics of speech in a sequence of static letters or symbols strung out in a line as a sequence of letters on a sheet of paper—or in any other static spatial display—it is useful to consider what is and what is not represented in the various writing systems of the world.

English Writing as Only Quasi-Alphabetic

Our own system of writing—the kind of writing that is represented on this page, for instance—is only quasi-alphabetic. That is, the symbols that we use to represent language correspond only in part to the distinctive sounds of speech. In our writing system, many of the distinctions that are possible are not made, some that are necessary are not made, and many distinctions that are made at the surface in our writing system do not represent any sounds whatsoever. For instance, "p" in "pneumonia" does not represent any sound at all and the "b" in "subtle" and "doubt" likewise does not represent any sound in either of those words.

Alphabetic Writing

If letters were to correspond as perfectly as possible to sounds, our system of writing would be fully alphabetic.

If letters were to correspond as perfectly as possible to sounds, our system of writing would be fully alphabetic. There are some languages, such as Spanish, that use a writing system much nearer a truly alphabetic one than English writing. But before showing how drastically English deviates from a fully alphabetic writing system, it is important to say just what is meant by alphabetic writing.

The Aim of a Perfect Alphabet

In principle, in a fully alphabetic system, there should be just one letter (or symbol) for each distinctive sound segment. That was the aim of the creators of the so-called International Phonetic Alphabet (IPA). It was the goal of its creators to try to come up with a system to represent the sounds of all the languages of the world so that for each distinctive sound there would be a distinct symbol.

The creators of that system stated their purpose this way:

> From its earliest days . . . the International Phonetic Association has aimed to provide "a separate sign for each distinctive sound; that is, for each sound which, being used instead of another, in the same language, can change the meaning of a word." (International Phonetic Association, 1999, *Handbook*, p. 27)

Many theoreticians and practitioners subscribed to the view that the goal of the International Phonetic Association was very largely achieved by the International Phonetic Alphabet. Both are commonly referred to by the abbreviation *IPA*.

What Is Represented in Alphabetic Writing

English writing conforms to an alphabetic system very imperfectly. However, it still serves to illustrate the **alphabetic principle**. In English writing, the letter "b" stands for the sound at the beginning of the word "beginning," the letter "p" stands for the sound at the beginning of the word "page," and so forth. To this extent the letters of our writing system correspond to what are called **phonetic segments** in speech and to **phonemic segments** of English.

If the given segment contrasts with others to signal a difference of meaning, the contrast is said to be phonemic, if not, any given characteristic signaled in the written segment is said to be merely phonetic—below the level of meaningful contrast. For instance, the /b/ and /p/ contrast in English, as in the words *bat* and *pat*, is phonemic. The contrast in question forms the basis for distinguishing those words and the words have different meanings. They are said to be a **minimal pair** because they differ only in the one phonemic segment which signals their difference of meaning—namely, the contrast represented by the letter "b" as contrasted with "p." However, the same phonetic contrast in another language—for example in Arabic—does not signal any difference in meaning. English listeners may notice that an Arabic "accent" in English is marked partly by the fact that words like "problems" tend to sound to us like "broblems."

The difference between a mere phonetic segment and one that is phonemic has to do with whether the given segment contrasts with others to signal (at least potentially) a difference of meaning.

Not All Phonetic Qualities Are Represented in an Alphabet

If we look a little deeper into the phonetic qualities of sounds in English—the **phonetic features** of any given segment that might be represented in an alphabetic system of some sort—we find that there are some that are not phonemic. For instance, if we consider the sound segments that are represented by the letter "p" in English, we discover that sometimes they are followed by a burst of air, and sometimes not. When we say the word "pat," for instance, a burst of air follows the release of the lips just prior to the onset of voice on the vowel that is loosely represented by the letter "a" in our writing of this word. This burst of air is technically referred to as the phonetic feature of **aspiration** and the "p" in question is said to be **aspirated**.

If we compare, however, the "p" of the word "spat," on the other hand, we discover that this one is not aspirated. There is no burst of air following the "p" in "spat." Yet we regard both of these sounds as instances of the same phoneme and we represent them by the same letter in keeping with the alphabetic principle. The feature of aspiration is not represented in English because it does not serve the phonemic purpose of distinguishing any particular meanings.

In another language, for example, in Thai—one of the languages of Southeast Asia spoken in Thailand—the phonetic contrast just described does signal a difference in the meaning of words. There are minimal pairs in Thai where the difference depends exclusively on whether a particular "p" is aspirated or not. Phonetically, if we express the phonetic aspect of the sound segment as aspirated or not in our writing, we need another written element or diacritic to show that the "p" in question is aspirated, or we need to use different letters for the contrasting sounds. Because the developers of phonetic alphabets were more influenced by English (and the Roman alphabet) than by Thai, they chose to represent aspiration by a superscript "h," as in $[p^h]$ by contrast with [p], rather than to use only two different letters to show whether any particular "p" is aspirated. This choice is arbitrary. If the developers of the IPA had been speakers of Thai, Arabic, or Chinese, the symbols chosen might have been very different from the ones seen in Figure 7–2.

In Thai the contrast between $/p/$ and $/p^h/$ is phonemic and, if we are following the alphabetic principle strictly, Thai requires two different letters for these phonemes. Or, to take another example, in English the contrast signaled in the letters "r" and "l" is phonemic because it enables us to distinguish words such as *led* and *red*, whereas the same phonetic difference in Japanese is not phonemic. English, therefore, requires two distinct letters for these sounds while Japanese could get by with only one. Such observations also help to explain and account for some aspects of foreign accents, for example, the tendency of Japanese speakers to confuse "rice" and "lice," not to mention all of the confusions that English speakers tend to fall into in trying to produce the sounds of Arabic, Japanese, Thai, and so forth.

What Is Represented in Other Writing Systems

In addition to letters corresponding to sounds in alphabetic writing, there are other writing systems that represent other units of surface form or meaning. For instance, syllables may be represented in what are called **syllabaries**—that is, in **syllabic writing**.

Written Symbols for Syllables

A major language that uses syllabic writing extensively is Korean. The American language of the Cherokee Indians was also written syllabically by the famed **Sequoia** [ca. 1776–1843] shown in an 1828 oil painting of him by Charles Bird King (Figure 7–4). See "Sequoyah" (n.d., retrieved March 3, 2009, from http://www.manataka.org/page81.html) and "Sequoyah" (2009, retrieved March 3, 2009, from http://en.wikipedia.org/wiki/Sequoyah) for the story of the Cherokee syllabary he invented.

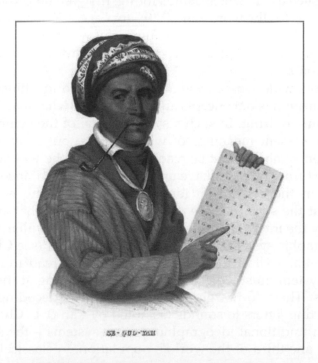

FIGURE 7–4. Sequoia and the syllabary of Cherokee. Portrait by Charles Bird King in 1828. Retrieved March 3, 2009, from http://en.wikipedia.org/wiki/Sequoyah. This image is in the public domain as its copyright has expired.

Sequoia was physically disabled at an early age by a hunting injury for which he was given his Cherokee name which means "pig's foot." In spite of his disability he is the only individual of history who is known to have single-handedly invented a widely used writing system. His syllabary helped to sustain the Cherokee language, which is estimated to have between 11,905 and 22,500 speakers today. During his lifetime, Sequoia's system became the basis for literacy in Cherokee and remains the preferred writing system for that language to this day.

In 1824 at New Echota, Georgia, Sequoia received from the Cherokee National Council the silver medal seen in the portrait. He is said to have worn it until the day of his death in 1843. As early as 1825, Sequoia's syllabary was the preferred writing system used for a translation of the Bible and many hymns also were translated into Cherokee (retrieved March 3, 2009, from http://www.ethn ologue.com/14/show_language.asp?code=CER). In honor of his achievement on behalf of the indigenous peoples of America, the great redwood trees of California are called Sequoias.

Logographic and Ideographic Writing Systems

Another approach to writing is to represent whole words in what is called **logographic writing**. English uses certain logographic symbols such as "I" which stands for the first person pronoun, "&" which serves for the word "and," "@" for "at," "©" for "copyright," and "¢" for "cents." Because the number of words in a language is very large, systems that directly represent words are cumbersome and not common.

> To the extent that Chinese writing is truly ideographic, its translation into speech forms in any language is more like paraphrasing than it is like reading from an alphabetic, syllabic, or logographic script.

A more widely used system is the sort used in Chinese where abstract meanings or concepts are expressed in what may be called **ideographic writing**. In such a system, some of the symbols used directly represent meanings of whole words, but in many cases, the written symbols must be read somewhat in the way we would read a text from one language and translate it simultaneously into another. In the case of an ideographic system, the words and phrases at the surface if we read aloud are somewhat arbitrarily chosen by the interpreter/reader. Because of the peculiar nature of an ideographic system of writing it can be argued (see Chapter 9) that essentially all of the persons who learn to read from such a writing system must work from the very beginning at the level of meanings. They do not go through a phonetic decoding process of converting letters to sounds (as noted by Pan & L. Chen, 2005). In fact, in traditional ideographic writing systems—the sort used by about one-third of the world's population, in classical Chinese writing and in common forms of Japanese and Korean writing as well—the direct conversion of written signs to speech sounds by sounding out the words is impossible. The written symbols of classical Chinese do not represent speech sounds at all.

English writing does not use many ideographic symbols as such but occasionally the dollar sign, "$,"may be used to indicate wealth, for example, in an animated cartoon in which dollar signs pop up where the character's eyeballs are supposed to be. Or a smiley face may be used to signify approval of some sort, for example, "☺,"or the opposite, "☹." We could translate or paraphrase the smiley in many different ways at the surface. We could say, "I approve!" "You have made me quite happy." "Thanks for cheering me up!" "You have made my day." "Wow!" "Super!" "I am sooooo glad you said that!" And so on. Another example of an ideographic sign in English would be a heart used to signify affection as in the writing on a tee-shirt or bumper sticker that says, "I ♥ New York"—where the heart symbol might be paraphrased as "love," "like," "am crazy about," "enjoy living in," "want to go to," "liked being in," and so on.

Unchanging Symbols for Segmental Sounds

Written records by their very nature are hypostatic—that is, they are relatively unchanging. They are static to the lowest limit of not seeming to move or change at all once they have been created. With reference to a given language, the written symbols are not only supposed to be formed in the same way each time they appear—for example, the letter "a" does not look like "a" on one appearance and then like "e" or "d" or any other letter on the next—but strings of symbols retain their distinctness and consistently have the same meaning and form from one occasion to the next. Because writing seems to be a relatively permanent way of recording and displaying linguistic forms and meanings, the idea that certain segmental elements of speech are also somewhat invariant naturally follows.

It was natural to suppose that all the sequences of sounds in all the languages of the world could be well represented in a single alphabet along the lines of the IPA. To a very great extent this goal has been achieved. The idea was also promoted by the fact that ordinary artifacts and the symbol systems of mathematics, music, art, architecture, photography, and sculpture also seem to suggest that hypostatic symbols can represent just about everything. At any rate, **structural linguistics**, especially under the leadership of thinkers like Leonard Bloomfield [1887–1949] in America, promoted the notion that speech can be reduced to a series of distinct, more or less discrete **segmental sounds** strung together like beads on a string—that is, that language could be reduced to a string of discrete letters written in a line.

We will have a good deal more to say about Bloomfield and his ideas about literacy in Chapter 9. Here, however, it is important to note that the idea that speech could be reduced to sound-letter correspondences was a gross oversimplification. In particular, though an alphabet as diversified as the IPA is a highly versatile system for representing certain aspects of the surface forms of any language, it encouraged linguists and literate people to underestimate the importance of meaning and the complexity of the processing leading from the surface forms of language—speech, manual signing, and writing—to the abstract conceptual realm of meaning.

Beyond the Segmentals

In addition to sound segments in the surface forms of speech, which can be represented by letters, there are also suprasegmental elements. These are represented in a considerable variety of additional elements in the IPA system as can be seen in Figure 7–2. Suprasegmental elements consist of the dynamic changes in voice quality (tone of voice), pitch, loudness, rate, and so forth.

Sometimes, theoreticians such as Raymond L. Birdwhistell [1918–1994] ("Kinesics," 2009, retrieved March 3, 2009, from http://en.wikipedia.org/wiki/Kinesics) proposed that ordinary human communication involved much more than just the suprasegmental aspects of speech. He argued that the study of articulate communication would have to include a much wider array of what were called **paralinguistic devices** such as distinct facial expressions, for example, smiling, grimacing, showing surprise, moving the head, trunk, gesturing with the hands, or even the whole body, and so on. Birdwhistell (1970) argued for a study of gestural systems that he proposed to call **kinesics**. He argued that there were distinct meaning-laden bodily movements that differentiated genders, ethnicities, social communities, and so on. He claimed that the greater part of the meaning in social settings is conveyed not by words, but by paralinguistic devices involving movement. His ideas did not achieve general acceptance, and he made the mistake of arguing that there are no universal human facial expressions. The latter idea was soon proved wrong (Ekman & Friesen, 1974, 1975).

Nevertheless, Birdwhistell and his successors helped to extend the boundaries of what was known to be important to the expression of meaning in human communication.

Louder Than Words

Significant movements that are commonly associated with speech or sign acts include pointing, nodding, waving hello or goodbye, drawing a breath to speak, sighing, hissing, whistling, grunting, snorting, and so on. The way we walk, move, talk, and the variations in facial expressions and body movements that we use, do tell a great deal about who we are and about our intentions in communication. According to the popular wisdom, it is said, in agreement with Birdwhistell that actions speak louder than words.

The Missing Boundaries

There has never been a sharp boundary between what was to count as a suprasegmental device in speaking as contrasted with any other action that might be performed by a producer or consumer of articulated signs. The boundary between what were called suprasegmentals and paralinguistic devices was always vague. But if we only look just a little farther—beyond the pointing, looking, grimacing, smiling, glaring, and so forth—to what is pointed out, grimaced at, and so forth, we discover that articulated signs connect with persons, events, and activities in the common world. Those other bodily elements, events, relations, and contexts of experience according to traditional approaches to speech and language were almost invariably considered outside of even the broadest sweep of the so-called paralinguistic elements.

All those other elements out there in the world of experience, including objects, events, spatial relations, and the like that might be referred to in linguistic discourse but that were not considered part of the surface forms of discourse were referred to as **extralinguistic elements**. Those elements fell into the realm of the so-called "material" or "physical" world.

Bloomfield's Exclusion of Meaning

Bloomfield and some of his successors held that meaning could play no role in linguistic analysis. The material world and its contents were too vast, according to Bloomfield, to be included in a linguistic analysis. For that reason the world and its contents were ruled out of bounds. What was left in bounds, by a kind of arbitrary declaration, consisted of the surface forms of speech as such —more specifically, whatever sound events occurred between the mouth of the speaker and the ear of the hearer. Bloomfield argued that the sounds of language could be analyzed and represented in a string of symbols—the letters of a special alphabet without any reference to meaning or to the vast world of ordinary experience. Bloomfield supposed that the world was too vast and the potential meanings too diverse to be called into play in linguistic analysis.

However, just as the boundary between speech and paralinguistic devices was uncertain, the boundary separating language from the "extralinguistic" realm of bodily persons, things, events, and relations in the material world was also a strange fiction. How could the material content associated with linguistic segments, words, phrases, and also with the "suprasegmental" or even "paralinguistic" devices of articulated language be entirely separated from them? Are the predicates associated with a person (e.g., female, human, adult) or other entity, (nation, sovereign, in America) or corporation (bank, international), not also associated with the actual stream of history in which that entity is involved? On what possible basis can

The boundary between what were called suprasegmentals and paralinguistic devices was always vague. But if we only look just a little farther—beyond the pointing, looking, grimacing, smiling, glaring, and so forth—to what is pointed out, grimaced at, and so forth, we discover that articulated signs connect with persons, events, and activities in the common world.

any action of any person be identified as such apart from the person performing the action?

Is it possible for there to be a dance without a dancer? (Here we take an example from Michael Tomasello in the summer of 2004 in Berlin, personal communication with J. W. Oller.) Similarly, how can there be a facial expression without a face or a successful act of referring without anyone to do the referring or anything to be referred to? The approaches to communication that propose to separate acts of communication from the world about which and in which we communicate are too narrow.

Referring as Part of the Grammar

Bloomfield and many of his successors excluded the process of pragmatic mapping from the study of language as being too difficult to account for. But we have shown why this is an error. We not only have to include referring terms but the objects under their scope of reference—both the agent that refers and whatever is referred to. This is essential to determine the meanings. We have to know what is referred to in words, phrases, clauses, and in acts of language use in order to begin to acquire a language in early childhood. Such knowledge is also essential to second language learning, and to the acquisition of literacy.

Bloomfield, however, excluded the meanings, purposes, intentions, decisions, and actions of communication which are produced, interpreted, and assessed by intelligent sign users. Can we suppose that a name such as *Abraham Lincoln* or a phrase such as *the American President who led the nation through the Civil War* does not reach out and capture under its scope the very individual referred to? Is it possible to understand the phrases in question and the dynamic discourse of the Civil War and all that has taken place since then without making the pragmatic connection to the person and the events that engulfed him and the nation implicitly referred to—the United States? Is it possible to understand or use those referring terms, *Lincoln*, the *Civil War*, and the *United States* in the normal way without to some extent actually signifying and conceptualizing the entities and events referred to by them?

When we talk about Abraham Lincoln we are not just stringing sounds together on a line because we speak English. In Chapter 12 when we come to the law and codes of ethics governing the treatment persons with communication disorders, we are talking about real people and actual events. Those real-world persons, events, and so forth, to the extent that our discourse is meaningful and true of what we say, must be included within the scope of grammar.

If the acts of speaking, signing, and using language in general occur in the real world and are performed by bodily persons in real time, then, there is no sensible basis for excluding from grammar the things, persons, events, sequences, and so forth that are referred

---

Bloomfield and many of his successors excluded the process of pragmatic mapping from the study of language as being too difficult to account for. But we have shown why this is an error.

When we use language meaningfully in the ordinary ways, the things, events, persons, and relations (and the intended combinations of all of them) are not incidental add-ons from some fictional "extralinguistic" realm. They are the essential elements of the linguistic discourse.

to in articulate language. It makes no sense to talk about the surface forms of articulated language without examining the intelligent volitional processes of intending, producing, interpreting, evaluating, revising, repeating, and using those surface forms to express meanings. As D. K. Oller (2000, p. 213) has observed, articulated language can be produced with the brain and limited intentions of a bird. A parrot or mynah can produce the surface forms of speech. However, to produce and comprehend the meanings underlying those forms requires a great deal more intelligence and abstract thought than a parrot evidently possesses.

Articulated language, for example, can be paraphrased, translated, interpreted, evaluated for truth value, summarized, elaborated, and so on, in ways that a parrot cannot begin to accomplish. If we asked a small child, say by about age 3, why he or she called the corn on the cob "corn," the child would say something like, "Because it is corn!" or "That's what it is!" but there is no evidence that the parrot can associate even one referring expression with its referent, much less can the parrot comment on such a pragmatic mapping relation. Yet, such associations form the essence of child language development and the indispensable foundation for abstract predications. Articulation without such meaningful intentionality and abstraction cannot reasonably be described as language use at all. So it follows that articulation involves the whole scope of grammar and whatever we may refer to in the world of experience.

WHY MEANING IS CRUCIAL TO ARTICULATION

In addition to the articulation of the surface forms of linguistic and even of iconic and indexical signs, there is the question of their meaning. With respect to meaning, as we will see, it is amazingly easy to overrate the importance of surface forms (the cover) and to under-estimate the role of meaning (as contained within the covers in the articulated discourse).

As we already saw in Chapter 4, meaning seriously outranks surface form in every aspect of linguistic processing. Attention to surface form without meaning can lead to the sort of imitation that a parrot is capable of producing, but unless the surface forms are articulated with respect to their meaning—that is, with comprehension of meaning—they are hardly different from meaningless strings of nonsense. To the extent that such performances by any parrot or other species are distinctively associated with different contexts of experience, they can be said to be meaningful, but to the extent that those surface forms are stripped of meaning—they cannot be said to provide a sufficient basis for language acquisition. No one can acquire a language by merely being exposed to its surface forms any more than a parrot or mynah bird can hope to understand and negotiate international treaties.

As the common proverb says, *"You cannot judge a book only by its cover"*—though every author/editor has met up with a few paid reviewers who seem to attempt it.

Articulation Involves More Than Surface Forms

When it comes to education, language acquisition, and to therapeutic interventions in communication disorders, the role of meaning can hardly be over-emphasized (see Badon, 1993; Badon, J. W. Oller & S. D. Oller, 2005; Hagoort & van Berkum, 2007; Nieuwland & Van Berkum, 2006; S. D. Oller, 2005, in press; Ozyurek, Willems, Kita, & Hagoort, 2007). With that in mind, it is obvious that changes in surface form can have only minimal impact on communication disorders that involve deeper levels of linguistic processing. Also, as we will see, the surface forms of speech, manual signing, writing, and all forms of intentional thought and reasoning are fundamentally dependent on the normal development of the language capacity. If that development is disrupted for any reason, depending on the severity and type of the disruption, deep language and learning disorders are the expected outcome.

It is interesting that speech-language pathologists often say that they feel most competent in dealing with articulation problems. They will often say something like, "I think I know how to treat articulation problems, but when it comes to the deeper issues of *language* I am much less confident." If we probe, we discover that the perceived difficulty in treating "language problems" encompasses the full range of the deeper pervasive developmental disorders including the whole autism spectrum and extending out to ADD/ADHD, Down syndrome, Alzheimer's, and so forth. It is no wonder that articulation problems are perceived as relatively more tractable.

Processes of articulation—that is, of differentiating the surface forms of signs—are like striking the right keys on the keyboard. We can notice articulation problems through our senses just as we can notice missteps, wrong key strokes, or errors we make ourselves when speaking, writing, or carrying out other intentional actions. They are at the surface and as a result, errors in articulation are more evident than problems at deeper levels of processing. However, it is important to see that articulation is involved in every motoric aspect of sign systems in general. Articulation is critical to the production and differentiation of all signs and it also is involved in their perception and in figuring out who or what is being referred to (Gallese, 2007; Hindmarsh & Heath, 2000; Nieuwland, Otten, & van Berkum, 2007; Nieuwland, Petersson, & van Berkum 2007; J. W. Oller, 2005). As we have already seen in Chapter 4, articulation is involved in every aspect of sign production. For instance, if we hit the keys on any computer keyboard in a random order, the result will be unintelligible. To get a particular sequence of letters, symbols, and operations from the computer—or to get a certain sequence of notes, chords, and harmonic results from a piano—the keys need to be struck in the right order. This is a matter of articulation.

Likewise, to figure out correctly who or what is referred to or pointed out in a complex predication, for example, *I'll meet you at the CC's near the Southside Bakery*, requires both articulation of the referring terms and their articulate linking with the intended referents. One of our interlocutors almost missed an appointment entirely by going to the Pizza Parlor that has the same name as the intended coffee shop. The articulation of the surface forms was nearly perfectly understood, but the connection to the intended referent was not. In understanding ordinary discourse, meaningful intentions count for more than surface forms. In fact, to the extent that communication is the goal of an interaction, the whole purpose of making distinctions in surface forms is to enable access to intended meanings. This is not to deny that people sometimes may deviate from the admirable purpose of making their meanings clear. Sometimes people avoid a painful subject by being obscure or by even lying about it, but even in inventing fictions, committing errors, or telling outright lies, human beings are still dependent in the final analysis on access to intelligible meanings. What is more, it has been demonstrated that all meaningful representations, at their basis, are completely dependent on ordinary true reports about the real world.

The Real World Is Special

There are various theories of language that take the material world seriously. There are **situation-based** models (Barwise & Perry, 1983; S. Kuhn & Cruse, 2007; Nieuwland, Otten, & van Berkum, 2007) and ones based on what is called **embodiment** (Gallese, 2007; Gibbs, 2003; Glenberg, 1997; Hindmarsh & Heath, 2000; Ignatow, 2007; M. Johnson, 1992; Lakoff & M. Johnson, 1983). In both situation-based and embodied approaches to language use the emphasis is on the contexts in which discourse typically takes place and the role of actual or imagined physical things, persons, and so forth, within those contexts.

It is possible, however, as Pylyshyn (2001) has argued, to make the mistake of giving the material world a rank that is higher than the level of abstract concepts. But such concepts cannot be produced without the intervention of intelligence (J. W. Oller, 2002) and that approach, as noted by Mahon and Caramazza (2008) is inconsistent with sound theory and is not necessary to account for the empirical data from discourse processing. The material world cannot outrank abstract concepts. This has been proved by the standards of Peirce's mathematical logic and is implicit in proofs developed by Peirce (1897) and the logician A. Tarski (1949, 1956). All those proofs show that although the "real" world enjoys a special place in the grand scheme of things, it cannot possibly generate the abstract concepts necessary to intelligence and language. In many cases we understand discourse by reference to how things work in the world, but we cannot do so without appeal to the sort of abstract transitive relations—for example, if A has a certain relation to B and B to C, then A must also have that relation to C—that utterly depend on

The fact that we language users have physical bodies and are perceivers of things and events does enable us to determine a lot about how things will work in the material world, but in the final analysis abstract concepts of language depend on the innate language capacity and cannot logically be constructed by accidental clashes of material objects.

prior existence of the innate human language capacity. However, embodiment theories are correct in asserting that there is no such thing as language acquisition, comprehension, or use in some merely possible world. All imagining about other universes either takes place in this real universe or—so far as empirical science knows—it does not take place at all.

The problems we deal with here are special because they are associated with real people in the real world and because all of us—as long as we live—are really at risk with respect to injuries, diseases, and disorders. The risks are real as are the institutions, clinics, schools, and the people in them. Governments, laws, codes of ethics, and moral obligations are important because the people are real and at risk. Bloomfield may have recommended the study of nonsense disconnected from our knowledge of real things, events, relations, meanings, contexts—disconnected from our valid knowledge and rational inferences about such things in the real world—but in the end, that plan leads to an impoverished theory of language.

Possible Worlds and Parallel Universes

There is a world of difference between the universe we actually live in and the merely **possible worlds** or **parallel universes** that science fiction writers and some philosophers are (or pretend to be deeply) concerned about. A valid theory of language must distinguish the real world from merely "possible" worlds.

Fauconnier (1985) and Bruner (1986) have come near the view that possible worlds are indistinguishable from the common one that all of us share for a time. Chomsky (1957, 1965, 1995) and some of his collaborators have pushed the idea somewhat harder. However, it is a remarkable pretense (a sophistry) to claim that some fictional world has the same status as the real world in which the inventor of the fiction actually lives.

We reject all such theories because they cannot possibly explain why it is that children are dependent on the real world to acquire language. Such theories cannot make the required distinctions between fictions, errors, lies, nonsense, and ordinary true reports. Also, empirical research shows that typically developing children begin to understand referring expressions that are true in the ordinary sense as early as six months. By the age of two to three years a typically developing child can distinguish a true representation of a game or tea party from pretending—a fictional representation. By the time the child gains another year or two of experience it will be possible to express the difference between imagining a fiction and an error resulting in a false belief. Within about one to three years later—roughly between years six and eight—a typically developing child will be able to express the difference between a false belief based on an error and a deliberately false report that is intended to deceive (see our review of the relevant literature in J. W. Oller, S. D. Oller, & Badon, 2006).

Without true references to the common world through ordinary truthful and conventional uses of words, language acquisition cannot occur. This has been proved in strict logicomathematical fashion (J. W. Oller, 2005 and it was suggested and/or proved by other logicians including Frege, 1879/1967; Peirce, 1897; and Tarski,

1949, 1956). In order for language acquisition to occur, some words must be truly mapped onto actual referents in real contexts of ordinary experience. Short of valid mappings of that kind, no language acquisition can occur. With reference to our discussion of articulation, it follows that valid linguistic mappings also require overtly articulated surface forms.

Bodily Action in the Real World

In understanding how the articulatory process of pragmatic mapping works in the production/interpretation of ordinary discourse, we also understand and explain the process of language acquisition. The articulate process of constructing comprehensible discourse is the very essence of language acquisition and use.

Stetson's argument (1945, 1951) that articulation plays a central role in language was correct. The same idea was independently stated by Vygotsky (1934/1978) who wrote about the "alloy of speech and action" which "has a very specific function in the history of the child's development; it also demonstrates the logic of its own genesis" (p. 30). Or as C. S. Peirce (1865/1982) put it in describing his own logicomathematical method of reasoning, the "logic itself" is its own "deduction and proof" (in Fisch et al., 1982, p. 340). The process of articulation is part and parcel of language use and acquisition.

Pragmatic mapping is utterly dependent, from start to finish, on real actions linking surface forms of language with bounded objects, bodily persons, events, relations, and so forth, in the course of ordinary experience.

DISORDERS OF ARTICULATION AND THEIR TREATMENT

In view of all the foregoing, it is not surprising that disorders of articulation actually range across all of the disorders that commonly affect the motor production of speech and language. Because they are manifested in the surface forms of speech and language, they are among the disorders most apt to be noticed by parents, teachers, and others, and they are the communication disorders most apt to be treated by speech language pathologists in schools or clinical contexts. In this section we review some of the common causes and treatments of articulation disorders beginning with the body and moving upward through the senses, motoric systems, and linguistic ones.

Physical Anomalies

The physical anomalies most notable in speech production are those affecting the articulators as we saw in Chapter 2. Most of those problems can be attributed either to genetics or to physical injuries that interfere with the articulation of the surface forms of speech. For example, as we saw there, a speaker with an unrepaired cleft palate may produce speech that is hypernasal. Also, an unrepaired cleft lip will result in difficulty in forming segments that require bilabial closure. In addition to these problems, many other disorders with a genetic basis affect the bones and other organ systems and impact articulation.

In many cases, genetic abnormalities impact multiple systems as is the case with **Smith-Magenis syndrome** (Bergmann, Morlot, & Ptok, 2007) which results in abnormal "facial appearance, infant feeding problems, low muscle tone, developmental delay, variable levels of mental retardation, early speech/language delay, middle ear problems, skeletal anomalies and decreased sensitivity to pain" ("Smith-Magenis Syndrome," n.d., retrieved March 3, 2009, from http://www.smithmagenis.org/WhatisSMS/overview_ssynd.htm). This disorder is supposedly caused in part at least by a single nucleotide polymorphism (SNP) at chromosome 17p11.2. The impacted systems not only affect articulation but go far beyond that. For reasons given from Chapter 1 forward, it is likely that other disorders and genetic SNPs may also commonly be associated with this syndrome. For all of those reasons, common articulatory problems may be indicative of more serious issues that may need attention, for example, in severe autism spectrum disorders. There are excellent reasons to suppose that many of the currently known communication disorders have multiple common causal mechanisms that interact in complex ways with genetic SNPs.

Sensory Loss

Even a mild loss of hearing can result, according to the research, in substantial losses in the clarity in speech (J. A. Jones & Munhall, 2000; Tremblay, Shiller, & Ostry, 2003).

At a level just above the bones, teeth, and organ structures that are deployed in the production of speech, there are disorders of articulation that are largely attributable to the inability to perceive the distinctions that are needed in the articulation of speech. It is commonly believed that the reduction in hearing acuity that can be caused by **otitis media**—middle ear infections and inflammation—can reduce hearing acuity so much that it affects the articulation of certain sounds (Lindsay, Tomazic, Whitman, & Accardo, 1999; Majerus et al., 2005). In fact, it is well known that hearing loss, depending on its severity, tends to increase the difficulty of acquiring the articulatory distinctions of speech (Nickisch et al., 2007).

Motor Difficulties

We discuss motor difficulties of a variety of kinds in greater detail in Chapters 6 and 8 along with their specific symptoms. In some instances, the level of damage in the nervous system can be determined by the nature of the symptoms. Depending on the nature and extent of the damage, or the generalized disease condition, speech and language may be affected. In the motor disorders that involve loss of muscle tone—in particular the condition known as **floppy child syndrome**—a generalized hypotonia affecting much or all of the child's body—the main difficulty may be limited to the muscles rather than in the central nervous system. On the other hand, certain kinds of hypotonia as seen in infantile autism, for example, see the video of Ethan Kurtz (at 46 seconds into the video) prior to his remarkable recovery, may accompany a generalized reduction in higher mental abilities.

At the stage of Ethan's disease condition where he is shown with his physical therapist in the video, Ethan's skeletal muscles are completely flaccid. While in that condition he showed no signs of being able to produce or comprehend articulate speech. However, his recovery after treatment with antifungal medication showed that his condition, which had lasted for approximately two years, had not prevented him from substantial language comprehension and acquisition. Contrary to the outward appearances of his condition, his recovery shows that his limitations were mainly motoric and that a lot of cognitive activity was still going on during what appeared to be periods of little or no cognitive progress.

Evan McCarthy, as reported by his mother (see McCarthy, November 10, 2007, at approximately 4:38 into the interview, retrieved March 3, 2009, from http://www.youtube.com/watch?v =zLJ9ez3pJIg&feature=related) gives an example of a time when she was devastated that Evan could no longer play the game of saying the sounds made by particular animals: for instance, on one occasion after he began to recover from his descent into severe autism, she asked him what sound a cow made. He was unable to respond, but about 45 minutes later showed up tugging on her dress to say, "Moo." She saw it as an important turning point in his recovery. Later, he brought up his memory of the period during which he could not talk. The two were having lunch when Evan said: "Mom, do you remember when I used to be shy?" She said she did and commented that he didn't really talk during that time. He said, "I know. I couldn't get the words out. I couldn't get my words out." She asked why and he said he didn't know, he just couldn't get them out.

Linguistic Difficulties Impacting Articulation

As we will see in Chapter 10, there can be problems owed to damage to the central nervous system resulting in motor apraxias of speech such as what is termed **Broca's aphasia** where damage especially to the left frontal lobe in the dominant hemisphere of the brain is apt to produce problems affecting articulation more or less directly. A problem affecting articulation at a still deeper level would be an agnosia preventing the naming of objects or persons

Some of the neurological systems that enable the production of fluent speech are also critically involved in the motor production of both signing and writing.

and, possibly, also preventing the comprehension of the corresponding nonverbal concepts—the iconic and indexical signs normally linked with the verbal (linguistic) symbols. These problems are evidently just as apt to affect the production of manual signed language as speech. It is to be expected that motor problems in the most central areas should also tend to impact writing along with speech (and/or manual signing) and evidently, as we will see in Chapters 8, 9, and especially in Chapter 10, this is usually the case—more than one modality is apt to be impacted. All these productive (motor) linguistic functions appear to be handled exclusively by the dominant (usually left) hemisphere of the brain as we will spell out in detail with a review of relevant research in Chapter 10.

THERAPEUTIC INTERVENTIONS

As we noted at the outset of this chapter, articulation problems are the ones that speech-language pathologists feel most comfortable in treating. However, because of the vast range of causes of articulatory problems, effective therapies likewise cover the full range from surgical interventions to correct cleft palate, for instance, to dietary regimens to correct metabolic imbalances, to the more common work known to speech-language pathologists who learn to demonstrate, measure, and help individuals produce articulatory movements.

Repetitive Modeling

On one Web site, the therapist recommends estimating the number of repetitions necessary to establish a new articulation and then setting aside as many tokens to reward the attempts as will, theoretically, be required to establish the new behavior. Such an approach supposes, wrongly we believe, that mere repetition is sufficient to produce an articulatory change.

The most common method is to model the articulatory movement and then encourage the individual undergoing therapy to attempt to repeat the modeled word or form. It is generally supposed that repetitive modeling and elicited imitations of the model by the client/student are required to instill new phonological habits. It is often supposed that repetition will cause the generalization of the desired articulatory movement or contrast to new contexts of experience and language use. Commonly clinicians use some kind of reward system, for example, cookie crumbs, M&Ms, tokens, or stickers that the individual undergoing treatment will work to obtain.

Usually, the attention of both the clinician and the person undergoing therapy are concentrating almost exclusively the surface contrast at issue. It is common to see a scenario like the following: the clinician says something like, "Now watch my tongue Sally and see if you can repeat what I am saying. Say, *train*, Sally, can you say *train*. See where I put my tongue when I say, *train*?" Then, perhaps, Sally will try to say *train* producing something like *tain* or *fain*. Will a hundred repetitions of this drill result in the desired change?

Generalization to New Contexts: Problematic

Interestingly, even if it is possible to get a child (or any client/patient) to produce an articulatory distinction in a clinical context, it may not generalize to contexts outside the clinic. For instance, after getting a child to say *ya, ya, ya yellow* instead of *lellow*, the next occurrence of the word in the natural discourse of the child is apt to be *lellow* still. As commonly noted by language teachers in many different contexts, practice in the artificial context of classroom and clinic often fails to transfer to the contexts in the larger world beyond.

Why is this? The answer has to do with the essential role of meaning in articulation.

The Language Acquisition Analogy

The problem presented often confronted in the clinical context is like the one facing a foreign language learner who is asked to notice the difference between say, [pan] and [pʰan] when the learner has no need for that distinction in his or her native language and is actually, for the present, unable to detect the difference in the spoken forms. How can the difficulty be remedied? Experience shows that many repetitions of the same task will often fail exactly as many times as they are attempted. They may never work.

If we want the currently inaccessible (unnoticeable) articulatory contrast to generalize to the myriad of contexts in the world outside the classroom/clinic, it is essential to take the intentions, purposes, and meanings of ordinary experience seriously. If the learner/client can be brought to a situation in which it is necessary to make the articulatory distinction that he or she is not yet making in order to achieve a desired communication purpose, it may become possible with the meaningful motivation to attend more closely, detect the distinction, and then even produce and generalize it. Here is an example based on an actual incident documented in the child language acquisition literature (e.g., by J. W. Oller, Badon, & S. D. Oller, 2006).

Harnessing the Pragmatic Motivation: Meaning Matters

At age three, a certain child known as Stevie accompanied his mom and dad to the Winrock mall in Albuquerque, New Mexico. The purpose was to buy Dad an overcoat for a trip to Madison, Wisconsin. So, Dad had coats on the brain, so to speak. On the way, they stopped at the sign of the golden arches for a delicious and quick meal. After two hours at the mall with a new overcoat in hand that cost Dad too much and was about one size too small, though it was the last one on the rack, they went back to the car. Dad lifted the three-year-old into the back seat. It was a blustery evening and Dad

It is common for clinician/teachers to try to instill articulatory distinctions through the use of minimal pairs dropped out of the blue— "Can you say *try* and *fie*, Sally? How about, *true* and *foo*, *tray* and *fay*, . . ." But suppose the child/individual undergoing treatment either cannot hear these distinctions, or commonly does not bother with them. How will the distinctions between the various surface forms be acquired and internalized? What is missing from such minimal pair drills? If we think about it, it is obvious that the meaningful motivation to make the distinctions in question is entirely lacking from the point of view of the person undergoing therapy. If the person does not or cannot make the distinctions in question, how will they be noticed and remembered based on surface forms alone?

made sure that the little red jacket was zipped and the little boy was buckled securely in his car seat in the back. As the family started down the road, Stevie announced, "I want my [kʰoʔ]." Dad replied, "You have your coat on, Son." The little boy said, "No, Daggy. I want my [kʰoʔ]." This exchange was repeated with increasing volume. Meanwhile, Mom reached over between the seats and handed the little boy his *coke*, which was beyond his reach between the bucket seats in the front of the car.

Dad now saw an opportunity for a redeeming linguistics lesson, alias speech therapy, to enrich the three year old's phonology. He said, "You mean you want your [kʰokʰ]" which he enunciated with a clearly aspirated [kʰ] both at the beginning and end of the word. Stevie repeated perfectly and with enthusiasm, "Yeah, Daggy, [kʰokʰ]!" Stevie called his Dad, "Daggy" on analogy with *doggie* which was one of his early words. His very first word had been "Chester," the name of the little dog that Stevie loved to torment.

Generalizing from Meaning Succeeds

The trip to Wisconsin came and went. A few days after returning to Albuquerque, one of Dad's doctoral students, now known as Dr. Jack S. Damico (the Doris B. Hawthorne Eminent Scholar and Chair at UL Lafayette), was visiting and Stevie was eating his crackers and peanut butter in the kitchen nook while Jack and his mentor, Stevie's Dad, were talking in the kitchen. Dad was telling about what would become known in the literature ever after as the *coke-coat incident*. When he reached the punch line, Stevie piped up from the other room and supplied it, "Yeah, Daggy. I want my [kʰokʰ]." It showed that the whole affair had made a lasting memory.

A few days later, on the way to the kitchen in the early morning Dad was greeted by Stevie with an observation. He said to his dad, "I call you Daggy, huh" to which Dad replied, "Yep. That's what you call me." Stevie continued, "But that's not your real name, huh!" Now, Dad was interested. There had been a conversation about names with reference to mom. Dad had explained how her name was *Mary Anne* but to Stevie she was *Mom*, "not *Mary Anne* because your mom is special to you. So that's why you call her *Mom* not *Mary Anne*." Dad expected Stevie to say, "Your real name is *John*." So, Dad asked, "What's my real name?" Stevie said, "Your real name is Daddy."

He had sorted out the articulatory distinction between [tʰ] and [kʰ] and also between [d] and [g]. We could say that the feature distinguishing the alveolar place of articulation from the velar had generalized to, it would seem, the whole phonological system. That is, three-year-old Stevie had not only solved the distinction between [kʰot] and [kʰok] but also between *daddy* and *daggy*, and all the other forms in the lexicon requiring an alveolar versus velar contrast. All of this brings us to the key question, why? Why did the generalization occur when it did and what precipitated the change?

The Pragmatic Motivation

It appears that the pragmatic motivation for the distinction between [kʰot] and [kʰok] was the fact that Stevie could not reach the *coke* from the place where he was buckled into his seat in the back. The pragmatic need for the distinction was promoted by the ambiguity that arose when his production of [kʰoʔ] failed to enable him to achieve his desired objective. He did not at first get the *coke* handed to him on the basis of that surface form. As a result, he was encouraged to enrich the surface form by adding the alveolar/velar contrast to the final segment. It is possible, even probable that the distinction would have eventually been added to his repertoire without the events that we are reporting here, but it seems likely that what caused the advance when it actually occurred, was probably the demand of a particular communication context which provided the occasion for a distinction in Stevie's phonotactic system that had not been needed much up to that point.

Meaning Matters
The upshot of the story is that meaning really does matter (as noted by J. S. Damico & S. K. Damico, 1993; S. D. Oller, 2005; Richard-Amato, 2003). It is the basis for the connection between the articulation of surface forms and the underlying purposes of communication. Meaning is the underlying pragmatic motivation for the differentiation of articulated surface forms and it is the basis for the deep relation between the phonetics of speech and the underlying phonological system of any particular language.

As in prior chapters, we found evidence with respect to articulation that language involves a complex layered mapping from intentions to surface forms.

SUMMING UP AND LOOKING AHEAD

In this chapter we considered why the surface forms of language, especially the conventional signs of speech, writing, and manual signing *must be articulated* at the surface in terms of discrete, distinct, and replicable signs that can be noticed, perceived, and interpreted. We also saw that the articulation of signs as a process can be considered from the different vantage points of their producers, consumers, and the material world of discourse in general. These distinct vantage points provide the basis for articulatory, auditory, and acoustic phonetics respectively. As in prior chapters, we found evidence with respect to articulation that language involves a complex layered mapping from intentions to surface forms. As in Chapters 3, 4, 5, and 6, we found additional evidence of disorders of different kinds and at different levels owed to peripheral versus central neurologic problems. As we will see in greater detail in Chapter 10, we have already noted here that the dysarthrias of speech, for instance, are notably different from articulation problems associated with aphasias.

Again, we found evidence that approaches to therapy which harness pragmatic motivations are more apt to succeed than procedures that focus attention exclusively on surface forms without meaning. In Chapter 9, we will find even more powerful evidence to show that deciphering the unfamiliar surface forms of printed symbols—as in learning to read and write printed words—is fundamentally dependent on access to meanings.

For all of these reasons, we also conclude that therapeutic interventions for articulation difficulties will work best when they enable the client/student to make use of the pragmatic connections of surface forms with meaning in whatever ways are possible. We know from prior research that meaning is crucial to discourse processing viewed from many different angles.

In articulation therapy, meaning matters. As we have seen in this chapter, the most important meanings are those associated with the well-being, feelings, and intentions of real human beings. It is because of our language capacity and all that it entails, including freedom of the will and moral responsibility, that it is important to treat human beings as persons—never as mere objects of study. In the following chapter, we consider another diverse class of movement disorders—ones that are associated with the production of "fluent" speech. In particular we focus on stuttering phenomena.

STUDY AND DISCUSSION QUESTIONS

1. Why is the differentiation of the dynamic surface forms of speech and manual signing dependent on movement?
2. What aspect(s) of the speech signal, in particular, cannot be represented at all in writing? Why is it impossible to represent these elements fully in writing?
3. Why does the articulation of speech necessarily involve all three positions of discourse and how do those positions relate to the three branches of phonetics?
4. What are the major classes of segmental sounds and how are they differentiated? What is peculiar about liquids and glides?
5. Why do analyses of conversation require multiple levels of transcription? Why do they typically incorporate moving pictures and sound recordings along with transcriptions?
6. What happens when you speed up the production of a sequence of syllables such as *op, op, op*? And if you slow it down gradually? Which syllable sequence can be produced at the faster rate *pa, pa, pa* or *op, op, op*? Why is this so?

7. What are some of the natural changes that occur when similar (and/or dissimilar) sound segments come into proximity with each other in the stream of speech?

8. What are the main differences between alphabetic, syllabic, logographic, and ideographic writing systems?

9. Why is it impossible to parse the ribbon of fluent speech without access to meanings?

10. If pragmatic mapping is included within the scope of grammar how can the expanded perspective enable improved speech therapy?

8

Fluency Disorders

OBJECTIVES

In this chapter, we:

1. Study the impact stuttering has had in the lives of individuals;

2. Discuss reasons to evaluate and treat the person rather than the stuttering;

3. Discuss assessment approaches and their relative strengths and weaknesses;

4. Explore the success of the **Lidcombe Program** for treating young children;

5. Discuss two treatment strategies for adolescent and adult persons who stutter; and

6. Describe three other fluency disorders and how they are different from stuttering.

KEY TERMS

Here are some key terms of this chapter. Many of them you may already know. It may help to review them. These terms are explained in the text and they are defined in the Glossary at the end of the book. They appear in **bold print** on their first appearance in the text.

absolute pitch	dys-	PET
acquired neurogenic	dysfluencies	phonemes
stuttering	electromyography	phonemic level of stuttering
acquired psychogenic	facilitating context	planum temporale (PT)
stuttering	fluency shaping	positron emission
asymmetry	function words	tomography
cancellation	heritability	precipitating factors
cluttering	hesitation phenomena	preparatory set
content words	incipient stuttering	processing malfunction
covert repair hypothesis	inter-rater reliability	models
cybernetics	intra-rater reliability	psychogenic stuttering
DAF	language disorder theory	pull-out
degree of freedom	Lidcombe Program	secondaries
delayed auditory feedback	masking noise	secondary behaviors
delayed side-tone	modular	speech-language pathology
demands and capacities	modules	stuttering block
model	monitor	stuttering events
developmental stuttering	monitoring functions	stuttering modification
discourse processing	monotone	stuttering severity index
disfluencies	monozygotes	Stuttering Foundation
dizygotes	monozygotic twins	syllabic level of stuttering
dizygotic twins	neurogenic stuttering	tachyphemia
dopamine	persistent developmental	twin studies
dual-tasks	stuttering	Wernicke's area

Imagine you knew exactly what you wanted to say, but whatever you tried, the words just stuck in your throat and mouth, or on your tongue. This is more or less the state of affairs for persons who stutter.

At one point or another, we have all "tripped" over our words, allowed our tongues to outrun our brains, or "drawn a blank." With stuttering, the problem is not in figuring out what you are going to say, but how to get the words that you have chosen out of your mouth. Marty Jezer says that he knows what he wants to say, but just cannot get the words out. In his book *Stuttering: A Life Bound Up in Words*, Jezer recalls how stuttering affected, not just his speech, but his entire life. He would often ride the subway home, but because he stuttered on the phrase "White Plains," the name of his stop, he would buy a ticket for the adjacent, "Hartsdale," several miles away. Then, he would walk home (Jezer, 1997, p. 10).

All this just to avoid stuttering. Other persons who stutter have reported ordering meals they do not like, giving false names, or not even speaking at all, just to avoid problem words or sounds that were difficult for them to say without stuttering. Why would they go to so much trouble? Kalinowski and Saltuklaroglu (2006; also see Stuart, Frazier, Kalinowski, & Vos, 2008) write that most persons who stutter have a deep-seated desire to hide the stuttering. Many people will go to great lengths to avoid stuttering or to do anything that would reveal the fact that they are prone to do so. Anxiety about stuttering avoidance can dominate a person's self image so much that they live in constant anticipation of failing to communicate (DiLollo, Manning, & Neimeyer, 2003).

Anxiety about stuttering avoidance can dominate a person's self image so much that they live in constant anticipation of failing to communicate (DiLollo, Manning, & Neimeyer, 2003).

THE MYSTERY OF STUTTERING

What criteria define a person who stutters as contrasted with someone who does not stutter? On the home page for the **Stuttering Foundation** (2009, retrieved March 5, 2009, from http://www.stutteringhelp.org/) the following persons (among many others) are described as persons who stutter.

Famous Persons Who Stutter

You may have heard of James Earl Jones. He was the voice of Darth Vader in *Star Wars*. At that page you will also find Winston Churchill, perhaps the most famous of all the British Prime Ministers, and one of the great figures of world history on account of his role in leading Britain during World War II. You will also find, John Stossel there—an investigative reporter for the news program *20/20*, and Carly Simon the singer, writer, and composer who won a 1989 Grammy for composing and singing "Let the River Run" which formed the major part of the sound track for the movie, *Working Girl*, starring Melanie Griffith and Harrison Ford (see and hear Carly Simon performing the song, retrieved March 25, 2009, from http://video.yahoo.com/watch/2033746/.V2164490).

Who Is "Bound Up in Words" and How Are They Released?

When was the last time you heard James Earl Jones "trip" over his words? When have you heard John Stossel repeating himself? Probably never. On the other hand, have you ever heard David Letterman trip over his words or repeat himself? Yet, David Letterman is not considered a stutterer. Why is this? What is it about the way a person talks that makes us think, "Oh she stutters," or "Bruce Willis is not a stutterer!"—but in fact he is. Willis said in a 2002 *Reader's Digest* interview (see "Bruce Willis," retrieved March 5, 2009, from http://www.rd.com/images/content/021102/bruce_willis_interview.pdf) that he discovered more or less by accident in a high school play that he didn't stutter on stage:

Bruce Willis on Stuttering

I had a horrible stutter . . . from the time I was 9 until . . . I was about 17. And a miraculous thing happened when I was in high school. I was doing this goofy play. It wasn't a goofy play, we just did it in a goofy way. *Connecticut Yankee in King Arthur's Court.* And when I got onstage, I stopped stuttering. When I stepped off the stage, I started stuttering again. And I went, "This is a miracle. I got to investigate this more."

What Counts as Stuttering?

Marty Jezer mentions several times in his book that he does not stutter when he does not speak. Einarsdóttir and Ingham (2005) have argued as Supreme Court Justice Potter Stewart might put it (see Silver, 2003, retrieved March 5, 2009, from http://library.findlaw.com/2003/May/15/132747.html) that stuttering, like certain other undesirable phenomena, is easy to recognize when you come across it and yet it is difficult to define precisely. Current research with toddlers of only 22 months shows that they can readily distinguish fluent from disfluent speech (Soderstrom & J. L. Morgan, 2007). It remains to say just how they are able to make these distinctions. It is even more difficult to say who will be a stutterer and on what occasions it will occur. One of our goals in this chapter is to consider the key symptoms of stuttering as they have been defined in the literature as well as how **stuttering events** have been singled out for attention, distinguished from fluent speech, and how they have been measured in the past. What is to count as a stutter? Does "ya-ya-ya-you" count as one event or four? Or are there only three stutters here?

Stuttering is a communication disorder and it can be debilitating. Having said that, it is nonetheless true that persons who stutter can benefit from the sort of good humor demonstrated by Marty Jezer in his book about stuttering. Another well-known expert on the subject, Walter Manning (2001) argues that humor about one's stuttering is a necessary component for effective therapy. No doubt many would say that coping with disorders in general can benefit from keeping a sense of humor.

Manning (2001), however, takes stuttering seriously and contends that treating the emotional and social disabilities that tend

Although there are jokes about stuttering—and though cartoon characters such as Porky Pig have been more or less defined by it (see "Porky Pig," 2009, retrieved March 5, 2009, from http://en.wikipedia.org/wiki/Porky_Pig)—the disorder itself is not funny.

to accompany it must be part of any treatment protocol for stuttering itself.

> . . . the disabilities associated with stuttering are like comments on a narrative, they are about the story, but they are not in the story line itself.

Emotional and Social Aspects

In the film, *Transcending Stuttering: The Inside Story* (2004), Taro Alexander describes his reaction to stuttering during a performance: "Oh my God, my career is over." In the same film, another young man, Steven Miller, considered quitting his high school football team when he had trouble calling the plays. However, after his team elected him captain he decided to keep playing. Dr. Phillip Schneider, the author, producer, and director of the film, describes stuttering like this: "The pain of stuttering is not in speech interruptions. That just takes a moment . . . What's painful is feeling different" (Schneider, 2004, "Transcending Stuttering," retrieved March 5, 2009, from http://www.onlineceus.com/continuingeducation/fluency/stut teringvideo.html).

How and why is it that the disabilities associated with stuttering are different from the stuttering itself? In what follows we will see that some of the disabilities associated with stuttering are like comments on a narrative, they are about the story, but they are not in the story line itself. Let's consider why and how this is so.

THE WORLD HEALTH ORGANIZATION CLASSIFICATION CRITERIA

The World Health Organization proposed a scheme for "The International Classification of Impairments, Disabilities, and Handicaps" back in 1980. This classification scheme was originally meant to bring a standardized terminology to diverse fields so that diagnosis, treatment, measurement of progress, and so on could be judged quickly and accurately. As the title implies, there are three classification criteria to be considered:

1. The *impairment*(s) is (are) the primary "abnormal" symptom(s).
2. The *disability* (or disabilities) associated with the impairment(s). A disability is a restriction or inability to do something in what could be called "the normal" way.
3. The *handicap* is a disadvantage that results either from an impairment or disability that keeps the person affected from fulfilling roles normal for that person's age, sex, background, and so forth.

Normalcy

Disorders are invariably defined in the final analysis as deviations from some norm.

Once again we are drawn back to the idea of normalcy. The norm may not be well-defined. It may just be a vague idea in the collective understanding of a community. Why does Justice Potter think he knows what obscenity is when he sees it in spite of the fact that he cannot give a hard and fast rule that every law enforcement officer and judge in the country could follow?

In fact, it is the deviation from what is expected in one way or another that seems to be the only (at least tenuously) agreed on aspect of stuttering. Stuttering is a kind of breakdown in fluency that falls outside the normal problems that everyone sometimes encounters. Almost all other aspects and descriptors that have been proposed to describe stuttering, however, are NOT agreed on. Again, we come back what Justice Potter might say: "Neither we ourselves nor any person who stutters can say exactly what stuttering is, but we recognize it as a disorder, and we are commonly able to recognize stuttering events when they occur."

Applying the WHO Criteria

In an attempt to standardize terminology regarding stuttering Yaruss (1998) applied the WHO classification scheme and provided the following descriptions for each criterion:

1. Impairment: Disruption of speech-language production typically characterized by certain interruptions in the forward flow of speech (e.g., unusually long or physically tense hesitations; repetitions of sounds, syllables, or words; or prolongations of sounds or articulatory postures beyond their usual duration), and including any associated audible or visible characteristics of those interruptions, if present (e.g., physical tension, nonspeech behaviors, and struggle in the speech musculature or periphery). The impairment itself is the aspect of stuttering that is noticeable from all discourse positions—but especially to observers in discourse position 3 (see Figure 6–1).
2. Disability: Limitations in an individual's ability to communicate with others or to engage in social or work-related activities, resulting directly from the individual's stuttering impairment, or from the individual's affective, behavioral, or cognitive reactions to the stuttering impairment. Disability is a function of how the individual who stutters may be constrained by the stuttering. The disability falls mainly to discourse position 1 (again see Figure 6–1).
3. Handicap: Disadvantages experienced by an individual, resulting from the stuttering impairment and associated disabilities, or from reactions to them (exhibited either by the individual or by those with whom the individual interacts), that *limit* the individual's ability to fulfill social, occupational, or economic

roles that would otherwise be considered normal and attainable for that individual (Yaruss, 1998, p 253). A fluency handicap arises largely on the basis of the actual reactions that may be perceived or only anticipated by the stutterer which have the effect of preventing certain interactions or cutting them short. Such a handicap is largely a constraint attributed by the person who stutters to his or her interlocutors in discourse position 2 (see Figure 6–1).

Yaruss describes the impairment as consisting of the noticeable symptoms of the disorder while disabilities result from reactions to the symptoms which are or seem to be outside the individual's intentional conscious control.

All Positions Considered

The description Yaruss provides of the *impairment* mainly concerns the speech signal itself and physical characteristics of stuttering as it might be recorded from the vantage point of an indifferent observer, that is, this description is mainly about the context of interaction as viewed objectively from a material point of view. This is the aspect of the stuttering event or sequence of them that can be regarded by observers watching a video clip after the fact. The description provided of the *disability* is mainly concerned with the viewpoint of the producer of the stuttering. How does that person react to the stuttering and how is that person affected by it as it is developing over time. The description of the *handicap* is mainly concerned with the reaction of other interlocutors, the logical position of the consumer. If the consumer is unwilling to listen to the stuttering for a sufficiently long time to enable the person who stutters to get the intended meaning across, the result of the stuttering can become a handicap. The degree of the handicap depends greatly on the reaction of other interlocutors to the stutterer and to the stuttering events.

Because stuttering affects all three of these positions of discourse, therapy for stuttering must deal with the whole communication process. The disorder cannot be treated effectively without taking context into consideration. Isolated events of stuttering are not apt to be informative. As we will see, treatment is commonly focused on the symptoms shown by the person who stutters (e.g., Prasse & Kikano, 2008), and often also on that person's ways of dealing with those symptoms, and somewhat less commonly on adapting the environment—including the parents, teachers, friends, children, spouse, and so forth—to accommodate the person who stutters.

What Is Stuttering?

It is uncontroversial to admit that stuttering is not well understood. Although experts and laypersons alike think that they know what

Yaruss's description of stuttering takes into account all of the positions of discourse—namely, producers, consumers, and the larger community in the whole context of interaction (including any other observers besides the intended consumer that may tune in).

Even expert judges differ with each other and have difficulty achieving consistency in saying whether certain instances really are or are not instances of stuttering.

stuttering is when they observe or experience it, this is not the same as saying that they agree with each other or that they are always consistent in their own judgments of what is and what is not stuttering. The research shows that the definitions of stuttering vary and that the judgments of what is and is not stuttering differ within and across individuals. Suttering experts and even the speaker of a recorded speech event may be uncertain if it involved stuttering or not. Nevertheless, there is some common ground in ideas about what stuttering is and it is useful to consider what is agreed on.

What the Experts Agree On
1. Like most communication disorders, stuttering has a significant genetic component.
2. Stuttering involves a loss of control of the speech signal.
3. There are some settings and processes that commonly enhance (or disrupt) the fluency of persons who stutter, and that commonly cause stuttering in persons who do not normally stutter.

In the sections that follow we examine each of these factors.

THE GENETIC FACTOR

Disorders tend to run in families. However, this is not evidence enough to claim that a disorder is genetic. Consider this illustration. Where we three authors live (in Louisiana and Texas), hunting and fishing are quite popular, and we can see that the enjoyment of hunting and fishing tends to run in families. Hunting and fishing are also more common among males than females. Does this make the enjoyment of hunting and fishing a genetic inheritance? Or is it learned through social experience? Behavior is not necessarily genetic. It may also be learned. In this chapter one of the key questions to be addressed is: To what extent is stuttering genetic rather than learned? To answer this question, we need to differentiate learned behavior from behavior caused by a genetic component. How can this be done?

Assessing the Strength of the Genetic Factor

One way to approach the question of genetic causation as contrasted with learning is through the study of persons who are known to have greater or lesser amounts of genetic material in common.

A General Hypothesis About Genetics

Shared genetic material is greater in identical twins than in fraternal twins, where it is greater than in mere siblings, where it is greater than in unrelated persons. If we use the symbol ">" to mean "share more genetic material than" we can write the general hypothesis like this:

identical twins > fraternal twins > siblings > unrelated persons

So **twin studies**—especially those comparing identical twins with fraternal twins—are particularly informative. This is not only true for stuttering, of course, as we will see in the following chapter about the **heritability**, for instance, of autism (as we saw in Chapter 5) or any heritable factor desirable or not.

Working backward from unrelated persons contrasted with siblings, here is the reasoning behind the general hypothesis we have just stated. Since we get our genetic inheritance from our parents, we know in advance that siblings (brothers and sisters), all else being held equal, must have more common genetic material than unrelated persons. Fraternal twins—dizygotic twins—are merely siblings of the same age. They have no more genetic material in common than siblings of different ages. But because fraternal twins are the same age, they are expected to be more alike than siblings of different ages on account of shared experience. But identical twins —**monozygotic twins**—have the limit of common genetic material. They have a common genome so they are genetically almost completely identical. Unless they are reared separately, they tend also to have essentially the same experience because they are of the same age and gender. They also tend to share many of the same preferences on account of all of these factors.

In fact, except for those disorders that are caused by physical accidents, communication disorders in general seem to have a substantial genetic component in most instances as is also the case for stuttering. Contrasts between identical twins, fraternal twins, siblings, and unrelated individuals, enable us to study the difference in the genetic component of stuttering, for instance, as contrasted with factors such as learning. We can reasonably suppose, for instance, that the environmental factors for fraternal twins are quite similar to those for identicals, so that *any differences observed in the tendency to stutter or not to stutter between these two groups should be more or less directly attributable to genetic inheritance.* With that in mind, if stuttering is made possible to a large extent by a certain genetic makeup, it follows that *the tendency for identical twins to both be stutterers (or not), should be higher than the same tendency for fraternals.* It is difficult to completely separate genetics from environmental factors even in

The experts and even the person who is the producer of a recorded speech event may be uncertain if it involved stuttering.

identical twins, of course, because persons with common genetic factors will tend to be susceptible to common injuries by environmental toxins, for instance. Nevertheless, it is possible in comparative studies of identical twins with fraternals (and siblings), to some extent, to tease apart the impact of genetics as distinct from environmental elements.

The Australian Twin Study

An important study on the genetic factor in stuttering was conducted in Australia by Felsenfeld et al. (2000). They studied 1567 pairs of twins plus an additional 634 individuals who were a part of a twin pair, but whose twin, for whatever reason, was not available. The twins were all between the ages of 17 and 29. Using self-report questionnaires and follow-up interviews the researchers determined the incidence of stuttering in the sample which included all of the twin pairs listed in the entire Australian Twin Registry—a substantial population. The basic research hypothesis was:

> If stuttering is primarily genetic, we should see a higher concordance (where both twins stutter or neither stutters) among identical twins (**monozygotes**) than among fraternal twins (**dizygotes**).

The authors were able to account statistically for approximately 70% of the variability in the tendency to stutter (or not) by genetic inheritance. Setting aside measurement error, the remaining 30% of the variability between the two groups could be attributed to undetermined environmental factors. This conclusion agrees with and explains the fact that stuttering runs in families. Stuttering appears to have a large genetic component.

Still, there is no way as yet to predict specifically who will or will not stutter, or to explain exactly why it occurs in the cases where it does occur. That is, we do not yet know just which genetic elements are involved or what additional **precipitating factors** may be involved. That is, we do not know in general why and how stuttering begins to express itself in particular individuals. However, research currently underway (e.g., Sanford, 2005) with the human genome leads us to believe that more specific genetic components involved in stuttering will no doubt be identified in the future. Also, the demonstrated general degeneracy of the genome owed to toxins, injuries, and the cumulative impact of errors over the long term, makes it a virtual certainty that stuttering instances, along with other disorders, barring intervention with new gene therapies, will continue to increase in coming generations. What is well established in the meantime concerning stuttering is that it is largely dependent on as yet to be determined genetic factors. In addition to those factors, a somewhat lesser role is played by experience (learning) and environmental factors.

LOSS OF CONTROL OF THE SPEECH SIGNAL

Most of the definitions of stuttering that have been proposed over the past 60 years have focused on some aspect of the loss of control of the speech signal itself that seems to be an underlying commonality in stuttering. It is a standard convention to distinguish such loss of control in stuttering events by calling them **dysfluencies** while controlled, intentional interruptions of the flow of speech—normal hesitations, false starts, restarts, midstream corrections, and the like—are termed **disfluencies**. This spelling difference is in keeping with the standard terminology for disorders where "**dys-**" is the prefix commonly used to distinguish abnormalities from phenomena that they may resemble but which are not considered to be abnormal. However, because the terms "disfluency" and "dysfluency" have the same pronunciation and nearly the same spelling—differing only in the letter "i" versus "y"—we prefer to use the phrase "ordinary disfluencies" where the phenomena remain under the intentional control of the speaker whereas "dysfluencies" is limited to "abnormal disfluencies." In common usage, the term "disfluency" is the more general one and includes the pathological cases—that is, abnormal disfluencies which are special instances.

Terminology, of course, is just the surface of the problem. The deeper issue is the content, not just what we are going to call it. As we will see, the experts and even stutterers themselves—some of whom are also experts in stuttering research—still have trouble telling consistently just which instances of disfluency are of the ordinary, normal kind, and which must be counted as abnormal. As we will see in the following sections, the surface forms of normal and abnormal disfluencies resemble each other so much that it is next to impossible for observers to tell them apart consistently on the basis of forms alone. This should not surprise anyone in view of the profound dependence of linguistic surface forms in general on deeper aspects of meaning and reference—semantics, syntax, and pragmatics (as we have seen especially in Chapter 4; also in Chapters 9 and 11).

A critical element in all of the widely known definitions of stuttering is whether or not the person producing the disfluent speech remains in control of the stream of speech or is falling under the control, to some extent, of other factors. With all that in mind, to see the complexity of stuttering it will be useful to examine some of the best known and most widely used definitions.

> The deeper problem is that any run-of-the-mill ordinary disfluency—that is, any hesitation, false start, or midstream correction—may not be readily distinguishable from a pathological dysfluency.

The Standard Definition

Wingate's (1964) definition is often called the "standard definition of stuttering":

The term "stuttering" means: I. (a) disruption in the fluency of verbal expression, which is (b) characterized by involuntary, audible, or silent repetitions or prolongations in the utterance of short speech elements, namely: sounds, syllables, and words of one syllable. These disruptions (c) usually occur frequently or are marked in character and (d) are not readily controllable. II. Sometimes the disruptions are (e) accompanied by accessory activities involving the speech apparatus, related or unrelated body structures [movements or gestures], or stereotyped speech utterances. These activities give the appearance of being speech-related struggles. III. Also, there not infrequently are (f) indications or reports of the presence of an emotional state, ranging from a general condition of "excitement" or "tension" to more specific emotions of a negative nature such as "fear," "embarrassment," "irritation," or the like. (g) The immediate source of stuttering is some incoordination expressed in the peripheral speech mechanism; the ultimate cause is presently unknown and may be complex or compound. (p. 498)

Right.

The "Standard" Definition Fails

The fact that stuttering is "complex or compound" cannot be disputed. It is obvious from what we know so far that stuttering is certainly both complicated and compounded by factors that may be coming from multiple sources including the speaker, the hearer(s), and the context of communication. However, the foregoing "standard" definition does little in helping us find a cause for stuttering or in explaining the systems that are involved in it.

Focusing on the Speaker's Viewpoint

Most definitions of stuttering deviate little from the "standard" description. Perkins (1990) differed by focusing on the speaker's perceptions of what is happening during the disfluencies rather than on the impressions made on the listener:

> The essence of stuttering, in my view, is not what is perceived by listeners as stuttering in the acoustical signal, but rather what occurs in the production of stuttered speech . . . Stuttering is the involuntary disruption of a continuing attempt to produce a spoken utterance . . . If the disruption is not involuntary to some degree, then it is not a stuttered disfluency. (p. 376)

While Wingate's definition focused attention on the second position of discourse (the receiver or consumer), Perkins' focused on the first position of discourse (that is, the speaker, the person who is stuttering). What is common to both definitions is the involuntary nature of the disruptions that occur in stuttering events. Both definitions stress that stuttering involves the loss of control of the speech process on the part of the speaker.

It's Not Your Fault!

F. H. Silverman, a long-time educator, practicing speech-language pathologist (SLP), writer, and himself a person who stutters, wrote in one of his books that it does more harm than good to convey to a person who stutters that he or she could stop the stuttering at will. He argues that this type of thinking conveys one of two messages, either the person chooses to stutter to satisfy some psychological need, or does not possess the strength of character to do what needs to be done to stop stuttering (2004, p. 216).

Marty Jezer describes the out of control feeling like this "[Persons who stutter] may know what to do and, even in the midst of a **stuttering block** [the sort of hesitation where speech stops and may be accompanied by grimacing, teeth clenching, or other gestures], may be thinking about what they ought to be doing to get through it. But thinking isn't doing. Unlike ordinary **hesitation phenomena** where a person voluntarily says "ummm, uh," and then may launch into a stream of speech only to stop, back up, and start again, and so on—in some cases with annoyingly high frequency —stuttering is not easily prevented or stopped by thinking about what it is that you are going to say.

Although hesitation habits can be adjusted without too much effort, stuttering is different. While hesitation devices are learned, can become habitual, and are at least somewhat automatic, beneath the level of conscious control, they do not fall completely beyond conscious and volitional control. However, they do fall near the boundary that separates conscious effort from habitual and automatic response. This fact, we believe, is suggested in the ancient Hebrew Proverbs recorded by Solomon. The following aphorism suggests the subconscious and remarkable nature of fluent speech: "The preparations of the heart belong to man, but the answer of the tongue is from the Lord" (Proverbs 16:1, *New King James Version of the Bible*). We understand this to mean that much of our use of the language capacity is, as Chomsky (1965) noted, many years later, outside of conscious and voluntary control.

We plan the meanings of what we say, and this planning involves conscious and volitional control. However, the normal fluency of our tongues in rolling out a sequence of syllables with a certain natural rhythm and intonation is ordinarily beyond our conscious control and is hardly short of being miraculous. Shakespeare (ca. 1599) described it this way in the words of his character, Hamlet:

"It is as if there were a decisive split, a cut cord . . . between mind and body, between brain and lips, mouth, tongue, larynx, and jaw" (p. 8).

Speak the speech, I pray you, as I pronounced it to you, trippingly on the tongue. But if you mouth it, as many of our players do, I had as lief the town crier spoke my lines. (Hamlet, III, ii, 1; retrieved March 5, 2009, from http://en.wikipedia.org/wiki/Speak_the_speech)

It is remarkable that normal language users are able to do what they do in fluent speech. If all systems are working properly, the words flow from the tongue at a surprisingly rapid pace with a degree of automaticity that is amazing. In pathological stuttering, this fluency is subject to one or possibly many sources of disruption.

Between Meaning and Sound

The threshold that separates normal hesitation phenomena from abnormal disfluencies involves a breakdown that seems to occur between the conscious intentional planning of what we have to say—that is the meaning—and the movements of the articulators that come into play in producing the stream of speech. A simple demonstration that this boundary, the threshold between thought and speech, exists, and that, to some extent, we work back and forth across that boundary is seen in the interaction between thinking and speaking. It is evident that we can reduce disfluencies by slowing down our rate of speaking and by being more deliberate about what we say.

FACILITATING CONTEXTS

A **facilitating context**, as the term "facilitating" is commonly applied with reference to stuttering, is one that either increases or decreases the likelihood of stuttering. For our own part, we prefer to distinguish contexts where stuttering is likely to increase from ones where it is likely to decrease. To do this, two terms are needed, but recall the complaint of LaPointe and J. Katz (2002; also Darley, 1967) that the terminology of communication disorders is not always systematic or precise. One individual wrote that "a facilitating situation is like giving candy to a child to get them to work harder." Actually, this description is headed in the right direction with respect to contexts that tend to induce more stuttering. Here are some descriptions of "facilitating" contexts paraphrased from various experts (also see F. H. Silverman, 2004; Manning, 2001; and Guitar, 2006 who provide similar lists) where stuttering is reduced, inhibited, or prevented.

Contexts in Which Stuttering Is Less Likely

For persons who stutter, some situations and tasks tend to decrease the likelihood of stuttering events. These typically include the following:

■ *Choral reading:* If a person who stutters simultaneously reads aloud the same passage along with one or more other persons, this activity usually induces perfect fluency. The same holds even if the two or more persons doing the task are all stutterers. The process seems to work like "drafting" in auto racing, cycling, or speed skating where the group can go faster together than they can go alone. The dynamic process of reading in unison normally results in seemingly perfect fluency even in persons who stutter. In choral reading the stuttering commonly disappears.

■ *Singing:* There are several famous musicians who stutter, including country singer Mel Tillis and the well-known Carly Simon. Because the music establishes the rhythm of the song lyrics and also specifies the pitch and the rhythms of the words to be uttered, the work of saying the words is reduced, making fluency easier to achieve. Stutterers typically do not stutter when they are singing.

■ *Speaking in time to a metronome:* Speaking in time to a metronome that provides an independent rhythm seems to work somewhat like reading in chorus or singing. By providing the rhythm, the metronome seems also to decrease the effort needed to produce a fluent stream of speech.

■ *Slowing the rate of speech:* Speaking about half as fast as normal will usually also induce greater fluency. Again, it seems that a reduced rate of speaking also makes the task easier and thus increases fluency. In fact, this should not surprise us since most complex tasks are easier when performed at a slower than normal pace.

■ *Speaking in any nonhabitual manner:* Another approach that seems to reduce stuttering is to deliberately use an accent, to drawl, mince words, speak with an intentional lisp, turn up the volume, or to imitate the manner of speech of someone else (such as talking like some well-known actor or politician). Somehow by shifting attention to any of these changes in the usual form of speech, the person who stutters will usually, at least temporarily, be more fluent. However, the beneficial effect of such effort tends to fade as the speaker becomes accustomed to the new way of speaking.

■ *Repeated practice:* If other factors are held equal, a passage that is read aloud repeatedly, or a speech that is practiced again and again, or even memorized, will tend to be produced more fluently on subsequent occasions. For persons who stutter, practicing a speech or reading a passage aloud multiple times will tend to reduce stuttering events on later productions of the same text or speech.

- *Speaking in masking noise:* Any steady sound in the background that is loud enough to make it harder for the speaker to hear what he or she is saying can serve as what is called **masking noise**. In experimental studies, and in many therapies, the sort of masking noise used is a lot like the constant whooshing that we commonly hear when the volume on the television is turned up but the channel selector is on an empty slot. The technical term for noise of this kind is *white noise*. Just as white light spreads across the entire light spectrum, white noise is spread across the whole sound spectrum. Because the presence of such noise, or any constant noise, in the background covers the sound of speech, it is called "masking noise." The surprising fact is that such masking tends to *reduce stuttering* in speech that is being produced by a person who stutters. Such observations lead theoreticians to conclude that stuttering involves a dynamic interplay of the motor and sensory feedback systems involved in speech production. However, because masking noise does not remove stuttering entirely, while choral reading and/or singing tend to do so, it must be supposed that other factors besides our ability to hear ourselves speaking must be involved in abnormal disfluencies. Another factor, as we saw most clearly in Chapter 4, is kinesthetic feedback from the movement of the articulators which is not masked by white noise. We can still feel our own movements even when we cannot hear ourselves speaking very well. Also, sound from bone conduction, as discussed in Chapter 3, and some auditory feedback may still be present even in masking noise.
- *Speaking to a child or pet:* It is commonly observed that persons who stutter tend to be noticeably more fluent when speaking with a child or talking to a pet. It may be supposed that this effect is caused in part by reduced stress. We are less anxious about the reaction of a small child, much less by a pet, than of peers, elders, or superiors. Reducing the potential stress and anxiety associated with any context of communication, often has the effect of increasing fluency for persons who stutter.

Contexts Where Stuttering Is More Likely

For persons who stutter, some situations and tasks tend to increase the likelihood of stuttering events. These typically include the following:

- Speaking on the telephone;
- Saying one's name;
- Telling a joke;
- Having to repeat a previous statement;

■ Anticipating an opportunity to speak in public, such as introducing yourself at a meeting or responding to long multi-part questions;

■ Speaking to a person in a position of authority; and

■ Trying not to stutter.

ARTIFICIALLY INDUCED STUTTERING

Perhaps the most interesting of the experimental findings with stuttering was the surprising and accidental discovery of artificially induced stuttering. We give this discovery considerable space before considering specific theories about the causation of stuttering in the next major section.

Delayed Auditory Feedback

There is one peculiar speaking situation—one that does not naturally occur in ordinary experience but that can be artificially created with recording and playback devices—that seems to fall somewhat near the border of situations that tend to produce stuttering and ones that tend to inhibit it. Like the McGurk interactions that we discussed extensively in Chapter 4, the impact of what is called **delayed side-tone** or, more commonly in our current literature, *delayed auditory feedback*, was also discovered quite by chance. Also, like the McGurk interactions, the effects of DAF are complex. The DAF effects reveal remarkable interactions across the motor systems involved in speaking and the sensory processes involved in our senses of hearing and touch in particular. Nowadays, DAF can sometimes be experienced on a cell phone where the speaker hears a delayed echo of his or her own voice. When the DAF is more noticeable than our own speech, some sounds and syllables tend to be repeated involuntarily as in "if-if-if ya-ya-ya" and some sounds and syllables are elongated as in "ya-ya-ya-yooooouuuuu."

Lee and Black in the 1950s

In 1950, Bernard S. Lee was not looking for a way to produce an artificial stutter in persons who do not normally stutter, but he stumbled onto one with accidentally produced DAF. Like the later cross-modal interactions discovered by McGurk and MacDonald, Lee and others became intrigued by what they discovered. It was known that an echo, or delayed feedback from a public address system, could interfere with a person's ability to speak fluently, but

We believe that artificial stuttering which is caused in the vast majority of fluent speakers when they are exposed to the phenomenon known as **delayed auditory feedback** **(DAF)** connects some of the best theories and helps to explain why choral reading, for example, tends to dramatically reduce the tendency to stutter.

the invention and manufacture of affordable tape recorders made artificial DAF a common experience in the year 1950. At that time anyone who purchased a tape recorder with a set of earphones could experience the brief delay between the time the tape passed the recording head and moved on to the playback head. What happened next was astonishing to Lee and just about everyone else who has ever experienced it.

Delayed Auditory Feedback

Lee (1950a) reported his observations on DAF in the following words in an article titled "Artificial Stutter" in the *Journal of Speech and Hearing Disorders*:

In the course of operating a magnetic tape-recorder, the writer found himself part of a new stuttering hybrid, half human and half electronic, and was encouraged to investigate the phenomenon further. (p. 53)

He found in listening to a recording of his own voice that was playing back about ¼ of a second after he recorded it, that he experienced a strange tendency to stutter. In describing his own experience and that of others, he noted that the DAF for some seemed to cause

a quavering slow speech of the type associated with cerebral palsy; others may halt, repeat syllables, raise their voice in pitch or volume; and reveal tension by reddening of the face. (p. 643)

Reporting additional detailed research on DAF a year later, another researcher who had become interested in stuttering induced by DAF, John W. Black, wrote:

With short delays [from .03 to .06 seconds], descriptions emphasize "a stretching out feeling." Longer delays [up to .18 seconds] may produce near traumatic effects that include the blocking of speech, facial contortions, the prolongation and slurring of sounds, and repetitions of sounds and syllables. Some of these effects are difficult for the subjects to describe and the reports usually refer to surprise and frustration. (1951, p. 58)

Lee noted that for speakers who do not normally stutter but who are induced to do so by DAF, trying to overcome the impact of DAF for "more than two minutes" is "physically tiring" (1950a, p. 53). All these descriptions of stuttering produced by DAF sound amazingly like present-day expert descriptions of stuttering by stutterers themselves and by researchers focusing their effort on understanding stuttering. The described symptoms especially resemble the descriptions by persons who stutter of their sense of losing control of the speaking process.

The Dynamic Role of Sensory Feedback in Motor Control

Citing the work of Norbert Wiener (1948) on **cybernetics**—the mathematical physics of self-controlling systems dependent on feedback loops—Lee (1950a, 1950b, 1950c) speculated that future research would discover at least four distinct levels of effects based on distinct feedback loops in speech production (also see Levelt, 1983, for a similar theory). Lee's theory included feedback loops at the level (1) of individual sound segments, **phonemes**, (2) at the level of syllables, (3) words, and (4) whole thoughts as expressed in sentences or clauses. In follow up research by Black (1951), the measure used to show the impact of DAF was "rate of reading"—that is, how long did take subjects to complete oral reading tasks with DAF ranging from zero to about one-third of a second. Black's research tended to confirm at least two of the levels of stuttering that Lee's proposed model predicted. Black wrote,

> the fact that the longest reading times occurred with delays of .18 second [180 milliseconds] suggests the possibility that the duration of the syllable may have an important bearing upon the effects of delayed side-tone. In normal reading, the mean duration of a syllable in the phrases [i.e., the ones Black used] is approximately .22 second [220 milliseconds].

Black's research also confirms the independent expectation that follows from Chapter 4—based on the layering, ranking, and integration of distinct sign systems—that multiple levels of stuttering can be distinguished.

Phonemes and Syllables

In fact, at least two levels of stuttering were distinguished experimentally and clinically by Black. His research with DAF not only showed a distinct **syllabic level of stuttering**, but also a **phonemic level of stuttering** as well. In the 1951 research paper, Black went on to say,

> . . . the disproportionate increment in the duration of a phrase that occurs when the readers experience a delay of .06 second [approximately 60 milliseconds] in their side-tone suggests that a delay that approaches the duration of a single phoneme may have special significance in retarding the fluency of speech. (p. 58)

All of these effects show that several distinct feedback loops—as proposed by Lee (1950a, 1950b, 1950c) and by Levelt (1983) following Wiener (1948)—are involved in the processes of producing fluent speech. The research also suggests that disruption of one or more feedback loops is probably a major causal factor in the stuttering of many persons who stutter.

Research on DAF since the 1950s has continued to accumulate. A search on the Web of Science on June 14, 2007 shows 183 hits for a search of ("delayed auditory feedback" OR sidetone OR sidetone). It reveals many interesting findings confirming that DAF commonly, though not always, produces stuttering in persons who are not usually dysfluent. The research shows that multilinguals are more susceptible to DAF effects in their second or third language than in their primary language (Van Borsel, Sunaert, & Engelen, 2005). Also, this effect evidently generalizes to a second "dialect" or later acquired variety of a person's native language. P. Howell, Barry, and Vinson (2006) found that DAF tended to cause speakers who had acquired a different dialect of British English to revert to the former native dialect.

A Piece of the Etiology Puzzle?

Lee himself (1950c, p. 54) suggested that the observed effects of DAF might help to explain why, at least in some cases, individuals stutter in the first place. He noted the observation of Bloodstein (1950) that choral reading is an activity in which stuttering typically ceases altogether even in severe stutterers and speculated that timing of auditory feedback was probably a factor. He supposed that choral reading produces naturally overlapping rates of phoneme-, syllable-, and word-level auditory feedback because the group of oral readers is never in perfect synchronization. As a result, in choral reading the person who might otherwise stutter—say, on account of DAF at the phoneme- or syllable-level—serendipitously is receiving auditory feedback smeared over a range of time segments corresponding to both of these units of speech. As a result, the known fact that choral reading tends to reduce or remove stuttering events altogether, may be explained, at least in part, by Lee's model of speech production which aimed to explain the impact of DAF.

More recently, Kalinowski, Saltuklaroglu, Stuart, and Guntupalli (2007; also see Stuart, Frazier, Kalinowski, & Vos, 2008) have defended the clinical use of a device called the SpeechEasy that employs "altered auditory feedback" (AAF). In their system, as Kalinowski and colleagues said in 2007, DAF is a

> derivation of choral speech (nature's most powerful stuttering "inhibitor") that can be synergistically combined with other methods for optimal stuttering inhibition. (p. 69)

Their approach raises the pitch of the feedback (Stuart, Kalinowski, Rastatter, Saltuklaroglu, & Dayalu, 2004) by 500 Hz and used a DAF of 60 milliseconds (.06 second), provided to the person who stutters through the SpeechEasy monaural (single ear) device. This method, according to Finn, Bothe, and Bramlett (2005), has not been sufficiently tested. The question is whether it really helps to reduce stuttering or not, and if so, why and how. One of the underlying questions is the one posed clearly back in the 1950s by Bloodstein,

Lee, Black and others: why is it that DAF produces stuttering in persons who do not normally stutter? In addition to this question, the more recent research raises the possibility that changing the rate of auditory feedback provided to the ears of some stutterers might help to reduce their stuttering. This possibility was alluded to by Lee (1950a, 1950b, 1950c) thinking along the lines of the choral reading effect and his own proposals for the role of auditory feedback in normal speech production. These ideas are all still under intensive investigation.

Differences in the Brain?

In an interesting study in *Neurology* in 2004, Foundas et al. proposed that adults who stutter and also have an anomalous anatomy in the part of their brains called the **planum temporale (PT)** were not only more likely to be more severe stutterers but were significantly more likely than stutterers without this anatomical anomaly to benefit from DAF. The PT is the cortical region just behind the auditory region that corresponds to **Wernicke's area** in the left hemisphere. Figure 8–1 shows what the PT looks like in a healthy brain (also see "Planum temporale," 2009, retrieved March 5, 2009, from http://en .wikipedia.org/wiki/Planum_temporale). Foundas et al. concluded that stutterers with a right shifted PT **asymmetry**—that is, where the PT on the right side of the brain is as great as or greater than that on the left side of the brain—were more severe stutterers but stuttered less under DAF. Because these portions of the brain are involved in auditory/semantic processing of speech and language, Foundas et al. supposed that perhaps this anatomical difference has some causal relation both to stuttering and to the impact of DAF.

However, it is interesting to note that the asymmetry of the PT has also been associated with phenomena as distinct from stuttering as the perception of **absolute pitch** (Keenan, Thangarai, Halpern, & Schlaug, 2001)—"the ability to identify the pitch of any tone in the absence of a musical context or reference tone" (p. 1402). Some musicians have that ability and others do not. For those musicians with absolute pitch (as contrasted with musicians and nonmusicians who do not have absolute pitch), Keenan et al. (2001) found that

> the left PT was only marginally larger in the AP group. The absolute size of the right PT and not the left PT was a better predictor of music group membership, possibly indicating "pruning" of the right PT rather than expansion of the left underlying the increased PT asymmetry in AP musicians. (p. 1402; retrieved March 5, 2009, from http://www.musicianbrain.com/papers /Keenan_AP_2001.pdf).

From studies like those by Foundas et al. and Keenan et al. it is evident that researchers are groping to try to associate gross measurements of the left and right hemispheres of the brain with specific functions.

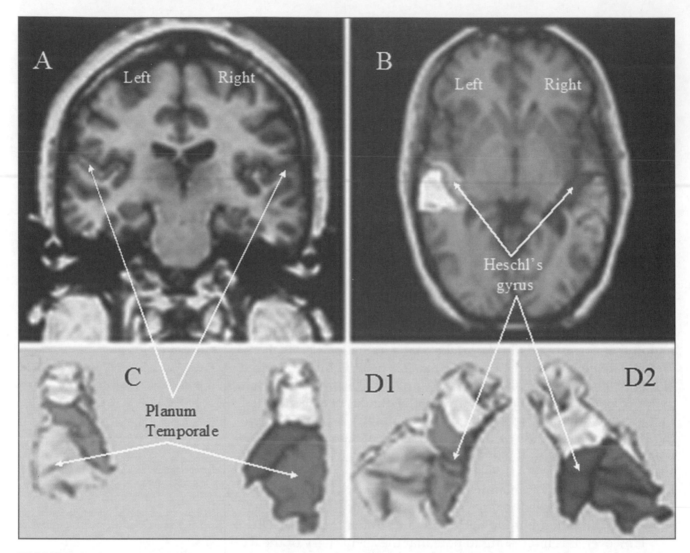

FIGURE 8–1. An inside (MRI) view of Wernicke's area divided between Heschl's gyrus (the cortical fold) just above and in front of the planum temporale (PT) and the PT itself in a healthy individual. From Y. Hirayasu et al., 2000, Planum temporale and Heschl gyrus volume reduction in schizophrenia: A magnetic resonance imaging study of first-episode patients. *Archives of General Psychiatry, 57*(7), Figure 1. Retrieved March 5, 2009, from http://www.spl.harvard.edu/pages/Special:PubDB_View?dspaceid=406. Copyright 2008 by Surgical Planning Laboratory. Adapted and reprinted with permission. All rights reserved.

Limited Explanatory Power

While some of the hunches proposed and tested may seem plausible, perhaps even correct after the fact, hemispheric asymmetries have only one **degree of freedom** (i.e., because they are based on just two sides of the brain there is just one logical chance of a contrast arising), so the conclusions along this line must be regarded as barely testable. Even when contrasts are found, they have limited explanatory power and little clinical utility.

In persons with persistent stuttering in adulthood, there is also research showing that short-term memory traces of the sounds produced in speaking last longer for persons who stutter than nonstuttering counterparts (Corbera, Corral, Escera, & Idiazabal, 2005). If we take account of the fact that DAF commonly produces severe and exhausting episodes of stuttering in persons who do not normally stutter (per Lee, 1950a, 1950b, 1950c), the finding of abnormally long and persistent memory traces for sounds in stutterers suggests a possible neurological basis grounded in the timing of sounds and syllables in at least some cases of severe stuttering.

DAF as a Remedy in Some Cases

There is abundant evidence that DAF almost universally, and certainly quite generally, produces stuttering immediately in persons who do not normally stutter. As for its impact on persons who stutter, the evidence is not the same for all individuals, perhaps for reasons just noted in reference to Foundas et al. (2004).

Impact of DAF on Stutterers

According to Fukawa, Yoshioka, Ozawa, and Yoshida (1988), the immediate impact of DAF for most stutterers, is the same as it is with nonstutterers. That is, DAF immediately causes more stuttering rather than less. They compared 40 stutterers and 40 nonstutterers and found that both groups were negatively impacted by DAF with stutterers being somewhat more affected than nonstutterers.

However, the research also suggests that in some cases of fairly severe stutterers, DAF can significantly reduce stuttering. Van Borsel, Reunes, and Van den Bergh (2003) concluded from a study of nine stutterers that repeated exposure to DAF over a three-month period without any other therapeutic intervention seemed to reduce stuttering. Kalinowski et al. (2007 and see their references) have concluded that DAF combined with an upward adjustment in pitch of 500 Hz can reduce stuttering in a person who stutters by as much as 80% (p. 71). Similarly, Stidham, Olson, Hillbratt, and Sinopoli (2006) reported results with "a bone conduction device" delivering DAF between 5 and 130 milliseconds (at the stutterer's discretion) used over a four-week time period reduced stuttering in 9 of the 10 patients who completed the study.

One way for nonstutterers to overcome the initial DAF-induced stuttering effect is for the speaker to just slow down. Slowing down, in general, as clinical experience confirms, helps many stutterers reduce the tendency to stutter. Evidently, they get better control of the speaking process and stutter less by consciously and deliberately speaking more slowly. Doing that also helps nonstutterers to

In any case, DAF effects for both persons who do and do not stutter suggest that stuttering, to some extent, involves a breakdown in the dynamic temporal coordination of speaking based in part on what we normally hear ourselves saying.

overcome the debilitating effects of DAF. Another way of defeating, or at least reducing, the effects of DAF is to disregard the sounds coming from the headset and to concentrate on the movements of the articulators—that is, to rely on motor-tactile (kinesthetic feedback) rather than auditory feedback.

THEORIES AND FINDINGS ABOUT THE CAUSES OF STUTTERING

We can argue that wanting *not* to stutter seems to be a factor in all of the speaking activities just mentioned in the preceding section where stuttering tends to be more likely for persons who are prone to stutter. It seems also to be the case that situations in which there is increased tension are also likely to increase normal disfluencies in many persons who do not normally stutter. In addition to whatever tension there may be, what else is it about these situations that causes disfluencies to be more likely? On the other side of the ledger, for situations and activities where disfluencies are less likely, besides a lessening of tension in some instances, what else is different in instances where stuttering seems to become less likely? Taking both the positive and negative instances together, what clues about the nature and causation of stuttering can be gleaned from situations or activities that make stuttering dramatically more or less likely?

Interestingly, theories about the causation of stuttering events and of the disorder as a phenomenon, are usually based on observations drawn from or related to commonly known facilitating/inhibiting activities. Of course, in addition to common observations about activities that tend to heighten or reduce the likelihood of stuttering episodes, there are other sources of information on which theories of causation commonly rely. For instance, there are experimental studies investigating possible causes and there are neurological studies of brain activity during fluent speech and during stuttering events.

In the following sections, we consider the most prominent—and, in our judgment, the most plausible—theories and "models" of stuttering. We will return to certain unsolved problems that all of theories of stuttering must deal with after we introduce several of the competing theories in the following sections.

Demands and Capacities

Among the most cited and plausible theories about the etiology of stuttering is the so-called **demands and capacities model**. This hunch was first put in its current form by C. Woodruff Starkweather (1987). According to his idea, capacities to speak fluently fluctuate with the relative demands of any given speaking situation. As demands for more and more complex structures grow with the increasing complexity of the child's experience, capacities need to advance to keep up. If they do not, Starkweather's hunch is that stuttering may be the result. As we will see below, this idea was more or less implicit in the writings of Oliver Bloodstein (1950, 2006). Bloodstein's earliest writings suggesting the basis for the Starkweather idea date back to the time of the discovery of the amazing effects of DAF in the 1950s by Lee, Black, and others. However, Starkweather extended the idea about demands to the expanding capacities of early childhood language. He argued that if the increase in demands happens to exceed the child's growth in processing capacities, it is to be expected that the child will begin to stutter. If the capacities do not subsequently catch up to the new demands of increasing complexity in linguistic structures, the stuttering may persist and become a disorder.

The demands and capacities theory is widely accepted as accounting for **developmental stuttering**—the kind that sometimes appears between years three and six but somewhere along the way commonly seems to correct itself. The child stutters temporarily and then seems to outgrow the stuttering. If developmental stuttering persists into adulthood it is termed **incipient stuttering** or, more transparently, **persistent developmental stuttering**.

> If developmental stuttering persists into adulthood it is termed **incipient stuttering** or, more transparently, **persistent developmental stuttering**.

The research discussed in previous sections of this chapter has focused on the incipient or persistent kind of stuttering but the demands and capacities model also fits that kind of stuttering well too. The activities/situations that make stuttering more likely or less likely, as described in prior sections, seem to fit the demands and capacities model well. Ones that enhance fluency also seem to be those that reduce the demands on the speaker—for example, choral reading, talking to a pet, and so on—while those seem to induce stuttering—such as speaking in a threatening context—also involve increased demands. Various other theories of stuttering involve key aspects of the demands and capacities theory.

Stuttering as a Disorder of Language

Bloodstein proposed the **language disorder theory** of stuttering. The reader can hear Bloodstein tell about his ideas in a digital recording ("The Nature of Stuttering," 1959, retrieved March 5, 2009, from http://www.mnsu.edu/comdis/voices/voices.html). Bloodstein, who has been publishing papers about stuttering for more than 57 years, argues that the onset of stuttering events tends to coincide with the anticipation of difficulties associated with particular linguistic forms. He argued (2006, pp. 186-188) that stuttering cannot merely be a speech disorder on the basis of several empirical observations based on clinical experience and research:

> For many researchers, clinicians, and theoreticians stuttering is often treated and regarded as a problem of speech. For instance, Yairi and Ambrose (2005) say that stuttering "is first and foremost a disorder of speech" (p. 84). But others, notably Bloodstein (2006)—the same Bloodstein cited by Lee (1950b)—argued that language processing is deeper than speech.

1. The first word of a syntactic phrase is more likely to be stuttered than a word appearing in another position (Bloodstein & Grossman, 1981). This observation shows that stuttering tends to occur at major word, phrase, clause, and conversation

event boundaries. This shows an involvement of language structures—syntax and meaning.

2. Early stuttering most often occurs on **function words** (Bloodstein & Gantwerk, 1967; P. Howell, Au-Yeung, & Sackin, 1999)—that is, on words like *on*, *to*, *the*, *a*, *my* and so on—while adults who stutter tend do so more often on **content words**—for example, *table*, *three*, *dog*, *go*, and so on.

3. In early stuttering by young children, the most common quality of words in stuttering is that they tend to be at the beginning of sentence (Throneburg, Yairi, & Paden 1994).

4. While adult stuttering is evidently the focus of Wingate's (1964) definition, early stuttering seems to involve whole word repetitions almost exclusively (Ambrose & Yairi, 1999; Bloodstein, 1960, 1974; W. Johnson & Associates, 1959). On this basis, it seems that the unit of structure that the child is working with is clearly at the word-level and this level can only be defined by language functions pertaining to syntax and meaning. It cannot be defined by phonological properties or articulatory movements of speech alone.

5. Children rarely stutter on utterances that consist only of a single word (Melnick, Conture, & Ohde, 2003). This fact suggests that it is the added burden of putting two or more words together in more complex phrase structures that induces developmental stuttering.

6. The earliest age reported for the onset of stuttering is 18 months, which coincides with the earliest advent of two-word phrases and the beginnings of syntactic complexity (Bloodstein, 1995).

7 & 8. Developmental stuttering is normally noticed between the ages of two and six years. This time frame brackets the ages during which syntactic development is advancing the most. Complex structures begin to develop with the two-word stage at about 20 months give or take a couple of months (J. W. Oller, S. D. Oller, & Badon, 2006) and the onset of developmental stuttering is rarely noticed much after age six when syntactic development, according to current theory and research, is nearing or has already reached the point of diminishing returns. After that, the child's attention shifts to pragmatic questions of what is true, appropriate, and/or a basis for valid inference. During the period from two to six, persons with developmental stuttering typically become persistent (incipient) stutterers or quit the developmental stuttering by about age six (Logan & Conture, 1995; Zackheim & Conture, 2003).

From the above observations, Bloodstein notes that incipient stuttering—the persistent kind of developmental stuttering that continues throughout a lifetime—develops while syntactic and morphological complexities are being acquired. Additionally, stuttering intensity, he argues, varies concomitantly with increasing syntactic and morphological complexity. Guitar (2006; hear him in a 1996 panel discussion on recovery, retrieved March 6, 2009, from http://www.mnsu.edu/comdis/voices/voices.html) claims that anecdotal evidence suggests that incipient stuttering varies not only with the complexity of utterances produced by the child but also with the complexity of utterances by the child's primary care giver(s). If the foregoing arguments are valid, then stuttering ought to be considered a disorder of language, at least during its initial stages. However, as we will see, incipient stuttering seems also to involve powerful emotional elements that tend to accumulate and intensify over time.

Modularity and Stuttering

Bosshardt (2006) summarized a decade of research leading him to conclude that language systems are **modular** and that stuttering involves distinct contributions from different **modules**—that is, language systems are differentiated into distinct and somewhat independent components. In proposing this idea, Bosshardt followed a tradition in cognitive psychology and linguistics beginning with Fodor (1983). Fodor elaborated on certain ideas from Chomsky (1957, 1965, 1972) and proposed that certain capacities are somewhat self-contained like the distinct organs of the body. The heart does not do the same work as the lungs or the brain, but all of them are interconnected.

With modularity in mind, Bosshardt argued that stuttering is the result of inadequate differentiation and coordination of distinct modules. He studied persons who stutter in contrast to a control group of nonstutterers on a speaking task carried out while comparing word meanings and forms. In one experiment, each participant was asked to make a two-pronged judgment about one pair of words while constructing a sentence using a different pair of words. If the first pair of words were in the same semantic category (e.g., *table* and *chair*), or if they were rhyming words (e.g., *hair* and *there*) the participant was to push a "yes" button, otherwise, a "no" button. At the same time the participant was supposed to construct a sentence with a different pair of words (e.g., *cake* and *yellow*) as in, say, "The yellow crayon fell into the cake." He called these experimental activities **dual-tasks**. Persons who stutter showed one of two outcomes when performing both tasks simultaneously. Either they stuttered more than in a speaking task without the simultaneous mental judgment, or they produced sentences that were less complex. He defined a less complex sentence as one containing fewer clauses, words, and so forth. For example, "She baked a cake" is less complex than "The tall slim gourmet baked a delicious yellow cake covered with chocolate frosting."

Bosshardt (2006) argued on the basis of this and similar studies that persons who stutter are more susceptible to interference across

The language module of human capacity, according to modularity theories, is itself a complex system of somewhat independent components.

distinct modules of processing, for example, from the demands of speech production while simultaneously performing cognitive judgments, than are persons who do not have the stuttering disorder. Clearly, the modularity theory has a lot in common with the demands and capacities model. As more modules of processing (capacities) are required to be activated at the same time, the demands of the task go up.

Process Malfunction Models

Some theories of stuttering fit in the class of **processing malfunction models**. Theories of this kind commonly focus on feedback and **monitoring functions**—that is, systems by which speakers check the accuracy of the surface forms and meanings of their own productions. One subclass of these theories proposes that the malfunctions in stuttering are motoric. In particular, stuttering is the result of a motor planning deficit or breakdown. Another subclass suggests that stuttering is due to a linguistic planning defect.

F. H. Silverman (2004) summarized 30 years of research on motor differences between persons who stutter and those who do not. One method of investigation uses **electromyography** where sensors are placed in key muscle groups to measure changes in the electrical potential of nervous impulses and muscle responses. Electromyographic studies indicate that there is a difference in the muscular activity in the throat, jaws, and lips between those who stutter and those who do not.

Brain scans with fMRI, and **positron emission tomography (PET)** also show (De Nil & Kroll, 2001; De Nil, Kroll, Kapur, & Houle, 2000; De Nil, Kroll, Lafaille, & Houle, 2003), again unsurprisingly, that during a stuttering event, the brain of a person who stutters looks different from the brain of a person who does not. More importantly, perhaps, the biochemistry is different in persons who stutter (Wu et al., 1995). In persons who stutter, more **dopamine** (Wu et al., 1997)—a neurotransmitter that is deficient in Parkinson's disease—is being used by many parts of the nervous system. Based on their PET studies, Wu et al. (1997) speculated that increased uptake of dopamine by the nervous system may be a causal factor in stuttering. Burghaus et al. (2006) carried this hunch a step further and showed that stuttering was increased in a Parkinson's patient by stimulation of the basal ganglia. They conclude that the circuitry in that region of the brain is therefore implicated.

The Covert Repair Hypothesis

Among the theories that propose a linguistic planning defect or deficit is the Postma and Kolk (1993) **covert repair hypothesis**.

They argued that stuttering is caused by processing errors that occur between planning what to say and carrying out the movements to say it. The repair theory is unassailable as a description, but everyone makes such adjustments somewhat covertly and not everyone stutters. To suggest the description as a theory of stuttering is like describing a train running off its tracks as a theory of why train wrecks occur. As a theory of stuttering the covert repair hypothesis only describes the problem without providing an explanation for it. It asserts that all of the covert activity, in some unexplained way, results in what appears at the surface as stuttering. By this theory, stuttering is a product of repairs gone amuck.

The theory does not explain why things go wrong, though it describes, in part, what may happen when they do. The covert repair theory has received a lot of attention. A Google search for "covert repair hypothesis" on March 6, 2009 returned 1,270 hits. The idea certainly has appeal. Say a person is speaking and an error occurs. That error can be phonological (*"p"* for *"t,"* *"st-"* for *"sp-,"* *"-vy"* for *"-cy,"* and so on), lexical/semantic (*"pear"* for *"apple,"* "bring me *the hose*" for "bring me *a glass of water*"), morphological (substituting *"pre-"* for *"per-,"* *"con-"* for *"in-"*), or pragmatic (*"thank you"* for *"good morning"*). In order to correct the error, the speaker may stop and say something like *"excuse me, I'm sorry, err, uh, wait, I mean . . . "* Then, the speaker may repeat the message with a revision.

A covert repair can occur under similar conditions. A motor plan is drawn up and the message is already going out before the monitor can register any error. There must be a lag between the registration of the error and the initiation of any repair. If the monitor finds an error, the message is halted, a repair is made, and the message is resent in its corrected form. However, in a covert repair, the monitor operates at a subconscious, more or less automatic level. The monitor halts the message and makes the repair without the speaker's being aware of the process. This repair mechanism can then find itself in a loop repeatedly producing failed motor plans evidenced either by complete halts in the flow of speech, or by repetitions of sounds, syllables, or words.

Postma and Kolk argue that this repair process—operating covertly—accounts not only for stuttered disfluencies but for other ordinary disfluencies as well. If an error is spotted before the message goes out, however, their model predicts that a stuttering block may occur. Depending on how much of the message is already out when the error is noticed, a phonemic, syllabic, whole word, or even a phrase repetition, will occur. What separates normal disfluencies from stuttering according to processing malfunction models is the individual's ability to create phonologically accurate articulatory plans. A logical inference from this theory is that we should expect more phonological errors among persons who stutter than those who do not. And, we do find more phonological errors in stuttered speech events.

Repairs, according to the covert repair idea, occur as the speaker discovers that the emerging speech does not match what was intended.

A Phonological Articulatory Deficit?

According to Louko, Conture, and Edwards (1999), 30% to 40% of children who stutter have phonological or articulatory disorders. But stuttered speech inevitably leads to more articulatory errors, so it is not a clear whether persons who stutter also have phonological disorders, or if the diagnosis of the phonological disorder is due in part to stuttering. Shenker (2006) writes:

> There will always be a place for stuttering treatments designed to eliminate or reduce stuttered speech. When those treatments are required, direct speech measures of treatment process and outcome are needed in clinical practice. (p. 355)

Judging whether chronic stuttering exists in the first place, and whether therapy has helped or not in cases where chronic disfluency has been diagnosed, requires accurate identification and measurement of stuttering events in addition to the detection and measurement of the emotional impact and other consequences of stuttering.

Generalizing to Expressive Communication?

If Bloodstein and those who see the diverse phenomena of stuttering as deeper than speech are at all close to the mark, it should be possible to find manifestations of stuttering in other forms of linguistic expression—for example, in manual signing, writing, typing, and even in silent reading. In fact, if bona fide examples of stuttering in manual signed languages could be documented, it would seem to clinch the case against the strong claims that stuttering is exclusively a phenomenon of speaking. It would also require a fundamental re-examination of some of the claims made for the modularity hypothesis. If stuttering should turn out to be a deeper semiotic manifestation of motoric expression, the distinct modules proposed by some theoreticians (e.g., Fodor, Chomsky, and others), would presumably have to be connected at a deeper level.

Snyder (2006) has done an intensive review of the literature on stuttering with that sort of hunch in mind. He noted the claim of Yairi and Ambrose that

> *stuttering* refers to the domain of motor speech production and its disruption by speech disfluencies. Physical, physiological, cognitive and emotional components, regardless of how frequent or intense they might be, would not be labeled as "stuttering" if they did not accompany a speaker's disfluent speech. (p. 19)

However, he came across a case of stuttering in a manual signed language by a deaf man who had learned English as a child and

ASL at Gallaudet University after becoming deaf. The man, referred to as GW, used a version of simultaneous speech and ASL, and stuttered severely in both systems. This observation caused Dr. Snyder to wonder if researchers had not perhaps overlooked many actual instances of manual stuttering in the past.

Stuttering in Other Modalities

The events that day with GW stuttering in both speech and sign, all in his own office, spurred Dr. Snyder to investigate further. The new interest and led him to review what turned out to be a long and substantial documentary record of stuttering phenomena in modalities other than speech—especially in manual signed languages. Dr. Snyder found many references by researchers dating back to Voelker and Voelker (1937) and including such well known authors on the subject of stuttering as Wingate (1970) and F. H. Silverman and E. M. Silverman (1971)—also see Whitebread (2004). Snyder (2006) also documents many instances of apparent stuttering in the tongue, lip, and breath control movements of flautists and trumpeters, and in the hands of pianists, violinists, and other musicians (Meltzer, 1992; F. H. Silverman & Bohlman, 1988; Snyder, 2006). He also found documentary evidence of stuttering in handwriting (Roman, 1959; Scripture, 1909). Dr. Snyder is currently conducting a national survey of his own to reassess the incidence of stuttering among users of manual signed languages.

If T. S. Kuhn's (1962) observations about scientific revolutions are applied—and we agree with Dr. Snyder that they seem entirely applicable to stuttering events in modalities other than speech—it is likely that manual and other expressive forms of stuttering are considerably more common than previously supposed. The fact is, as Kuhn pointed out, we tend to overlook things that we are expecting *not* to find. The phrase that comes to mind is "hiding in plain sight." It turns out that even when something unexpected is perceived superficially it tends to be dismissed as if it had never occurred.

For instance, when a certain Caucasian linguist who spoke both Cantonese and English from early childhood approached a Chinese gentleman in Hong Kong to ask directions to a certain restaurant, the Chinese man threw up his hands and protested loudly in Cantonese that he did not understand a word of English. Then, as he walked away, the linguist (Thomas Scovel, personal communication to J. W. Oller) overheard the Chinese man saying to his friends, "That's strange, it sounded like that foreigner was asking directions to a certain restaurant"—which, of course, was the case. The Chinese man had heard, processed, and understood, and yet not fully believed that he was actually hearing something he

If the modality of music is also found to involve stuttering as the research literature suggests, it would appear that musical expression probably does involve a level of meaning that is profoundly associated with linguistic prosody as some theoreticians have suggested (Freeman, 2000; Reybrouck, 2004; M. Silverman, 2007).

didn't expect to hear. So his conscious mind dismissed what he had actually perceived correctly. It was as though he had heard it plainly at a subconscious level and yet simply did not believe he had heard it at all in his conscious experience.

Dr. Snyder supposes, and we agree, that something similar has probably happened with respect to stuttering in modalities other than speech. All highly skilled (linguistic) expressive motoric acts, according to a general theory of signs (see J. W. Oller, S. D. Oller, & Badon, 2006), should be equally susceptible to whatever may be going wrong in stuttered speech events. It remains to find out what is going wrong and where. Perhaps as Dr. Snyder supposes, the whole field of research and theory concerning the diverse phenomena of stuttering is ripe for a major paradigm shift. We believe that this is the case.

TESTING THE THEORIES

When it comes to assessment and especially measuring factors believed to contribute to stuttering phenomena, the interplay of theory and fact is problematic. It seems that the most important aspects of stuttering, such as its emotional consequences and its impact on planning and execution of skilled movements, exist beneath the surface. If stuttering is as deep a semiotic phenomenon as we suspect that it is, affecting many different expressive modalities, it will probably turn out that stuttering events are like the tips of icebergs above the water while the greater substance lies beneath the surface. There are also some interesting theoretical inadequacies of the theories of stuttering proposed to date.

A Profound Circularity

Consider the demands and capacities model and how readily it can be adjusted to fit the apparent surface facts. When we see an increase in stuttering it is easy enough to say, "Well the demands exceeded the capacities." When stuttering seems to decrease or disappear, it is just as easy to suppose, "See there! This only goes to show, the capacities must have caught up to the demands." A similar circularity can be found in reference to the modular theories of stuttering and at least some aspects of their competitors. The idea of a give-and-take balancing act between demands and capacities —or distinct modules, covert processes, and so forth—is easy enough to understand and appealing. It seems plausible to suppose that some sort of interaction between distinct systems has gotten out of balance when stuttering events occur.

Also, if suitable measures can be found, how will they account for experimental effects produced by DAF? Unless DAF can be construed as a strange demand factor, or as a factor that somehow reduces an existing capacity, it would seem that DAF provides a prima facie ("on its face," i.e., plain and simple) refutation of the demands and capacities theory. It also requires some mental gymnastics to fit the demands and capacities theory to phenomena involving choral reading, singing, speaking to a metronome, and the like. How do these activities reduce emotional or cognitive demands? Or how do they enhance existing capacities? It may be possible to develop plausible arguments in each case, but they must be contrived. They are not readily evident and clear explanations do not flow logically from any of the existing popular theories.

DAF as Fundamental

With respect to the phenomena just noted, the demands and capacities model fares no better or worse than the modularity, and process malfunction theories. All of them merely contrast stuttering with nonstuttering in one respect or another without adequately explaining what causes stuttering or how to measure the hypothetical factors that increase or decrease the likelihood of stuttering events. However, all of the previous problems are upstaged in part by the empirical evidences pertaining to delayed auditory feedback. The observed results from DAF research must be explained.

How can the various theories account for DAF, masking, and other experimental effects on stuttering? For instance, the covert repair hypothesis suggests a role for feedback of various kinds. Feedback is the essence of the comparison of what is intended with what is emerging. By contrast, any theory that does not implicitly or explicitly take feedback into account, will run into difficulty in trying to explain how or why masking noise usually tends to increase fluency in persons who stutter. But in the case of the covert repair hypothesis, if the masking noise is sufficiently loud, presumably, the internal processing of any disrupted feedback will be covered up to the point of becoming unnoticeable so that it cannot interfere much (or possibly at all) with speech production. The covert repair hypothesis can then account for the impact of masking noise on the assumption that the noise prevents the noticing of the disrupted feedback that leads to the stuttering. But what is the covert repair hypothesis going to do to account for the effects of DAF?

In any case, theories of the causation of stuttering will remain incomplete until DAF effects are explained. Meantime, there are other problems to be solved such as determining the severity of stuttering in cases where it occurs.

It seems essential to discover the specific neurological basis for the impact of DAF and also for the internal disruptions in persons who stutter.

The Measurement Problem

Measures of demands and capacities—ones that might enable researchers to put them on a common scale—do not exist and are not easy to imagine.

What are the independent measures of the interacting factors, for instance, of the so-called "demands and capacities model"? If we want to assess their ratio in order to predict stuttering, what exactly are the measures of the demands as contrasted with the capacities?

The demands on speakers in producing speech involve a vast complex of potential factors some of which will be present on a given occasion and some not. But there is no way to predict in advance just how the mix will shape up. So, in predicting or explaining who will stutter and when, which factors are to be taken into consideration and how will the choices be made? The capacities involved are equally complex and are neither fully understood nor even fully known. So, how will they be measured so that the relative availability of only partly understood capacities can be judged against the requirements made by the elusive and not always present demands? Figuring the interactions between the demands and the capacities requires measuring one or several of each and then getting them on some common scale. But how will the ratio be determined if we cannot measure the demands and the capacities separately? And, how does the changing ratio account for their observed interaction? In the clinical, theoretical, and research literature on stuttering, the judgment of the ratio of demands to capacities is actually assessed, for the most part, by whether or not stuttering tends to increase or decrease. The inference to the relative strength of demands and capacities is based on the observed occurrence or lack of it of stuttering.

Demand factors include the complexity of the subject(s) under discussion in any given speaking context: How many people are involved? How active is each one in competing for the floor (so to speak)? Where is the interaction taking place—at home in the kitchen or before an intimidating audience in a formal setting? How well do we know our interlocutor(s), the subject, the language we are using? How much time do we have to get our point across? And so on and so forth. These factors and a host of others contribute to the "demands" element in the demands and capacities model.

We find similar complexity on the capacities side. What capacities are involved and how do we measure them? There are sensory capacities, motor abilities and skills, and language skills of various kinds. Across and within the various systems, as we have seen in earlier chapters, there are rankings, layering, and interactions. Also, each of the separate systems can be broken down into subsystems. For all of these reasons, just how the demands and capacities interact remains to be worked out. What is needed is a more detailed theory of normal speech and language development, and a better understanding of how the processes of speech perception and production develop over time. In other words, how does speech unfold in the short term, say, from a single second or less to a 30-second sound-bite and how do the capacities to generate a fluent sound-bite develop over the long term, say, from conception to maturity or during any given span of weeks or months in between?

Assessing the Severity of Stuttering

Severity of stuttering has generally been measured by comparing the number of stuttered words or syllables to the total number of spoken words or syllables. Such a comparison yields a proportion or percentage, say, of stuttered units. Although estimates vary, most authorities put the threshold for "stuttered" speech some-where between 3% to 10% of the total number of speech events of a given kind (Guitar, 2006; F. H. Silverman, 2004). This is because of the fact that fluent individuals are apt to produce borderline dis-fluencies. These are sufficient to classify nonstutterers on existing subjective scales as "mild" stutterers (Yaruss, 2006). Because of this finding and other failings of such scales, their validity has been challenged (Franic & Bothe, 2008). Typically, a language sample is collected through some elicitation procedure such as picture description, retelling a story, counting backward from 100, reading a list of words, repeating words, phrases, or sentences, reading a paragraph aloud, participating in an interview, or some combina-tion of tasks such as one or several of these.

The third edition of the *Stuttering Severity Instrument* (*SSI*) is probably the best example of the types of measures that have been applied. In the case of the language sample, first a transcript of the patient's speech is drawn up, or at the very least a total word count. Next, the total number of single sounds, syllables, and word repe-titions, as well as the number of hesitations, prolongations (drawing out of a sound), and blocks (stoppage of sound production and often airflow as well) are added up. This total is then used to com-pute a **stuttering severity index**. However, this process is not as straightforward as it sounds.

Although on the surface, the methodology appears sound, questions have been raised about its reliability and more impor-tantly its validity. Roger Ingham and his colleagues have questioned the reliability of the proportion of stuttered syllables to total sylla-bles (Cordes, 1994, 2000; Cordes & Ingham 1995a, 1995b; Ingham & Cordes, 1992). They showed that **inter-rater reliability**—a mea-sure of the degree of agreement between two or more judges—on measures that require counting of instances is often quite low. This is particularly so when the raters come from different geo-graphic locations or more importantly when they were trained at different universities or clinics. The main question is what counts as a stuttering event. The call may seem simple. It seems easy enough to say that any marked repetition, hesitation, prolongation, or block should count as a stutter. The problem, however, is that

The only behavior that actually looks and sounds significantly different from most ordinary disfluencies is a block, and usually a block only looks different from an ordinary hesitation if it is accompanied by what are called **secondary behaviors**, which include grimacing, teeth clenching, and the like.

people who do not stutter sometimes repeat sounds, syllables, words, phrases, or sometimes hesitate or prolong a sound, so that it becomes difficult to say whether any given instance is stuttering or just an ordinary disfluency.

Ingham and Cordes (1992) demonstrated that even trained professionals have difficulty distinguishing an abnormal dysfluency and an ordinary hesitation (also, Franic & Bothe, 2008). W. H. Perkins (1990) showed that even the person speaking—the person doing the stuttering or hesitating—may have difficulty separating their own stutters from stuttering-like disfluencies. The upshot of this discussion is that even experienced judges—including persons who stutter and professionals who treat stuttering—do not agree with each other or even with their own prior judgments in some cases when it comes to singling out particular instances of abnormal stuttering as contrasted with ordinary run-of-the-mill disfluencies.

A related question that complicates the situation is how to count repetitions. For example, is "b-b-b-butter" a single stutter or four? Most authorities (Guitar, 2006; F. H. Silverman, 2004; Wingate, 1964) would count it as a single stutter. However, it seems transparently true that a prolonged staccato stutter such as "b-b-b-b-b-b-butter" is more distracting than a much shorter "b-butter." To this end, Cordes and Ingham (1999) proposed a method for measuring stuttering severity which involves dividing a recording into 3 to 5-second intervals, and then labeling those intervals as containing a stuttered speech event or not. They claim to have achieved higher levels of interrater reliability as well as **intra-rater reliability**—agreement across distinct events judged repeatedly by the same rater on different occasions—with this method. The question for any given segment is whether it contains a stuttering event or not. The problem of counting all individual instances within any 3 to 5-second segment is thus removed.

The Deeper Validity Issue

Whenever a measure has limited reliability, it is necessary to question its validity as well. This is essential because a completely unreliable measure cannot achieve any validity at all. Sometimes researchers suppose that there is a tradeoff between reliability and validity such that more of one means less of the other. That is not true. Low reliability necessarily (and always) means low validity at best and as reliability approaches zero, validity also vanishes. But validity requires more than mere reliability. It is possible for a measure to give the same results on different occasions and still for it to be completely invalid, inappropriate, and useless for the purposes to which it is applied. Many examples of widely used but invalid measures can be found in the so-called "scientific" literature. For instance, in the speech sciences it is possible to get very accurate measures of syllable length, voice volume, fundamental voice frequency, and many other phenomena, but the applications of such measures to the basic phenomena of stuttering may be about as relevant as highly accurate measurements of shoe-size and hair length are to the assessment of human intellect. The validity question absolutely transcends and supercedes the reliability question.

The validity question absolutely transcends and supercedes the reliability question.

What to Measure: Events or Fears

To the extent that validity in measurement is achieved, it requires that the measure actually be a measure of whatever it is supposed to be measuring. Like a distant echo of Dr. Schneider's sentiment about the pain of "feeling different," Manning (1996, in a panel discussion retrieved March 5, 2009, from http://www.mnsu.edu/comdis/voices/voices.html) has argued that counting stuttering-like disfluencies (or measuring their surface properties) neglects the greater part of the stuttering pathology. Kalinowski and Saltuklaroglu (2006) argue that the stuttering events themselves are only about 20% of the problem. Stuttering events come and go, sometimes they are more frequent, sometimes less, but the fear that stuttering can happen at anytime is always there.

Jezer (1997) writes about fluent and nonfluent times throughout his life in several places in his book. A young man quoted by DiLollo, Manning, and Neimeyer (2003) put it like this: "Okay, so when is this gonna all come falling down on me? Okay, when am I gonna? I always knew that my speech pattern would get worse and would, you know, begin to struggle again eventually. So I was sort of waiting for, you know. I still have the fears . . . I knew eventually that my fluent day or my fluent time of speaking was going to be over soon" (p 178).

The validity and reliability issues in the counting or measurement of stuttering events also make it difficult to tell when a given therapy is helping or not. One of the problems is how to separate variability in the disorder from changes brought about by the therapy? Another problem is that reduction in the number of stuttering events may even be accompanied by an increase in the anxiety about the possibility of stuttering at any moment. Is a therapy that has this result effective or not? Counting stuttering events may give the appearance of improvement owed to the therapy when, in fact, the number of stuttering events is merely owed to fluctuation that would have occurred without the therapy.

More importantly, the greatest reservation about counting stuttering events is that these events only represent the aspect of the disorder that is noticeable by someone other than the person who stutters. The observable surface events—those that can be perceived by persons other than the stutterer—only represent part of the picture. Recalling the World Health Organization criteria for stuttering, it is important to keep in mind that its outward manifestations in visible and audible attempts at speaking do not tell the whole story. How the speaker feels about these events, or the possibility of their occurrence, and how listeners react must also be taken into consideration. For these reasons, various attitudinal scales have been developed along with assessment procedures. A good resource along this line is *Clinical Decision Making in Fluency Disorders* (Manning, 2004).

TREATMENT OF STUTTERING

The treatment of stuttering has commonly been differentiated both by the age and maturity of the persons treated, and by where the treatment approach focuses attention. The main distinction in therapies has to do with the age of the stutterers—children being contrasted with adolescents and adults—and the secondary distinction has to do with where attention is focused in the therapy itself—whether on instances of stuttering or on instances of relatively fluent speech.

Common and Different Elements

Generally, adults who stutter are treated differently than children because the children have not yet experienced the full impact of long-term stuttering.

To some extent, the therapies in all cases are similar. All of them are concerned with distinguishing fluent speech from stuttering, and all are concerned with enhancing the speaker's ability to achieve fluency and to escape the undesirable emotional and other consequences of long-term involuntary stuttering.

Early stuttering in children, according to (Ambrose & Yairi, 1999; Bloodstein, 1960, 1974; W. Johnson & Associates, 1959), mainly involves involuntary hesitations on whole words. According to their claims, if incipient stuttering sets in as the child matures and progresses into adulthood, the stuttering may increasingly involve false starts and pauses at major linguistic boundaries—for instance, between syllables, words, phrases, and clause structures.

However, theoretically well-informed linguistic studies of stuttering at any age are largely missing from the literature. Most of the studies have been done by clinicians trained by other clinicians—per the requirements of the American Speech-Language and Hearing Association's approach to certification and licensing. The fact that clinicians tend to rely on clinical experience and to depend on other clinicians more than anything else is suggested by the subtitle of Yairi and Ambrose (2005) concerning early childhood stuttering: *For Clinicians by Clinicians*. As a result of such thinking, studies of stuttering phenomena that are deeply informed by linguistic theory and by general theoretical semiotics have yet to be carried out.

The existing work by clinicians and those who train them is heavily influenced by attention to surface forms as is encouraged by the ASHA curriculum and standards for training and licensing of speech-language pathologists. However, the work of individuals such as Snyder (2006) suggests that deeper and more powerful approaches to the study of stuttering phenomena are underway. This is healthy for the theoretical side as well as the practical. Clinicians have much to contribute to the testing and improvement of existing theories and to new theory-building. For the interdisciplinary impact to occur, however, it is essential, as ASHA has often noted, for clinicians, researchers, and theoreticians to interact (see the article on "Cross-Talking" by Jeanette Hoit, 2006, p. 102), Editor of the *American Journal of Speech-Language Pathology*. She affirms that

> Speech-language pathology seems to be a natural partner in research endeavors that call for the collaboration of scientists from a variety of different disciplines. Fortunately, many successful examples of interdisciplinary collaboration can be found in our scientific community, and the importance of such collaboration is recognized by the American Speech Language Hearing Association. (retrieved March 6, 2009, from http://www.asha.org/members/phd-faculty-research/interdis-collab/module1)

Secondary Behaviors

Over time children who stutter may become adolescents and are more and more apt to be impacted by the long-term effects of stuttering. As a result, adolescents and adults tend to be affected by what are termed *secondary behaviors*—sometimes referred to merely as **secondaries** in the literature. Secondaries are concomitant behaviors—usually distracting and ineffective as means of communication—that occur during or just prior to a stuttering event. They may include facial grimaces, repeated and sometimes prolonged eye blinks, foot stomping, tongue extrusion, teeth clenching, balling up of the fists, or any action that the speaker may stumble upon either intentionally or unintentionally in trying to get the words out. Secondaries are generally judged to be ineffective attempts to compensate for, prevent, or halt a stuttering event. As a result, they tend to come to be habitually associated with stuttering events. Secondaries are common in adolescent and adult stutterers and are accompanied by and possibly caused by emotional reactions that are not entirely observable. Childhood stuttering tends not to manifest these secondaries, presumably because children who stutter are not yet so keenly aware of the impact that stuttering has on others and they have not yet become fully aware of the social stigma that may be associated with stuttering.

Secondaries are concomitant behaviors—usually distracting and ineffective as means of communication—that occur during or just prior to a stuttering event.

An interesting study by Bajaj (2007) made a systematic comparison of 22 children with stuttering (CWS) against 22 fluent peers in kindergarten through second grade on "morphological, syntactic, and narrative abilities" but found that CWS group "did not differ significantly from their typically fluent peers" (p. 227). Evidently, it takes some time and socialization before really significant differences can appear in children who stutter. It seems that it is only after some awareness of the social stigma associated with stuttering settles in that secondary behaviors tend to appear and instead of reducing the social stigma of stuttering, they tend to make it more severe.

Early Intervention

It seems to be almost universally agreed that early intervention is desirable in most communication disorders if not all because the treatment of children is simpler than treatment of adolescents or adults and because earlier treatment is expected to be more successful.

Especially for the reasons given in the preceding section, early intervention in stuttering is probably best just so long as the intervention *does not increase the stigma of stuttering and promote the development of secondary behaviors*. On the one hand, an argument for avoiding early intervention in stuttering is the possibility that the therapy itself may tend to promote undue attention to the stuttering events and thus potentially increase the likelihood of causing incipient stuttering to develop along with undesirable and distracting secondary behaviors.

The fact that early treatment is generally considered to be more effective, on the other hand, is not only expected on account of the fact that secondary behaviors are theoretically and empirically later developments but because early treatment takes advantage of the normal direction of growth and development. The sooner the difficulty is detected, the easier it will be to correct it and forestall its potential long-term consequences. It is easier in general to shape the linguistic behaviors of children on account of the fact that children have not yet achieved all the complexities of adult communication behaviors. Therefore, it should not surprise us that therapies for children who stutter are generally judged to be more successful and are somewhat less complex than therapies for adults. This, of course, is not to say that the phenomena of stuttering are ever simple. They are not simple at any age.

The main reason that early intervention is apt to be more effective is precisely because development over time provides advantages to the therapy. Some have argued that it also makes measurement of effects owed to therapy difficult to distinguish from effects owed to normal growth and development of the child. Of course, this is true, but such a difficulty of measurement is not an argument against early intervention. The main effect and advantage of early intervention is like swimming faster when going with the current, or running with a good strong wind to your back. Development over time, as we have already noted, often results in improvements that may or may not be caused by therapy. On the other hand, if the goal is to enable the child to get downstream as efficiently as possible, why not take advantage of the current of normal growth and development that is already flowing in that direction? Early intervention makes all the more sense and is all the more reasonable when we take account of the fact that it gives therapy a leg up. If our goal is to help children succeed as communicators, why would we not use every reasonable advantage to achieve this goal?

Treatment of Children

One of the best known, and reportedly one of the most successful programs for treating young children who stutter (see Bernstein & Tetnowski, 2006) is the *Lidcombe Program* developed primarily by Mark Onslow and his colleagues (Lewis, Packman, Onslow, Simpson, & M. Jones, 2008; Onslow, Costa, & Rue, 1990). This program gets its name from a suburb of Sydney, Australia where it was developed. Because of it known successes, the Lidcombe Program has been widely adopted as the therapy of choice for children (Guitar, 2006; Kalinowski & Saltuklaroglu, 2006).

Operant Conditioning

At its basis, the Lidcombe Program relies on the behavioral theory of B. F. Skinner (1957) and more particularly on his theory of operant conditioning. According to Skinnerian theory, in the case of the Lidcombe Program for stuttering therapy, if desired behaviors which consist of fluent speech events are rewarded whenever they occur, and undesired behaviors which consist of stuttering events are either not rewarded, on account of the fact that involuntary stuttering is itself a punishing experience, fluency should increase and stuttering events should tend to disappear. As fluency is reinforced, its likelihood should increase, while as stuttering events are intrinsically punishing events, they will tend, in Skinner's terminology, toward extinction. They will diminish toward a limit of not occurring at all.

> According to Skinnerian theory, in the case of the Lidcombe Program for stuttering therapy, if desired behaviors which consist of fluent speech events are rewarded whenever they occur, and undesired behaviors which consist of stuttering events are either not rewarded, on account of the fact that involuntary stuttering is itself a punishing experience, fluency should increase and stuttering events should tend to disappear.

The Primary Caregiver as Therapist

In addition, the Lidcombe Program trains the primary caregiver(s) to take over the role of an on site clinician for the child who stutters. The caregiver is trained by a qualified clinician to recognize disfluencies (unambiguous stutters), to model slower fluent speech, and to reward spontaneous fluent speech. Caregivers are also instructed to address the level of the child's conversational development. This means avoiding overly complex subjects and ideas that are beyond the child's understanding. They are instructed to allow the child time to respond to questions and to provide comments that encourage the child to talk more about whatever may be the current conversational topic. The caregiver is to value what the child says and never to dismiss it as irrelevant, or childish. For every negative reinforcement the care giver should provide five positive reinforcements. In short, caregivers are trained to be desirable conversational partners. Finally, to accomplish these objectives the Lidcombe Program requires that caregivers spend at least 5 to 30 minutes every day in conversation with the child.

To ensure validity of judgments about progress, throughout the therapy, stuttering assessments are always made by at least two individuals. This usually consists of the primary care giver (usually one of the child's parents) and the qualified clinician. The evaluation of improvement is done by counting stuttering events and also considering ratings of fluency. To determine just which aspects of the program were having an impact, Harrison, Onslow, and Menzies (2004) proposed a research paradigm that could determine the relative contribution of each aspect. In their preliminary investigation, they measured the reduction of percent of stuttered syllables as the dependent variable. They found that parental reinforcement of fluent speech reduced the percent of stuttered syllables more than it reduced parent ratings of stuttering. Could the actual impact of positive reinforcements on stuttering events have been greater than the parents themselves were able to realize? Or did parents have more difficulty than expected in distinguishing fluent performances from dysfluent ones? Another question bound to come up was whether the Lidcombe Program resulted in greater improvements than could have been achieved without intervention or by some other program, say, one without parental involvement?

Critical Examination of Lidcombe

With those questions in mind, it is unsurprising that the Lidcombe program has been critically examined by researchers. Kalinowsk and Saltuklaroglu (2006) have argued that the recovery rate for the Lidcombe program, at about 80%, is not very different from the observed spontaneous recovery rate without any treatment at all, which is also about 80%. The underlying question is whether there is a significant difference in the spontaneous rate when carefully contrasted with the rate observed in the Lidcombe Program for a substantial number of comparable individuals. Operant conditioning, as applied in the Lidcombe Program, is not the only strategy at issue. The Lidcombe Program also relies on two other commonly used treatment strategies for reducing stuttering. These are (1) slowing down the rate of speaking and (2) reducing the complexity of utterances. With that in mind, the deeper question for contrasts between distinct methods is whether the Lidcombe Program would have its effect without the operant conditioning component? Would it have its effect without the slowing of speech? Or without reducing the complexity of speech? All these questions are difficult if not intractable on account of the seemingly unsolvable problems of finding comparable participants across different treatment programs.

Those difficulties aside, other therapies that include caregivers as part of the treatment based on the demands and capacities model, for instance, report success rates indistinguishable from those of the Lidcombe Program. Franken, Kielstra-Van der Schalka, and Boelens (2005) made such a comparison, and found no differences between the two approaches. The remaining question is whether the failure to find any differences was because the approaches are equally successful or because neither of them actually produces a result different from what would be expected without any treatment at all.

In answer to criticisms voiced against Lidcombe, it has been countered that it also improves overall behavior (Woods, Shearsby, Onslow, & Burnham, 2002), achieves significant success in less than 12 weeks (Kingston, Huber, Onslow, M. Jones, & Packman, 2003; an outcome also claimed for a demands and capacities model by Franken et al., 2005), and despite reducing the complexity of language inputs results in increased complexity of speech along with fewer disfluencies (Lattermann, Shenker, & Thordardottir, 2005). Of course, it is to be expected that the complexity of utterances produced by children will normally increase as they grow older irrespective of any therapeutic intervention. So the controversy over which program to choose, or which therapy is most likely to produce the desired outcomes, remains unresolved.

HOW IMPORTANT IS SURFACE FORM?

A Caveat for Therapy

One thing that can be said for sure, based on both theory and research about language use and acquisition is that programs of treatment for stuttering or other communication disorders need to keep in mind that the surface forms of speech serve the purpose of meaningful communication. It is common in stuttering therapy, however, to direct attention toward surface forms to the extent that they become an end in themselves while the deeper meaning and fundamental purpose of communication may be obscured or sometimes lost altogether. This result is like making the process of road construction more important than, say, the roads and bridges themselves.

Communication through language serves to enable connections between people. If stringing sounds and syllables together in a stream of fluent speech becomes an end in itself, it is like making the preparation of a meal more important than the enjoyment, nourishment, and satisfaction of the people who will consume it. Tools are perfected for their uses. Fluent speech is desirable and important only to the extent that it serves the purpose of meaningful communication and enabling desirable and useful relationships between people. Speech therapy can often result in an interesting shift of attention to qualities of surface forms that make them the main purpose for speaking. This is especially evident in stuttering interventions where it is possible to create bigger problems than we are trying to solve. The tendency for stutterers and even sometimes for experts in the treatment of stuttering to develop distracting secondary behaviors such as grimacing, teeth clenching, foot stomping, and so on shows that excessive concern with surface forms is obviously and by a long shot the most pathological aspect of dysfluent speech in adults.

Developing Social Concern

A recent study by Bajaj, Hodson, and Westby (2005) showed that children who stutter at ages 5 and 6, ones who have been exposed to some socialization and perhaps informal intervention by their teachers and to more or less intensive therapy in some cases, are already in the process of developing a greater interest in surface forms of speech than their fluent peers have. In fact, children with stuttering in the study in question demonstrated that they have already developed a fundamentally different concept of what constitutes a good communication partner than their "fluent" peers.

> Bajaj, Hodson, and Westby (2005) found that the children with stuttering tended to define good speakers as ones who use "turtle talk"—a learned term for speaking slowly—and who do not "trip over their words." These and related descriptors were used by children who stutter as contrasted with fluent non-stuttering peers who tended to define good speakers as kids who were funny, honest, and nice. The nonstutterers tended to put the emphasis on relationships, truthfulness, and cooperativeness rather than on surface forms of speech.

Although Bajaj (2007) found that the 22 children with stuttering did not differ significantly from 22 fluent peers in the language abilities measured, the qualitative analysis of narratives written by the two groups showed one contrast that we believe is especially revealing. Bajaj, Hodson, and Westby (2005) found that the children with stuttering tended to define good speakers as ones who use "turtle talk"—a learned term for speaking slowly—and who do not "trip over their words." These and related descriptors were used by children who stutter as contrasted with fluent non-stuttering peers who tended to define good speakers as kids who were funny, honest, and nice. The non-stutterers tended to put the emphasis on relationships, truthfulness, and cooperativeness rather than on surface forms of speech. The children with stuttering, on the other hand, had been socially trained to regard a "good talker" in terms of the rate of speech and the avoidance of stuttering.

Keeping Meaning in Mind

The implication of this research—especially in the light of what we already know about secondary behaviors—is that the natural focus on meaning and the deeper purposes of communication is being shifted to the speech forms through which communication of meaning is achieved. Also, it is evident that this shift is largely because of the social reactions to stuttering, including whatever therapy or intervention is being attempted by parents, teachers, and others. In light of the vast research literature in **discourse processing**, first language acquisition and second language teaching shows plainly that successful communication depends in the final analysis on the accessibility of meaning.

No doubt the idea of "turtle talk" can be a good thing and a step toward effective communication. However, in Chapter 4 especially, and throughout this book, we see evidence from experimental research and from sound theory that surface forms of speech normally play a subordinate role. The McGurk interactions show that meaning is the highest ranking and most powerful system in guiding communication. Similarly, the dramatic effect of delayed auditory feedback in causing artificial stuttering shows that directing attention to surface form in an unnatural way can be the cause of certain kinds of stuttering. For all these reasons, therapies and interventions that deal with the surface forms of stuttering are especially prone to promoting some of the very behaviors they seek to prevent.

When the focus shifts entirely or primarily to surface forms, the results can be the opposite of what we are hoping and trying to achieve. We can teach children to sound out letters in a way that prevents them from understanding the story they are reading (see the discussion of "instructional dyslexia" in Chapter 9). We can teach a child who stutters to focus on the surface forms of speech— for example, through "turtle talk" or other surface changes—to such an extent that the child may commonly lose track of any meaning that might have been in view at the beginning of the turtle talking. The rational deterrent, if there is one, to early intervention in developmental stuttering by children is the evidently real possibility that sufficient focus on the stuttering events themselves may even precipitate the development of secondaries and/or possibly encourage the persistent variety of developmental stuttering.

It is essential, therefore, in any therapy, to keep the underlying purposes of communication in mind. All efforts in stuttering intervention, or for any communication disorder, at the end of the day, should serve the purposes of effective communication. Ineffective secondary behaviors such as grimacing, teeth grinding, foot stomping, and the like are extreme examples of behaviors that evidently arise as natural, though undesirable and unproductive outcomes, of focusing attention on the surface forms of stuttering events. When that occurs, the stuttering itself disrupts and even takes over the whole of the discourse effort. In the meantime, the meaning and the desired relationships can be tragically lost and the secondaries themselves inevitably become obstacles rather than paths to effective communication.

Surface forms either serve the purposes of meaning or no purpose at all.

The therapy must not make the production of fluent surface forms so important that the "turtle talk," or whatever, becomes the end in itself or the primary focus of social attention. There is a genuine danger that therapies themselves can help to create additional problems rather than solving the ones they are aimed at alleviating.

TREATMENT FOR ADULTS AND ADOLESCENTS

The most commonly employed approaches to stuttering treatment for adolescents and adults usually focus at first, and sometimes almost exclusively, on stuttered speech forms. In the sections that follow we deal with several such procedures. One of the most commonly used approaches undertakes the task of changing the stuttering behavior into fluent speech and another approach that begins with the stuttered forms aims to get control of them by stuttering on demand. These are very different approaches in spite of the fact that these, along with various others, share the emphasis on gaining control of the surface forms of stuttering—one approach aims to gradually change the stuttered forms into fluent speech and the other seeks control of the stuttered speech in order to "stutter more fluently."

Fluency First, Naturalness Later

In the approach called **fluency shaping**, the objective is first to gain control of the speech signal by changing or distorting it in some way. For instance, shaping may involve streeeetchiiiing iiiiit ooooouuuut into very long syllables, and then, later, gradually speeding up this distorted "fluent speech" to make it sound more normal. The objective is to enable fluency by first removing or reducing the stuttering as much as possible and then gradually reshaping the fluent surface forms to get them to sound natural. The theory is that this can be done in gentle steps while retaining the fluency achieved by whatever means may work. The presumption is that naturalness can be achieved after the surface stuttering is removed.

> With fluency shaping the idea is to start with distorted fluent speech and remove the distortion. In the case of stuttering modification the idea is to gain voluntary control over stuttering (regarded as a distorted form of fluent speech) and then make it more fluent through voluntary adjustments.

A somewhat different approach is **stuttering modification**. It involves gaining conscious control by stuttering on purpose. The idea is that a person who stutters intentionally will be able to gradually modify the stuttering itself to make it more fluent.

Theoretically, it is possible to use both of these approaches simultaneously, or in some combination, in a program of therapy. Both of these approaches and variations on both themes attend primarily to the production of surface forms of stuttering.

Beneath the Surface

With adolescents and adults (as with children), in addition to dealing with stuttering events as such, the clinician must keep the meaning, emotions, and background consequences of stuttering and therapies into account. With adults who may have developed secondary behaviors and related disabilities or handicaps, this aspect of therapy may be the more important part. In many cases, the most successful therapies seem to focus on the secondaries more than on the "primary" more superficial stuttering behaviors. Kalinowski and Saltuklaroglu (2006) argue that the secondary behaviors and associated disabilities and handicaps are 80% of the disorder while the stuttering itself accounts for only about 20% of the disorder. They argue that persons who stutter have learned much about how to survive, and because of the shame and stigma associated with stuttering, they have learned subtle ways to hide and avoid revealing themselves.

Skillful Avoidance

It is not unusual for the original fluency breaks to be so well-disguised that their stuttering behavior is not apparent even to sophisticated listeners" (Manning, 2004, p. 268). Peter Ramig (2002, p. 259; hear him in a 1996 recording him retrieved March 5, 2009, from http://www.mnsu.edu/comdis/voices/voices.html), for instance, tells how he ended up as a marine in Vietnam because he "danced" around his stuttering "by avoiding words and circumlocuting, creating the misperception that I was a fairly fluent speaker" which, according to the interviewing physician showed he was well-suited for the military. If he had revealed the full extent of the disorder, he would have been released from the draft because, as Ramig reported, the psychiatrist said, "Son, stuttering is a very good reason to avoid the military."

Walter Manning (1996) tells in his own personal story that he was rejected as a volunteer for military service on account of his stuttering (retrieved March 6, 2009, from http://www.mnsu.edu/comdis/voices/voices.html). The fact is that the surface forms of stuttering can be controlled to a very great extent while the real problem remains beneath the surface. We need to keep this fact in mind as we consider the therapeutic approaches to changing and/or controlling stuttering events.

Fluency Shaping

Fluency shaping involves beginning with facilitating contexts such as speaking in rhythm with the tick tock of a clock or a metronome and/or just deliberately slowing the rate of speech. These are two of the most common techniques leading in to a fluency shaping approach. Another technique is to make "soft contact" between articulators. Instead of a hard sounding "d-" on "dog," the speaker would be instructed to touch the tongue to the gum ridge lightly in producing the "d-" and the clinician might demonstrate the "soft contact." Another technique is to initiate words with breathy "h-" after each pause in speaking or before making any new articulatory gesture at the beginning of an utterance. Still another whole class of techniques it to introduce an accent, speak in a monotone, raise or lower the pitch, and so on. Once the client is able to speak fluently using one or more of these techniques, the speech can then be "shaped" to sound more normal. That is, the rate of speech can be gradually increased in small steps, normal prosody can be reincorporated, and so on.

However, the "fluent" speech does not sound normal. Try this experiment. Clap your hands (or tap a pencil) at a rate of about twice per second (120 beats per minute), or slower, and read this sentence saying one syllable with each clap of your hands.

> ## Strange Speech Forms
>
> Click here to listen to a <u>Fluency Shaping</u> example on the DVD of the sort of speech that might be produced where each syllable is spoken at a given rate and with nearly the same pitch and stress as every other syllable. Does the speech produced by this method sound natural to you? Probably not, because that is not a normal way to produce speech. Most people speak at a rate of 130 to 200 words per minute (Arons, September 1992) though super-fast-talkers like John Moschitta (2009, retrieved March 5, 2009, from <u>http://www.videosift.com/video/Worlds-Fastest-Talker-John-Moschitta</u>) and Fran Capo (May 7, 2008, retrieved March 5, 2009, from <u>http://www.youtube.com/watch?v=aZb6iBmHqkY</u>) achieve rates up to about 3.5 times the middling average.

*Speech sounds odd when each syllable is given equal weight and when it is spoken on a **monotone**. The oddity does not go away just because the speech presented in these strange ways may be intelligible. It can be intelligible and still be very strange.*

Also, at least in English, not every syllable (much less every sound segment) is of the same length, nor does each syllable receive equal stress. Neither are syllables typically produced on the same pitch. The variability of pitch, timing, and stress together are called *prosody*. When the prosody is changed, the speech is harder to understand and in some cases may not even be recognizable. John Moschitta and Fran Capo, for instance (listen to them on the links in the preceding paragraph), are difficult to understand when they are speaking at their fastest rates. Notice that their prosody is less variable than in speech produced at a normal rate. Also, check out the exercise showing the importance of <u>Stress Placement</u> on the DVD. In that exercise, common English words are read first with stress placed on a syllable that is not usually stressed. See if you can recognize the words in list one. Compare them with the same words in list two. Isn't the second list easier to understand? A favorite line is, "You're putting the em-PHA-sis on the wrong syl-LAB-le."

For these reasons, the major complaint against fluency shaping is that speakers who use this class of techniques sound as though they are droning or chanting, but not actually speaking. In fact, Kalinowski and Saltuklaroglu (2006) argue that most listeners prefer listening to stuttered "normal" speech than to "fluent" slow speech that has been drained of its prosodic information.

Stuttering Modification

At the basis of stuttering modification therapies is the objective of gaining voluntary control of stuttering events. The key component of most definitions of stuttering is that the disfluencies result from a loss of voluntary control on the part of the speaker. So, some clinicians have supposed that even if speakers cannot control *when* they are going to stutter, perhaps they can control *how* they stutter when stuttering events occur and they can thus gain some voluntary control over the stuttering process. It is a kind of "if you can't beat 'em, join 'em" strategy. The Van Riper (1973) method is the best known and most definitive of the class of stuttering modification therapies.

Charles Van Riper is not only one of the first practitioners, some say he is "the founding father," of the field of **speech-language pathology**. Minnesota State University has preserved a classic recording of Dr. Van Riper from 1957 (retrieved March 6, 2009, from http://www.mnsu.edu/comdis/voices/voices.html). Certainly, his work on stuttering is still widely cited as a landmark approach to stuttering therapies. The Van Riper method (1973) is a hierarchal system that involves first training the speaker to "cancel" a stutter, "pull-out" of a stutter, and finally to engage in a series of "preparatory-set" behaviors that will prevent a stutter from taking place.

The **cancellation** is used during the middle of a stutter. The speaker is instructed to stop speaking, think about what happened, and then try again. This action is always a negative reinforcement (punishment) tending to reduce the likelihood of further stuttering. The goal in this step, however, is not to eliminate stuttering, but to restart stuttering on one's own terms. The control achieved by this action is reinforcing in a positive way because it leads to sounds coming on the speaker's own terms.

The **pull-out** is the next technique taught. Like the name implies, the speaker is instructed to recover during the middle of a stutter by using some variation on changing the rhythm of the stutter (for example b-b-bat would become b–b–b–b-bat) prolonging the stutter and deliberately repeating certain sounds. Once again, the emphasis is not on eliminating or preventing the stutter from occurring, but gaining voluntary control of the stuttering.

Van Riper says, "Take control of the stutter and never do it the same way twice" (van Riper, 1991, retrieved March 5, 2009, from http://www.mnsu.edu/comdis/isad7/papers/bridgebuilders7/vanriper7.html).

In another venue in 1957, Dr. Van Riper told how he stuttered so badly in his teenage years that one summer he pretended to be a deaf-mute so that he would not be expected to speak. He worked as a farm laborer that way, but was miserable. Finally, he decided to go home even though he was, in his own thinking, not wanted there. Along the way, he stopped to rest under a tree where a farmer was plowing a field. Later a man came along in an old car and stopped to talk with the farmer. Van Riper noticed that the old man had a funny way of speaking and wondered if he were a stutterer. He ended up hitching a ride with the old man and stuttered uncontrollably when the man asked his name. The old man laughed and Charles became angry. He wrote:

> I could have killed him! Seeing my anger, he said, "Take it easy, son. Take it easy. I'm not laughing at your stuttering. I've been a stutterer all my life and I used to jump around and make faces like you do but I'm too old and tired to fight myself now so I just let the words leak out. And they do! [Hear a slightly different version of this story, Van Riper, 1957, retrieved March 6, 2009, from http://www.mnsu.edu/comdis/voices/voices.html]

The insight that came to Van Riper that day was that "that I should learn how to stutter." In fact, that insight defined the rest of the illustrious career of Charles Van Riper as a student of his own disorder. Late in his life as a theoretician and clinician, still a stutterer, he would nevertheless report that he had learned "how to stutter" so that "most of my listeners do not even recognize that I've stuttered when I do and I probably stutter as much now as I ever have but it's no big deal anymore." The key was "learning how to stutter," and gaining voluntary control over the involuntary phenomenon. Van Riper believed that by breaking up the patterns of the stuttering, he and his thousands of clients could stop "practicing" stuttering and start practicing fluency.

The Preparatory Set

The **preparatory set** is a more advanced technique that has speakers engage in behaviors that they know will lead to fluency even before the stutter occurs. These behaviors are not necessarily those found in the fluency shaping paradigm. They may also include techniques like stuttering on purpose before the expected stutter occurs. Barry Guitar (2006) has developed his own style of therapy based loosely on the Van Riper method, and Walter Manning (2004) argues that persons who stutter prefer stuttering modification methods over fluency shaping methods. However, stuttering modification has its detractors as well.

The two major complaints about stuttering modification therapies are that they are not as easy to implement as fluency shaping procedures—that is, it takes longer to achieve results—and the

An excellent study of voluntary stuttering is the dissertation by Heather Grossman (2008). She provides results from clinical and experimental approaches that encourage voluntary control of stuttering events.

stuttering behaviors, though brought under some voluntary control, are not eliminated. Once again, when considering that the loss of voluntary control is the most essential defining element of stuttered speech, and given that most people prefer stuttered speech over a monotonic droning, stuttering modification therapies may indeed seem a lot more appealing and reasonable over the long run just as Manning argues. They can also lead to something that shaping strategies give up on at the outset: voluntary control. Such control over stuttering events can evidently lead to a kind of self-acceptance that is liberating in itself. It certainly seemed to be for Charles Van Riper. He may not have overcome his stuttering entirely, but, his attitude was, so what. Everyone has difficulties to deal with. Van Riper's was stuttering and like the old man that gave him a lift that day, Charles Van Riper was able to come to terms with his disorder and to gain a good deal of control over it by learning how to stutter. In the talk by van Riper ("Voices: Past and Present: Charles Van Riper," 1957, retrieved March 6, 2009, from http://www.mnsu .edu/comdis/voices/voices.html) you can judge for yourself just what degree of fluency he achieved.

OTHER FLUENCY DISORDERS

Stuttering is not the only fluency disorder that is generally recognized in the literature. There are three others including **neurogenic stuttering**, **psychogenic stuttering**, and **cluttering**. We look at each of these in turn, briefly describing the major behaviors associated with each of them, and we also consider how they are differentiated from each other and from the more common varieties of stuttering that we have already discussed above.

Neurogenic Stuttering

Neurogenic stuttering is also often called **acquired neurogenic stuttering**. It is most different from developmental and incipient stuttering in its origin. Neurogenic stuttering is known to be caused by an injury to the brain. It can be caused by a physical blow to the head, by internal bruising of the brain caused by a sudden stop, by a chemical injury (that is by some kind of poisoning), or by a disease impacting the brain. The most common behaviors associated with neurogenic stuttering is repeating sounds, syllables, or words. Depending on the extent of the injury the individual may or may not be aware of the disfluencies that occur. Similarly, the prognosis for recovery depends on the extent of the injury.

Neurogenic stuttering can also be differentiated from developmental or incipient stuttering in several ways. The first is that developmental or incipient stuttering rarely manifests after ages 6 to 8, while neurogenic stuttering commonly has a much later time of onset. The neurogenic variety typically occurs in older children and more commonly in adults. Usually the brain insult associated with the onset of neurogenic stuttering can be determined after the fact or has been identified on or before the time of onset.

Another distinct feature of neurogenic stuttering is that most of the facilitating contexts that either increase or decrease stuttering behaviors in other cases seem to have little to no effect on persons with neurogenic stuttering. For instance, Balasubramanian, Max, Van Borsel, Rayca, and Richardson (2003) describe a case of a man with acquired neurogenic stuttering showed no advantage in fluency during choral reading nor with delayed feedback or frequency altered feedback. Because of such evidence, it is believed that the causes of developmental stuttering are fundamentally different not only in onset but also in kind from neurogenic stuttering.

Psychogenic Stuttering

Psychogenic stuttering is also sometimes called **acquired psychogenic stuttering**. Similar to neurogenic stuttering, it can begin in adulthood, but psychogenic stuttering is usually associated with a traumatic emotional event. In some cases the causal event may be known to the person experiencing the disorder. In other cases it may be inferred. The distinctness of stuttering of the psychogenic kind, however, is that it is caused by a psychological rather than a neurological trauma. The primary behaviors that are manifested in psychogenic stuttering, however, resemble those of neurogenic stuttering and have the same peculiarity: psychogenic stuttering like the neurogenic variety is less susceptible than developmental or incipient stuttering to the facilitating activities that normally work with other kinds of stuttering.

Cluttering

> The majority of disfluencies associated with cluttering seem to be the result of the excessively fast rate of speech, but see the videos (hyperlinked earlier in this chapter) showing superfast talkers Moschitta and Capo who do not seem to stutter at all.

Cluttering is a fluency disorder that is characterized by excessively fast speech, it is also called **tachyphemia**.

The majority of disfluencies associated with cluttering seem to be the result of the excessively fast rate of speech, but see the videos (hyperlinked earlier in this chapter) showing super-fast talkers Moschitta and Capo who do not seem to stutter at all. It is also interesting to note in passing that Winston Churchill, according to D. Weiss (1964, p. 58), was supposed to be a stutterer of the cluttering kind. However, the Churchill Center posts an article claiming that, in fact, he never stuttered at all though he did have a lisp (http://www.winstonchurchill.org/i4a/pages/index.cfm?page id=100 retrieved March 6, 2009).

Some argue that cluttering is more of a language processing disorder than a speech disorder (St. Louis, Raphael, Myers, & Bakker, 2003; St. Louis, Myers, Faragasso, Townsend, & Gallaher, 2004). The key difference between cluttering and stuttering, according to those who claim to be able to tell the difference, is that those who clutter are rarely aware of the disfluencies in their speech, while those who stutter usually notice when they produce disfluent speech (F. H. Silverman, 2004).

SUMMING UP AND LOOKING AHEAD

Stuttering is characterized by repetitions of sounds, syllables, words, and/or phrases, by hesitations, prolongations of sounds, and blocks. However, stuttering in adults also commonly includes secondary symptoms, such as grimacing and clenching, and very often involves a strong emotional component that can be even more debilitating than the disfluencies that may be evident (or not) at the surface during speech production. Assessment of stuttering by means of counting the number of stutters per 100 syllables, for example, is the most common method despite the fact that the rate of stutters per unit of speech is highly variable. The counting of stuttering events also does not take into consideration the strong emotional component especially impacting speakers and also, in many cases, their listeners. For these reasons, assessment should focus not merely on the speech itself, but on the overall communicative intentions, needs, and desires of the individual who stutters and of the persons with whom the stutterer typically interacts. Treatment options should emphasize communicative effectiveness in all respects—not just the surface forms of stuttered utterances. Finally, neurogenic stuttering, psychogenic stuttering, and cluttering (tachyphemia) must also be taken into consideration. Despite the core symptoms looking similar on the surface, the etiology of the latter varieties of dysfluency as well as their differential responsiveness to facilitation or inhibition mark these varieties as distinct from developmental stuttering and persistent developmental stuttering. In the following chapter, we move on to consider developmental and other disorders associated especially with the acquisition of literacy.

STUDY AND DISCUSSION QUESTIONS

1. What are some of the ways that individuals who stutter may compensate or cope with the disorder?

2. How much of the stuttering disorder is evident in stuttering events that a listener might observe? What aspects of the disorder are not observable by interlocutors of the person who stutters?

3. What is your reaction to cartoon characters like Porky Pig after reading this chapter? What is different, if anything, about your view of what stuttering is like from the inside out? What might be done in the early grades to enable children who are naturally fluent, nonstutterers, to be more accepting of other children who are possibly at risk of becoming persistent developmental stuttering? What about educating parents, teachers, pediatricians, and other caregivers about stuttering? What should the key objectives be, and how could they best be achieved?

4. Why is it important to take all three positions of discourse—producer(s), consumer(s), and the physical world—into account when dealing with stuttering? What peculiar elements must be considered for each one of these logical positions that may help us in understanding what stuttering is and in preventing, curing, or treating it?

5. What evidences are there that stuttering is affected by genetic factors? By the same token, how can you show that stuttering is not entirely genetic and that it involves learned behaviors in at least some cases and in some fairly common respects?

6. Have you experienced delayed auditory feedback in a setting that caused you to stutter? What about in the other "facilitating contexts" listed in this chapter? Which of them, if any, cause you to engage in a greater or lesser number of hesitation phenomena?

7. What is the difference between phoneme level and syllable level stuttering? Based on your own observations and experience with DAF, for instance, what examples of the distinct manifestations of stuttering at the phoneme and syllable level can you offer?

8. Why is counting stuttered events problematic as a measure of the severity of stuttering? For example, what aspects of the stuttering disorder can it measure and what aspects does it leave undiscovered? How does the widely used *Stuttering Severity Instrument* proposed by Yaruss compensate for the difficulty of counting individual stuttering events?

9. How do secondary behaviors help to reveal the emotional side of stuttering from the speaker's point of view and how might they also be influenced by listener reactions, or perceived/imagined reactions?

10. What are some of the advantages of early intervention? At the same time, why are some of the methods commonly used with adults and adolescents probably not appropriate with very young children? What, in particular, are the dangers of focusing too early or too intensely on instances of developmental stuttering, say, between ages 3 and 4?

11. If the basic findings claimed for Charles Van Riper's solution to the problem of persistent developmental (incipient) stuttering were applied to early childhood, developmental stuttering, what should be the proper attitude of peers, parents, teachers, and others to stuttering events? Contrast the implications of Van Riper's thinking with approaches that stress shaping paradigms, for example, "turtle talk." Where do very young children get the idea that stuttering is stigmatized?

12. What conclusions can be drawn about the etiology of developmental stuttering from neurogenic, psychogenic, and the "cluttering" variety of dysfluency? Why are choral reading effects, delayed auditory feedback effects, and frequency altered feedback effects probably important to our understanding of the causation of developmental and incipient stuttering?

9

Literacy and Dyslexia

OBJECTIVES

In this chapter, we:

1. Discuss and critique competing theories of literacy;
2. Consider why babies can begin to read as soon as they understand spoken or signed words;
3. Review definitions of dyslexia and related disorders;
4. Consider why literacy is primarily about meanings and intentions only superficially about surface forms of print or writing;
5. Demonstrate that reading involves the process of pragmatic mapping as illustrated by Helen Keller;
6. Contrast difficulties with surface form versus brain damage;
7. Review research showing that dyslexia responds best to attention to meaning;
8. Discuss research showing that literacy acquisition is like acquiring a second language; and
9. Consider the special problem of acquiring literacy in a second language/dialect.

KEY TERMS

Here are some key terms of this chapter. Many you may already know, but it may help to review them. These terms are explained in the text and they are defined in the Glossary at the end of the book. They appear in **bold print** on their first appearance in the text.

"acquired" disorders
acquired dyslexia
alexia
allophones
alphabetic principle
balanced bilingualism
canonical babble
chronological narrative order
cycle of abstraction
decoding
discrepancy approach
discriminated symbol
dysgraphia
epigenetic disorders
extrinsic factors
hypostasis
hypostatic symbols

intrinsic factors
jargon
language learning impaired
learning disability
literacy modality
LLI
meaningful sequence
negative inertia
neurolinguistics
onset
phonemic awareness
phones
phonetic transcription
phonics
phonological awareness
pragmatic isomorphism
prescinded symbol

prescinding
psycholinguistics
reading readiness
receptive repertoire
rime
semiotics
sensory aphasia
sequential (episodic)
    organization
sociolinguistics
speech to text
stroke
temporal integration
    threshold
trilingualism
variegated babble
word recognition

Is it true that the author of $E = mc^2$, the inventor of the lightbulb (Thomas Alva Edison), and the script writer that created the Rockford Files, Baretta, 21 Jump Street, and 40-plus TV series, not to mention his movies, DVDs, and 12 best-selling novels (Stephen J. Cannell), all shared the disorder of dyslexia? Is it also true that dyslexia enhanced their successes?

Was Einstein Dyslexic?

It is interesting that different experts think Albert Einstein had various disorders. Dyslexia was only one of them (for example, Berninger, 2000; also Cannell himself, "Dyslexia Videos, Article and Resources," 2006, retrieved March 5, 2009, from http://www.cannell.com/dyslexia.php). After his death in 1955, different experts diagnosed him with autism and/or Asperger syndrome (according to Simon-Baron Cohen in an interview with Muir, 2003), and probably ADHD (Elster, 2000). In "Young Stutterers Fight Prejudices," (2005, retrieved March 5, 2009, from http://www.dw-world.de/dw/episode/0,1569,1683498,00.html) he was listed along with Marilyn Monroe and Winston Churchill as a stutterer. Which of these stories, if any, are true?

Was Einstein dyslexic? It probably does not matter much whether he had any of the above disorders, but the description and diagnosis of any given case depends a great deal on the prior definition of the various disorders. So what exactly is dyslexia?

The published research on dyslexia is as uncertain as its definition. It is said to involve, "reversing letters and/or numbers," "inability to remember or understand sequences," "faulty short-term memory," and "not knowing left from right." It is said to be a "life-long condition," "a genetic condition," a special form of "brain damage," or a "developmental brain abnormality." These are some of the phrases you will hear in the story of Stephen J. Cannell about his life with dyslexia at "Dyslexia Videos, Article and Resources," (2006, retrieved March 6, 2009, from http://www.cannell.com/dyslexia.php). In this chapter you will also learn about a young girl whose parents were told that she was "hopelessly dyslexic." They should encourage her to "work with her hands." They consulted special education teachers, diagnosticians, speech-language pathologists, pediatricians, and several clinics. We will see how she overcame "dyslexia" after nine years of apparent failure to understand even a single printed word. How is it possible to go from a genetic form of permanent brain abnormality (e.g., Lyon, Shaywitz, & Shaywitz, 2003) to what appears to be normal literacy?

Is it possible to overcome a life-long genetic condition fairly suddenly by merely changing an instructional method? Along the way we deal with what literacy is, how it is like acquiring a first or second language, or a new way of representing one or both. We see that literacy can be acquired by children who are also acquiring the language in which they are learning to read and write. We present evidence (see Aleka Titzer on the DVD) that normal babies just beyond the milestone of **canonical babble** can learn to read and act out the meanings of printed words.

ACQUIRING LITERACY

Everyone who knows how to read and write is a kind of expert in the process. We all think we know how we did it. Those of us who were taught our ABCs either in public schools or by teachers who went to such schools, may have some very strong and deep-seated ideas about how we became the experts that we are. It is somewhat the same with our experience as language learners. All of us are experts to a high degree. There are no computer programs for language comprehension, for literacy, translation, paraphrasing, explaining texts, illustrating stories, or reporting narratives that can compete with a normal, ordinary, literate user of any human language. It is true that we are all experts, but how did we become this way? When did we start? Is it necessary to wait until school age to begin to acquire literacy? Should we wait even longer as some have pro-

In actual fact, the ordinary language user knows more about language than it has been possible for the professional experts to figure out.

By the middle of the baby's fifth month of life, usually he or she has already reached the zone of proximal development (ZPD) for discovering the surface forms of a vast range of spoken or manually signed symbols.

posed? What is the earliest and best time to begin to acquire literacy? What does the relevant research and theory actually show?

A Surprising Prediction About Reading Readiness

In our *Milestones* book (2006) we included a review of the research evidence showing that by the time babies begin to respond to their own name, by about 4.5 months (Werker & Tees, 1999) they are demonstrating the ability to distinguish its surface forms—its sounds, rhythms, intonations, and mouth shapes (see Kuhl Meltzoff, 1982; M. L. Patterson & Werker, 1999, 2003)—from all the other symbols that are being presented at different times by the persons that interact with the baby. The baby is, at that time, already cooing and gooing and beginning to form syllables and/or manual signs. For instance, the baby will use the pick-me-up gesture as an effective command.

Within a matter of days or weeks, the normally developing baby will reach another important milestone known as canonical babbling (D. K. Oller, 1975, 1980; Petitto & Marentette, 1991)—that is, babbling of the repetitive, rhythmic, syllabic kind that is often accompanied by hand banging or even clapping (Ejiri, 1998; Ejiri & Masataka, 2001). The babbling will typically become enriched, moving from repeated syllables, "bababa" to distinct syllables "badaga" and so on. This step marks the baby's normal progress in gaining motor control over the surface forms of speech.

Progress in Comprehending Language

Meanwhile, the baby is also making progress in the meaning department. By about the ninth month, give or take a month or so, the normally progressing baby will not only respond to his or her own name, but will also demonstrate comprehension of that name and quite a few other referring terms. The baby will show understanding, for instance, of the names of other persons by looking to them when their name is spoken by someone else. At this stage, the baby will also demonstrate by actions the answers to verbal questions about distinct persons, pets, or event/actions such as: "You want to go to Mama?" "Oh, you want to go to Dada?" "You want to come to Pop?" "Want to go bye-bye?" "Want me to pick you up?" "Want me to put you down?" "Where's Mama?" "Where's Dada?" "Where's Mimi?" "Where's Ashley?" "Can you give me the ball?" And so on.

If the baby can do the sorts of things just described, for example, by going to get an object that was talked about but that is not present, the baby is demonstrating comprehension of abstract linguistic signs. When the baby reaches this stage, it follows that the baby is ready to acquire printed signs—to begin reading words with comprehension.

This hypothesis is a necessary (logicomathematical) conclusion that flows directly from the theory of abstraction. The hypothesis in question also has the beauty of being both surprising and testable. And, as we will see from a video of a baby demonstrating comprehension of many printed words before the baby can say those words, it also has the virtue of being true. We will discuss in some detail the crucial empirical evidence showing that the hypothesis is true—*that babies can learn to read printed words with comprehension before they can produce those words in speech.* We will show that a baby can learn to read printed words as soon as that baby can understand the first few spoken words referring to persons, actions, things, and the like. The theory of abstraction shows that the advance to the earliest pragmatic mapping capabilities occurs by about the baby's seventh postnatal month which is about three to six months before the baby is able to produce its first intelligible word in speech—something that normally occurs about the end of the baby's first year of life. To see how the surprising prediction about literacy flows from the theory of abstraction, especially because of its importance to certain theories of literacy that it demolishes—it will be useful to show how the hypothesis in question is derived from the theory of abstraction.

As soon as the baby demonstrates the milestone of mapping a spoken or manually signed symbol onto its intended logical object—which may be an action like toddling away while waving bye-bye to the adult calling the baby's name!—the baby is capable, theoretically at least, of associating a printed symbol with a demonstrable meaning.

The Theory of Abstraction

The theory of abstraction correctly predicts the necessary sequence of steps leading to the development first of meaningful icons, then of indexes, and finally of linguistic symbols (just as laid out earlier in Figure 1–3). The steps involve repeated applications of what is called the **cycle of abstraction**.

Discrimination is the process of finding boundaries and thus creating iconic representations; **prescinding** is the process of representing movements of icons and thus constructing indexes; and **hypostasis** is the process of defining abstract concepts which form the semantic basis for linguistic representations—the meanings of words.

The theory of abstraction leads to the discovery of a dense sequence of finely graded sign systems leading up to the discrimination of the gross sounds, rhythms, and intonations of spoken syllables necessary to the name-orienting response as observed at about month 4.5 in normal infants. The steps spelled out in detail in the *Milestones* book lead through a series of icons to a series of indexes and then on to the first strictly linguistic signs in a finely graded series of steps.

None of the steps can logically be skipped over because each higher level of signs, as we saw in Figure 1–3, depends on the formation of one or many signs at the level just preceding the higher one. Each successive level is a necessary scaffolding for the next. Here we focus on how the baby proceeds forward from the discrimination, of its own name, for instance—or any other salient surface form of a linguistic sign—to genuine readiness to understand printed words.

The cycle begins with the baby's discriminating of certain bodily persons and objects, followed by **prescinding** them from their locations and actions (either by moving them or moving around them), and then **hypostasis** which involves separating them still further from the contexts in which they were first encountered.

From the Discriminated Symbol to the Hypostatic Symbol

The discrimination of the baby's name is normally followed by the infant's gaining additional motor control over syllabic rhythms. One of the key milestones in the predicted sequence is the baby's realization that certain syllables, such as the sounds of his or her own name, or of highly frequent words such as "mama," "dada," "baba," and so on, are often repeated. As the baby is beginning to discriminate the sounds of such syllables, it becomes possible to single out the most common and salient one of all—typically the baby's own name (as noted by Werker & Tees, 1999, and others). At first, the baby cannot know what that word means, but comes to realize that *this* sequence of sounds is common. The baby must think—not in the surface forms of words but in the discriminatory act of recognizing the repeated sequence of sounds—something like this:

> Whoah! I've heard that sequence a lot! That one is familiar! It must be important! There is something valuable here! It is often repeated in my presence when people are talking to me and looking at me! Hmmm! I better pay attention to that sequence!

The result is what is termed a **discriminated symbol**—in this case, the baby notices that its name is distinct from other sound sequences (or possibly manual signs for a deaf infant) that are commonly produced by others.

This realization is prerequisite to the baby's new behavior of orienting—that is turning and usually looking directly at the person who says the baby's name in the baby's presence. As we saw in Chapter 5 in discussing developmental disorders, this step marks a critical gain that is lost in regressive forms of early childhood autism. Meanwhile, as we have seen in this chapter, and as the theory of abstraction correctly predicts, the baby continues to work toward motor control of the surface forms of speech through progressively more complex babbling. As increasing success is attained, the baby achieves what is called canonical babble, as in /bababa/. This development cannot precede the discriminated symbol because the baby cannot repeat a sequence of sounds or actions intentionally until that sequence of sounds or actions can be discriminated. If it could not be discriminated by the baby, the baby could not notice much less produce the repetition. When the repetitive babbling occurs, however, the baby has achieved what is called the **prescinded symbol**. Soon after that the baby will move on to increasingly diverse and **variegated babble**, as in /bamagadza/ and so on.

Sometime after the attainment of the baby's first prescinded symbols as manifested in syllabic utterances—usually by about the seventh month—the baby will also discover the meaning of his or her own name. Typically, soon after other pragmatic mapping relations—referring terms for persons, actions, and so forth—will be

As the baby is beginning to discriminate the sounds of such syllables, it becomes possible to single out the most common and salient one of all—typically the baby's own name (as noted by Werker & Tees, 1999, and others).

solved by the child. The first linguistic signs of this higher kind are **hypostatic symbols**. Hypostasis, the highest stage of abstraction, is the process of mentally carving out and separating the conceptual meaning of a referring term as that term is associated with whatever it may refer to. It is as if the meaning of the referring term—the person, action, or whatever that it refers to—were highlighted in experience so that it becomes distinct from everything else in the contexts where it may be found. It is the process by which the meaning is noted and set apart from other meanings, as if it were extracted from its context so that it could be recognized in any context in which it might be found.

Reading Readiness Reinterpreted

The theory of abstraction shows that as soon as a baby has a receptive repertoire of just a few hypostatic symbols there is nothing standing in the way of that baby's understanding of printed words. The baby is already at the ZPD where the comprehension of printed forms is within range. By this time, the normally developing baby has already solved many pragmatic mapping problems. Such a problem has been solved multiple times for every distinct spoken symbol in the baby's growing receptive repertoire of words for persons, things, and actions. As surprising as it may seem—especially to theoreticians and experts who supposed that **reading readiness** cannot begin much before the first grade (by around five to seven years of age)—the theory of abstraction predicts that the baby is actually ready to begin reading printed words by about the seventh month after birth, give or take a month or so.

As surprising as it may seem—especially to theoreticians and experts who supposed that **reading readiness** cannot begin much before the first grade (by around five to seven years of age)—the theory of abstraction predicts that the baby is actually ready to begin reading printed words by about the seventh month after birth, give or take a month or so.

Aleka Reading at Nine Months

Meet Aleka Titzer
Next have a look at the <u>Aleka and Friends</u> video (just click on the expanded Table of Contents entry on the DVD). Keep these questions in mind: (1) Does Aleka know the meaning of more than one or two printed words? (2) Does she differentiate the meanings of those printed words plainly? (3) Does she come up with the demonstrations on her own? (4) Does Aleka sound out any of the words? (5) Does Aleka say any of the words out loud at all? (6) Is Aleka converting print to speech? (7) Is Aleka getting the meaning of words from the print? (8) Is Aleka performing a pragmatic mapping of print to meaning? (9) Does her dad say the word before or after she demonstrates the meaning?

On the video demonstration (beginning at 26 seconds into the sequence), we see nine month old Aleka with her father Dr. Robert Titzer, demonstrating that she understands printed words. He shows her a word on a flash card with large letters and she looks at the word and then demonstrates its meaning. When he shows her the word "foot" she grabs her own foot and moves it around. When the word is "pointing" she demonstrates the meaning with a pointing gesture, and so on. A little later on the same video demonstration, we see Aleka at the age of three years and two months reading out loud the story of "The Three Little Pigs" and the Big Bad Wolf who is threatening to blow the house down. We can understand her surface forms of speech if we know what the story is and her dad tells how at that age she reported that she felt as if she herself was "in the story." On the same video there are demonstrations by other children reading well before the traditional age of *reading readiness*.

Enter the Big Bad Wolf

If Aleka Titzer at age three were playing the part of Little Red Riding Hood we might expect to find the traditional linguist Leonard Bloomfield as the Big Bad Wolf. It was he and his followers who insisted that reading readiness would have to come at the stage of life where children are at least able to understand what is called the **phonemic** or **alphabetic principle**—the complex mapping of letters onto the distinct sounds of the language in which the reading is to be done. This theory of reading (Bloomfield & Barnhart, 1961), and of reading readiness, led to the supposedly scientific approach to the teaching of reading grounded in linguistics and later known as **phonics** (also see "Phonics Basics," retrieved March 6, 2009, from http://www.pbs.org/parents/readinglanguage/articles/phonics/pbasics.html). That approach involves teaching children sound-to-letter correspondences through explicit rules. There are many variations but the underlying rules are essentially equivalent to the familiar ones where "A is for /æ/ as in *apple*; B is for /b/ as in *bat*; C is for /k/ as in *cat*" and so on.

With complications owed to phonetics (Ball & Müller, 2005; Ladefoged, 2001) and phonology (Chomsky & Halle, 1968; Gough & C. H. Lee, 2007; Pike, 1947) the correspondence of sounds to the letters in a comprehensive and well-designed alphabet is the basic idea underlying the International Phonetic Alphabet (2007). Bloomfield's followers and proponents of his ideas ever after would suppose that reading readiness could not be attained much before the age of six years. The idea was that teaching of literacy should wait at least until the child was old enough to understand sound-to-letter correspondences.

It is interesting that literacy, according to the whole class of theories that would follow from Bloomfield forward, was basically about surface forms of language divorced from their meaning. It was about the sound emanating from the speaker's mouth and impacting the hearer's ear. Bloomfield himself would contend that reading consists of converting text to speech and writing the reverse (Figure 9–1). He supposed that the teaching of reading could best be accomplished by focusing attention exclusively on sound-to-symbol relations using nonsensical forms so that the children learning to read would not be distracted by meaning (Bloomfield & Barnhart, 1961).

Little Red Riding Hood portrayed by Aleka Titzer might have turned the tables on the Big Bad Wolf played by Leonard Bloomfield.

Bloomfield himself would contend that reading consists of converting text to speech and writing the reverse (Figure 9–1).

Little Red Riding Hood with Aleka Titzer

Imagine the surprise of the Big Bad Wolf disguised as a harmless and well-meaning school teacher to find Aleka reading words with comprehension months before she could even say those words out loud and about five years before what phonics advocates believe is the proper age of reading readiness.

The Big Bad Wolf might have said, "What a huge leap you have made my dear!"

And innocent Little Red Riding Hood might have responded, "The better to show you how language really works, Dear Teacher. The better to demonstrate the incompleteness of Dr. Bloomfield's theory. My, what big errors he made!"

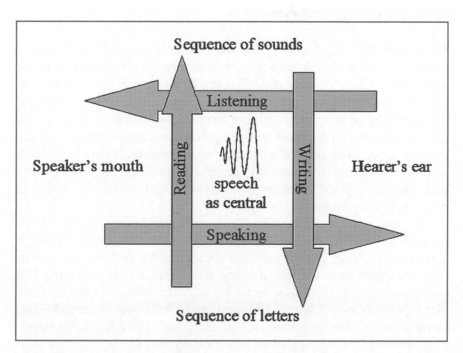

FIGURE 9–1. Bloomfield's view of reading as converting print to speech.

The Incompleteness of Phonics

Baby Aleka could not be reading by converting print to speech because Aleka could read many words she could not yet say out loud at all. So, we should make a note that Bloomfield's theory of reading was incomplete at best. However, keeping in mind that his theory was the foundational starting point for methods of reading instruction based on sounding out words, we need to consider the consequences that such instruction will lead to. According to Bloomfield and followers, it is not possible for a child to read—at least not according to the theory of phonics which Bloomfield can be credited with having invented—until the child knows sound-to-letter correspondences.

According to the standard theory, children must develop what is called **phonemic awareness** or **phonological awareness** (Gough & C. H. Lee, 2007; Torppa et al., 2007). The sort of awareness in question is supposedly demonstrated in tasks like the following: The child might be asked to say a word that starts with the same sound as "cat" begins with (where the child is supposed to say something like "car" or "camp" and so on), or to say a word that begins with the last sound in "jump" (for instance, "put"), or a word that rhymes with "kite" (say, "tight"), and so on. However, the proponents of this kind of phonological knowledge will be surprised because a baby at seven to nine months cannot do any of these things yet, but as the theory of abstraction predicts, the baby can read. Consider why this is necessarily so.

Pragmatic Isomorphism

The pragmatic map the baby has to form for each and every meaningful symbol that goes into what is commonly called the **receptive repertoire** (Chiat & Roy, 2007; Rivera & Zawaydeh, 2007) is logically the same kind of relation that is required for understanding the meaning of a printed symbol or a sequence of such symbols. The two kinds of pragmatic maps—which admittedly differ at the surface, one consisting of a spoken word and the other a printed sequence of letters—underneath are the same. They have **pragmatic isomorphism**. Their meanings are determined by the same kinds of mapping relations.

Figure 9–2 shows the sort of mapping that is required in both instances—that is, for the baby to understand its own name (or someone else's) or for the baby to understand a printed symbol in relation to whatever thing, action, or person it may refer to. The important point to make here is that the two mapping relations (shown as "A" and "B" in Figure 9–2) are essentially the same in form. They are isomorphic. They each have the same shape and systematic mapping structure of different surface forms onto distinct meanings. In each case the symbol is represented as a

The pragmatic map the baby has to form for each and every meaningful symbol that goes into what is commonly called the **receptive repertoire** (Chiat & Roy, 2007; Rivera & Zawaydeh, 2007) is logically the same kind of relation that is required for understanding the meaning of a printed symbol or a sequence of such symbols.

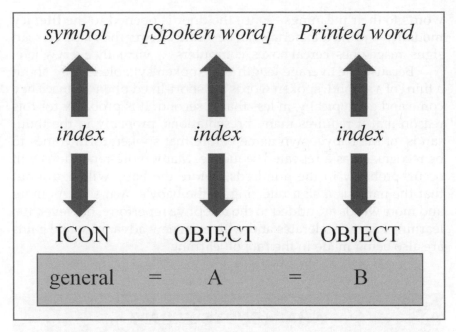

FIGURE 9–2. The pragmatic mapping relation in a symbol that signifies (refers to) an object (icon) through an indexical act.

word—spoken in the case of "A" and printed in the case of "B." In each case, the connector is an indexical act and the logical "object" referred to or signified is the same. For instance, in the case of Aleka Titzer, the foot is the same foot whether it is referred to by her father's spoken word *foot* or by a printed form of the word "foot."

As a result, the mapping relations that hold between speech and the world or between print and the world require similar mental actions on the part of the baby.

A Subtle Difference

There is, however, a difference between the process of understanding a spoken word as contrasted with understanding a printed one. It is more difficult in principle to discriminate one spoken word from another than it is to discriminate printed symbols. A printed symbol sticks around and we may usually examine it for as long and as often as we like. However, for the baby at seven to nine months of age—a baby who does not yet produce any spoken words on its own—the occurrence of any given spoken word is intermittent, fleeting, and totally outside the baby's volitional control. Someone else has to produce the spoken word in order for the baby to notice it. Of course, Aleka didn't make up her own flash cards and Dr. Bob Titzer did introduce Aleka to the cards and the demonstrated meanings in a kind of instructional game that he played with her. However, once Aleka, or any individual, begins to go from the printed

When Aleka reads the word *foot* and demonstrates her understanding by grabbing her FOOT and moving it around with her hand, she could as easily be responding to a spoken command—*Show me your foot!*—as to the printed word FOOT.

words to their meanings—once the door is opened to the **literacy modality**—printed materials can be found all over the place: on road signs, magazines, cereal boxes, computers . . . virtually everywhere.

Because the average length of a spoken syllable is only about a third of a second, spoken words are short-lived phenomena. They come and go, typically, in less than a second. It is probably for this reason that it requires many presentations, probably in the thousands, of the baby's own name before that spoken form comes to be recognized as a repeated sequence. Many more repetitions will occur, probably in the hundreds, before the baby will figure out that the name is a sign referring to the baby's own self. As more and more words are added to the receptive repertoire, however, the learning curve accelerates and with each new advance while gains are also being made in the rate of learning.

WHAT IS "DYSLEXIA"?

The definition of dyslexia varies depending on the source and some of the most authoritative sources end up saying that no definition is really possible. In 1995, Elaine Miles, writing for the first issue of the British journal *Dyslexia* argued that "dyslexia is not the sort of concept that can be summed up in a single formula" (p. 37) for which reason she argues it might be best to talk about a "description" rather than a "definition." Although she supposes that this would not affect the validity of the concept, she says that "the detailed wording of descriptions [of dyslexia] still presents a problem, as research on dyslexia involves many different disciplines" (p. 37).

From Orton to the International Dyslexia Association

The Orton Dyslexia Society was founded in 1949 in honor of Samuel T. Orton, a neurologist who studied the reading difficulties associated with the term *dyslexia*. Today the organization is called the International Dyslexia Association (IDA). In 2002—53 years from the time of origin—the Board of Directors, at least (but not the membership) came to agreement on the following definition of *dyslexia*:

> Dyslexia is a specific **learning disability** that is neurological in origin. It is characterized by difficulties with accurate and/or fluent **word recognition** and by poor spelling and **decoding** abilities. These difficulties typically result from a deficit in the phonological component of language that is often unexpected in

relation to other cognitive abilities and the provision of effective classroom instruction. Secondary consequences may include problems in reading comprehension and reduced reading experience that can impede growth of vocabulary and background knowledge. (IDA, 2007, retrieved March 6, 2009, from http:// www.interdys.org/ewebeditpro5/upload/Definition_of_ Dyslexia.pdf)

Probing the IDA source for more information on the "Neurological Basis" of dyslexia we found the following:

The conjecture explored here [retrieved July 11, 2007, from http://www.interdys.org/servlet/compose?section_id=5&page_id=47 but removed since] is that there is a disruption of the cerebral architecture during gestation that sets in motion a cascade of events resulting in reorganization of neuronal circuits and networks. This reorganized anatomical substrate is not optimally organized for language acquisition and does not flourish in the typical environment/education system.

Further along in the same section it comes out that certain neuronal connections that are not expected are found in the autopsied brains of individuals with dyslexia. There is also some speculation that there is a genetic basis for the abnormalities found.

The British Dyslexia Association

The British Dyslexia Association (BDA) wrote in 1989:

We define dyslexia as a specific difficulty in learning, constitutional in origin, in one or more of reading, writing and spelling and written language, which may be accompanied by difficulty in number work. It is particularly related to mastering and using written language (alphabetic, numerical and musical notation) although often affecting oral language to some degree. (as quoted by Miles, 1995, p. 40)

Today, under the link labeled "What is dyslexia?" at the BDA Web site we find the following definition:

Dyslexia is a specific learning difficulty which is neurobiological in origin and persists across the lifespan. It is characterized by difficulties with phonological processing, rapid naming, working memory, processing speed and the automatic development of skills that are unexpected in relation to an individual's other cognitive abilities. These processing difficulties can undermine the acquisition of literacy and numeracy skills, as well as musical notation, and have an effect on verbal communication, organization and adaptation to change. (BDA, 2009, retrieved March 6, 2009, from http://www.bdadyslexia.org.uk/aboutdyslexia.html)

The "learning disabilities" (LDs) included under the umbrella of dyslexia cover a lot of ground but there is not much that is specific in the definition. Terms like "difficulties," "deficit," "unexpected," and "effective instruction" are hardly specific descriptions of any unique disorder.

The Learning Disabilities Online Definition of Dyslexia

At Learning Disabilities Online (LD Online), which claims to be "the world's leading website on learning disabilities and ADHD," we find a somewhat broader definition of dyslexia:

> A language-based disability that affects both oral and written language. It may also be referred to as reading disability, reading difference, or reading disorder. (LD Online, 2007, retrieved March 6, 2009, from http://www.ldonline.org/glossary)

Seymour (1986) suggested that it made sense to refer to a child as "*dyslexic* if basic reading functions were impaired" (as quoted by Miles, 1995, p. 38). In 1991, the *Special Education Handbook* defined dyslexia as "difficulty with reading" (see Miles, p. 38).

The National Institute of Neurological Disorders and Stroke

A reasonably comprehensive definition is offered by the National Institute of Neurological Disorders and Stroke (2007b):

> Dyslexia is a brain-based type of learning disability that specifically impairs a person's ability to read. These individuals typically read at levels significantly lower than expected despite having normal intelligence. Although the disorder varies from person to person, common characteristics among people with dyslexia are difficulty with phonological processing (the manipulation of sounds) and/or rapid visual-verbal responding [reading aloud and the like]. (retrieved March 6, 2009, from http://www.ninds.nih.gov/disorders/dyslexia/dyslexia.htm)

The Controversial Discrepancy Definitions

The definitions of dyslexia, or of learning disabilities in general and reading disability in particular, generally refer to an unexpected difference between a measure of ability and a measure of achievement. For instance, Shaywitz, Escobar, Shaywitz, Fletcher, and Makuch (1992) defined "reading disability" as a discrepancy between

> the level of reading ability predicted on the basis of intelligence (ability) and the actual level of reading achievement. (p. 146)

The **discrepancy approach**, as just defined in the immediately preceding quote, has also been applied in the definition of mental retardation. However, because of the fact that IQ tests are deeply influenced by language/dialect proficiency (see Chapter 11) just as reading comprehension is—the idea that intelligence can be sharply distinguished from language/dialect proficiency and all the other abilities that are linked to it is simply false. It is refuted by sound theory and by the research summed up in Chapter 11 (also see Yan & J. W. Oller, 2007).

Challenged in the Courts

The discrepancy approach has also been challenged by sensible people and judges in the courts. In Chapter 12, the most important cases spelling out the controversy are: *Hobson v. Hansen* (1967), *Diana v. Board of Education* (1970), *Parents in Action on Special Education (PASE) v. Hannon* (1980), *Larry P. v. Riles* (1979/1984), and *Crawford v. Honig* (1994).

The consensus seems to be that IQ tests in General American English cannot reasonably be used as a basis for determining who is or is not mentally retarded. By implication, those tests should not be used to determine anything other than proficiency in a particular language/dialect—that is, in General American English. Nevertheless, the current definitions of dyslexia by the IDA and the BDA still appeal to the discrepancy method at least indirectly. It is contained in the part of the definitions that refer to the difference between what is positively "expected" in skills and abilities (on the basis of IQ scores) and what is not observed (on the basis of reading performance). That is, when reading performance is low relative to IQ, then a learning disability is diagnosed.

The reverse logic is never applied: High performance on language/dialect tests accompanied by low IQ scores has never been proposed as a definition of "over-achievement" or anything like it. Why not? Because it cannot happen. Since IQ tests measure language/dialect proficiency more than anything else (see Chapter 11), low scores in one language/dialect battery (say, an IQ test) with high scores in another battery (say, a reading test) would normally indicate that the individual just had a bad day on one of the test batteries (in this case, the IQ test).

Why Discrepancy Judgments Are Often Wrong

Low scores, for reasons discussed in greater detail in Chapter 11, are a lot less trustworthy than high scores. There are many ways to get a low score. On a machine scored answer sheet, for instance, if the test taker loses track of the numbering, one error may lead to a whole series of additional errors even when the test taker knows the correct answers. There are also many other ways to make a poor showing on any test or assessment procedure.

For these reasons, substantial differences in test scores should be interpreted with great care and any discrepancy to be used in a

Anyone can have a bad day for lots of different reasons and when it happens the test administrator does not necessarily know which reason applies. By contrast, to have an exceptional run of luck where lots of items or procedures are handled very well is vanishingly unlikely.

Understanding complex communications does not come about by accident. Failing to comprehend complex linguistic constructions, however, could easily be due to some accident or other.

diagnosis should be confirmed from multiple angles with multiple measures before it is taken as a basis for determining any particular diagnosis. Generally high scores are more informative than low ones because high scores are less likely than low ones to be the result of something other than whatever we are trying to measure. Multiple successes in complex communications do not come about by accident for reasons we discussed in detail in Chapter 3 with reference to Braille writing. For instance, readers would not be able to guess the meaning of this sentence without reading and understanding it. Readers would not be able to guess such a meaning if the sentence were written in an unknown language, or if it consisted of a string of nonsense syllables, and so on.

For that reason, success in complex communication processes is a great deal more informative than failure. As a result, discrepancy approaches, which depend on judgments of what someone has failed to do on one or more tests, are apt to lead to mistaken diagnoses.

VARIETIES OF DYSLEXIA AND DISORDERS IN GENERAL

The word "dyslexia" is based on the Greek root meaning "to speak" —as seen in *-lex-* —and the prefix *dys-* from the verb meaning "to break." The term "dyslexia," as we have seen in the definitions of the two preceding sections of this chapter, is commonly used as a cover term, an umbrella, for all kinds of literacy difficulties but especially difficulties in reading. As with disorders and disabilities in general, there are theoretically three varieties of literacy disorders:

- First, there are *genetic disorders* that are present at or before conception. To the extent that any variety of dyslexia may involve genetic brain abnormalities, it belongs in this first category. Genetic disorders, however, tend to spill over into the second kind and may be symptomatically indistinguishable.
- The second kind are **epigenetic disorders**—where genetic tendencies interact with factors such as nutrition, socialization, hygiene, rest, and risk factors such as disease, injury, and combinations of these. Deep literacy disorders are commonly epigenetic. They are rarely discovered until after the age of 7 to 9 years when a child is expected to be reading independently and writing with considerable success. Stephen J. Cannell's dyslexia condition, for instance, as he understands it, was not discovered until he was 35 years old (Cannell, 2006).
- Third, there are so-called **"acquired" disorders** that can develop suddenly where the known cause is something like a head injury, a disease, or poisoning by drugs or other toxins.

Acquired Versus Unacquired Disorders

When literacy is acquired normally but something happens to cause a sudden regression to a pre-literate stage of development, or to demolish previous gains altogether, the condition is commonly referred to as **acquired dyslexia**.

The most extreme version of such an acquired dyslexia results in the condition called **alexia**—where a person cannot understand print at all. This condition is sometimes called "word blindness" or "text blindness" and, where it occurs, it is often associated with a more general form of the condition known as aphasia—where some or all of the ability to speak and use language is lost. The loss is often attributable to a particular event such as a **stroke**, head injury, or some other cause of brain damage. One source describes "alexia" as

> an acquired type of **sensory aphasia** where damage to the brain causes a patient to lose the ability to read. ("Sensory Aphasia," 2009, retrieved March 6, 2009, from http://en.wikipedia.org/wiki/Alexia_%28disorder%29)

It is possible, in theory, for a person to be born with the damage that would cause the special aphasia known as alexia in later life, but on account of the fact that literacy is not usually acquired until sometime after the first grade (after about the age of five or six years), alexia can hardly be diagnosed as a developmental or genetic disorder.

Less extreme losses of literacy, "acquired dyslexia," in some instances, can also be special forms of aphasia. We will have more to say about aphasia in Chapter 10. For instance, in forms less extreme than complete alexia, dyslexia—whether "acquired" or "genetic" —is often said to include the condition known as **dysgraphia**:

> . . . a neurological disorder characterized by writing disabilities . . . [causing] a person's writing to be distorted or incorrect . . . despite thorough instruction. . . . Children with the disorder may have other learning disabilities [e.g., dyslexia], however, they usually have no social or other academic problems. Cases of dysgraphia in adults [the "acquired" kind] generally occur after some trauma. In addition to poor handwriting, dysgraphia is characterized by wrong or odd spelling, and production of words that are not correct (i.e., using "boy" for "child"). The cause of the disorder is unknown. [NINDS, 2007a, retrieved March 6, 2009, from http://www.ninds.nih.gov/disorders/dysgraphia/dysgraphia.htm]

It is useful to consider why neurologists refer to the kinds of disorders that are produced by extrinsic events or injuries as "acquired." Usually we think of "acquisition" in relation to intentional activities like acquiring a business, a new language, or a new

With an acquired form of dyslexia, the person affected seems to be going along quite normally when all of a sudden a **stroke** or head injury, or perhaps a disease or toxic chemical exposure, produces neurological damage and skills that were formerly in place are lost.

car. So the term "acquired" does not quite capture the intended meaning—as if folks were out their trying to get themselves injured or to cause themselves to have strokes. Of course, that is not what the neurologists mean to suggest by using the phrase "acquired disorders." Nevertheless, it needs to be noted that the phrase "acquired disorders" is what in less technical **jargon** is called a "near miss"—close, but no cigar. The verbal attempt fails to capture important aspects of the intended semantic target. Even the genetic disorders that a person may get from parents are "acquired" in a weak sense, so the phrase in common use, misses on that score also because the genetic kind of disorders are supposed to contrast with the "acquired" ones.

Sharpening the Focus: Extrinsic Versus Intrinsic

The goal of contrasting "acquired" disorders with the presumably "unacquired" ones is to distinguish disorders that can be attributed to **extrinsic factors** from outside the individual as contrasted with **intrinsic factors** from inside the person.

The point of the "acquired" versus "unacquired" distinction—the real target—if we think about it, can be brought into sharp focus.

At a limit on the intrinsic side, we have the genetic makeup of the individual and at a limit on the extrinsic side, we have everything that impinges on the person from the outside world—the food, social exchanges with other persons, the nurturing, interactions, quarrels, diseases, injuries, and so on. In between these extreme limits, there is an intimate interaction which consists of what today we call epigenetic phenomena. For our own part, we believe that the interactions—in the common ground—are the most interesting kind because that is where communication has its impact. That is where therapeutic intervention can occur, and that is where we can—as teachers, researchers, and clinicians—make a positive difference for persons with and without disorders.

CAUSING DYSLEXIA

In addition to all of the foregoing kinds of literacy disorders, there is also a widespread form of dyslexia that can only be called instructional dyslexia. It consists of a halting, inefficient, letter by letter approach to reading that tries to make sense of text one letter at a time. The result is something like a melody that proceeds one note at a time and where every note is punctuated by silence on both sides—before and after each note. It is difficult to hear the melody or any harmony in music produced by such a method. However, playing a melody one note at a time is still more meaningful than sounding out text one letter at a time.

Dyslexia Caused by Instruction

The *instructional dyslexia hypothesis* is the prediction that *normal intelligent individuals who are highly proficient in one or more languages and who are capable of normal interactions through speech and language will show primary symptoms of dyslexia if they are instructed exclusively in phonics and if they do not use any other method of learning to read.*

Individuals with instructional dyslexia may conceivably have additional genetic, epigenetic, or other extrinsically caused disorders and disabilities, but instructional dyslexia can be and is commonly caused by the exclusive application of strict phonics methods of instruction. It will be useful next to see why meaning is neglected in those approaches.

Meaning as a Distraction?

The linguist who promoted the basis for phonics to educators worldwide but especially in the United States was none other than the Big Bad Wolf himself, the American linguist Leonard Bloomfield (1933; Bloomfield & Barnhart, 1961). He argued, as proponents of phonics and its various elaborations still argue today (see "Elaborating Phonics: Phonological Awareness" below), that his method was strictly scientific. In fact, it was based on an impoverished theory of linguistics.

Bloomfield's Grand Error

As noted in Chapter 7, Bloomfield had the strange notion that it was possible to analyze language completely without any reference to meaning. He supposed that meanings were so rich and that the universe of all the meanings that might be expressed was so vast that it was necessary, in principle, to dispense with the analysis of meaning, because, it would be impossible to take it into account in any case. His method in teaching literacy aimed to remove attention as far as possible from the meaning of printed texts. The main goal of Bloomfield's phonemic theory of literacy—and the basis of phonics in all its varieties—has been to teach sound-to-letter correspondences. Even at the time of this writing phonics remains the most widely used and defended method of literacy instruction in American public schools today.

Babies Solve the Meaning Problem

It did not seem to occur to Bloomfield that by about the age children begin to walk—about one year after birth—they succeed in solving the foundational problem that he supposed was too difficult for adult linguists. By about 12 months of age, give or take a couple of months, normal children succeed in analyzing meaning. They parse up the world of experience into meaningful objects, persons, event sequences, and so forth, to solve the fundamental pragmatic mapping problem. By the age of four to seven years the normal child has unraveled the mystery of language to the point that essentially all the syntax, semantics, and most of the pragmatic systems of language have been conquered.

From there on, for normal children it is just a matter of adding to the knowledge base with an increasingly rich vocabulary and more detailed, abstract, and general information. It also did not occur to Bloomfield that the discovery of the meanings embedded in print is vastly more important than converting those printed forms into spoken words. Of course, literate persons can usually read aloud whenever they want to, but a huge amount of print processing, the vast majority, largely happens without converting printed text to spoken words. Imagine how tired you would get if you had to read everything out loud.

When the focus is shifted, as it is in phonics approaches to literacy, from meaning to the surface forms of print as they relate to the surface sounds of speech, certain symptoms that are typical of dyslexia will follow.

Reading aloud is a special skill that literate people also incidentally acquire, but as Aleka Titzer demonstrated in the video, converting print to speech is not essential to the comprehension of printed forms.

Pragmatic Mapping Is Required

The sure fire method to produce *instructional dyslexia* is to do exactly what we are doing with the phonics method in most American schools. Of course, that is not what is intended, but it is what is happening. How can we be certain? There are several ways to show that phonics instruction, provided it is pursued vigorously and exclusively —where it is the only method of reading that is being attempted by the persons being taught—will produce instructional dyslexia with algebraic certainty in all the children who use that method exclusively. The symptoms match the most common variety of developmental dyslexia—slow halting oral reading, inability to spell, difficulty in making sense of ordinary texts, a general dislike for reading, a sense that "I am just not good at reading and I cannot spell or recall the correct spellings of words. I am a dunce for sure!" And so forth.

Success in Language and Literacy

The key in all cases of successful language acquisition and in successful acquisition of literacy is the pragmatic mapping of symbols to their meaningful content—that is, the meanings intended by writers and commonly understood by successful readers. When success occurs, the symbol is correctly linked with its intended meaning and vice versa. The pragmatic map is completed. The surface forms of print must be connected through pragmatic mapping with meaning. There are three essential elements: (1) printed symbols, (2) pragmatic relations, and (3) meanings or content.

Phonics Is an Incomplete Theory

If three bricks were required, the phonics theory would be two bricks short of a full load. What ensures that phonics as a theory of reading is incomplete is that it only looks to the surface forms of letters and their relations to the surface sound segments of syllables. It is superficial from start to finish. We might ask why this emphasis was promoted.

Leonard Bloomfield (Bloomfield & Barnhart, 1961) argued that children learning to read would only be distracted by attending to meaning. For that reason, he supposed, it is essential to concentrate only on letter-to-sound relations. As a result, phonics approaches set aside the mapping of print to meaning—along with morphology, lexicon, syntax, semantics, and pragmatics. Phonics puts all the initial emphasis on letters in relation to surface phonology. To be fair to the phonics proponents, they do argue that meaning will be discovered in the process of converting print to speech, but looking back to Aleka is it true or false that the discovery of meaning requires converting print to speech? In fact, she cannot yet say the printed words that she is able to read with comprehension. She demonstrates her comprehension without speaking by displaying the meanings of printed words and phrases through her actions. She goes from print straight to the meaning.

Or, to generalize the argument to the reader's own experience, say you read this sentence with comprehension. Do you have to read it out loud in order to know what it means? What about a phone number? Take the number 505-983-2268. If you look at this number do you need to repeat it over and over to recall it if you want to write it down or dial it? Or take a word problem in simple arithmetic: "Bill had ten dollars but he gave two of them to Sally." Do you need to say the words out loud to know how much money Bill had left?

If you were strictly trained in phonics, you should answer *yes* to each of the foregoing questions. If you received the basic phonic training at any point in your early education, you are probably experiencing some of the residual effects of phonics even now. Most readers trained in phonics are relatively slow readers even if they are highly skilled ones. Slow readers are typically slow because they are reading somewhat as if they were reading aloud. Fast read-

To be fair to the phonics proponents, they do argue that meaning will be discovered in the process of converting print to speech, but looking back to Aleka is it true or false that the discovery of meaning requires converting print to speech?

If reading is converting print to speech, how is it possible, then, for anyone to read with good comprehension at more than ten times the rate of the world's fastest talkers?

ers, on the other hand, can read with comprehension many times faster than they can speak. Recall Stephen J. Cannell's statement that he can only read at about 200 words per minute. Consider that many fast readers can achieve rates between 3,000 to 10,000 words per minute with excellent comprehension. The comprehension of such fast readers is generally better than readers who are moving along at 300 to 500 words per minute.

How is really fast reading, with excellent comprehension, possible if print must be converted to speech to get to its meaning? Really fast talkers speak at only about 300 words per minute and at that rate are difficult to comprehend. There are, of course, extreme "speed talkers" like John Moschitta, and Fran Capo, whom we met in the previous chapter. Capo can talk at about 600 words per minute and Mocchitta at about 500 words per minute. See them for yourself at http://www.youtube.com/watch?v=aZb6iBmHqkY and http://www.youtube.com/watch?v=NeK5ZjtpO-M (both retrieved March 6, 2009). However, the intelligibility of anyone speaking at more than 300 words per minute is questionable at best. If reading is converting print to speech, how is it possible, then, for anyone to read with good comprehension at more than ten times the rate of the world's fastest talkers?

The phonics theory is incomplete to begin with. It is like a rocket with only a fuselage but no engine and no fuel to make it fly. Worse yet, the part of the theory that has supposedly been worked out in detail—the part that G. Reid Lyon (1997; retrieved March 6, 2009, from http://www.readingrockets.org/article/221) and others consider to be the "scientific" phonological part—concerning sound-letter relations—is demonstrably mistaken. The mapping relations of sounds-to-letters in written English are imperfect. The relations of letters to sounds cannot be deciphered at all in most cases without reference to higher levels of structure and meaning. But those higher levels of structure and meaning—the engine and the fuel in the rocket metaphor—are precisely the elements that are ruled out by the phonics method. What is more, in elaborations of the Bloomfieldian tradition along the lines of phonological and phonemic awareness—as we will see below in the section on "Elaborated Phonics: Phonological and Phonemic Awareness"—fare no better.

Phonics Is an Incorrect Theory

For the distinct sounds of spoken English, according to any rational analysis—see Crystal (1987), *The Cambridge Encyclopedia of Language*—there are multiple ways to represent any given sound in letters of the alphabet and any given letter can usually represent more than one sound. For instance, the vowel in *peach* can be spelled as *e, ee, ie, ei, ea, y, i,* and *oe*. At the same time, a letter, for instance, *c*, can represent the consonants /k/ as in *can*, /s/ as in *city*, /ts/ as in *fancy*, not to mention part of the initial cluster of sounds, /tʃ/, in *chain*, and so on.

The theory of phonics is flawed because no one can figure out how to pronounce any reasonably lengthy sequence of letters in English on the basis of the letters alone. The theory is not just fundamentally incomplete with respect to meanings—not to mention the pragmatic mapping of symbols onto those meanings and vice versa—it is fundamentally incorrect in the very limited part of the English writing system that it claims to explain. The claims of the theories underlying phonics are largely incorrect with respect to phonology and the production and comprehension of speech. We have already provided the basis for the critique of Bloomfieldian phonetics, phonics, and phonology in Chapters 4 and 7 where we showed on the basis of experimental studies and sound theory that movements, vision in addition to hearing, and especially meaning have to be taken into consideration in ordinary speech perception. As we saw in those chapters, a simple string of letters cannot fully represent what is going on in ordinary speech production and perception. Much less is it adequate to explain the full depth of what happens in acquiring and using literacy skills.

Reading One Letter at a Time?

In reading a musical score, it might be argued that the note played is the meaning of the note written. However, written letters and the meanings of words cannot ever be said to coincide quite perfectly with each other. Written letters, as we will see, do not even agree very well with the sounds they are supposed to represent and more importantly, even if they did, as in a fully phonetic spelling system, sounding out a complex text letter by letter does not result in very intelligible speech. Try reading a novel, or the instructions about how to bake a cake or put a tricycle together by sounding out each letter of the text one at a time. It is tedious in the extreme. It is exhausting to read ten words in that way, much less a whole book, and reading words one letter at a time does not result in a very intelligible form of speech.

Beginners taught to sound out letters one at a time are confronted with the additional difficulty that English spellings are considerably less than 50% predictable on the basis of sound-to-letter relations. The fact is that sounding out words one letter at a time will cause the primary symptoms of dyslexia. This fact can be demonstrated in several ways. Except for the hypothetical "brain abnormalities" associated with definitions of dyslexia given in the first section of this chapter, a strict adherence to phonics in reading will cause all the symptoms described in definitions given by the leading dyslexia associations—especially, IDA and BDA. This is not to deny that there are dyslexias caused by brain injuries from a variety of sources, but it is to say that many cases of "dyslexia" which are commonly attributed to "brain damage" of some sort are actually owed to mistaken theories of how language works and of how literacy can be instilled.

Nowhere is the failure of theories of phonics more clear than in attempts to produce fully functional *text to speech* (TTS) and **speech to text** (STT) computer systems. The history of phonetic approaches to building TTS and SST computer programs shows the utter inadequacy of basing them on sound-to-letter correspondences.

The main symptoms of dyslexia are a necessary consequence of applying rules of phonics diligently. Yet phonics approaches require children who cannot yet read and write to do something that skilled linguists and highly complicated computer algorithms cannot do well even with the assistance of a vast memory system accessible at near the speed of light. Nowhere is the failure of theories of phonics more clear than in attempts to produce fully functional *text to speech* (TTS) and **speech to text** (STT) computer systems. The history of phonetic approaches to building TTS and SST computer programs shows the utter inadequacy of basing them on sound-to-letter correspondences.

Converting Print into Speech (and Vice Versa)

One of the best empirical demonstrations that dyslexia can be caused by a strict phonics approach to literacy comes from attempts to get computers to do just a small part of what phonics aims to teach children to do in beginning reading classes.

The Stanford Experiment: Speech to Text

A team at Stanford University in California, Hanna, Hanna, Hodges, and Rudorf (1966), first spelled 17,000 English words phonetically. They used phonetic spellings to reduce the complexity of the problem up front. Phonics approaches to the teaching of reading usually work with ordinary English spellings which are only quasi-alphabetic—phonetically they are very imperfect. So children are confronted with a more difficult problem in using phonics than Hanna and company tried to solve.

Then, Hanna et al. used a complex inventory of phonological rules to convert the words back to their original spellings. They succeeded in achieving correct spellings in only about 50% of the words. Would we consider a person who misspelled every other word as having achieved normal literacy? Suppose an adult misspelled, on the average, every other word. Does this not sound like a symptom of dyslexia? According to the definitions (or descriptions) of dyslexia given by the experts and professional organizations cited earlier in this chapter (notably the Orton Society, the IDA, and the BDA), persistent and uncorrectable misspellings are one of the key symptoms of dyslexia. However, applying the phonics approach not only cannot correct the spelling errors in question, in the research by Hanna et al. applying phonics to the English writing system is a certain way to cause about 50% of the words encountered to be misspelled. A strict approach to phonics will produce a huge number of spelling errors. Therefore, is it not reasonable to suppose that phonics certainly can produce the symptom of chronic and uncorrectable misspellings?

The research by Hanna et al. shows that phonics fails about 50% of the time as a method of explaining even the surface spellings of words. But aren't sound-letter correspondences what the phonics method is supposed to explain best? Instead, phonics is a guaranteed method of producing individuals who can only spell about half the words they may want to write down or to try to sound out if we reverse the task.

Reversing the Task: Text to Speech

Hanna et al. simplified their problem from the start by using a **phonetic transcription** of the 17,000 English words in their list. They started with phonetic renderings of English speech forms and tried to convert them to written text according to English spellings. They were working from speech forms (in theory at least) to text (STT). So, what happens if the task is reversed and the object is to convert printed text to speech (TTS). The latter was a project undertaken by Ainswort (1973), and followed up more recently by El-Imam and Don (2005) and by Damper and Marchand (2006). Interestingly, as Damper and Marchand note, "pronunciation of words from their spelling alone is a hard computational problem, especially for languages like English and French where there is only a partially consistent mapping from letters to sound" (2006, p. 207). Ainswort's program with 159 rules—many more rules than are taught in most beginning reading programs—was designed for TTS, but succeeded only in producing text that was about 70% intelligible.

Ainswort's program used essentially all the sound-to-letter associations that could be mustered plus a good deal more. His system consisted of many more rules than beginning readers are typically taught in phonics instruction and was supplemented by rules going beyond phonics. However, his results were so unsatisfactory that essentially all researchers since his time have used much more information about the language to be converted from TTS than can be found in sound-to-letter relations. Again, phonics fails as an exclusive program for reading. In the case of Ainswort's results, sticking strictly with phonics is a certain way to produce terrible reading comprehension—another standard symptom of the most widespread cases diagnosed as dyslexia.

Was the Problem Just English Spelling?

English is a notoriously difficult language to spell because of its seriously unphonetic spelling system (as we noted in Chapter 7). However, the problem of going from print to speech requires a great deal more than sound-to-letter correspondences even in fairly phonetic spelling systems such as are found in Arabic (as noted by El-Imam, 2004). In follow-up work, El-Imam (2008) has demonstrated that intonations must be added with natural rhythms and flow—the sort of thing that is not represented in the surface forms of letters at all—in order to achieve natural sounding and highly intelligible speech. However, such pragmatic components of speech forms are not found in "sound-to-letter" correspondences.

Referring to the difficulty created by multiple pronunciations for a given letter sequence or multiple spellings for a given sound or sound sequence, El-Imam wrote in 2004, "For standard Arabic (SA) these problems are not as severe as they are for English or French but they do exist" (p. 339).

In fact, if all those problems could be solved, a strict phonetic transcription still fails as a basis for a successful text to speech conversion (El-Imam, 2008). Hanna et al. (1966) also showed that it fails 50% of the time in converting good phonetic spellings back to ordinary textual spellings. For all of these reasons, the most up-to-date attempts to get computers and/or robots to produce intelligible speech are using vastly more complex programs than can be devised on the basis of phonics approaches to literacy (T. E. Moore, 2007).

Sound-to-Letter Rules Alone Fail

When the computers must do what beginning readers are asked to do on the basis of phonics alone—to sound out the words based on their spellings, or vice versa—they fail.

Hooked and Crooked on Phonics

Damper, Marchand, Adamson, and Gustafson (1999) showed that rules of pronunciation based on spelling (sound-to-letter correspondences) succeed in a correct reading or spelling for only about 26% of the new words encountered. Imagine trying to get a child to read by following the sorts of rules that fail 74% of the time on new words and according to Hanna, et al. (1966) that fail 50% of the time in trying to spell out known words? How can the child be expected to succeed in converting more than half the new words in a text to the intended spoken forms by a method that fails with 74% of the new words that are encountered?

We are not saying that phonics rule systems are useless, but we are saying that they are not sufficient by themselves. They may be fine to use as supplementary reading aids after the child is already doing some successful reading, but phonics approaches are a bad place to begin and end.

As a result of the extensive research and experimentation, no current TTS or SST system uses only rules concerning sound-to-letter correspondences. In fact, Hanna et al. (1966) and Ainswort (1973) had already realized the need to incorporate extensive lists of whole words, idiomatic phrases, and a good deal of information about prosody. More recently it has become clear that syntax, semantics, and pragmatics are all involved along with prosody in making sense of printed texts (especially El-Imam, 2008). Because of such advances, by incorporating higher level information, TTS and SST systems have been greatly improved and are becoming more and more adequate. However, they could never have achieved anything close to their present levels of success on the basis of phonics alone.

Less Than a 50% Success Rate

By sounding out words, a success rate of only about 50% or less is attainable. At that rate even a highly familiar text is hardly intelligible. Consider the following one, for instance:

> Four XXXXXXX and XXXXXX years XXXXXX our XXXXXX
> brought XXXXXX on XXXXX continent XXXXX nation XXXXX
> in XXXXXX and XXXXXX to XXXXX proposition XXXXX . . .
> shall XXXXX a XXXXXX birth XXXXXX freedom, XXXXXX that
> XXXXXX of XXXXXX the XXXXXX by XXXXXX people XXXXX
> the XXXXXX shall XXXXXX perish XXXXXX the XXXXXX.

Did you recognize the Gettysburg Address? The rest of its words can be found at the following Web site ("Gettysburg Address," 1863, retrieved March 6, 2009, from http://showcase.netins.net/web/crea tive/lincoln/speeches/gettysburg.htm). It is difficult to comprehend any text, even a familiar one, when half of its words are made unintelligible. If 50% of the words in a text are misspelled, it will be a lot less intelligible in nearly all cases. As a consequence, a strict adherence to phonic rules is certain to produce yet another of the primary symptoms of dyslexia: failure to understand what is read.

More of the Same Method Will Produce More of the Same Results

There is only one other major symptom of common dyslexia remaining to be demonstrated to be a consequence of phonics instruction. It is the failure to progress in spite of exposure to literacy instruction. Some have argued, as we saw earlier, that such failure to progress is because of "reorganization of neuronal circuits and networks" that occurred before or during gestation—perhaps because of brain injury or perhaps because of genetic errors. Or so the standard theory goes according to the professional organizations—the Orton Society, the IDA, the BDA, and so on. It is because of the alleged brain damage supposedly involved in the most common diagnosis of dyslexia that it is often claimed that dyslexia is bound to be a persistent, life-long condition.

However, another explanation—a simpler, more consistent, and more comprehensive theory—is that *failure to progress in spite of being exposed to intensive phonics instruction could well be caused by the persistent application of phonics in trying to get someone to acquire literacy.*

> If phonics is both the cause and the remedy for instructional dyslexia, both the theory and the research are clear: *instructional dyslexia will persist.* In fact, more phonics for persons with instructional dyslexia just digs them deeper into the hole they are already in.

All of the Primary Symptoms

It comes out, then, that all the main symptoms of the most common form of dyslexia can be produced by phonics. What is more, instructional dyslexia also assures that the discrepancy approach to diagnosis will show a person with instructionally induced dyslexia to be dyslexic: The person who has instructional dyslexia will seem to perform in literacy tasks at a level far below what the person appears to be able to do on the basis of, say, an oral IQ test or a conversational interview. So, it comes out that all the primary symptoms of dyslexia can be produced by the method of instruction that is the one most widely used in the United States today: All the symptoms of dyslexia can be produced by an exclusive diet of phonics in the schools.

Is it possible that the method of instruction itself is the main culprit in producing so many children who are poor readers and who appear to be dyslexic? Could we be seeing a massive experiment in progress that is inadvertently producing the very condition for which it is supposed to be the best possible—according to some, the only—remedy? We will return to these questions, but first it is important to consider the fact that the solution that is recommended for the widespread occurrence of dyslexia according to the IDA and BDA is—believe it or not—more phonics.

So why are we trying to use phonics methods, sounding out words based on phonological rules, to teach reading in American schools? Or stranger still, why would anyone claim that more of the sound-to-letter training would remove major symptoms of dyslexia? Not only have proponents of phonics methods not recognized the error of their ways even in the face of instructionally induced dyslexia in many children, they have insisted that the dyslexia in most cases is actually owed to genetically induced developmental brain damage and that the best cure for such brain damage is more intensive phonics. Proponents of phonological theories of dyslexia suggest subtle ways of ramping up to a fuller understanding of the challenging sound-to-letter relations of English spelling and phonology. With that in mind, they have proposed some more elaborate theories of phonics which we consider next.

ELABORATED PHONICS: PHONOLOGICAL AND PHONEMIC AWARENESS

The theory of phonological awareness aims at the smallest segments of print.

The idea, as explained by proponents, is to take speech segments apart and then put them back together. Chard and Dickson (1999) explain phonological awareness as

the understanding of different ways that oral language can be divided into smaller components and manipulated . . . sentences into words and words into syllables (e.g., in the word "simple," "sim-" and "-ple"), **onset** and **rime** (e.g., in the word "broom," "br-" and "-oom"), and individual phonemes (e.g., in the word "hamper," "h-," "-a-," "-m-," "-p-," "-er"). Manipulating sounds includes deleting, adding, or substituting syllables or sounds (e.g., say "can"; say it without the /k/; say "can" with /m/

instead of /k/). (retrieved March 6, 2009, from http://www .ldonline.org/article/6254)

Snow, Burns, and Griffin (1998) describe what is meant by the awareness of phonemes as "the sounds of speech as distinct from their meaning" (p. 51). They say that when the child realizes that "words divided into a sequence of phonemes, this finer grained sensitivity is termed phonemic awareness" (p. 51).

The Elusive Phoneme: Is It Real?

Technically speaking, a phoneme is a class of countless different sounds whose manifested members—the ones that can be said and heard, which are commonly called **phones** or when they vary depending on context **allophones**—are regarded as the same by a speaker of the language in question. Now, if you already think the idea is abstract, complex, and a little on the difficult side for a preschooler or a nonreader, you are correct. The world's best linguists and psychologists are still struggling to understand the idea of what constitutes a phoneme and whether the concept corresponds to anything real. Edward Sapir's famous 1933 paper on the psychological reality of the phoneme is still controversial. For instance, see the discussion by Chomsky and Hornstein (2005) arguing that in the final analysis "psychological reality" just means truth in a particular area of investigation but Chomsky (p. 107ff) continues to maintain (as he did earlier in Chomsky & Halle, 1968) that there is not enough evidence to justify such a conclusion for the elusive concept known as the phoneme.

Most literate individuals do not usually come up against the question of what a phoneme is until they get into a stiff college course in linguistics. That course is always bristling with many other technical terms pertaining to morphology, lexicon, syntax, semantics, pragmatics, **semiotics**, and a bunch of formerly hyphenated terms like **psycholinguistics**, **sociolinguistics**, and **neurolinguistics**. For most literate college students in their first course in linguistics the real disappointment (or excitement depending on interests) does not set in until they learn that all of these formerly hyphenated terms and the fields of study they associate with each other are essential to figuring out what the phoneme is.

The proponents of teaching phonemic theory—also known as the *alphabetic principle*—to pre-literate children are taking on a task that, for one inescapable reason, challenges highly literate adults in college and the best abstract thinkers in the world. The fact that language can be used to talk about language and about all the other phenomena in the universe shows that it must be equally or more abstract and complex than those phenomena or it could not be used to represent their complexities. Therefore, we may conclude—and a much more detailed and rigorous proof can be given, though none is needed to show—that language is complex, period.

If language is more complex (or at least as complex) as whatever it can be used to fully represent, it follows that language is the most complex phenomenon within our universe.

The reason that the idea of phonemes is difficult to grasp is because there is no simple way to define such an abstract idea. The false idea that phonemes are simple comes from what appears to be a one-to-one mapping between a sound like /k/ for instance and the letter "k." Such a mapping illustrates the alphabetic principle in its simplest form: one letter for one sound. It sure seems simple when we put it like that. But the simplicity is deceptive. The trick is that we must know the target sound in advance in order for the alphabetic principle to work. The problem, then, is how do we know any phoneme in the first place?

Phonics Fails Even with Alphabetic Systems

Recall that Hanna et al., to get their system of rules to convert sounds to letters correctly just 50% of the time, had to start with "phonetic" descriptions of the sounds. The speech they were converting to print had already been converted to a system of segmented individual sounds represented by letters of an alphabet. However, their system of rules (alphabetic rules!) failed to work about 50% of the time in mapping their phonetic representations into the letters of actual items in their list of 17,000 words.

"Well," someone might say, "that's because English is not very faithful to the alphabetic principle. The system would work with a language like Spanish, or Arabic, where the spellings are more phonetic." But the defender of the alphabet, as Little Red Riding Hood might point out about now, forgets that Hanna et al. started with phonetic transcriptions of the 17,000 words in their list. She might go further to point out that the Big Bad Wolf (Bloomfield) and his friends keep trying to make English spelling the bad guy when it is the theory of phonemes that is the real culprit. El-Imam (2004) and El-Imam and Don (2005) showed that writing systems such as those found in Arabic and Standard Malay which follow the alphabetic principle more closely than English are still not susceptible of TTS and SST on the basis of simple phoneme rules. And, recall Damper et al. (1999) who showed that for new words, phoneme rules work only about 26% of the time.

Attempts to make out that the phoneme is simple end up with definitions that are, in the end, plainly false—just as it is obviously wrong to say that modern English adheres very closely to the alphabetic principle. It is false that English represents each of its phonemes with just one letter and each letter represents just one phoneme. In fact, a deeper problem for proponents of the alphabetic principle (and phonics in all its elaborated varieties) is that no one can say just how many phonemes there are in English until we pin down a particular variety of English. But even then, the problem of which phonemes to represent is not solved. In General American English, for instance, even something as simple as the number of vowels cannot be pinned down with any certainty. For some speakers of General American English, words like *caught* and *cot* are rhymes as are *pin* and *pen*. For others, even *full* and *fool, cull* and *cool* are rhymes. So, the number of vowels to be represented in General American English, a relatively homogeneous dialect spoken across much of America and around the world, cannot be determined very exactly.

Meet the Real Abstraction: The Phoneme Himself

For the advocates of the alphabetic principle, the oddities of English spelling are not the central difficulty. The phoneme itself is the central problem. There is a long-standing debate about whether or not the concept of the phoneme is valid.

No one has been able yet to improve much on the argument for the psychological reality of the phoneme as it was put many years ago by Edward Sapir (1933). The concept of the phoneme has a certain psychological abstract reality—English speakers, for example, believe that /l/ and /r/ are really different phonemes as in *leak* and *wreak*, *light* or *right*. We do not, however, distinguish between the /p/ of *pit* and the one in *spit*. But speakers of Japanese regard /l/ and /r/ as the same phoneme and Thai speakers hear the /p/ of *pit* as an entirely different phoneme than the one in *spit*. In English, we distinguish words like *plaque* and *black*, and yet Arabic speakers do not bother to distinguish /p/ and /b/ in that position. For English speakers, /p/ and /b/ are different in those words, but for Arabic speakers they sound the same.

In 1973, Foss and Swinney, however, showed that it takes longer for adult college students to identify a phoneme in a spoken utterance than to handle two syllable words, or single syllables (retrieved September 19, 2008, from http://lcnl.ucsd.edu/LCNL_main_page/Publications_PDF/1973_Foss_Swinney.pdf). As Foss and Swinney (1973) observed,

> The same signal will be perceived differently in different linguistic environments and, in some cases, quite different signals will be perceived as being identical . . . speech decoding processes cannot be simple ones. (p. 246)

How true. Even the simplest imaginable one-to-one sound-to-letter correspondences are highly abstract and depend on deep mental processing that is anything but simple.

As we saw in Chapter 4 the motor elements in the inner ear can increase or decrease the strength of a certain aspect of a sound by as much a 100 times (Santos-Sacchi, 2003). Is it any surprise that Sapir was correct in supposing that the sounds of human perceptual systems are tuned to the particular language/dialect that we acquire? With that in mind, it should not surprise us to discover that the production and perception of any single phoneme—whatever it may be—is only a tiny part of the larger process of making sense of language. The rich systems that connect the various components of the sign hierarchy (see Chapter 4) enable the psychological reality of a unit that may be called the phoneme. However, to track him down, we must first know his habits and hangouts. It's

Why are phonemes harder to notice and process than syllables or whole words? The obvious conclusion that is sustained by the research on discourse processing is that we tend to understand whole texts on the basis of their meanings while the analysis at the level of phonemes is something that comes after the meanings have already been discovered.

tough detective work for pre-schoolers who have not yet been admitted to college.

Time to Tell Phonemes Apart? Sensory Integration Theory

Undoubtedly, one of the simplest ideas in many years that has been proposed about phonemes concerns the amount of time it supposedly takes to tell one from another. The idea comes from Dr. Paula Tallal (n.d.), a neuroscientist at Rutgers University, Newark, New Jersey (retrieved March 6, 2009, from http://cmbn.rutgers.edu/researc h/tallal.aspx). It is certainly one of the most interesting and amazingly simplistic controversial ideas ever associated with the phonological awareness movement. It also involves a fairly long chain of inferences. Let's see if we can follow them from their beginning up to the present.

Some Long Leaps of Inference

To begin with, Dr. Tallal reported that some infants take longer than others to tell the difference between two simple acoustic signals such as a low beep followed by a high one. The time interval she focused on was the one between the beeps. She and colleagues at Rutgers reported that some infants (at about six months of age) need hundreds of milliseconds, say, 200 to 500, to notice a difference between two distinct acoustic events—for example, a low followed by a high beep—whereas other infants are able to perform this discrimination in less than 50 milliseconds. In following the same infants over time, she reports that the infants who required the longer time intervals in order to make the discrimination were also slower in language acquisition than the infants who required less time. She called the time interval in question the **temporal integration threshold**.

Dr. Tallal noted that the slower infants, the ones with the higher threshold, were likely to come from families with a history of disorders and were more likely to be diagnosed later on as disordered themselves. The latter inference was supported by research contrasting matched groups of normal typically developing (N) children with children who had been diagnosed as having some language impairment or disorder (D). She reports that her research got the predicted outcome: The N group performed discriminations with shorter intervals between tones than the D group.

For reasons that ought already to be obvious, it is a long leap of inference from a time interval between pure tones—low beep, pause, high beep—to the idea that what is being measured is the time it takes a language user to perceive a shift from one phoneme to another in the processing of speech. One obvious difference, besides the fact that speech sounds are not beeps, is that the change from one phonemic segment to the next within a stream of speech is not normally marked by a pause. We do not say, "/k/ [pause]

We do not say, "/k/ [pause] /æ/ [pause] /t/" when mentioning that, "Pete's cat just jumped through the window into Andy's truck and then out the other side." There are no pauses between the phoneme transitions. Recall de Saussure's remarks about the ribbon of speech that is produced without distinct boundaries between sound segments.

/æ/ [pause] /t/" when mentioning that, "Pete's cat just jumped through the window into Andy's truck and then out the other side." There are no pauses between the phoneme transitions. Recall de Saussure's remarks about the ribbon of speech that is produced without distinct boundaries between sound segments.

However, the long leaps of inference, like the first leap of Pete's cat, do not end in with just one jump from pure tone beeps to phonemes. Dr. Tallal and her colleagues, notably Dr. Merzenich who was doing neurophysiological studies with monkeys, discovered that with "intensive training, monkeys could gradually improve their identification of faster and faster sounds" and in doing so Dr. Merzenich and colleagues found in the brains of the trained monkeys that the "specific auditory regions had reorganized and significantly expanded their neural circuits" (retrieved March 6, 2009, from http://www.newhorizons.org/neuro/tallal.htm). Hmmmm.

From Monkey Brains to Human Language

Having already generalized from pure tones to phonemes—a small step for some humans but a giant leap for any monkey—it was presumably easy to go right on to infer that

> if we could create a computer algorithm to acoustically disambiguate the rapidly changing acoustic cues within ongoing fluent speech, this might help **LLI [language learning impaired]** children process, and thus consistently represent, phonological cues in syllable, word and sentence context. (from the same Tallal Web site not updated since 1998)

How this might be done is not explained in any detail anywhere, but it supposedly forms the basis for therapy recommended for everything from dyslexia to autism by the neuroscience team at Rutgers. We are told, however, that there are:

> listening exercises designed to explicitly train on-line [real time] phonological discrimination and language comprehension using acoustically modified speech (same site).

So we have come full circle back to the notion of phonological awareness and its exclusive role in treating dyslexia. The basic idea, Dr. Tallal explains, it is to speed up processing time which is, she says,

> a fundamental goal of both speech and language therapy for language impaired children, as well as phonological awareness training for reading impaired (dyslexic) children (same site).

Is it true that speeding up the processing time required to discriminate pure tones—high versus low, for instance—will improve literacy or cure the sort of brain damage that some (e.g., the Shaywitz's, Lyon, and others) are claiming is the cause of supposedly widespread dyslexia? We believe it is far more likely that the sorts

It is extremely unlikely that training aimed at speeding up the time it takes to notice contrasts between different pure tones would improve language comprehension or the overall cognitive abilities associated with literacy. The theory proposed has so little to do with language processing that it is unlikely to provide the slightest help in curing any complex communication disorders.

of differences between normal individuals and persons with severe disorders as measured in Tallal's laboratory, supposing only that the measurements are valid, are owed to causes such as toxicity, disease, and genetics.

Needed: Critical Thinking and Fresh Insights

We have taken the trouble to go through the litany of variations on the phonics theme ranging from phonological awareness, the alphabetic principle, the psychological reality of the phoneme, to "intensive sensory integration training" that has been developed from studies of pure tone beeps and monkey brains so that our introductory students will see that their own wisdom and fresh insights are greatly needed in the study of communication disorders.

It is, we believe, essential to enable newcomers to the study of disorders to see just how easily unworkable false theories can be promoted and widely accepted.

Clearing the Way for Hope

The upshot of the excursion so far has been to show, that the essential remedies proposed for standard, run-of-the-mill dyslexia, are largely what is causing it in many, though probably not all cases. Sudden onset dyslexia caused by a blow to the head would be one of the exceptions. However, many cases diagnosed as genetic brain damage are virtually certain to belong in the category of instructionally induced dyslexia. In the following section we deal with cases where the diagnosis of hopeless lifelong dyslexia turned out to be wrong.

CURING INSTRUCTIONAL DYSLEXIA

Training in phonics and in phonological awareness, sound-to-letter relations, and all the "blending" of separate sounds and letters to try to get normal sounding speech, will certainly produce the symptoms of dyslexia in any normal child who can be persuaded, or forced, to use such methods exclusively. That sort of phonological training, to the exclusion of any other methods that might conceivably enable him or her to make sense of some meaningful text, is sure to produce all the symptoms of dyslexia as we have seen earlier in this chapter. The reasonable conclusion from the research with SST and TTS systems—not to mention sound theory concerning how discourse processing normally works—is that a steady and exclusive diet of phonics will make any normal child dyslexic.

Some Bad News and Some Good News

We have heard the bad news that phonics can cause instructional dyslexia, but finding this out is good news because it leads to reasonable hope.

The Good News
If instructional dyslexia can be caused by misguided instruction, it can be cured by using better methods of instruction based on a more complete understanding of language, language acquisition, and literacy. If directing attention away from meaning and focusing it on surface form causes instructional dyslexia, then directing attention back to meaning ought to cure it.

Overcoming the Inertia of a Negative Self-Image

Many individuals who have a curable form of instructional dyslexia are like a boy we knew. We will call him GW for short and to protect his identity. He told his Aunt B, after being held back in two grades, "It ain't no use, Aint B. I cain't read." By this time, GW was a foot taller than any other child in the third grade and there was a good reason why—he should have been in the sixth grade except for starting school late and being held back twice in the second grade. When he went to live with Aunt B and Uncle J, they got him admitted to a third grade class on the promise that somehow he would learn to read, write, and do his numbers up through multiplication and long division. He had what we are calling instructional dyslexia and he didn't get over it without a change in instructional methods. He also had some self-image issues that created some **negative inertia**. That is, he didn't think he could learn at all. He was roughly in the state of mind described by Stephen J. Cannell on his Web site at 26 seconds into the presentation on "Dyslexia in Childhood" (retrieved March 6, 2009, from http://www.cannell.com/dyslexia.php?vid=2). He says,

> I was never told by my parents or my teachers that I was stupid, which I've heard other people with this condition have said, "Oh, I was told by my teachers, I was stupid." I never got that. I got this other thing, I wasn't applying myself. Uhmm. But I knew I was stupid. I knew there was no other answer that I could come up with that was responsible for all these D's and F's . . .

A critical obstacle to curing instructionally induced dyslexia is the notion in the affected person that,

> I can't do this. I am a non-reader. I don't understand words. When I look at a page of print, I choke. My eyes want to close on their own. I can't keep them open. I can't think of anything but getting out of this situation.

A person affected by instructional dyslexia soon gets the idea that reading is something they just can't do.

Stephen J. Cannell was often told he was lazy, but he knew that was not correct. No one was telling him he was stupid, but he reached that conclusion on his own. We know that his own conclusion also was not true, but he reached it just as certainly as water runs downhill.

Stephen J. Cannell tells that when he was being held back for three different grades, the teachers never told him he was stupid. He learned later, however, that other individuals with instructional dyslexia commonly get that line a lot. In his case they didn't tell him he was stupid. They just told him that he didn't work very hard or apply himself. More about that in a moment. For Stephen Cannell, however, for them to tell him he was stupid would have been completely redundant. He had already reached that conclusion on his own. He explains that being a football star in high school was all that saved him from a completely awful self-image. When he went on campus he was somebody because he could out-run all the high school competition in California and just about everywhere else on the football field.

Tanking Tests

Football successes kept him from the total depression that comes with the conclusion that me, myself, and I—never mind Irene and Jim Carrey—are all just plain stupid. Cannell says he knew this had to be true every time he "tanked a test." It even happened multiple times after he (and his mom) had spent many extra hours studying so it wouldn't happen again. On one memorable occasion, when he asked a pal in the parking lot after the history exam, "Hey, how much time did you spend studying for that A?" and the friend said, "None, really. I just glanced at it in the parking lot." That's when he knew he was stupid. He didn't need anyone to tell him. He just knew it. But lazy? Far from it. Laziness was not a problem for Stephen J. Cannell—not then, not ever.

Mr. Cannell is a guy who worked a regular job, went home at five and made it a habit to write till 10 pm every night for five years before he sold a single manuscript. This is a guy who still gets up at four o'clock in the morning everyday of the week, Saturday and Sunday included, to write for five or six hours. He says,

> You'd be surprised how much forward motion you can get out of a career if you're willing to put that much energy into it. (hear him tell how to treat people and how to build a career; retrieved March 6, 2009, from http://www.cannell.com/video QA.php?s=9&k=84f011ccbe88f676c6aeaa73929104fc)

Stephen Cannell is not lazy and he is nothing if not persistent. He married a girl he met before they entered high school and he is still married to the same woman—way to go, Steve and Marcia!—almost four decades later. Does he sound like a lazy guy who never learned how to apply himself when he was going to school?

Some Relevant Facts

So, let's see. He wasn't stupid, wasn't lazy, what about the idea that he is the victim of genetically induced brain damage? Or could it be that Stephen J. Cannell, like a lot of other students who took the phonics approach seriously, became a victim of a misguided approach to instruction? Frankly, we think that Stephen J. Cannell has described symptoms of his own dyslexia that are consistent with instructionally induced—phonics produced—classical Bloomfieldian dyslexia. But, we do not intend to challenge his diagnosis as such. What we do intend to do is to show how instructional dyslexia can be cured. We know that instructional dyslexia is curable just as certainly as we know that Stephen J. Cannell did not get to be a successful script writer, novelist, and one of the most creative minds in Hollywood by being stupid. We know that he didn't create his own company and eventually compete successfully as a private owner against Metro Goldwyn Mayer (MGM) and Universal Studios by being stupid or lazy.

We are equally certain that it also is not true that genetically induced brain damage can be cured by phonics or that instructionally induced dyslexia dooms individuals to a lifelong (genetic) condition.

> Instructional dyslexia is not a form of brain damage. It's just the unfortunate result of a very misguided approach to the teaching of literacy.

Going to School on Success

In golf tournaments, the player who gets to putt last, they say, has an advantage. That player gets to see how the other player's shot rolls toward the hole. They say that the person who takes the later shot "goes to school" on the other person's experience. As for the theories that turn out to be wrong, we can learn from them too, but we just don't want to rely on them, or to subject people to methods of instruction that don't produce success. We are always aiming for success. When it comes to successful language acquisition, language teaching, and literacy, there is a great deal of research providing a basis for testing the competing theories. Some of the theories come up winners, others losers. As teachers, caregivers, clinicians, researchers and theory builders ourselves, we want to put our money and effort on the winners.

In the research on discourse processing there are many lessons about what makes processing easier, memory more accessible, text more intelligible (or less), words more recallable, syntax easier to process, meanings more accessible, and so on. What is more, there are general principles that can be counted on across essentially all of the contexts, populations, languages, and modalities that have ever been studied (J. S. Damico & S. K. Damico, 1993; Krashen, 2004;

> Many of the principles that hold in first language acquisition also hold in second language studies and in literacy instruction.

Principles of Literacy Instruction

Principle (1) *Use stories*. Narratives where one event leads to another are foundational. In real life things don't just happen higgledy piggledy. (Using nonsense to teach reading dispenses with this principle and all those that follow. Phonics cannot, therefore, benefit from any of them.)

Principle (2) *Use true reports of actual experience*. These are easier to generate and understand than fictions—not to mention errors, lies, and nonsense.

Principle (3) *Demonstrate and act out meanings*. Actual content whether it is known through experience, dramatization (acting out), or vicariously through demonstration, is more intelligible and memorable. We say: *Actions speak louder than words* but the subtext is that actions often reveal real intentions more accurately than the surface forms of words. Meanings are clearer when we see the action.

Principle (4) *Get client/students personally involved*. This can be done through meaningful conflict, doubt, and surprise, and difficulties of central actors in the story line. All these things make any story, text, or task more interesting.

Principle (5) *Work at the ZPD*. When challenged, intelligent interpreters/producers of discourse tend to work at the highest level of representation of meanings and intentions of which they are capable. This is where we need to focus our client/learner's attention.

Principle (6) *Use multiple modalities to display the meaning*. The more I know about the meaning of a text—as shown, for instance, in different modalities of processing such as seeing, hearing, acting out, and experiencing the content—the easier it will be for me to decipher it, to unpack its surface forms, to map those forms onto their meanings, and, in general, to become able to understand, produce, and creatively manipulate those surface forms. This last principle holds even if the text or discourse is in a language/dialect that I don't know yet. Recall the old adage: *Tell me and I will forget, but show me and I will remember*.

The principle that telling is less effective than showing is universal. The expression of it in this aphorism, "*Tell me and I will forget, but show me and I will remember*," we owe to our inspiring friend, Craig Winter. It is just one of the many take-home messages that we got from him. It has a distinctly oriental ring to it, and yet, it fits the western world as well as the eastern.

S. D. Oller, 2005). Among them are these general principles (which we will number so you can easily see how they connect with the success stories to follow in the next two sections):

Every one of the bulleted principles just stated has been shown to be valid in experiments with discourse processing and language acquisition in multiple contexts of experience (J. W. Oller, L. Chen, S. D. Oller, & Pan, 2005). The principles stated also get results in difficult cases, for instance, in individuals who are diagnosed with disorders such as dyslexia.

The Case of GW

GW (whom we mentioned earlier) was taller than any other third grader and physically advanced above his peers, but he couldn't read, write, or do simple arithmetic. He was facing the huge obstacle of a negative self-concept that was just about exactly the size and shape of the image he saw in the mirror whenever Aunt B got him to brush his teeth and comb his hair—that would be every day before school. But school was not going well.

The reports were consistent, GW could not read.

He was far behind his peers and it looked like he was going to fail another year. Unless something drastic happened he would be held back for another shot at the third grade next year. He'd only been put in the third grade rather than the second on account of the fact that his younger cousin DR was in that grade and in that classroom. It was hoped that GW would somehow be able to catch up.

It took a while, but it happened.

Here is the story of GW's eventual complete recovery from instructional dyslexia.

Every night after school, Aunt B would read a particular story that GW liked in a storybook that was handy. It was a narrative (Principle 1) about characters that GW identified with and events that involved significant conflicts (Principle 4). The first time through Aunt B read the story all the way to the end and then asked questions about it (Principle 6). The next time, Aunt B would point to the text and occasionally pause for GW to guess the next word or sentence. It might be something like, "That day Tom was supposed to . . . "

And GW might inject, "I know, Aint B. Whitewash the fence. That's what they were gonna do. But he got one of his friends to do it by bribin' him with an apple core."

And so it went night after night with an hour or more of instruction for GW every single day after school until one night, after a few weeks, it seemed that the light went on. It was true that GW knew much of the story by rote at this point and that he knew every significant fact in it from start to finish. What was more, he also had begun to pick apart the surface forms until they were also almost completely decipherable without assistance. When he took the book in his own hands and began to read the story out loud, there was a sneaking suspicion that maybe GW was just reciting from memory (Principle 6). There was no doubt he could do that for many of the lines of the text. But, the clincher was that he could turn the page at the end of the oral reading of the familiar story and he was able also to read the next one, and, in fact, he could read any story in the book.

He also overcame, to a great extent, the cumulative negative inertia of four very unsuccessful years of trying to learn to read. He never slipped back to the dyslexia of those early years and it was obvious that his condition was neither life-long nor any form of genetically caused developmental brain damage.

Within a few weeks, GW had overcome instructionally induced dyslexia by diligent attention to meaning with a little help from a mature and skilled reader.

The Case of RM

When RM's parents first started taking her to clinics, pediatricians, and speech-language pathologists, she was only about two years past the ideal age of "reading readiness" according to the standard theories—she was already seven years old. Her brother, JM, just two years older than her, had been reading for four years by this time. By the time she was eight, R was diagnosed with dyslexia. Interestingly, the programs attempted with her up to that point were all of the phonics variety. She not only did not seem to understand phonics, but it seemed to have a seriously negative impact on her ability to think at all when looking at the letters of a word. She could not read the word "the."

They Said It Was "Genetic"

Her parents were told that R's condition was genetic and that her brain was affected. She would never be able to read, write, or do arithmetic. Those kinds of abstract skills were out of reach for R, forever. Her parents were advised to help her prepare for a career "using her hands." They were told that she would probably never be able to read. R seemed to have a form of extreme dyslexia—the kind sometimes called "alexia" or "word blindness." She did not seem to be able to recognize different letters or any single word, no matter how familiar and ordinary. She could not read or write her name.

Being well-educated, reasonably well-off middle class individuals in the beautiful hills of San Diego, California with its high density population and ready access to clinics and specialists of every known stripe and degree, R's parents were not about to give up without seeking a second, third, fourth, and however many opinions it might take to find a specialist who could give them some hope. During the course of the search, R's mother was diagnosed with an aggressive cancer early in R's ninth year. The prognosis for mom was terminal—the illness might last for a few weeks or, at most, a few months.

Diagnosis: Hopeless

By this time, R's mother believed that R was "hopelessly dyslexic" and knew that she herself (R's mom) did not have long to live. When we met R's mom, however, her foremost concern was not for herself but for whether or not R might have any hope of becoming literate, completing an education, and living a normal life. During the course of a conversation with R and her older brother J, the most striking facts were that she was able to hold her own on any subject. She talked about her home, how she liked living in San Diego. She pointed out where she and her family attended church and in all respects seemed to be a highly fluent speaker of English with no sign whatever of the sort of genetic developmental "brain damage" that her parents had been told was keeping her from learning to read. We did not talk about reading that day, but her mom reported that her favorite stories included such classics as *Beauty and the Beast*.

Normal Speech and Language

On the first encounter with nine-year-old R, it was evident that there was nothing in R's behavior to indicate that her language abilities were not normal. They were right where they should be in terms of expected milestones of vocabulary, syntax, semantics, pragmatics, social skills, world knowledge, and the evident recall of recent or distant events. Her ability to report a narrative sequence, and so forth, was normal. As a result, there was no hesitation in our suggesting a plan of action very much like the one described above for GW. The added elements included video viewing of a story like *Beauty and the Beast*, or some particularly meaningful part of it; reading of the movie script; reading the story in a text form; asking follow up questions to each version to establish the major facts of the story line. For instance, R's mom was encouraged to ask, "And then, what happens? Why does Belle go to the castle?"

Multiple Passes Through Familiar Material

The plan was to cycle through the viewing of and discussing of the video and the repeated readings of the various text forms while going deeper into the story on each reading, always seeking on each pass to get farther into the material. The key is to get to know the event sequences while becoming more and more acquainted with the printed words, phrases, and surface forms to the point of over learning—near memorization. R was to become so familiar with the story that the meaning could be used as a scaffolding to support the deciphering of the surface forms of the printed story line.

First, the names of main characters, for example, Belle, Beast, Ludovic, and so forth, would become both familiar and recognizable wherever they appeared in the story line. Then, key relations would be developed, major events, scenes, and so on. Once again, the plan was to keep recycling and going deeper on each pass until R was able to read names of characters, then whole phrases, then whole lines, and finally the whole text on her own.

Business took one of us to San Diego about once every six months over the next year and a half. On each trip, there would be a request for a report about R's progress. About halfway through the first six months, R's mother got the good news that she was evidently in remission from her cancer. But by the next trip to San Diego, the bad news was that R had made no progress in the early going and mom had given up.

Another Round of Discouraging Prognoses

R's mom and dad had been to see a couple more specialists, including a pediatrician in whom they had a lot of confidence. Mom had given up on the tutoring program we had devised. However, during a weekend trip to the hands-on science museum with R's whole family at Balboa Park, R's mom got encouraged to try again.

Six months later, essentially the same conversation was repeated. Mom had again become discouraged with the reading sessions and just didn't think it was ever going to take. R knew and seemed to understand the stories that mom was working on with her, but R was not showing any sign that she could read on her own.

The Light Goes On

Then, about a year and a half into the process, as in GW's case, the light finally came on. R's dad had mentioned some bad news about the cancer coming back and that work was not all that he had hoped either, but, "By the way," he said on the way to the airport, "R read for the first time this week."

He told how R's mom had started to read a familiar story to R, a couple of weeks before. R had said, "Mom, I think I can read that story myself." She took the book and managed to read the whole story with hesitations on only a couple of words.

The critical thing was that the next story was one they had not studied.

While she was reading, as her mom reported later to dad, it occurred to mom that R had merely memorized the text. Mom's heart sank like a rock. But about the time R got to the end of the story, when mom's heart had hit the bottom of the Pacific Ocean, R turned the page and said, "And, mom, I think I can read the next one too." And so she did.

Then, her father reported that R had told her mom she wanted to call dad and read to him over the phone. She did, and on the way to the airport that day, he told how R had read every word of the poem titled, *The Charge of the Light Brigade* by Alfred Lord Tennyson [1809–1892] (retrieved March 6, 2009, from http://poetry.eserver.org/light-brigade.html). It starts like this,

> Half a league, half a league,
> Half a league onward,
> All in the valley of Death
> Rode the six hundred. . . .

And so it goes for 265 words. R's mother died later that year, but R went on to graduate from college and, according to all accounts, completely overcame her dyslexia.

ACQUIRING MULTIPLE MODALITIES AND LANGUAGES

We have already seen that babies can learn to read before they can even speak intelligibly. Before they can even say their first word, normal infants, by about seven to nine months can understand many spoken words. The theory of abstraction shows why this accomplishment already exceeds the representational basis needed for understanding printed words. What is more, at a very early age, the research shows that normal babies can about as easily acquire two or even three languages as one (Swain, 1972). Should it surprise us to discover that with teaching methods that respect the pragmatic processes children use to acquire one or more languages also enable them to acquire literacy in a new language?

That is to say, with pragmatic methods of instruction that rely on meaning and the general principles of discourse processing described earlier in this chapter, children can learn to read in English when their home language is Hottentot, or in Thai when their home language is Mandarin, Hmong, or some other language. Acquiring another modality for processing—adding printed words to an existing repertoire of spoken words—or acquiring a whole new language/dialect are similar processes at their foundations. All of them in all combinations depend on the kind of pragmatic mapping process that Helen Keller engaged in with the assistance of Annie Sullivan. All of them involve the comprehension of content prior to the association of that content with new ways of representing it—for example, in print rather than speech, or in English rather than Hottentot.

In the sections that follow, we will show the logical, fundamental dependence of each of the processes we have just described, on the pragmatic mapping relation by which distinct symbols are mapped onto known content.

Print as Another, Easier Modality

Reviewing and expanding on what we noted earlier in this chapter, spoken words are more difficult to discriminate, recall, and recognize on a subsequent presentation than are printed words. An average syllable of English (or any spoken language) takes less than half a second to produce, but the same word, say, *hand*, if it is printed can be perceived, discriminated from everything around it, and refreshed by re-examining the word as many times as we like by looking away and then back again at the printed word. It sticks around a lot longer than the half second it takes for someone to say it out loud.

The theory of abstraction shows why the baby who can move her hand when asked, "Can you show me your hand?" is also able to perform the same action in response to a flash card displayed where she can see it that happens to have the word *hand* printed on it. The theory of pragmatic mapping shows that the mental processes involved are logically isomorphic. It is a logical certainty that an individual who has the necessary sensory and mental resources to perform the pragmatic mapping involved in understanding a spoken word and map it onto the sort of action involved in demonstrating that she knows what is meant by her "hand" is also able to perform the simpler mapping involved in associating a printed word with the same action. We do not need to perform a brain scan or any sort of anatomical study to take this argument all the way to a certain and necessary conclusion. It is more certain than saying that a banker who can make change (without a calculator or computer) can also count.

Therefore, GW, RM, and all normal persons who can perform such mappings of spoken words, have the necessary resources to do so with print. Or putting the argument the other way around, any mental or sensory deficits that would make impossible the mapping of the printed word "hand" onto an action by a baby of displaying her own hand, would also make impossible the more difficult pragmatic mapping of the same action onto the spoken word *hand*.

This finding alone empirically refutes the strongest claims of the theories of phonics, phonological awareness, and all of the methods of reading instruction that insist literacy instruction must begin with converting letters to sounds and print to speech. All those theories are mistaken and are empirically disproved by Aleka Titzer all by herself.

By three years and two months, Aleka could read fluently the story of *The Three Little Pigs*. And she was not alone in this as seen in her friends in the video. She could report that in reading a story she felt she was in it. Her comments as reported by her dad, and her actions, animation, and ability to talk about the meanings of what she was reading, all show that she was already reading very much like an expert adult reader and she was doing it by age 3.

Adding a new modality—print—to an existing one—speech—is possible for babies and it is logically possible for anyone who can understand speech. If this is so, there is something fundamentally incorrect about standard theories of dyslexia.

> As demonstrated by Aleka Titzer, with a little help from her dad, Dr. Robert Titzer, it is evident that it really is possible for babies to understand printed words before they can produce spoken versions of those words on their own. The baby can actually read printed words before being able to say them.

Becoming Multilingual/Multidialectal

Linguists and language students never cease to be amazed at little children who easily do in a foreign language/dialect what seems difficult to us as adults. The adults often comment that it is humbling as well as amazing that the little children in, say, Tokyo, speak perfect Japanese with little effort while adult foreigners struggle with simple expressions like "hello," "please," and "thank-you." All over the world adults complain that they feel like helpless children when confronted with the need to express themselves in a foreign language. One Farsi speaker complained that he is a poet and professor of literature in his native language. And yet when he tries to express himself in English, he is reduced, almost to the level not of a child, but as he put it, of a fool—a person who appears to have no good ideas because he can't express them well enough or fast enough. He noted that he might not still have an audience when and if he ever gets around to saying what he means in English. Imagine trying to get an advanced degree under those kinds of conditions. It isn't easy. But for children it all seems to be child's play. They seem to make language acquisition easy. How do they do it?

What is more, they can do it with two, three, or perhaps even more languages simultaneously if given the opportunity. Several things, however, are required in order for a child to acquire two or more "first" languages (Swain, 1972). They must have access to model speakers of both languages on a fairly regular (usually a daily) basis, and they must have both the opportunity and the social need to communicate in both languages. Relatively **balanced bilingualism**—where the individual is equally proficient in both languages—is rare. Balanced **trilingualism**—where a person is equally at ease in three languages—is rarer still, but it does occur. Examples in the field of applied linguistics include Claire Kramsch, professor of German at the University of California at Berkeley, and William F. Mackey, professor emeritus at Laval University in Quebec. All that is required, evidently, is access to the needed native models and the social demand to use all three languages about equally. However, all skilled multilinguals report that there are situations in which one of their several languages is preferred.

Even for multilinguals who are far from equally proficient in their several languages, the preferred language is not always the "first" or "native" language. In a certain context one of the languages of lesser proficiency may be preferred. For instance, we know a multilingual man whose native language is English, but who also speaks Spanish, French, and German. He learned and studied Judo in Spain but competed in other combative sports in the United States. Interestingly, but unsurprisingly, whenever the subject of Judo comes up it seems awkward to him to talk about it in any of his several languages other than Spanish. All of the terminology is accessible in Spanish but requires tedious work to translate to English much less would he consider talking about Judo in French or German. What does such a common experience show us? Simply that the language we acquire in particular contexts of experience is mapped into those contexts so completely that it becomes permanently associated with them, and they become associated with the surface forms of that language. The association is so complete, in genuine language acquisition, that when we go into the situation again, we find the language is there too.

As J. W. Oller, Sr. (1965) put it in the "Introduction" to the Spanish program, *El español por el mundo* (*Spanish for the world*),

> the moment a student can react automatically [in the foreign language] . . . to a given situation . . . he "knows" the foreign language used in *that* situation. The proper procedure then is to immerse the student in the world in which this language is used, a world inhabited by people about whom he knows and cares. This sharing . . . establishes the *sine qua non* [without

which not] for the teaching of the language, the desire of the students to learn to communicate with the people of that language. (p. ix)

Adding a Language/Dialect and a Modality

It is also possible to acquire literacy—to add the print modality to speech—while at the same time acquiring a new language. Obviously, putting both tasks together makes for a more difficult teaching and learning experience. However, theory, research, and practice all show that it is not only *not impossible*, but acquiring literacy in a second language can be done in very difficult socioeconomic conditions. It has been accomplished, for example, by Hottentot children (Australian aborigines; see Hart, Walker, & Gray, 1973) in English (see J. W. Oller, Walker, & Rattanavich, 1993; Rattanvich, Walker, & J. W. Oller, 1992), by the Hill Tribe children of northern Thailand in Thai. Read the success stories about the Rotary Lighthouse literacy programs in these difficult parts of the world (retrieved March 6, 2009, from http://www.cleliteracy.org/).

Briefly put, the requirements for acquiring literacy and a second language simultaneously are the same as those for both of these tasks if they were performed separately. The most important element without any competition is meaning. We need a meaningful structure to work from and the meaning must be made comprehensible to the learners—nonsense does not work well in any context and here it will not work at all. It should also be noted at this point that assessment and diagnosis of disorders, a subject we deal with

> If literacy can be achieved in a second language by largely nomadic groups in places like the drug infested and war torn area of the Golden Triangle (see Figure 9–3) formed by Thailand, Burma (now Myanmar), and Laos, it can be done in any part of the world.

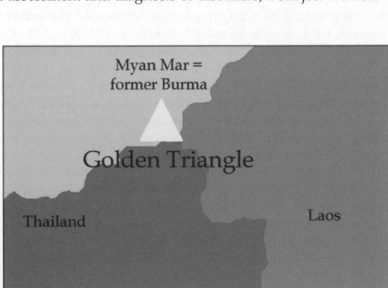

FIGURE 9–3. The Golden Triangle of Southeast Asia inhabited by the Hill Tribes who speak at least nine distinct languages that are not native to any of the three countries.

intensively in Chapter 11, is more difficult when we are dealing with the dual task of both second language acquisition and the acquisition of literacy. The standard definitions of dyslexia, unfortunately, will identify every learner as dyslexic in the early stages of acquiring both literacy and a second language simultaneously. Is it any wonder, then, that minority language/dialect users are more apt to be diagnosed with a reading disorder/disability than majority language/dialect users? At the same time, consider just how strange it would seem to propose to a person who does not know a word of the target language—say, it is English—"Just sound it out Sophal! Just ask yourself what sounds the letters make." It will not matter how loudly and plainly the teacher says these words, or writes them, if Sophal does not understand them, the instruction will fail.

Phonics is an unworkable approach to teaching a foreign language while at the same time building literacy in that same language. It is exactly like proposing to teach a preliterate child to read and write in Igbo, say, by teaching them the phonics of Igbo in Igbo. It won't work. Why? Simple. Because the child does not understand Igbo.

The Advantage of Narrative Structure

The key is to start with facts that the child already knows. This is best done with stories about experience rather than abstract lessons in linguistics presented in an unknown language/dialect. Since experience unfolds as a narrative, it is always best to use materials for teaching language and literacy that respect the sequence of experience. All activities, games, dramatizations, reports of activities, not to mention stories about real experience, tend toward the sequential narrative form. There are logical reasons for this. The simplest reason is simplicity itself.

The standard definitions of dyslexia, unfortunately, will identify every learner as dyslexic in the early stages of acquiring both literacy and a second language simultaneously. Is it any wonder, then, that minority language/dialect users are more apt to be diagnosed with a reading disorder/disability than majority language/dialect users?

Chronological Organization: The Simplest Reason

All human beings throughout the world tend to report events in a **chronological narrative order** on account of the fact that this is the simplest possible arrangement. Consider this: if events 1, 2, 3, and so on appear in that order and they are reported in symbols, say, A, B, C and so on, is there any simpler way to achieve the pragmatic mapping of the events than to map A to 1, B to 2, and so on? It can be strictly proved that there is absolutely no simpler way. So, human beings everywhere prefer a simple chronology over more complicated ways of representing the event sequences of experience.

For that reason, it is unsurprising that research with language processing and acquisition, universally sustains the conclusion that, all else being equal, simple sequential narratives are easier to comprehend (Mandler & Goodman, 1982; Speer & Zacks, 2005; Thorndyke, 1977; Trabasso, van den Broek, & Suh, 1989; Zwaan, 1994), produce (Claus & Kelter, 2006; Kelter, Kaup, & Claus, 2004; J. W. Oller & Obrecht, 1969), recall (Radvansky, Zwaan, Federico, & Franklin, 1998; Wolman, van den Broek, & Lorch, 1997), or any combination of these (Magliano, J. Miller, & Zwaan, 2001; Speer, Zacks, & Reynolds, 2007). If the same textual material is presented in a scrambled or otherwise disconnected form, in bits and pieces, or if matched segments of material dropped out of the sky are presented instead of a sensible narrative (J. W. Oller, 1994; Zacks, Speer, Swallow, Braver, & Reynolds, 2007)—the disrupted narrative structure is harder to process and to learn from.

We Know More About Narratives in Advance

The research, in general, has to come out as it does in favor of narrative structures because of what we know about ordinary stories in advance. We know a great deal about how sequences of events are arranged in experience (Kintsch, 1978; Mandler & Goodman, 1982; J. W. Oller, Sr., 1965; Thorndyke, 1977; Speer, Zacks, & Reynolds, 2007). We know quite a lot about what can happen and what cannot happen. As a result, the meanings of narratives are more coherent and easier to process.

To demonstrate this to yourself, consider the fact that A comes before B in the alphabet just as 1 comes before 2 in counting. Next, try to produce a random sequence of either letters or numbers out loud as fast as you can. Try mixing letters and numbers. Or try producing out loud a random list of words as fast as you can. Compare the results of all these experiments with saying the alphabet in sequence, counting as fast as you can, or telling what you did all day starting from breakfast. In each of these comparisons, which anyone can make, the sequential productions in chronological order (the basic narrative structure) is more fluent. It is more productive. It is easier to recall. It is easier to understand.

Nonsense is not only meaningless, it is more difficult to produce, recall, and to learn from. We cannot comprehend or learn anything much from nonsense—that is why it is called nonsense. Nonsense can only be used to illustrate surface forms. They are very useful when connected to meanings, but otherwise, they are just nonsense, period.

More importantly, for researchers and consumers of research who depend on measurement in the sciences, it has been strictly proved (J. W. Oller & L. Chen, 2007) that the very possibility of doing any valid measurement of any kind is utterly dependent on

The research, in general, has to come out as it does in favor of narrative structures because of what we know about ordinary stories in advance. We know a great deal about how sequences of events are arranged in experience (Kintsch, 1978; Mandler & Goodman, 1982; J. W. Oller, Sr., 1965; Thorndyke, 1977; Speer, Zacks, & Reynolds, 2007).

the kind of **sequential (episodic) organization** found in ordinary experience. Summing up the argument very briefly, if we could not tell that event A precedes B which comes before C, for instance, we could not validly differentiate any pair of events—A versus B, or B versus C, or A versus C—whatsoever. We could not represent any event truly or correctly. Much less could we take any valid measurements involving scales of that are more complex than the judgement that this is A rather than not A (i.e., B, or C, or whatever).

Measurement in the sciences, and in any kind of experience, utterly depends on the kinds of transitive relations found in the kinds of sequences of events that make up a narrative. They are essential to the kinds of true statements we make in reporting what happened or what we did in an experiment, or a simple recipe. This conclusion has been demonstrated and proved logically and mathematically in a variety of ways (see J. W. Oller & L. Chen, 2007; J. W. Oller, L. Chen, Pan, & S. J. W. Oller, 2005; Peirce, 1897; Tarski, 1936/1956, 1944/1949). Take a simple recipe as an example. Emeril Lagasse, or America's sweetheart of beer and pretzels, Rachael Ray (retrieved March 6, 2009, from http://en.wikipedia.org/wiki/Emeril_Lagasse and https://www.rachaelraymag.com/), might report a recipe this way: "A, first you get certain mate-rials; then, B, you heat water in a pan till it starts to bubble, . . . " and so on.

> Measurement in the sciences, and in any kind of experience, utterly depends on the kinds of transitive relations found in the kinds of sequences of events that make up a narrative.

Meaningful Sequence
Simple stories (narratives) are the best basis for teaching languages and literacy on account of their richness of meaning and because their events are arranged in a **meaningful sequence**.

Usually, we report the events in a story more or less in chronological order—that is, in a temporal order where if A precedes B it is reported before B and so on for all the events in the sequence.

So, temporal order is a kind of transitive relation. Similarly, if event A causes B, then A will tend to be reported first for both temporal and causal reasons. But transitive relations also include things such as equality where if A = B and B = C then A = C, where time and place play no necessary part. Transitive relations also fit many spatial instances where if A is to the left of B, and B is to the left of C, then, we can infer that A is to the left of C. This spatial relation, however, does not involve either time or causation. So, transitive relations are general, abstract, and the basis for all kinds of transitivity and thus for reasoning. In narratives, time sequence is foundational and forms the basis for our discovery of causation and also for the inferences we form about causal relations. Both the content and the sequence of narratives are foundational.

In this chapter we have discussed evidence showing that it is virtually certain that the most commonly recommended treatments for dyslexia are the primary cause of many cases of reading difficulties or failures.

SUMMING UP AND LOOKING AHEAD

In this chapter we have discussed evidence showing that it is virtually certain that the most commonly recommended treatments for dyslexia are the primary cause of many cases of reading difficulties or failures. Reading difficulties produced by nearly exclusive attention to letters and their abstract relations to sounds—the more exclusive the attending, the more severe the difficulties—are mistakenly being diagnosed as "dyslexia." Research with SST and TTS shows that reading aloud by sounding out new sequences of letters generates speech that is only about 50% intelligible. Spelling by phonics, going from sounds to letters, similarly, result in misspelling about 50% of the words attempted. Individuals trained to read exclusively by sounding out letters, will have all the primary symptoms of dyslexia. Many such cases are incorrectly being diagnosed as having genetically induced "brain abnormalities."

Sound-to-letter correspondences alone do not give good results in SST and TTS even if we start from the best phonetic spellings. It is even less effective in English because our spelling system is very far from using one letter for each phoneme. It is even more difficult to sound out unknown words in English for this reason than it is in phonetically spelled languages—but intelligible discourse cannot be produced by that method even with a phonetic spelling as the starting point. A more complete theory, however, shows why meaning is the solution to the reading problem. It is possible for a baby to understand printed words as soon as the baby can understand spoken words. The critical mental operations involve pragmatically mapping printed symbols correctly onto persons, actions, relations, and sequences of events in the world of experience. This can be done by normal infants at about seven to nine months of age—five or six months before the baby can say any spoken words out loud. Also, instructional dyslexia can be cured by changing from strict phonics to pragmatics.

The research evidences show, just as it is possible for children to become bilingual when they are babies, or to acquire literacy as infants, it is also possible for children to acquire a new language and literacy at the same time. Meaning must be attended to throughout. Nonsense should generally not be used and linguistic analysis of phonemes, phonological awareness, and all of the sound-to-letter relations of the alphabet, are best acquired in the context of stories we already understand. An exclusive diet of sound-to-letter relations will produce instructional dyslexia. To cure it, we need to enrich the diet to include meaningful stories that children can understand. Then, later on, when they do become able to talk about abstract sound-to-letter relations, they will be ready for a course in linguistics, and they will be able to understand phonetics and phonemics.

An exclusive diet of sound-to-letter relations will produce instructional dyslexia. To cure it, we need to enrich the diet to include meaningful stories that children can understand.

STUDY AND DISCUSSION QUESTIONS

1. Why would someone like Albert Einstein be a candidate for so many different disorders?
2. Why can't fully intelligible speech be produced by babies before they are able to understand any speech forms?
3. In the videotape of Aleka reading the flash cards, how many times does dad say the word before Aleka demonstrates comprehension of it?
4. Why is understanding speech logically more difficult than the discrimination, recall, and repeat recognition of print?
5. How do the standard definitions of dyslexia incorporate the discrepancy approach to defining disorders in general?
6. Why not define "giftedness" in terms of a discrepancy between unexpectedly low scores in language/dialect proficiency accompanied by high scores in math and reading, say?
7. What are the main differences between intrinsic (genetic) disabilities and extrinsic (acquired) disorders?
8. What elements are left out of play in a strict application of phonics—sound-to-letter and letter-to-sound—teaching of literacy?
9. What is wrong with the statement that "English basically has an alphabetic writing system"? Suppose someone says, "English strictly adheres to the phonemic principle."
10. What kinds of inferences are involved in supposing that measuring the threshold of perception for a gap between two beeps will enable the diagnosis of reading disabilities?
11. What scaffolding elements enabled GW, RM, or other persons you know of who had severe reading difficulties to overcome them?
12. Why is adding another modality to our language skills somewhat like adding another language? What are the similarities and differences? Why would you not propose a method like phonics for teaching, say, Mandarin to English speakers?

10

Adult and Neurological Disorders

OBJECTIVES

In this chapter, we:

1. Discuss neurological disorders owed to injuries, disease, toxins, or some mix of them;

2. Differentiate extrinsic, intrinsic, and autoimmune neurological disorders;

3. Discuss different injuries to the central nervous system and loss of distinct sign systems;

4. Analyze the theory of the "gene pool" and show why eugenics is not a viable option;

5. Consider the different types of aphasia on the basis of the sign systems they impact;

6. Discuss Alzheimer's, Parkinsonism, and degenerative neurological disorders; and

7. Discuss exacerbating neurotoxins known to contribute to dementias.

KEY TERMS

Here are some key terms of this chapter. Many you may already know, but it may help to review them. These terms are explained in the text and they are defined in the Glossary at the end of the book. They appear in **bold print** on their first appearance in the text.

acquired immune deficiency
  syndrome
adrenoleukodystrophy
adult "neurogenic" disorders
agenesis
agnosias
AIDS
amyotrophic lateral sclerosis
aphasic jargon
apoplexy
arcuate fasciculus
arrhythmia
asymptomatic
auditory illusions
autoimmune disease
autopsy
Broca's area
CAT
childhood aphasia
cloning
commissure
commissurotomy
computed axial tomography
conduction aphasia
congenital disorders
contralateral pathways
coronal
CT
cytoarchitecture
deceptive representation
degenerate
delusional experiences
dementia pugilistica
epileptic seizures
excitatory
expressive aphasia
false representation
fictional representation
fMRI

functional hemispherectomy
functional MRI
Gauss
germ cells
global agnosia
global aphasia
gustatory
hemispherectomy
hemorrhagic strokes
HIV
human immune virus
human immunodeficiency
  virus
imperfect
inhibitory
intracerebral hemorrhage
ipsilateral pathways
ischemic stroke
lateralization hypothesis
legal sanity
localization hypothesis
Lou Gehrig's disease
magnetic resonance imaging
mechanical injuries
mesothelioma
MRI
multiple sclerosis
myelin
nanotechnologies
neologisms
olfactory
peritoneum
peritonitis
portmanteau
positrons
prosopagnosia
radioactive tracers
real-time processing
receptive aphasia

reflex arc
retrotransposons
sagittal
schizophrenia
secondary injury
semantic aphasia
sensory alexia
sensory asignia
sensory dyslexia
short-term memory
simian virus 40
sleep-walking
somnambulism
splenium of the corpus
  callosum
split-brain experiments
stroke
subarachnoid hemorrhage
subcortical motor aphasia
subcortical sensory aphasia
supplementary motor area
SV40
syphilis lesion
TBI
telegraphic
threshold of coherence
threshold of insanity
tip of the mind
tip of the tongue
  phenomenon
transcortical motor aphasia
transcortical sensory aphasia
traumatic brain injury
true narrative representation
tubulin
unity of conception
Wernicke's aphasia
word deafness

In this chapter we deal with disorders that usually become symptomatic after some maturity. Many can occur at any stage of development, but some only occur in mature or aging adults. It follows that adults are more apt to have disorders than children because damage accumulates over time. Because of their longer time of exposure, adults have a higher exposure to accidents. If there were, say, 1 chance in 100,000 of being injured on any day, after one year, a child is up to 365 chances in 100,000, and by age 85, an adult is up to $(365 \times 85)/100,000 = 31,025/100,000$ or 3.1 chances in 10. The longer we live, the greater the accumulation of damage from injuries is likely to be.

COMMUNICATION DISORDERS OF ADULTS

Between extrinsically caused and intrinsically caused disorders there are many interactions. Factors on the inside interact with factors on the outside. In the real world, genetics and environmental/social factors, are not neatly separated.

Unless a childhood disorder can either be cured in childhood, or unless it is fatal, we are bound to find mature individuals with developmental disorders of the types discussed in Chapters 2–9.

A Comment on Terminology: *Neurological* Versus *Neurogenic*

In this chapter we consider what are commonly called **adult "neurogenic" disorders**, but we generally refer to them as "neurological" for a reason.

Neurogenic: A Problematic Term

"Neurogenic" suggests a cause in or by the nervous system. The root "*neuro-*" refers to the nervous system, especially the brain and spinal cord. The term "*-genic*" is from the root shared by other words such as "genes," "genesis," and "genetic" having to do with the beginnings of things. But neurological disorders can begin in any system related to the nerves and do not always begin within much less are they *caused by the nervous system*. They can be caused by any kind of injury or damage to the nerves and may have almost any imaginable source and may begin in any system related to the nervous system. However, *all of the body's systems are related to the nervous system*.

We discuss the most common adult neurological disorders, their known or suspected underlying causes, and their correlated anatomical aspects as studied by clinical neurologists. We ask what adult and neurological disorders reveal about human communication systems and vice versa. Although no one would be apt to undergo brain surgery for the sake of research, when serious neurological disorders arise, they often provide a natural laboratory for the study of human communication systems. And, as we will see, diagnosing and understanding the nature of a disorder is often crucial to discovering methods of successful treatment and, in some cases, ways of curing and/or preventing the disorder in question.

Survivable Childhood Disorders Become Adult Disorders

Children that survive become adults. As a result, congenital, developmental, or even acquired childhood disorders, tend to become adult disorders later on. Temple Grandin, a PhD and professor of animal husbandry at the University of Colorado with high functioning autism (retrieved March 7, 2009, from http://www.templegrandin.com/), often stresses that enabling the transition to employment is a crucial goal of intervention in long-term disorders like autism.

Corky in the 1990s series, *Life Goes On*, was played by a real child with Down syndrome named Christopher Burke (retrieved March 7, 2009, from http://www.nndb.com/people/380/000086122/). Children with disorders, unless they die or are cured, become adults with disorders, and adults present special challenges and needs that they did not have as children. Among them is the need for self-sufficiency and employment or long-term institutional care.

Corky was just a character in a forward-looking socially advanced sit-com as a child, but Christopher Burke became an adult with Down syndrome ("Life Goes On," 2009, retrieved March 7, 2009, from http://en.wikipedia.org/wiki/Life_Goes_On_(TV_series).

Diverse Causes of Adult Disorders

As we have seen in earlier chapters, it is common to make a distinction between what are described as "acquired" disorders—ones with extrinsic causes—and ones that are believed to be genetic (intrinsic). Commonly, an additional distinction is made between **congenital disorders**—ones present from birth that may be either genetic or "acquired"—and ones that are described as *developmental*. The class of "developmental" disorders and conditions are generally taken to be ones that develop after birth and that may be caused by some combination of internal genetic and extrinsic environmental factors. However, developmental conditions can certainly begin to appear in the womb, or anytime after conception. Such "developmental" conditions should be thought of as epigenetic in most cases because they invariably involve interactions between genetic systems and other factors.

Genetic disorders are commonly known to be triggered by injuries from outside the organism just as certainly as a brick falling on someone's head can be an extrinsic cause of a head injury. For instance, the cumulative damage to nerves in the case of **adrenoleukodystrophy** (ALD)—a genetic disorder—is triggered by long chain fatty acids that build up over time preventing the normal functioning of **myelin**. The buildup, however, can be blocked by certain other acids as discovered by a banker named Augusto Odone and his wife. Their son, Lorenzo, had ALD. An award winning movie was made about the discoveries and advances brought to the medical field by this highly motivated couple with no background in medicine. Augusto was awarded an honorary doctorate for his work ("The Myelin Project," 2009, retrieved March 7, 2009, from http://www.myelin.org/en/cms/?14). The medicine Dr. Odone researched and developed was called *Lorenzo's Oil*. The movie staring Susan Sarandon as Michaela and Nick Nolte as Augusto Odone tells the essentials of this amazing true story (G. M. Miller & Enright, 1992; Odone, 2009, retrieved March 7, 2009, from http://en.wikipedia.org/wiki/Lorenzo's_oil).

Disorders with significant genetic components can occur at any point from conception to maturity and even in advanced old age. Disorders may be associated with external events, such as cumulative blows to the head, or they may be triggered by disease, toxins, or combined injuries. An example of the extrinsic type of injury is seen in Mohammad Ali with **dementia pugilistica**, a disorder caused by repeated brusing of the brain as it is jarred by punches to the head. Certain neurotoxins are also known to trigger Parkinson's disease. Among them are the methamphetamine drugs (Volz, Fleckenstein, & Hanson, 2007).

There is no sharp boundary between genetic and acquired disorders. Genetic disorders, however, can also express themselves at any point in life—well after maturity. Also, in spite of the fact that genetic factors are inherited, those factors themselves may exist solely because of an extrinsic injury to the **germ cells** of former generations. The germ cells, of course, are the gene carrying components of our parents, grandparents, and so forth, right on back. The most common adult neurological disorders are known to involve significant genetic components—especially Alzheimer's and Parkinsonism. In fact, essentially all neurodegenerative conditions have significant genetic components. In addition, such disorders are also known to be triggered, exacerbated, or in some cases caused outright by toxins (Atianjoh, Ladenheim, Krasnova, & Cadet, 2008).

Disorders from Injuries

It can be argued that essentially all disabilities and disorders are the result of injuries of one kind or another. We do not usually think of diseases, toxins, and their interactions with biochemicals as producing injuries, but they do. It is just that the injuries are at the atomic and molecular levels of our bodily systems and are sometimes not readily noticed or easily detected even with complex medical tests. But as Harman (1956) argued, and as he and others subsequently demonstrated, even minute quantities of toxic chemicals do damage that tends to accumulate over time. Those injuries are the main causes of aging and the eventual death of the individual.

An example of the extrinsic type of injury is seen in Mohammed Ali [1942–present] (see "Mohammed Ali," 2009, retrieved March 7, 2009, from http://en.wikipedia.org/wiki/Muhammad_Ali) who has the condition known technically as dementia pugilistica—a form of Parkinson's disease caused by blows to the head.

With that in mind, it can be argued that essentially all degenerative conditions, including genetic ones, are the result of injuries.

Biochemical injuries may originate in toxic chemicals from outside the organism—for example, smoke released from a refinery containing heavy metals. They may come from a particular disease agent that gets into the body from outside, for example, the disease agents that cause tetanus or botulism (see Chapter 5). Or, toxins may be released from one part of the body into another as a result of some other injury. An example would be a burst appendix which can produce a general infection known as **peritonitis**—inflamation of the sack called the **peritoneum** that contains the intestines. Or a penetrating injury in the brain, for instance, may cause the release of multiple neurotoxic chemicals and oxygen-free radicals that are normally safely contained within cells. Once released they can make the primary injury worse through what is referred to as a **secondary injury** (Marion, 1999, p. 5).

Known Causes May Be Diagnostic

We ordinarily think of sudden (traumatic) physical events as the sources of extrinsic injuries. In the medical profession, these are sometimes referred to as **mechanical injuries**.

Traumatic Injuries
An injury or loss can also have emotional or psychological consequences owed to shock. An event such as a blow to the head can be the obvious cause of a subsequent loss of **short-term memory**. For instance, after arriving at the Emergency Room the child asks, "Dad, where are we?" The father answers, "We're at the hospital. You had a fall from your bike. We're going to see a doctor in a couple of minutes." In a few moments, the child asks again, "Dad, where are we?" The same answer is provided. He may repeat the same question several times in the space of a few minutes in spite of the fact that the question has been answered each time in the same way. Because of the repetition of the same question, it is evident that the previous answers did not transfer from short-term memory to long-term memory.

When a known injury produces a sudden change in behavior, it is reasonable to suppose that the injury—say, the head injury preceding loss of short-term memory—probably caused the loss of memory. When symptoms can be closely linked with a likely causal event, it is often reasonable to infer a causal relation. We can often correctly diagnose the causal relation on the basis of the known traumatic event which is followed by the observed symptoms. If the symptoms have never appeared before but do appear suddenly

When a known injury produces a sudden change in behavior, it is reasonable to suppose that the injury—say, the head injury preceding loss of short-term memory—probably caused the loss of memory.

following the trauma, it is not unreasonable to infer that the trauma has probably caused the symptoms. When a likely cause occurs in close temporal proximity with what appear(s) to be an outcome(s) probably produced by it, we generally look for additional confirmations before we can be reasonably certain of causation. In the case of the head injury in question, the multiple questions demonstrate that the blow to the head has probably caused the loss of memory. As in the case of ordinary communication, when multiple observations made by different observers on multiple tasks and/or occasions agree, the likelihood of an incorrect inference of causation diminishes rapidly toward a vanishing point.

In some cases, it is possible to pinpoint the location and nature of the injury. By doing so we may discover that certain neurological processes come under the control of distinct areas of the brain. To the extent that this is true, injuries to different parts of the brain and nervous system provide a basis for discovering and mapping the functions of the brain.

MAPPING BRAIN FUNCTIONS

The idea that different parts of the brain control different functions can be traced to an inference about the loss of the ability to produce fluent speech in a patient that could still understand language. After the individual in question died, Paul Broca [1824–1880] (see "Broca's Aphasia," 2009, retrieved March 7, 2009, from http://en.wikipedia .org/wiki/Paul_Broca) performed an **autopsy**—he cut open the brain of the late Mr. Leborgne and found a **syphilis lesion** destroying the area labeled in Figure 10–1 as "Broca's area." The autopsy showed damage in the left frontal lobe of the brain.

Subsequently, the loss of fluent speech became known as *Broca's aphasia* (Broca, 1861; for details see Goodglass & Geschwind, 1976)—also **expressive aphasia**.

The discovery of the brain region that came to be known as **Broca's area** marked the beginning of efforts to map brain functions onto particular regions of the brain. In Broca's aphasia, speech production is commonly described as **telegraphic**—where function words such as *the*, *a*, *of*, *and*, plural marking (e.g., the "-s" on "cats"), tense (e.g., the "-ed" on "walked"), and the like tend to be omitted whereas content words consisting of nouns, verbs, and descriptors tend to be retained. For instance, "Weather cool, not rain, see soon, come see" might mean "The weather is cool. It isn't raining and I hope to see you again soon. Come see me."

The discovery of the brain region that came to be known as **Broca's area** marked the beginning of efforts to map brain functions onto particular regions of the brain.

The Laternalization and Localization Hypotheses

The discovery of Broca's area, confirmed an idea from an earlier, less well-known researcher named Marc Dax [1771–1837]. Dax had

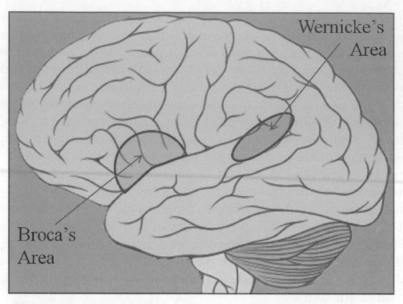

FIGURE 10–1. Mapping brain functions in the left hemisphere for fluent speech (Broca) and comprehension (Wernicke).

proposed in 1836, a quarter of a century before Broca, that language/speech functions were located in the left side of the brain (Dax, 1836/2009, retrieved March 7, 2009, from http://en.wikipedia.org/wiki/Marc_Dax). Dax also had relied on evidence of damage to the left side of the brain after a patient who had lost language ability had died. Dax's idea may be called the **lateralization hypothesis**—the notion that the language function is handled by the left side of the brain. If we look down on the brain from the top with the front of the brain oriented toward the left of the page, as shown in Figure 10–2, we can see that the brain is divided into what appear to be almost equal halves. These can be split right down the middle, into what are called the left hemisphere and the right hemisphere roughly in the way that a pecan can be broken into two halves.

The structures on the left side seem to be mirrored, more or less, on the right. But this appearance is deceptive because the two sides of the brain are not equal. The lateralization hypothesis suggested that the functions of the brain are not distributed evenly between its left and the right-hand sides. In fact, the language functions tend to be handled by the dominant hemisphere which in right-handed individuals, owing to the fact that the left hemisphere is neurologically connected to the right side of the body, is the left hemisphere. The right hemisphere, correspondingly, is usually the subordinate half of the brain and is always connected to the left side of the body. It follows that the dominant hemisphere is also the one that handles the most basic language functions. As we will see, it is the dominant hemisphere that evidently is also the primary control center for volitional action and thought.

The idea that language functions were distributed to the left side, Dax's hypothesis, seemed to be confirmed by Broca's finding

The lateralization hypothesis suggested that the functions of the brain are not distributed evenly between its left and the right-hand sides.

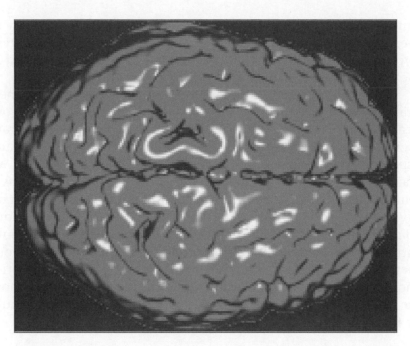

FIGURE 10–2. The left and right hemispheres of the brain viewed from the top downward with the front of the brain oriented toward the left side of the page.

in the autopsy of Mr. Leborgne. In Figure 10–1, we see a drawing of just the left side of the brain. If the face of Broca's patient were drawn into the picture, he would be looking to the left side of the page. His back would be to the right side of the page. To find Broca's area in your own brain, probably, you should look to the area just a few centimeters above and a few centimeters in front of your left ear. We say "probably" because the speech area in some left-handers and in some women in particular may be located in the right brain. In a very few, it may be distributed to both the right and the left hemispheres (for an excellent summary with references; see Derakshan, 2003 and also see "Lateralization," 2009, retrieved March 7, 2009, from http://en.wikipedia.org/wiki/Lateralization_of_brain_function).

Broca's conclusion was that he had discovered the area responsible for the production of speech. Mr. Leborgne could only say the word "tan" and for that reason, got the nickname, Tan. In his 1861 paper, Broca did not mention the earlier lateralization hypothesis of Dax. However, he knew of Dax's work, as he later noted in 1877 (Dax, 1836/2007). In any case, Broca's finding seemed to confirm the lateralization idea, which suggested a division of labor between the left and right hemispheres. However, his finding suggested that lateralization was just a gross and global manifestation of a much finer gained division of labor within parts of the brain. To thinking individuals, Broca's finding suggested the possibility that there were more specific areas with still more specific functions throughout the brain. This idea would come to be known as the **localization hypothesis**. Simply put, it is the idea that particular functions

Broca's finding suggested the possibility that there were more specific areas with still more specific functions throughout the brain. This idea would come to be known as the **localization hypothesis**.

can be attributed to highly focused brain areas. It was, as is easy to see, a natural extension and refinement of the global lateralization hypothesis. Both ideas have turned out to be correct only in part in the light of more advanced investigative procedures.

It is evidently true that it was the syphilis lesion in Leborgne's brain, which was in fact on the left side, that caused him to lose nearly all of his capacity to speak. It is also true that different brain regions have somewhat distinct functions. However, as is in many aspects of sign systems, things begin to get interesting when we consider the holistic interactions across distinct regions and systems of the brain and the entire body. Although there are important divisions of labor in the brain, the idea that particular functions could be strictly localized to particular regions of the brain would turn out to be an over-simplification. It violated Einstein's famous dictum (see George Wills, 1979, p. 100) that scientific theories should be "as simple as possible but no simpler." However, before the oversimplification could be revealed, additional evidence would be found in favor of the localization hypothesis.

> Although there are important divisions of labor in the brain, the idea that particular functions could be strictly localized to particular regions of the brain would turn out to be an over-simplification.

Wernicke's Aphasia

Not long after Broca's discovery, another researcher, Karl Wernicke [1848–1905] identified a different area in the left hemisphere which he associated with the ability to comprehend speech (Wernicke, 1874/1977). Persons with **Wernicke's aphasia**—also sometimes referred to as **receptive aphasia** or **semantic aphasia**—may retain the ability to speak fairly fluently but lose the capacity to make sense of or to produce ordinary novel discourse in their own native language. An example of speech from a person with Wernicke type aphasia might sound something like this:

> "You know that smoodle pinkered and that I want to get him round and take care of him like you want before" meaning something like: "The dog needs to go out so I will take him for a walk." (National Institute on Deafness and Other Communication Disorders, 1997, retrieved March 7, 2009, from http://www.nidcd.nih.gov/health/voice/aphasia.htm)

Or here is another example from Gardner (1975). The patient was asked how he ended up in the hospital and responded:

Example: Wernicke-Type Aphasia

Boy, I'm sweating, I'm awful nervous, you know once in a while I get caught up. I can't mention the tarripoi, a month age, quite a little, I've done a lot well, I impost a lot, while on the other hand, you know what I mean. I have to run around, look it over, tribbin and all that sort of stuff. (p. 68)

Loss of Coherence in Wernicke's Aphasia

Interestingly, persons affected by the Wernicke type of aphasia often not only do not understand the discourse of others, but are unaware of their own tendency to produce what is called **aphasic jargon**—incomprehensible stretches of discourse.

As in the examples just given in the section above, in addition to its general incoherence and lack of meaningful sequence, aphasic jargon is usually characterized by multiple **neologisms**—that is, nonexistent and uninterpretable new word-forms such as "smoodle," "pinkered," "tarripoi," "impost," and "tribbin." These nonsense words conform to English phonology, but have no determinate meaning. To supply a possible meaning for any of them, we would be forced to rely heavily on the context of the discourse—for example, the fact that the person puts the leash on the dog that is scratching at the door and starts outside—or the mere resemblance of the surface forms to other existing words. For instance, we might ask ourselves if "smoodle" could be a word suggesting the need to let the dog out by combining forms such as "pooch," "piddle," "poodle," "puddle," "muddle," "smudge," and so on. But in doing this we may be guessing wildly. In fact, in some cases persons who produce the aphasic jargon may themselves be unable to detect the fact that anything is wrong in the syllables strung together and may be struggling and largely unable to make sense of what they are trying to think of, much less to say.

As we noted in Chapter 9, the meaningful sequence of ordinary discourse is foundational to its comprehensibility. When that sequence is disrupted dramatically, the discourse loses its essential quality of coherence. It is interesting that jargon aphasia resembles deliberately created nonsense. It actually has some of the same properties. The most famous example was the Jabberwocky created by Lewis Carroll in *Through the Looking-glass, and What Alice Found There* (1871). There Humpty Dumpty explains that " . . . *slithy* means *lithe* and *slimy* . . . You see it's like a ***portmanteau***—there are two meanings packed up into one word." Perhaps Carroll, whose real name was Charles Lutwidge Dodgson [1832–1898], had observed aphasic jargon. There are hints of it in his coining, for instance, of the term *portmanteau* (retrieved March 7, 2009, from http://en.wikipedia.org/wiki/Portmanteau). In any case, he created the most widely known example in the English language in his *Jabberwocky* (retrieved March 7, 2009, from http://en.wikipedia.org/wiki/Jabberwocky).

Meaningful Sequence and Memory

Aphasic jargon, however, is not intentionally created nonsense. But it is just as difficult to make sense of. In the curious psychological process of trying to figure ourselves out, we learn that nonsense is not only difficult to understand, it is also difficult to recall. This fact

It is interesting that jargon aphasia resembles deliberately created nonsense. They actually have some of the same properties.

was illustrated in an interesting way by a predecessor of Lewis Carroll who may have been the source of inspiration for Dodgson's *Jabberwocky*. That other humorist was Samuel Foote [1780–1846] (retrieved March 7, 2009, from http://en.wikipedia.org/wiki/Samuel_A._Foot). Foote once attended a public lecture where the speaker—a certain Charles F. Macklin [1690–1797] (see Cousin, 1910; also Macklin, ca. 1797, retrieved March 7, 2009, from http://en.wikipedia.org/wiki/Charles_Macklin)—boasted that he could memorize any text of up to 100 words having read it only once.

Macklin was a noted actor and boxer who lived more than a century and is said to have become even uglier after his many fights than he was before. Foote wrote the following text handed it to Mr. Macklin written on the back of cloth napkin at a public dinner. Foote asked Macklin kindly to read it once aloud and then repeat from memory the following 100 words:

> So she went into the garden to cut a cabbage-leaf to make an apple-pie; and at the same time a great she-bear, coming down the street, pops its head into the shop. What! no soap? So he died, and she very imprudently married the Barber: and there were present the Picninnies, and the Joblillies, and the Garyalies, and the grand Panjandrum himself, with the little round button at top; and they all fell to playing the game of catch-as-catch-can, till the gunpowder ran out at the heels of their boots. (Oxford University Press, 1980, p. 216)

Macklin, who had successfully defended himself in a murder trial—acting as his own lawyer after killing a man by poking him in the eye with his cane—was unable to prevail against Mr. Foote. Macklin could not repeat the text from memory after reading it only once. The point was made that discursive memory depends a great deal on the ordinary meaningful sequence of common events. It depends on the episodic organization, the normal chronological narrative structure of experience.

Novel Construction Impaired in Wernicke's Aphasia

The person producing the jargon aphasia may or may not have any clear meaning in mind and may even be unable to formulate a coherent meaningful sequence in thought. In the most severe cases the person affected may not be able to speak at all and may also be unable to show any comprehension of language whatsoever.

In some cases the ability to engage in routine conversation such as greetings, leave takings, and small talk, say, about the weather, may remain intact. However, the individual may falter if asked to formulate a response to a question that requires a novel construction. For instance, one of the patient's we worked with who had a Wernicke type aphasia when asked, "How are you today Mr. T.?" was able to say, "Oh, I'm fine, how are you?" However, when asked something like, "Did anyone stop by to see you, Mr. T.?" he

In jargon aphasia both the meaningful sequence of events in experience, and the understanding of that sequence, as well as the ability to use meaningful sequence in constructing discourse is either lost or impaired.

might say, "I . . . I . . ., I don't know. You wouldn't try to trick me, would you?"

For all the foregoing reasons it is sensible to argue that Wernicke's aphasia is primarily a disorder of the highest levels of syntax, semantics, and pragmatics. It interferes with the ability to comprehend, and thus to construct, coherent meaningful discourse. Aphasia of this kind is clearly a language/linguistic/cognitive disorder as distinct from lower order motor-speech problems of the sort we discussed and illustrated in Chapter 5. It is a higher order problem than the kind of aphasia displayed by Mr. Leborgne, Broca's patient, where comprehension of language was more or less left intact but the ability to speak fluently was almost completely lost.

REFINING THE IMAGES OF THE BRAIN

The idea that inevitably followed from the findings of Broca and Wernicke was simple: *Every distinct area of the brain must have its own special function.* This hypothesis was carried farther by Korbinian Brodmann [1868–1918] (Figure 10–3) than by anyone else. In 1909, he wrote one of the most important reference works in the history

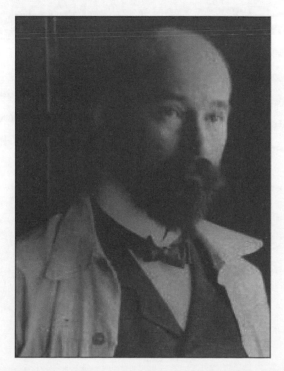

FIGURE 10–3. Korbinian Brodmann [1868–1918] the clinical neurologist best known for anatomical maps of the human brain. Retrieved March 7, 2009, from http://www.ibro.info /Pub_Main_Display.asp?Main_ID=96. Image in the public domain due to expired copyright.

of neurology providing a detailed mapping and numbering system for regions of the brain as shown in Figure 10–4 that is still widely referred to today.

Brodmann's System of Mapping

Brodmann's system was deeply based in anatomy. He argued that all theories of physiology and functions needed to be grounded in the study of the actual tissues themselves and in the study of their architecture. As noted by Harvard neuroanatomist Jeff Lichtman

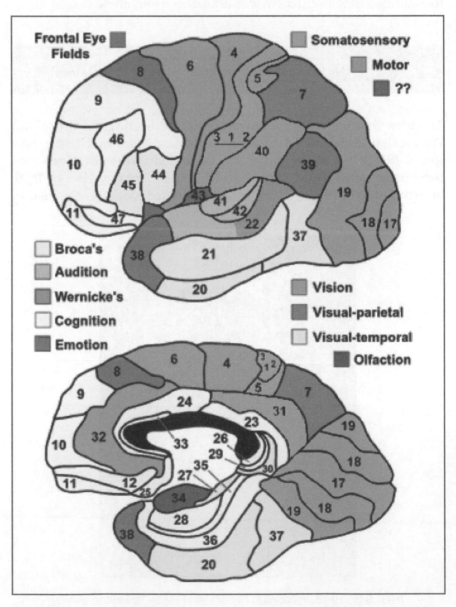

FIGURE 10–4. Colorized diagrams of Brodmann's areas. Retrieved March 7, 2009, from http://spot.colorado.edu/~dubin/talks/brodmann/brodmann .html. Copyright © 2007 by Professor Mark Dubin. Reprinted by permission. All rights reserved.

(2003), Brodmann quoted another neuroanatomist (a certain Dr. Gudden) as having said, "Faced with an anatomical fact proven beyond doubt, any physiological result that stands in contradiction to it loses all its meaning . . . So, first anatomy and then physiology; but if first physiology, then not without anatomy" (Brodman, 1909/2003, retrieved March 7, 2009, from http://www.extremeneuroanatomy.com/synapse_resolution.htm). Brodmann's numbering of areas of the human brain are still the ones most widely used today by neurologists and anatomists, more than a century after his first works were published. Dr. Lawrence Garey, who translated Brodmann's "Localization in the cerebral cortex," in 1994 and commented in 1999 that Brodmann's "famous 'maps' of the cerebral cortex of man, monkeys and other mammals must be among the most commonly reproduced figures in neurobiological publishing" (Garey, 1999, retrieved March 7, 2009, from http://www.worldscibooks.com/medsci/p151.html).

Figure 10–4 shows the detail of Brodmann's maps with the elaboration of the areas identified earlier by Broca—Brodmann's areas 44 and 45—and by Wernicke—Brodmann's areas 22, 41 and 42 (also see "Brodmann's Areas," retrieved March 7, 2009, from http://en.wikipedia.org/wiki/Brodmann_area). Brodmann's method for finding and differentiating the 52 distinct regions of the human brain that he identified was based on cell structure—technically termed **cytoarchitecture**—as determined by staining the cells of actual brains. Unfortunately, his maps of human brain areas, some complained, were often based on nonhuman brains. Nevertheless, Brodmann's areas, with certain elaborations through the addition of letters to some of his numbers, for example, the division of section 23 into 23a and 23b, remain the most common basis for researchers and clinicians in referring to particular regions of the brain today. However, far more detailed maps have been constructed based on actual internal views of the brain. Vastly more detailed studies can be found today based on living human brains (see Zapawa & Alcantara, n.d., retrieved March 7, 2009, from http://www.med.wayne.edu/diagRadiology/Anatomy_Modules/brain/brain.html; also see Figure 10–17 later in this chapter).

Modern Marvels: Enhancing the View of the Inside

By the time Brodmann published his work on brain areas in 1909, photography had been in use for three quarters of a century. The first relatively permanent photograph was produced by Louis Daguerre in 1828 (retrieved March 7, 2009, from http://inventors.about.com/library/inventors/blphotography.htm). But photographs only showed reflected light and could not picture the inside of the body. In 1896, Wilhelm Conrad Röntgen [1845–1923] produced the first x-ray image of his wife's hand. Figure 10–5 shows an x-ray image also produced by Röntgen. Until then, to get a photograph of the bones of the hand, would have required removal of

Brodmann's method for finding and differentiating the 52 distinct regions of the human brain that he identified was based on cell structure—technically termed **cytoarchitecture**—as determined by staining the cells of actual brains. Unfortunately, his maps of human brain areas, some complained, were often based on nonhuman brains.

To map the inside of the brain, into the 1930s doctors and researchers were still using highly invasive procedures—for example, ones involving opening the skull and probing brain tissues (Penfield & Boldrey, 1937). Röntgen's x-ray pictures permitted views of the inside of the human body without cutting the body.

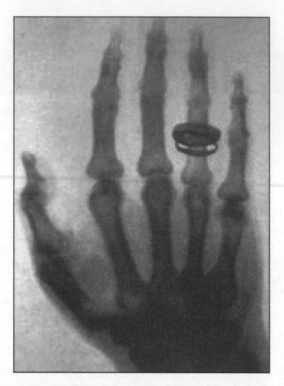

FIGURE 10–5. An x-ray picture of Albert von Kolliker's hand taken by Wilhelm Röntgen in 1896. Retrieved March 7, 2009, from http://en.wikipedia.org/wiki/Image:Roentgen-x-ray-von-kollikers-hand.jpg. Image in the public domain due to expired copyright.

the flesh from the hand. There were no living volunteers for that procedure and, even fewer individuals were willing to permit photographs of the inside of their heads.

In 1901, the harmfulness of radiation was not fully understood, but the usefulness of the pictures created by x-rays won Röntgen the first ever Nobel Prize in Physics (Röntgen, 1901, retrieved March 7, 2009, from http://nobelprize.org/nobel_prizes/physics/laureates/1901/rontgen-bio.html). Unfortunately, x-rays are not harmless and, as is well known, many of the early experimenters died of cancers that were produced by overexposure to radiation as did Röntgen himself.

After the discovery of x-rays (see Figure 10–5), one of the major advances was **computed axial tomography** (**CAT** or **CT**; see "Computed tomography," retrieved March 7, 2009, from http://en.wikipedia.org/wiki/Computed_tomography). The term "tomography" comes from the Greek words for "slice" (*tomos*) and "record" (*graph-*), as in a drawing or written description. The term "axial" was included in the descriptor because the original scanners captured x-ray images in a particular orientation. In 1979 Godfrey Newbold Hounsfield at a lab in England sponsored in part by the Beatles, and Allan McLeod Cormack at Tufts University, in the

United States shared a Nobel Prize for the independent development of CT scanning. The first CT scan was made in 1972. The initial images took about two and a half hours to process. The technique required the patient to hold still for several minutes at a time while each slice of the body was being x-rayed. A horizontal CT slice of the brain at eye-level is seen in Figure 10–6.

The development of positron emission tomography (PET) came just a few years after the first successful CT scans were produced. In 1975, Michael Phelps and others (see Cherry, Sorenson, & Phelps, 2003) developed PET. It involved injecting a radioactive material into the patient's bloodstream. Subsequently, the radioactive material emits particles called **positrons**. These are the antimatter counterparts of electrons. When they meet up with an electron, they destroy each other in a miniature explosion that releases two other particles called photons—the primary form of the energy we see as light. The release of the photons can be detected as a burst of light and recorded by mechanical sensors. The intensity of the light in different regions of the scan can then be shown as seen in Figure 10–7.

What the PET scan shows is differences in the concentration of the radioactive material in different body tissues, mainly the blood. Whereas x-ray images and CT enhanced x-rays were based on beams radiated from outside the body passing through the inside (see "Positron Emission Tomography," 2009, retrieved March 7, 2009, from http://en.wikipedia.org/wiki/Positron_emission_tomography), the PET procedure involves radiation moving outward from

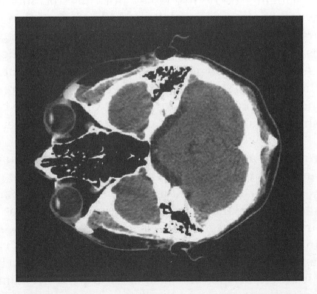

FIGURE 10–6. An axial CAT scan of the head at eye-level. Retrieved March 7, 2009, from http://en.wikipedia.org/wiki/Computed_tomography. Posted by Andrew Ciscel at http://www.flickr.com/photos/ciscel/124548696/. Reprinted as licensed under the rules of Creative Commons Attributions 2.0 Generic.

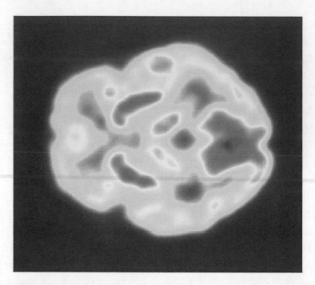

FIGURE 10–7. A black and white conversion of a typical PET horizontal slice of a human brain viewed top down (person looking toward the left of the page)—on the DVD in the colored version, red areas show maximal concentration of radioactive positrons and blue minimum. Retrieved March 7, 2009, from http://en.wikipedia.org/wiki/Positron_emission_tom ography#_note-0. Copyright © 2005 by Jens Langner. Image placed in the public domain by its creator Jens Langner February 2, 2006.

inside the patient's body. It enables not only the monitoring of blood flow to various regions of the body, but by attaching **radioactive tracers** to particular body chemicals that are injected into the blood, it is possible to monitor the amount of that chemical in particular tissues after a sufficient time-lapse (usually about an hour) to allow the body's tissues to absorb the chemical. An area of great interest and the focus of much research is, of course, the brain. Figure 10–7 shows a single axial slice of a human brain generated by a PET scan.

Neurologists and anatomists think of the three dimensional space occupied by the human body (especially the brain) when it is stationary, in terms of just three distinct perpendicular planes. Any slice parallel to the plane of rotation around the body (as seen, for instance, in Figures 10–6 and 10–7) is termed "axial." Since all slices pictured in the initial CTs were of this kind, it was called "computed axial tomagraphy" (CAT). From computer data generated by a CAT, however, it is actually possible also to produce a two-dimensional image in any orientation (see the three planes illustrated later in Figure 10–17). Also, it is possible to produce a three dimensional image of a particular region of the body as shown in Figure 10–8 where the CT technology is combined with PET. Click on the hyperlink in the caption of Figure 10–8 to see a moving three-dimensional image on-line.

Any slice parallel to the plane of rotation around the body (as seen, for instance, in Figures 10–6 and 10–7) is termed "axial." Since all slices pictured in the initial CTs were of this kind, it was called "computed axial tomagraphy" (CAT).

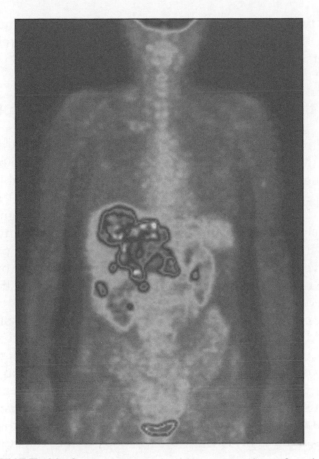

FIGURE 10–8. A black and white conversion of a richly colored (see DVD) combined PET and CT x-ray image. Retrieved March 7, 2009, from http://en.wikipedia.org/wik i/Positron_emission_tomography#_note-0. Copyright © 2006 by Jens Langner. Image placed in the public domain by its creator Jens Langner May 22, 2006.

The brighter portion of the image seen in Figure 10–7 is produced by PET while the background of the body and skeleton are CT images. A moving three-dimensional version of Figure 10–7 can be created by combining many slices of both PET and CT images simultaneously (see "Applications," 2009, retrieved March 7, 2009, from http://en.wikipedia.org/wiki/Positron_emission_tomogra phy#_note-0).

Both x-rays and PET images involve exposing the person pictured to nuclear radiation. The PET procedures involve the additional invasive procedure of putting the radioactive tracer element inside the bloodstream. The main differences are that x-ray images, whether or not they are enhanced by CT, register differences in tissue density, while by contrast, PET images show the relative concentration of the radioactive tracer in a particular region. Both procedures can be useful in detecting the abnormalities and distinct

PET and CT can be combined to produce simultaneous views. They show the relative density and distribution of body tissues and organs along with blood flow and chemical uptake by various organs at the same time.

kinds of tissue damage that may be involved in communication disorders. Nevertheless, for studies of neurological problems in particular, less invasive procedures are desirable.

Kicking the Resolution of the Image Up a Notch: MRI

With the invention of the technique called **magnetic resonance imaging** (**MRI**), much more detailed examination of the brain and monitoring of its processing functions has become possible (see H. Damasio, 2000; also "Magnetic Resonance Imaging," 2009, retrieved March 7, 2009, from http://en.wikipedia.org/wiki/Magnetic_reso nance_imaging). MRI can be done without injecting any foreign material into the blood and without subjecting the patient to radioactive exposure. Figure 10–9 shows the exterior of one of the older MRI machines and Figure 10–10 shows an MRI slice inside the brain of a living human being.

MRI pictures typically show more detail in the soft tissues than could possibly be obtained by either CT enhanced x-rays or with PET, or with both CT and PET combined. Because of their sensitivity to different densities and structures right down to the level of atoms, the MRI procedure can be adjusted to show an almost miraculous degree of detail in the living human body. By augmenting the MRI pictures with injected tracers, in a manner similar to PET scans, remarkably clear pictures of body tissues can be obtained.

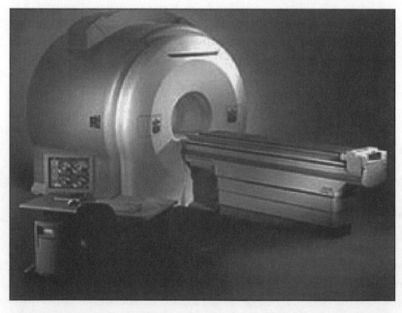

FIGURE 10–9. An MRI scanner. Retrieved March 7, 2009, from http://rst.gsfc.nasa.gov/Intro/Part2_26c.html. United States National Aeronautic and Space Administration publication. Image in the public domain.

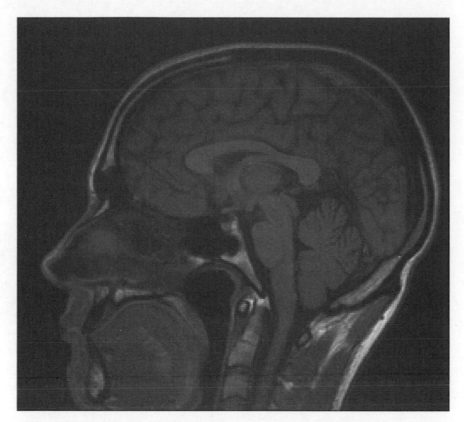

FIGURE 10–10. A relatively noninvasive MRI vertical slice down the middle center of the inside of a living person showing the inside of the head and skull. Retrieved March 7, 2009, from http://en.wikipedia.org/wiki/Magnetic_resonance_imaging. Image placed in the public domain by its creator Cajolingwilhelm March 27, 2007.

For example, Figure 10–11 shows an image of the blood vessels in a human head.

How is this possible? An MRI machine consists of multiple components of which a central part is a powerful magnet. The earth's magnetic field, measured in a unit called a **gauss**—named after the mathematician Johann Carl Friedrich Gauss [1777–1855] (Gauss, 1855/2009, retrieved March 7, 2009, from http://en.wikipedia.org/wiki/Carl_Friedrich_Gauss)—has a strength of .5 gauss. The main magnet used in modern MRI machines, of which there are thousands in the world today, produce a magnetic field in the 5,000 to 20,000-gauss range. A magnet at the upper end of this range can pick up an automobile.

The first MRI of a human body was produced in 1977. The machine was bulky, incredibly expensive, and the images were not very good. However, it was evident that the technique had great potential in diagnostic applications. Current systems use a main magnet to create a highly homogeneous magnetic field within which (inside the magnet) the human brain, say, or the whole body,

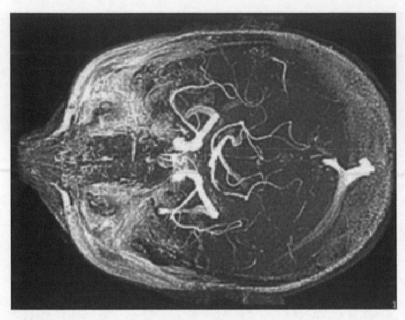

FIGURE 10–11. An axial MRI of blood vessels in the head. Retrieved March 7, 2009, from http://rst.gsfc.nasa.gov/Intro/Part2_26c.html. United States National Aeronautic and Space Administration publication. Image in the public domain.

can be fitted. Inside the main magnet there are three less powerful magnets at right angles to each other to enable construction of three dimensional images. A radio pulse generator also sends a signal intermittently through a slice of tissue that can be selected within the magnetic field to be pictured. The interactions between the magnets and the atoms in the material to be pictured—say, a particular part of the human brain (as in Figures 10–10 and 10–11) —create distinct resonant frequencies in those atoms as they are impacted by the radio pulses. The variations in their resonance in response to the radio pulses can be registered and displayed in very tiny cubic pixels in a three-dimensional space, or in squares in a two-dimensional display as seen in Figures 10–10 and 10–11. Interestingly, the cubic pixels are called *voxels*, which is as Dodgson would have said a portmanteau derived from the phrase "volumetric pixels."

And Another Notch: fMRI

*A key goal, still off in the future, has been to step up the speed of imaging systems until we can see what is going on inside the brain during **real-time processing**.*

Which areas of the brain are involved when a person is reading a novel, viewing a film, carrying on a conversation, conducting an interview, and so on? MRI technology has been miniaturized and speeded up to the point where researchers are attempting what is called **functional MRI**, abbreviated as **fMRI**. Their primary objective is to speed up the processing of images to the point that detailed neurological processes can be observed while those processes are actually taking place (see Columbia University, retrieved March 7, 2009, from http://www.fmri.org/fmri.htm). Presently, it is possible to monitor blood flow to different regions of the brain with fMRI, and by doing this to infer that where there is greater uptake of oxygen (judged by more blood with a tracer in it), there must be more brain activity going on. However, the fastest acquisition of fMRI pictures still comes up well short of the standard 30 frames per second for motion pictures on television or 24 frames per second at the movies. Mayer, Xu, Pare-Blagoev, and Posse (2006) comment:

> Although functional magnetic resonance imaging (fMRI) has arguably become the most ubiquitously used imaging modality, questions remain about the reproducibility of the observed patterns of activation and *the acquisition time required* [our italics] to achieve statistically significant and reproducible maps. (p. 129)

According to the Columbia University Web site (2009), the acquisition time that they report is in the range of 30 images per 90 seconds. However, only about one third of the 30 images obtained within a given 90 second run are on the task of interest—for example, performing the function of saying a particular word. They note:

> During a typical functional imaging series, 30 images are acquired in a 90 second run where the initial and last 10 images are baseline conditions and the middle 10 images (30 seconds) are acquired during a task. (retrieved March 7, 2009, from http://www.fmri.org/fmri.htm)

This means that fMRI images being produced with the equipment at Columbia University in 2008 are, according to their Web site, 270 times slower than ordinary digital video cameras. Considering the fact that it takes only about half a second to produce a single syllable word, if it requires 90 seconds to get just 10 images of the brain, there is no way that the highly delicate movements of speech could possibly be captured in the fMRI film produced by such a machine in 2009. Much less could they keep up with the rapid production of a meaningful sequence of words in ordinary discourse.

The modern marvels have come far, but they still have a ways to go to get up to speed with speech—so to speak—and there also remain all the challenges of the multiple mental processes going on simultaneously during the production of discourse.

GROSS RELATIONS BRAINS, SIGNS, AND FUNCTIONS

Starting from the gross distinctions between the functions of the two hemispheres of the brain, it is possible to show the broad outlines of the major sign systems and processes that we have already introduced in previous chapters. Those systems emerge independently from the research on neurological disorders that impact the brain. In particular, the different aphasias which are generally associated with the left hemisphere are instructive, but there are also certain cognitive losses that are associated with damage to the right hemisphere. Just as Broca, Wernicke, Brodmann, and others had supposed, the gross functional distinctions between the work done by the left hemisphere and that done by the right have generally been sustained. In this section, we show that the main systems of signs discussed in earlier chapters—and in the process of pragmatic mapping—are all actually found in the major anatomical structures and functions of the brain.

The Basic Components in a Successful Pragmatic Mapping

At the foundation of language acquisition and use is the pragmatic mapping process. It involves connecting known facts of experience with abstract symbols of language. That is, known facts about persons involved in meaningful events and sequences of events, on the one hand, are systematically mapped into sequences of symbols manifested in experience in speech, writing, or manual signs (and vice versa). The linguistic signs consist of the words, phrases, sentences, and higher structures of discourse that may be spoken, written, read, heard, merely thought, or some combination of these.

In Chapter 3 we discussed the method by which Laura Bridgman learned that the raised print that Dr. Howe taped to the key was a symbol for a key (see Figure 3–1). She had to discover the pragmatic mapping of the word onto the object. Or, recall the explanation of Helen Keller about how she acquired the word *water* as spelled out in her hand by Annie Sullivan while the water from the pump was running over her hand (see Figure 3–4). Helen Keller had to discover the relation between the spelled out word "w-a-t-e-r" with one hand while the other was experiencing the flow of the WATER.

The necessary starting point for language acquisition is the pragmatic mapping relation described in Figures 3–1 and 3–4. This has been shown by strict logicomathematical arguments beginning with C. S. Peirce (1897), by empirical research and by clinical applications much of which we have discussed and cited in earlier chapters. All complex language-based representations (especially words, numbers, and notations) are known to be derived from this simpler referential kind by abstraction, elaboration, and recombination. The most elaborate and complex metaphors, fictions, fantasies, lies, and all kinds of derived nonsensical forms, have their point of origin in simple referential relations like the one seen in a name as related to the person that is named. Three essential elements are present in every such successful act: First, there is the known fact; for example, the recognizable person or event singled out for attention in the act of referring. Second, there is the act of associating and mapping the representation (known through our senses) onto the refer-

> The simplest form that any successful pragmatic mapping act can take is a referential act of naming or referring to a distinct person or event.

ring term. Third, there is the production of the referring term (say, a name) in a sequence of motor actions (and/or thought processes) whereby the referring term is mapped onto the fact signified.

The Brain Anatomy of Pragmatic Mapping

In Figure 10–12, we abstract the pragmatic mapping process and show how it also happens to correspond to the gross anatomy of the brain and to the primary distribution of distinct functions to the left and right hemispheres. Michael Gazzaniga (2000) succinctly sums up the gross division of labor that is characteristic of the human brain, with

> the left hemisphere specialized for language and speech and major problem-solving capacities and the right hemisphere specialized for tasks such as facial recognition and attentional monitoring. (p. 1923)

In between the two hemispheres is a huge bundle of intricately distributed nerve fibers connecting the two sides of the brain and enabling the vast majority of the communications that take place between the two hemispheres. That bundle of fibers is called the "corpus callosum"—which translated into English from Latin means the "calloused body." In addition to its other functions, it provides relatively rigid junction holding the hemispheres in place.

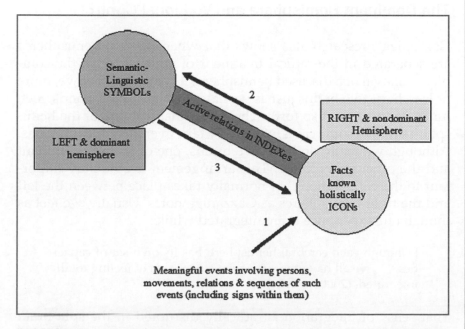

FIGURE 10–12. The pragmatic mapping relation through active indexes linking the facts of experience, known mainly through icons and their holistic relations, with linguistic-semantic symbols.

The major functions of the corpus callosum are represented in our diagram, Figure 10–12, in the tube connecting the left and right hemispheres with arrows going in both directions.

J. M. S. Pearce (2007) confirms the major elements and their functions as described by Gazzaniga and he adds that it was

> Michael Gazzaniga, who investigated patients subjected to surgical division of the corpus callosum. These so-called "**split-brain experiments**" established the role of the corpus callosum in inter-hemispheric information transfer. (p. 250)

The division of labor between the left and right hemispheres and the communication between them through the corpus callosum are plainly suggested and experimentally demonstrated by Damasio et al. (2004).

Evidence of the division of labor between the two hemispheres and the communication between them mainly through the corpus callosum comes from H. Damasio, Tranel, Grabowski, Adolphs, and A. Damasio (2004). Examining data from damage to particular regions of the brain in the left and right hemispheres along with data from subjects without brain damage, they showed that retrieval of words referring to tangible objects was dependent on distinct regions in the left temporal lobe whereas the retrieval of holistic concepts of those same objects depended on corresponding regions of the right hemisphere. The division of labor between the left and right hemispheres and the communication between them through the corpus callosum are plainly suggested and experimentally demonstrated by Damasio et al. (2004). Their work independently and quite indirectly shows the anatomical validity of the broad outline of pragmatic mapping theory.

The Dominant Hemisphere and Volitional Control

Gazzaniga's research also shows that when the two hemispheres are separated in the radical treatment of epilepsy, or in the complete removal of a diseased hemisphere, it comes out that we, more or less, have two brains just as we have two eyes, ears, hands, feet, lungs, kidneys, and so forth. The fact is that just one of the hemispheres can, in some cases, effectively take over all of the functions. Although we really do have two brains, one of them is dominant and the other subordinate. This arrangement is evidently important to the cooperation that normally takes place between the left and the right hemispheres as Gazzaniga notes. Usually, we feel as though our experience is an integrated whole:

> [T]hough each cerebral hemisphere has its own set of capacities, . . . we all have the subjective experience of feeling totally integrated. (2000, p. 1923)

That sense of integration is radically disrupted in the split-brain operation where the left and the right hemispheres can no longer communicate via the corpus callosum.

However, as Reggia, Goodall, Shkuro, and Glezer (2001) have pointed out, there is a long-standing controversy about whether the information being passed back and forth between the two hemispheres has the purpose of causing mental or other actions or preventing them. They comment that it has been unclear whether communications across the corpus callosum are "primarily **excitatory** or **inhibitory**" (p. 465). Their review and modeling suggest that, when either hemisphere is damaged, the communications from the other tend to be excitatory, but when all is well, the communications seem to be inhibitory—allowing each hemisphere to do the work it is best equipped to do. Interestingly, research with motor signals —ones causing or preventing movements of the body—by Derakshan (2003) suggests that the direction of the flow of traffic is from the dominant—usually left hemisphere as shown in Figure 10–12 —to the subordinate hemisphere. He explains that the excitatory influence from the dominant to the subordinate hemisphere is normally devoted to

> volitional movements occurring on the nondominant side. Thus, it is the directionality of callosal traffic that is responsible for cerebral asymmetries seen in the motor realm. (p. 538)

Thus, right-handed individuals not only tend to throw with their right hand and kick with their right foot, but they also do volitional planning such as figuring out what move to make next in a game of baseball or chess, with the left hemisphere. The right hemisphere, in the mean time, is getting its main instructions from the left through the corpus callosum. The patterns differ somewhat across the sexes, but the basic dominance of the left hemisphere appears to be similar across men and women (Schmithorst & Holland, 2006). However, as we have seen throughout this book, it is hardly surprising that things can go wrong. When they do, there is much to be learned from the symptoms involved, and from the sign and the brain regions that are affected.

Although both hemispheres tend to be involved in all complex mental processes and activities, there are advantages if one side or the other is clearly in charge.

Moving Out from Experience to Imagination

Looking back to Figure 1–3, the top half of the diagram corresponds to the mind's representation of the past in *memory*, the present in *consciousness*, and the future in *expectancy*. In order for the higher systems to work normally, the systems beneath them need to be in place and they need to be functioning more or less normally. If a representation is merely imagined, we do not call it experience. We call it fantasy or imagination. If it is both imaginary and yet mistaken for real experience, something actually happening rather than merely being imagined, we do not call it imagination only, but dreaming, or possibly delusion or hallucination. It is only hallucination if the person experiencing it and mistaking it for fact is awake. If we take a further step beyond hallucination to the point where the representations either become completely chaotic, random, unrecognizable, or nonexistent altogether, we would not be

From valid ordinary experience, it is a short step to imagination, a significantly further step to dreaming (while asleep), yet another to hallucination.

talking about meaningful experience, but confusion or nonsense. If even the confused representations were to vanish entirely, then, we would be describing a state of complete unconsciousness, or perhaps material death.

When a person hallucinates, elements of imagination are represented as if they were real. It is comparable to a situation where a person is experiencing elements of reality along with dreamed elements while the person doing the representing is awake. To move from hallucination to a completely confused consciousness where nothing makes sense at all requires a further step away from ordinary valid experience. As we have already noted, to get to the theoretical point where consciousness itself vanishes, presumably, requires yet another step even beyond merely confused representations. That step would lead to the theoretical vanishing point where representations are no more.

Degrees of Incompleteness in Representations

In thinking through this series of steps away from ordinary, usually valid, wakeful, experience, it is relatively easy to see that the valid and true representations of ordinary experience provide the gold standard against which all other representations must be compared and judged. Imagination is less valid than actual experience because imagination is about at least some things, persons, or events that are not real. Imagination may include references to many actual persons, places, and events, as when we plan a vacation, but it also includes things that are not yet and perhaps never have been or ever will be real. However, imagination tends to be harmlessly incomplete—logicians would say **degenerate** and grammarians would say **imperfect**—when compared against ordinary valid experience (a true representation of events unfolding over time). Imaginations are relatively less harmful or dangerous than reality and they are usually not regarded as true of reality. We do not take imagination as representing events that are presently real.

The Usefulness of Imagination

Imagination is very useful to us because it enables us to explore the future by what are, in effect, virtual experiments. We can easily imagine what would happen if we stepped off the cliff, or walked out onto the track in front of an on-coming train, or other less harmful activities, say like writing a book, or pursuing a degree in speech-language pathology. Imagination helps us to understand what may have happened in the past, or what may happen in the future. Dreaming, no doubt, is also useful in allowing us to sort through memories and, so long as actual bodily movements are suppressed while we are dreaming, it is relatively safe.

When bodily movements are not suppressed during sleep, the result called **sleep-walking** in common speech, or **somnambulism**, can be dangerous. We know a man who dreamed he was diving into a pool of water just before he actually leaped head first into the dresser from the end of his bed, as witnessed and later reported to one of us by his slightly mortified (but later amused) wife. The same man when he was a teenager managed to waken all of his companions at a summer camp to get them to help him find a non-existent skunk under one of the beds. They had the lights on, the covers lifted off the floor, and were on hands and knees searching for the skunk before they realized that the boy who reported having seen it was sleep-walking.

Delusional Experience: Mistaking Imagination for Fact

Somnambulism is a disorder akin to the extreme hallucinatory experience portrayed—though not entirely accurately—in the film about John Forbes Nash [1928–present] who is shown in real life in Figure 10–13. He actually experienced **auditory illusions** of voices of persons, some of whom never existed and were only products of his mind. In the film, *A Beautiful Mind* (Howard, Goldman, & Nasar,

Somnambulism is a disorder akin to the extreme hallucinatory experience portrayed—though not entirely accurately—in the film about John Forbes Nash [1928–present] who is shown in real life in Figure 10–13.

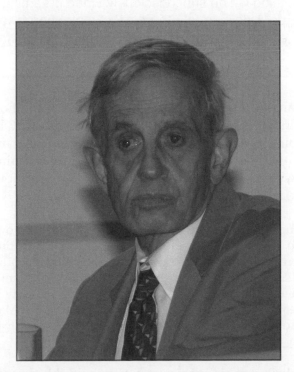

FIGURE 10–13. John Forbes Nash, winner of the Nobel Prize in Economics in 1994, at a meeting on game theory at the University of Cologne in Germany in 2006. Photo by Elke Wetzig. Retrieved March 9, 2009 from http://en.wikipedia.org/wiki/John_Forbes_Nash. Reprinted under the http://en.wikipedia.org/wiki/Wikipedia:Text_of_the_GNU_Free_Documentation_License GNU Free Documentation License, Version 1.2.

2001; also Universal Studios and Dreamworks, 2001) starring Russell Crowe as Nash (retrieved March 7, 2009, from http://en.wiki pedia.org/wiki/A_Beautiful_Mind_(film)), the illusions are presented as wakeful dreams, where Nash has conversations with persons whom he thinks he sees and hears but who are not real. In actuality, according to his own account in a PBS interview (view a video record of an interview with Nash, 2002, retrieved March 7, 2009, from http://www.pbs.org/wgbh/amex/nash/sfeature/sf_nash_ 07.html) the hallucinations were strictly auditory, though he did believe them to be real experiences. Only later, did he come to recognize the voices as **delusional experiences**—ones that were created in his own mind but that he wanted to believe were real. His delusional experiences are symptomatic of mental disorders under the general term **schizophrenia** (2004, retrieved March 7, 2009, from http://www.schizophrenia.com/diag.php#diagnosis).

Confusing Imagination with Reality

From the point of view of the pragmatic mapping process, the hallucinations Nash experienced either put imaginations in the place of facts or intermingled facts with imagined fictions. The problem is not so much in creating the imagined events. It is something we do subconsciously when dreaming and we can also do it deliberately to some extent when awake. The difficulty arises because of Nash's regarding the imagined events as if they were real.

There are many varieties of schizophrenia, but all of them, by definition, involve delusional experiences of some sort. In the film, Nash's coping with his disorder is portrayed as having been helped greatly by modern medicines, but in fact he claims that the medicines were not the source of his eventual restoration to a semblance of normal experience. He says:

> The drugs I think can be overrated. All of the drugs now continue to have some bad side effects. There would be times in between when I would stop taking drugs and I would not immediately go under any regimen. So I don't know. I am lucky to have come out of mental illness at all, but certainly in the later years I had no drugs (J. F. Nash, 2002, retrieved March 7, 2009, from http://www.pbs.org/wgbh/amex/nash/sfeature/ sf_nash_07.html).

In fact, he attributes his success in coping with his disorder mainly to rational thought. He was able to determine rationally that some of the voices he was hearing were creations of his own imagination. He compared the incomplete pragmatic maps of voices without faces and bodies, against ones where the voices were connected with bodily persons. Because some of the voices he was hearing did not come from bodily persons while others were coming from bodies he could also see, he knew that he was hallucinating some of the voices and was even able to determine which voices were imaginary.

In thinking through J. F. Nash's case, and essentially all forms of what is loosely termed "schizophrenia"—a term so loose that it included childhood autism from 1943 until 1979—we can see why such cases receive special attention in psychiatry. The danger in believing things to be real when they are only imagined is not difficult to appreciate. At one time, Dr. J. F. Nash, for example, left his young child in the bath in the care of imaginary individuals whom he had invented. We are reminded of a recent news report about a small child that drowned in the tub while mother was distracted with another task (see Rillos, 2002, retrieved March 7, 2009, from http://www.topix.net/forum/city/dateland-az/TQBL1KS5GGSAEVSLR).

The disordered (abnormal) representation can never be simpler, more complete, or more consistent with the facts than a valid, ordinary true representation—for example, that the baby is in the tub and that no one is speaking to Mr. Nash—of the same actual facts of experience. To discover that his imaginary representations were not real, in the movie John Forbes Nash was portrayed as conversing with other persons. In real life, according to his own account, he was able to determine that the voices he sometimes heard were not real because they were not accompanied by visual representations of bodily, visible, tangible, moving persons. The voices represented things in ways that were not consistent with his memories of recent valid experience and that were not consistent with facts on hand that he could investigate by seeing and touch in addition to hearing. For Nash, according to his reports, the vivid illusions he sometimes experienced were mainly auditory ones and they were not as coherent as portrayed in the movie, *A Beautiful Mind*.

> A failure to represent things the way they really are can be life threatening. There is no situation where any disordered representation of common facts of experience—for example, whether the baby is in the bath water, or whether someone is standing there telling John Nash to leave the room immediately—is better than an ordinary true representation of the same facts.

Pathological Lying

Among the many forms of confusion about what is real or merely imagined, there is another disorder, or at least a behavioral symptom of a disorder, that goes a step farther. It involves a willful, deliberate, intentional form of deception which succeeds so well that the person engaging in the deception becomes ensnared in the mental trap laid to deceive others. The deceivers with this disorder succeed in deceiving themselves. Popularly, this disorder is called *pathological lying*—and technically *pseudologia fantastica* and *mythomania*. Although it has not yet been incorporated as one of the categories in any of the versions of the *DSM-IV-TR* (2000), psychiatrist Dr. Charles C. Dike and his colleagues have suggested that perhaps it ought to be considered as a category. Whether it is included or not in future *DSMs*, it is clearly a departure of an abnormal kind from ordinary truthful representation, or ordinary imagining. It is

> One of the defining traits of pathological lying is that it often seems to involve story embellishment, for no particular purpose or gain.

deviant behavior and whether or not it is recognized as such by psychiatry, it is seen as deviant in ordinary experience, the market place, and in the courts. Also, it is logically distinct in a strictly formal way from true reporting, fictionalizing, making an honest mistake, or from even ordinary lying. Also, the strictly formal, logical distinctions first proposed between such linguistic performances in some of our own work from 1993 forward have been demonstrated empirically in experimental studies using fMRI (Langleben, et al., 2002). The latter work has been cited 94 times on the Web of Knowledge in follow up studies at the time of this writing on March 7, 2009.

The Case of Judge Couwenberg

In August 2001, the California Commission on Judicial Performance recommended removal of Judge Patrick Couwenberg for lying to the Commission. He had made quite a few claims about himself that proved to be completely false—that he had won a purple heart in Vietnam, that he had earned a masters in psychology, and that he had participated in covert operations for the U.S. Central Intelligence Agency, though he had never done any of these things (Dike, Baranoski, & Griffith, 2005, p. 342). Eventually, he was removed from the bench.

In fact, many different varieties of pathological lying seem to exist and have been documented historically in many interesting cases over the last 100 years. In our earlier book on *Milestones* of normal speech and language, we mentioned the Baron von Munchausen [1720–1791] who according to Dike and colleagues was an actual cavalry officer, not merely the invention of the fiction writer Rudolph Erich Raspe [1737–1794]. They point out that the Baron, was not only the inventor of tall tales (e.g., the most famous one of lifting himself by his boot straps), but that he also believed his own inventions. One thing that is certain about pseudologia fantastica is that it tends to mingle with disorders that involve delusions. According to Dike and colleagues, this happened with the Baron and also with the California judge. The judge was under oath before the Commission and gave every impression that he himself believed his false stories—that is, he was delusional, a pathological liar.

If we ask why the Commission recommended his removal, the answer has to do with the logical and formal differences, as well as the practical differences in the actual consequences, of true reports about known facts as contrasted with fictional reports of imagined or possible facts; erroneous reports where fictions of one kind or another are mistaken for facts; and deliberate lies where known errors are represented as if they were facts. It might be an error, for instance, for Judge Couwenberg to claim that he won a purple heart in Vietnam if he did not know that in fact he never even served in Vietnam. But because he knows he never served in Vietnam his claim is a lie. But it seems that his memory was almost as much influenced by his story-telling as by his actual experience. This seems to be a characteristic of pathological lying in general. In that case, the judge may well have come to actually believe the lies he invented. As Dike, Baranoski, and Griffith point out, pathological lying is subtle, and, needless to say, deceptive. Logically speaking, in the case of what is called "pathological lying," it can be strictly proved beyond any doubt that the deception is certain to be most damaging to the deceiver who is, in such cases also self-deceived.

Do Pseudologues Believe Their Own Inventions?

Perhaps the most difficult question, and perhaps the most important with respect to the diagnosis of pathological lying, is to find out just when and how the person inventing the false stories begins to believe them and to what extent that person is willfully and knowingly inventing the false stories in the first place or to what extent the person is compelled to do so by metabolic imbalances, toxins, disease, or brain damage that is beyond the person's control. For instance, in one of the well-documented examples used by Dike and colleagues, a student of a certain distinguished Professor Ellis observed, "He seemed so genuine. Perhaps it was a fantasy he came to believe himself," (Dike, Baranoski, & Griffith, p. 242).

What has been agreed, at least since Healy and Healy (1926), is that pathological lying is typified by "falsification entirely disproportionate to any discernible end in view," and that it "may be extensive and very complicated, and may manifest over a period of years or even a lifetime" (Dike, Baranoski, & Griffith, 2005, p. 243).

Is the Misrepresentation Intentional?

As to whether pseudologues are willful liars or whether they become so entrapped in their own stories that they can no longer distinguish them from reality is an open question. There is good evidence, however, that there is a vague threshold of pathology where the person inventing the fictions begins to have difficulty differentiating the facts that he or she has actually experienced—as represented in perceptions and memories—from the invented fictions that he or she has only represented. The person afflicted by such a pathology may intermittently waiver between representing actual events recalled and fictional scenarios that have been reported as truths. In many cases, as Dike and colleagues demonstrate with well-documented cases, the pseudologue may appear to many as a paragon of forthrightness and integrity, defending inconsistencies as if anyone disagreeing with him had, as an afflicted person once put it, "lost all respect for the truth." The pseudologue is apt to say things like, "It's time someone said what is really going on here . . . " and, after covering an inconsistency with an angry denial and an accusation of other persons, he will defend the outburst by saying: "You know me, I was just venting. Let's talk about something else."

In his recorded interview, Dr. John Forbes Nash (2002) suggested that his own delusions were partly brought on by wishing that he were more prominent, more famous, and more successful as a mathematician than he could reasonably claim to be.

In his recorded interview, Dr. John Forbes Nash (2002) suggested that his own delusions were partly brought on by wishing that he were more prominent, more famous, and more successful as a mathematician than he could reasonably claim to be. However, as his illness progressed, his delusions seem not to have been entirely under his control. As a result, it is easy to see that psychiatrists are in a difficulty to say whether a given case of pseudologia fantastica is willful or not. There evidently is an element of willfulness at the beginning of the pathological delusions—trying to protect against a deep inner insecurity. But in pathological lying, volition becomes subordinated to the stories already told until any actual memory the pseudologue may have of what really happened, or even of what is possible, can be overwhelmed. It may not ever occur to the pseudologue, for instance, that what he or she claimed may be logically impossible because of the contradictions that it contains. When the contradictions are made apparent to the pseudologue, however, an angry outburst or flight from the situation is predictable. It is logically because of the covering up or running from the inconsistency rather than dealing with it that delusional pathology sets in. It can overwhelm reason as well as reality. Thus, simply put, pathological liars become victims of their own deceptions.

Legally Responsible?

As Dike, Baranoski, and Griffith (2005) note, the deeper question of law and ethics is whether the pseudologue does or "does not know that what he or she is doing is wrong" (p. 348). Because pathological liars "usually have sound judgment in other matters" it is difficult to argue that such a diagnosis, even if it existed, would reach the "**threshold of insanity** in most jurisdictions" (p. 348).

However, Dike and colleagues suggest that neuroimaging might be used as a basis for determining debilitating neurological conditions. He supposes that in some cases it might absolve some pathological liars of responsibility for their actions (p. 347). In fact, before Dike et al. published their probing questions about pathological lying, the logical and formal distinctions between lying and telling the truth had already been empirically demonstrated with fMRI comparisons by Langleben et al. (2002). More recently, after the thoughtful questions of Dike, Baranoski, and Griffith (2005) were published, Abe, Suzuki, Mori, Itoh, and Fujii (2007) reviewed the experimental research contrasting acts of lying with truth telling with both fMRI and PT scans and found striking differences in the neurological systems involved in intentional deception as contrasted with truth-telling. One of the applications of that work by Spence, Kaylor-Hughes, Brook, Lankappa, and Wilkinson (2008) may provide a way to vindicate innocent persons who have been convicted in a court of law. The distinction hinges on the fact as predicted by the theory of true narratives that lying is more complicated and involves more brain activity, different regions, and longer latencies than truthful reporting of ordinary memories of facts.

SIGN SYSTEMS, RANKS, AND INTEGRATION

The German neurologist, Ludwig Lichtheim [1845–1928], in 1885 (see D. Smith, 2009) had already roughly distinguished the three major sign systems we described above in Chapter 1. He did it by describing the symptoms of distinct kinds of aphasia. In particular, his system distinguished three major interrelated elements in the production and comprehension of speech: In the sensory domain, Lichtheim focused his attention mainly on (1) the auditory systems—to which we would add systems of vision, smell, touch, and taste. He also referred to (2) a motor component; and (3) a semantic/conceptual component. As we will see, his incomplete system of distinctions nevertheless anticipated the differentiation of brain functions accounted for in the theory of pragmatic mapping (see Figure 3–1) and as later described by Gazzaniga as we saw above with reference to Figure 10–12. Lichtheim attributed his distinctions to discoveries made by Broca and Wernicke respectively concerning representational functions that were evidently distributed to different regions of the brain. Today, we can know a good deal more about the motor control systems of the left hemisphere and how it communicates with the right. We also know a good deal more about the semantic/conceptual systems as they are involved in mapping linguistic elements in the left hemis-=phere onto conceptual elements in the right—the pragmatic mapping process. Lichtheim's diagram, which we have modified only slightly for the sake of comprehensibility, is shown as Figure 10–14.

On the basis of the hypothesized relations between the different components of the language system, which are shown in Figure 10–14, Lichtheim predicted eight different types of aphasia. All of these kinds of aphasia and a few others besides, not to mention combinations of these, had either already been documented at the time of Lichtheim's analysis or were documented later on. They exist in varying degrees of severity depending on the nature and extent of damage to the brain.

We might expect that a theory proposed in 1885 would have been greatly improved by 2009, but Lichtheim's ideas, though expanded on and refined by his successors, are still the standard categories commonly referred to in the medical profession (see França, 2004;

The line between **legal sanity** and *in*sanity under the law—like the boundary between willful intentional behavior and an illness that overwhelms the will and the mind—is one that lawyers and psychiatrists find difficult to draw.

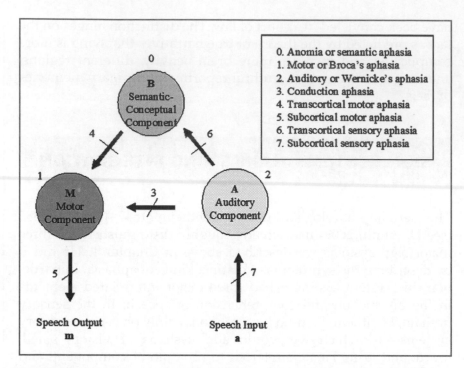

FIGURE 10–14. "Lichtheim's House". A diagram expanded from *Brain*, 7(4), 436. Retrieved March 7, 2009, from http://www.smithsrisca.demon .co.uk/PSYlichtheim1885.html . Adapted and reprinted with permission from Derek Smith. Original image is in the public domain due to expired copyright.

Fuller, 1993; Weems & Reggia, 2006). Concerning his simple system, Lichtheim (1885) wrote the following explanation:

> The **reflex arc** consists in an afferent branch aA [speech input to the auditory component], which transmits the acoustic impressions to A [the auditory component]; and an efferent branch Mm [from the motor component to the linguistic output], which conducts the impulses from M [the motor component] to the organs of speech; and is completed by the **commissure** (arcuate fasciculus [see Figure 10–14; and path numbered 3 in his diagram]) binding together A [the auditory component] and M [the motor component]. When intelligence of the imitated sounds is superimposed, a connection is established between the auditory center A, and the part where concepts are elaborated, B [*Begriffen* in German, meaning, the *semantic* or *conceptual* component of the diagram].

In the sections that follow, we consider the types of aphasia that Lichtheim described on the basis of his model, and how we would modify the model to conform better to current theory. As we go through the eight distinct varieties of aphasia that he described, it will be useful to keep in mind that in the next major section, we will discuss ways that aphasias and a host of other neurological disorders are commonly caused. As we work through Lichtheim's diagram, it is also useful to keep in mind that he is referring mainly to disorders caused by damage to the dominant hemisphere of the brain. We will meet other disorders, typically associated with the nondominant hemisphere later in this chapter.

Anomia or Semantic Aphasia (0)

It seems that Dr. Lichtheim ranked the disorders much as we would rank them based on the most up-to-date theory and research. He numbered the different categories beginning with the most severe and pervasive type of aphasia at 0 and progressing to the least common at 7. We will point out places where the order seems to need adjustment. However, the meaning/conceptual system certainly belongs where he has placed it at the highest rank by all accounts. That is where we find it in "Lichtheim's house" (also see the discussion and links created by Derek Smith, 2007).

From a conceptual point of view, as we have argued in the theory of abstraction, the kinds of meaning represented at the top of Lichtheim's house are at the upper limit of abstractness and generality. There is nothing more abstract or general than the semantic concepts underlying words, phrases, and linguistic forms in general. There cannot logically be any system higher than semantic concepts fully general and fully abstract. By fully general we have in mind the fact that any abstract concept, say, of "light" as contrasted with "darkness," or "gold" as contrasted with "dirt," or "something" as contrasted with "nothing," can be applied to absolutely any conceivable thing that might be represented by that concept that might have ever existed in the past, might be existing in the present, or at sometime might exist in the future of any observer. General semantic concepts also apply to anything that might somehow be represented in some fantasy or fiction. By fully general we mean applying to any and all possible or imaginable instances of whatever the concept might represent. By fully abstract we mean that the concept of whatever any given concept may be a concept of has no properties that could not be found in all the instances of whatever that concept may be a concept of. That is, if the fully abstract concept were say of a "horse," or say "a pot of gold," or "sailing," or "the aged mother of Dr. Lichtheim," to be fully abstract it should not include anything whatever that is not common to all the possible instances that might be represented by that concept.

In its milder forms the anomic type of aphasia resembles the common **tip of the tongue phenomenon** where we know a name, word, phrase, or concept, but for the life of us, we cannot quite get to it. In severe cases, there is a generalized inability to access

Consider the fact that if the linguistic semantic/conceptual system is effectively wiped out, the individual so affected ends in a state of zero capacity to communicate. Intelligence and social capacities are certain to drop to a theoretical zero as well. Based on what research teaches us about the role of meaning in discourse processing, Lichtheim has placed the conceptual element right where it belongs: at the top.

In its milder forms the anomic type of aphasia resembles the common **tip of the tongue phenomenon** where we know a name, word, phrase, or concept, but for the life of us, we cannot quite get to it.

concepts. In mild cases, the person will be able to recognize the name, word, phrase, or concept if someone else says it, or writes it, but may not be able to do so without prompting. In some instances, the person may be able to repeat the otherwise inaccessible sign after someone else produces it, but in severe cases, the meanings and signs for them may remain inaccessible even with prompting.

Motor or Broca's Aphasia (1)

The Broca type aphasia is one we have already encountered and have described earlier in this chapter. In Lichtheim's diagram, Figure 10–14, it is represented in the motor component and he ranks it as second—perhaps because of the order of its historical discovery by Broca after cases of complete anomia had already been observed. We would rank it as third in importance behind Wernicke's aphasia which Lichtheim placed third in his system. Individuals with mild Broca's aphasia seem dysfluent when attempting to string syllables together that formerly would not have presented any particular difficulty. Typically, a person with Broca's aphasia can understand the speech, writing, and/or signing of others more easily than he or she can produce speech, writing, or signing. Because the affected person can understand language in its spoken and/or written forms, he or she is apt to be aware of, and dismayed, by the loss of ability to perform linguistic motor tasks fluently. It is often possible to remember having done so in the past and to be astonished at the inability to do so in the present. In severe Broca's aphasia, the capacity to speak may be lost altogether.

Auditory or Wernicke's Aphasia (2)

Lichtheim placed Wernicke's aphasia third in his list, possibly because it was discovered after Broca's aphasia. However, in our own theoretical system of ranking signs (as discussed in Chapters 1–4 especially), Wernicke's aphasia is the more severe kind both from an intellectual and social point of view. It leaves intact the capacity to string syllables together more or less fluently, but it disrupts the capacity to produce or comprehend coherent meanings. The family of a person with Wernicke type aphasia may feel unable to reconnect with their loved one. Whereas comprehension at least remains intact with Broca's aphasia, in moderate to severe cases of Wernicke's aphasia, the possibility of sharing news, for example "Did you know that Aunt Lois died last week?" or hopes for the future, for example "We think the doctors will let you get out of here and go home in just a few days," may be just out of reach. In some cases of Wernicke type aphasia a written message will be understood when a spoken one is incomprehensible. For this reason, Wernicke's aphasia is sometimes called "auditory" aphasia.

Evidently, Lichtheim supposed that "auditory" aphasia was owed to damage to brain systems dedicated to the processing of signals delivered specifically to the ears. Assuming that is the case, we should also predict and discover other kinds of sensory aphasias associated with visual processing of signs as in reading— a strictly or primarily **sensory alexia** or **sensory dyslexia**—or in comprehending manual signs by the Deaf. At the Seventeenth Meeting of the Annual Convention of Instructors of the Deaf a report was given by Dr. Charles W. Burr of an adult signer who had been deaf from birth but lost her capacity to use signs or to understand them after "a bout with **apoplexy**" (1905, p. 338)—where the term, as applied in 1905, probably meant a stroke. Presumably if such a disorder occurred it might be called **sensory asignia**. If a strictly sensory form of Wernicke's aphasia were to occur at all, presumably, it would be indistinguishable from what is called cortical deafness or CAPD. Usually, however, Wernicke's aphasia involves generalized difficulty in managing linguistic concepts across the board.

Conduction Aphasia (3)

In what is poorly named **conduction aphasia** meaning transfer from the sensory system to the motor system—as in a task where the individual is asked to repeat a word said by a clinician, or to read aloud, or to write from dictation—the patient generally encounters difficulty or is completely unable to perform the task. This particular difficulty might better be described as "reception-to-production aphasia." The term "conduction" supposedly was used to suggest the transfer of information previously written or spoken by someone else into speech or writing to be produced by the individual with the disorder.

Meanwhile, the ability to understand speech, to speak spontaneously, to write one's own ideas as in a letter, to carry on a conversation, or to read silently with comprehension may remain more or less intact. The difficulty in this distinct kind of aphasia seems to be in the coordination of information in transferring it from the senses to the motor systems. It is as if the two little homunculi (seen in Figure 1–8) are not cooperating fully. In particular, the sensory homunculus is not handing over the information received so the motor homunculus can do his work. However, the motor homunculus is able to do fine on his own if he is getting the information about what to do from the conceptual system rather than the sensory homunculus. Individuals with the aphasia in question will

To our knowledge there are no recorded instances of loss of the capacity to understand manual signs while retaining the capacity to produce them.

have difficulty reading aloud, repeating, or writing down the words, phrases, or sentences of a message given to them to pass on to someone else.

A computer generated diagram of the bundle of nerve fibers—the **arcuate fasciculus** (Latin for an "arched bundle")—believed to be involved in this kind of aphasia is shown in Figure 10–15 (Digital Anatomist Project, 1995, retrieved March 7, 2009, from http://www9.biostr.washington.edu:80/cgi-bin/DA/PageMaster?atlas:Neuroanatomy+ffpathIndex/3D^Pathways/Arcuate^Fasciculus+2). The bundle in question consists of a mapping of neurons from what is called Wernicke's area to Broca's. The fibers form a kind of wide ribbon-like arch wrapping inward toward the center of the left hemisphere from Wernicke's area around to Broca's. Four views are presented showing the fibers and linked areas in question from different angles.

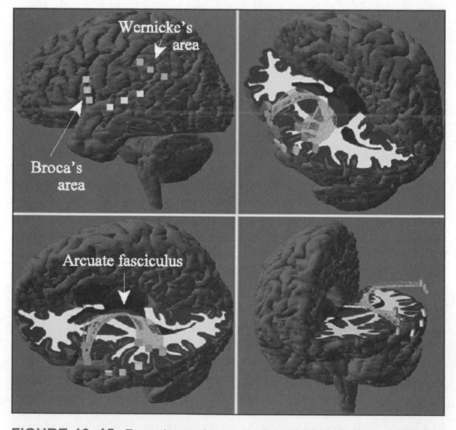

FIGURE 10–15. Four views of the arcuate fasciculus connecting Wernicke's with Broca's area—the area damaged in conduction (sensory reception-to-motor production) aphasia. Retrieved March 7, 2009, from http://www9.biostr.washington.edu/cgi-bin/DA/imageform. Copyright © 1995 by the Digital Anatomist Project, University of Washington. Adapted and reprinted with permission. All rights reserved.

Transcortical Motor Aphasia (4)

The damage that seems to produce what is called **transcortical motor aphasia** is generally in the area above and somewhat in front of Broca's area but may also extend beneath it. The central region of Broca's area, however, is typically not damaged. A. R. Luria [1902–1977] also described this kind of aphasia (Luria, 1966, p. 126). It seems to involve what is known as the **supplementary motor area** (Brodmann's area 6—see Figure 10–4) and the parietal area in the dominant hemisphere. It may be supposed that it is only because Wernicke's area remains intact and the arcuate fasciculus is untouched that persons with this disorder are able to repeat, read aloud, and write from dictation (Brookshire, 1997, pp. 141–142). However, if asked a question that requires complex sequencing and planning they are unable to perform as normally expected. Comprehension, on the other hand, and ability to repeat verbal material is relatively unaffected.

Subcortical Motor Aphasia (5)

It is doubtful whether this variety of motor difficulty—**subcortical motor aphasia**—which does affect speech, should be called "aphasia" at all. It typically involves damage to the area in front of and below what is called Broca's area. Speaking ability is evidently affected because of the partial or complete paralysis of the dominant side of the body—caused by damage to regions of the brain beneath the cortex but involved in the execution of movements. If the condition does not impact the comprehension or production of language as such, but only the power to move the speech muscles, many believe that it should not be called aphasia, but rather "dysarthria" (as discussed in Chapter 5). However, because of the diffuseness of the kinds of damage that may cause either one of these conditions, it is common for them to overlap to some extent. Also, damage to one area, for reasons discussed in Chapter 1 concerning comorbidity, can easily spill over into the other. Brain damage rarely has sharp boundaries.

Transcortical Sensory Aphasia (6)

McCaffrey (2001) refers to **transcortical sensory aphasia** as "an extremely rare form of fluent aphasia" (retrieved March 7, 2009, from http://www.csuchico.edu/~pmccaffrey//syllabi/SPPA336/336u nit8.html). What is believed to happen in this kind of loss is destruction of Brodmann's areas 37, 22, and 39 (see Figure 10–4). The damage is believed to leave the main speech, signing, and writing areas—Wernicke's, Broca's, and the connecting arcuate fasciculus—intact while effectively destroying the areas that enable meaningful conceptions and connected thoughts to be formed or understood. What is left is a person who can speak, read aloud, or write, but without making sense of the output. Goodglass and Kaplan (1983) note that the most definitive aspect of transcortical sensory aphasia is the ability to repeat words, phrases, and even complex sequences such as a prayer or poem. Because of this ability to repeat sequences, evidently showing good communication between Wernicke's and Broca's areas through the arcuate fasciculus, the person with this type of aphasia may seem to understand much more than they do. As they echo what they hear their interlocutor saying, they may seem to understand language and be contributing, at least by agreement, to the conversation. However, a person with this particular syndrome will be unable to read, write, or understand the meanings of language in any modality.

Subcortical Sensory Aphasia (7)

In **subcortical sensory aphasia** the individual affected may hear the sounds, syllables, words, phrases, and so forth, perfectly well but be unable to interpret them. This condition is also called **word deafness**. The difficulty appears to be specific to words and yet the condition, if it exists, is not well documented. Strohmayer in 1902 described 12 cases including a patient who, after having a pain in his right ear, had a loss of memory. Strohmayer may have been the last physician to actually diagnose someone with this supposed condition when he described:

> a man of thirty-six years, who had a luetic [syphilis] infection eight years before, six years after this noticed loss of memory and rapid intellectual fatigue. He then had [three] epileptic attack[s followed by] . . . pain in the right ear and . . . weakness of memory . . . When examined there were found several syphilitic manifestations, and it was noted that the patient heard badly and that he did not understand spoken words although he could hear faint sounds easily. Written speech he understood very well. (p. 163)

Subsequently, Dr. Strohmayer diagnosed "focal symptoms of subcortical sensory aphasia in the sense of Wernicke-Lichtheim" (p. 163). Theoretically, it would seem that this last, rare, type of aphasia is akin to what are called CAPDs which we discussed in Chapter 3. The lesion is somewhere between the ear and the sensory cortex dedicated to hearing and the processing of speech. However, because the damage is likely to affect both motor (efferent) fibers descending to the ear as well as sensory (afferent) fibers ascending from the ear, ones that are evidently uniquely involved in speech processing, it may be reasonable to suppose that this type of aphasia actually exists. If it does, it must be either rare or diagnosed as something else.

In **subcortical sensory aphasia** the individual affected may hear the sounds, syllables, words, phrases, and so forth, perfectly well but be unable to interpret them. This condition is also called **word deafness**.

UNDERSTANDING APHASIAS AND OTHER DISORDERS

Language and the Whole Brain

Aphasias are the most important disorders of the dominant hemisphere of the brain (Figure 10–16). We have seen, however, that to make sense of language in the normal way, we rely on both hemispheres. We must connect abstract representations expressed in strings of words or symbols—a function of the major or dominant hemisphere—with the facts of ordinary experience. Knowing the facts of experience, through integrated holistic perceptions, is a primary function of the minor or nondominant hemisphere. Connecting the two hemispheres is the corpus callosum with all of its power to transmit information back and forth between the two hemispheres.

Anatomical studies are now being conducted with a predictive MRI technique at the level of the neurological pathways within the corpus callosum (Zarei et al., 2006; also see Taber & Hurley, 2007).

There are also neurological pathways from the sensory systems that cross directly to the opposite hemisphere. These are called **contralateral pathways**—meaning "opposite side" as contrasted

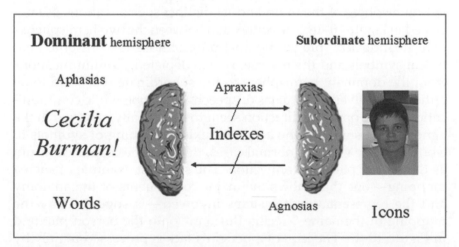

FIGURE 10–16. Pragmatic mapping of words (such as a name) onto their objects (such as the person named) and the major classes of communication disorders. Photograph of Cecilia Burman (at the right side of the figure) retrieved March 7, 2009, from http://www.prosopagnosia.com/. Reprinted with permission.

When we understand ordinary experience as it unfolds over time, or when we tell someone about a sequence of events that we have experienced, or when we report or understand any narrative in a film or novel, we are normally using both hemispheres of our brain, and especially the corpus callosum, that connects them.

with **ipsilateral pathways** meaning "same side." Beneath the whole system as Sperry (1981) noted, some communication is also possible between the two hemispheres through the common brain stem beneath them that they both share. Together all these connections, but especially those in the corpus callosum, provide the essential basis for our being able to make sense of what is going on in experience by representing sequences of events in spoken, written, or signed words and vice versa.

The connections are crucial to our being able to make sense of sequential representations in order to interpret, say, a novel into a sequence of events that we visualize. Sometimes, like the three-year-old Aleka Titzer, we find ourselves feeling as if we are participants in the scenes. When we understand ordinary experience as it unfolds over time, or when we tell someone about a sequence of events that we have experienced, or when we report or understand any narrative in a film or novel, we are normally using both hemispheres of our brain, and especially the corpus callosum, that connects them.

Assuming that this global distribution of functions is more or less correct—as it has been described by Gazzaniga (2000) and other neurologists, and as the process of pragmatic mapping has been defined since at least 1975—three major classes of disorders can be distinguished. There are the *aphasias*—disorders involving loss of language abilities. Then, there are the **agnosias**—loss of access to or knowledge of facts associated mainly with the minor hemisphere. Finally, there are the *apraxias* of speech and action. The latter involve the loss of ability to produce the articulate associations of language (or intentions) with facts (including faces or persons) through speech, writing, or signing.

The first class of disorders can be roughly associated with the left hemisphere of the brain and its distinct specializations as suggested in Figure 10–16. The connection between the two hemispheres, and the indexical (pragmatic) mapping of holistic icons onto analytical symbols and the reverse, is also depicted. Communications from the dominant hemisphere to the subordinate one seem to be critically involved in apraxias of speech and action while communications in the opposite direction seem to be critically involved in the agnosias. Presumably, the active indexical mapping of symbols to icons and vice versa, in normal cases, involves the corpus callosum as the central paths of connection. The simplest example of such a mapping—one that shows the major components of the anatomy and the representational systems involved—is suggested by the mapping of the name "Cecilia Burman" onto the person pictured in Figure 10–16. The icon of a person's face is processed mainly by the right hemisphere. By contrast, the assertion about who the picture represents, that the person is "Cecilia Burman" is processed mainly by the left hemisphere. To make this connection requires communication between the two hemispheres through the corpus callosum as shown in Figure 6–4 (Chapter 6) and later in Figure 10–20.

The Unified Brain: Major Functions Can Go Left or Right

The fact that all the functions in the brain can be performed to a considerable degree by either hemisphere was shown dramatically in a series of **hemispherectomy** or "split-brain" experiments that won neurologist Roger W. Sperry [1913–1994] a Nobel Prize in 1981. In those cases, one of the hemispheres is completely removed or rendered incapable of direct communication with the other hemisphere. Normally, such a radical treatment is only done in cases of life-threatening diseases such as recurrent **epileptic seizures** that are believed to be caused by, or that always begin, in one of the hemispheres.

The radical surgeries, where one hemisphere is effectively shut down or completely removed, show that essentially all functions can be handled by an undamaged but single hemisphere. Sperry and colleagues showed that the right and left hemispheres can both perform tasks that are known to be the specialty of the opposite hemisphere. Sperry put it like this in his Nobel lecture of 1981 describing certain outcomes of the split-brain experiments:

> Each brain half . . . appeared to have its own, largely separate, cognitive domain with its own private perceptual, learning and memory experiences, all of which were seemingly oblivious of corresponding events in the other hemisphere. . . . The speaking hemisphere [the dominant one] in these patients could tell us directly in its own words that it knew nothing of the inner experience involved in test performances correctly carried out by the mute partner hemisphere [the minor one].

The fact that all the work can sometimes be done fairly well by just one of the hemispheres is evident from such studies.

> We must bear in mind in considering the specializations that are lateralized in a whole brain, that all the functions can to a considerable degree be performed by either hemisphere.

Using Only Half His Brain

In one dramatic case, reported by A. Smith (1966; A. Smith & Sugar, 1975), after surgical removal of a whole hemisphere the patient was able to complete a college education, attend graduate school, and do better than average on all kinds of standardized tests including the kinds of language proficiency tasks in IQ tests (also see Sperry, 1981).

Many cases have been treated and studied since then. A search for "hemispherectomy" on the Web of Knowledge on April 1, 2009 turned up no fewer than 758 hits, with 51 of them having been published in 2009. If the **functional hemispherectomy**—removal or disconnection of one hemisphere—is performed early on, it is apparently the case that the remaining hemisphere can largely, if not completely, take over the functions of the hemisphere that is shut down or removed (see Loddenkemper et al., 2007; Paiement et al., 2008).

However, Backlund, Morin, Ptito, Bushnell, and Olausson (2005) showed that sensations pertaining to the detection of spatial and directional differences are probably diminished in persons with just one hemisphere. Backlund et al. speculated that telling differences in space may depend on "spatially and temporally precise afferent [sensory] information . . . in a distributed cortical network [i.e., one that involves information in accessible to both hemispheres]" (p. 332). In Chapter 3 we showed why detection of differences in direction and location of a source of sound, for instance, is dependent on the distance between the ears and evidently on an internal construction of the three-dimensional space outside the body. To do that kind of spatial processing in particular, it seems likely that two distinct hemispheres may be required. Distinctions in timing and sequence, with respect to sensation, also appear either to require or to be enhanced by having both hemispheres intact.

It is almost as if we have two brains—both of which can perform all, or nearly all, the functions that are needed by the body. Normally, the minor hemisphere does part of the work under the direction of the major, but in emergencies, to some extent, some or all of the functions can be taken over by either hemisphere. This is especially true if the loss of one hemisphere occurs very early in life.

Specialization Lateralized: Symbols, Left, Icons, Right

Bearing all the foregoing facts in mind, it still holds that broad classes of distinct disorders can be associated, more or less distinctly, with the specialization of the left or the right hemisphere. As suggested in Figure 10–16, aphasias are typically—almost but not quite exclusively—associated with the dominant, usually, the left hemisphere while right brain counterparts, the "agnosias" are associated with the minor (nondominant)—usually the right—hemisphere. But we must keep in mind that none of the disorders in question can be rigidly distinguished with respect to either hemisphere.

What is more, the most pervasive disorders commonly involve both hemispheres and the connections between them. Early in development, and probably as written in the genetic material itself for any given individual, the left hemisphere is programed to take charge of control functions and to assume the main responsibility for language and sequential (temporal—time based) reasoning. Meantime, the minor hemisphere, usually the right, specializes in holistic processing of the spatial kind.

As suggested in Figure 10–16, aphasias are typically—almost but not quite exclusively—associated with the dominant, usually, the left hemisphere while right brain counterparts, the "agnosias" are associated with the minor (nondominant)—usually the right—hemisphere.

The Unity of Coherence

It is also important to bear in mind that in all comprehension and conceptualization—from ordinary communication to scientific theory building—conceptual unity, common understanding, and agreement is normally the goal. Even if we are reporting a dream or a fantasy, we normally try to make our report coherent enough that our interlocutors will be able to know what we are talking about. As we have seen throughout this book, and especially in Chapter 9, experience normally unfolds over time a lot like a story—like a narrative. As a result, narrative structures in language are foundational.

When the story fits the facts of experience, we say the story is a **true narrative representation**. If some or all of the facts in a given story are merely imagined, we call it a **fictional representation**. If some of the facts are inadvertently misrepresented, or if the representation does not fit them well, we describe the result as some kind of error, a **false representation**. If the falseness is intentional and is intended to deceive someone else, we call that a lie—a **deceptive representation**. Ones that just don't make any sense at all, we call *Bloomfieldian phonics*. Just kidding. We call them nonsense.

The important thing to keep in mind in classifying neurological disorders is that for any representation to be recognized as representing anything at all, a certain amount of coherence is required. The representations must, to some extent, agree with what they represent and the agreement must be accessible in some way. In Figure 10–16, for instance, the picture of Cecilia Burman needs to be a picture of the person that goes by that name, and the person that goes by that name needs to be the person in the picture. Otherwise, coherence breaks down. If the major and minor hemispheres both have access to the correct mapping of symbols—say, the assertion, "That's Cecilia Burman!" when in fact the person pointed out is indeed the person that goes by that name the assertion is coherent to a limit. It is a true narrative representation.

In ordinary true reports about facts, an optimal amount of coherence is achieved. The symbols do not claim any more about the facts—the icon(s) at hand—the picture, say, of Cecilia Burman as she looked at age 32—than the icon(s) deliver(s). The icon really is a picture of Cecilia Burman. When this kind of agreement exists between the two hemispheres, we can say that the unity of coherence has been achieved. When it does not happen, we describe the representation as incomplete or incoherent. Disorders always involve incomplete, sometimes quite incoherent representations.

Aphasias (Left), Agnosias (Right)

As shown in Figure 10–16, if the words (or abstract symbols of thought and language) do not get linked appropriately with the facts

To make sense of what is going on in the world, we must make our representations fit our ongoing experience of the world as events unfold over time.

The key to a complete and coherent representation—according to the theory of pragmatic mapping—is to get the symbols to agree with the icons through indexes that connect them appropriately.

(the concrete icons of experience and/or imagination) the class of disorders implicated are aphasias. Because aphasias are associated with the dominant hemisphere they are usually to the left as shown in Figure 10–16.

If the problem involves information about the concrete icons, a different class of disorders, the agnosias, are indicated. As the processing of holistic icons (real or imagined) is largely the specialization of the minor hemisphere, they are usually associated with the right hemisphere. However, the distinctions are not rigid for reasons we have noted above, and most of the difficulties, as usual, lie in the middle ground where the pragmatic connections must be made through appropriate indexes. Also, it is in that middle ground where teaching and clinical intervention must operate to help out in cases where some of the neurological functions are damaged or lost.

Expanding on and Generalizing Lichtheim's Aphasias

When the dominant hemisphere is damaged, often, we may get one or more of the aphasias identified by Lichtheim and his successors. The type depends in part on where the damage is located, but even more so on how extensive the damage is (as noted by Luria, 1966). The most severe cases of aphasia—which may involve combinations of the eight kinds elaborated on by Lichtheim—is termed **global aphasia**. It may be caused by extensive damage to the dominant hemisphere of the brain, or by focused destruction of the language areas only.

Although the aphasias associated with speech processing—receptive and productive processing—are the better known and more commonly studied varieties, as seen in the elaboration of Lichtheim's eight categories above, more specific types of aphasia do occur that seem to impact other modalities of processing differently. We dealt with the major literacy disorders in Chapter 9, including, "acquired alexia" or "word blindness" and "acquired dyslexia" as well as "agraphia"—loss of ability to write. All of these conditions are types of aphasia and are guaranteed to accompany global aphasia because reading, writing, manual signing, verbal thinking, and any form of reasoning that depends on general language abilities is bound to be lost if those general language abilities are lost. In other words, it is a strict logical necessity that global aphasia must be accompanied by alexia, agraphia, and a host of other conditions that flow from the complete loss of language abilities.

Generalizing Lichtheim's Diagram

Although Lichtheim's "house" diagram was focused on speech, as are most studies of aphasia to this date, it is reasonable to suppose that approximately the same varieties of aphasia ought to be found in manual signing and in literacy. Also, in view of the logicomathematical proofs developed by others and ourselves showing that even the most extremely imaginary fantasies and fictions at their basis are dependent on pragmatic mappings—the same kind being common to speech, sign, and writing (for example, see Figures 1–9, 3–1, 9–2, 10–2, and 10–6)—it is certain that loss of the power to perform pragmatic mapping must affect all modalities of processing that require access to meaning through symbols. This result is assured in advance by the strictest forms of logicomathematical reasoning and it suggests that Lichtheim's house should be generalizable to other modalities.

To the extent that Lichtheim's diagram is correct for aphasias impacting the speech modality, it must also apply to literacy, manual signing, and the abstract thought processes that depend on words and the concepts underlying them.

What Is Agnosia?

The term agnosia—means "the absence or lack of knowledge" and can be translated from the Greek as "not known." The word *"a-gnosia"* consists is the Greek negative *"a-"* plus the root *"gnosia"* meaning "knowledge." The one thing that the different forms of agnosia have in common is that they universally involve some breakdown in the holistic determination of just what sort of things, persons, spaces, scenes, and contexts of experience are at hand. The agnosias involve the interpretation, recognition, and holistic understanding of things—where by the word "things" we intend to include persons, places, settings, and anything that can be perceived or imagined. A "thing" in this sense is any logically possible or conceivable entity.

To the extent that lateralization of functions actually occurs, the agnosias involve the special capacities that are assigned primarily to the minor hemisphere. From the point of view of the theory of pragmatic mapping and the distinct specializations of the hemispheres, the agnosias are the counterparts of the aphasias. We suggest this in Figure 10–16 in the directional arrows at the center of the brain, where the corpus callosum connects the left and right hemispheres. We use Lichtheim's convention of drawing a slash through the connecting arrow to suggest a breakdown. The different kinds of aphasia are associated primarily with the special capacities that are the province of the dominant (usually, right) hemisphere.

In the vast early literature on the aphasias, the communication of the dominant hemisphere with the subordinate one is not prominently discussed.

Although Lichtheim's model remains the most commonly referred to standard for categorizing different kinds of aphasia, it makes no mention of any connection with the subordinate hemisphere. All the focus is on the dominant hemisphere as if language abilities had little or nothing to do with holistic representations of the world of experience.

H. Damasio et al. (2004), by contrast—and many other studies could be mentioned here—showed that the distribution of symbolic (linguistic) concepts in the dominant hemisphere corresponds to a similar conceptual differentiation of iconic (holistic) ones in the nondominant hemisphere. However, the general tendency to overlook or omit consideration of the nondominant hemisphere with respect to language processing is consistent with the fact that most researchers in American linguistics and related areas (e.g., literacy studies) have been taught to think about language in terms of its surface forms—letters, sounds, syllables, and so forth. Readers will easily see that this omission of the real world of experience and holistic representations of it—the essential work of the subordinate hemisphere of the brain—is consistent with the Bloomfieldian theory of speech and reading. Bloomfield was certainly not the only theoretician to neglect the world of experience and its conceptual representations in icons and indexes.

Meaning Still Rules

Meaning is by far the dominant element in the actual perception, production, acquisition, and use of linguistic representations. Surface forms are superficial. That is why we call them "surface" forms.

As all three of us have argued in various publications (Badon, 1994; J. W. Oller, Sales, & Harrington, 1969; S. D. Oller, 2005) ranging across almost half a century, and as the vast research on language acquisition and discourse processing confirms (see our review in *Discourse Processes*, J. W. Oller, L. Chen, S. D. Oller, & Pan, 2005), surface forms are superficial and must either be connected with meaning through coherent pragmatic mappings to real or imagined conceptual representations at a deeper level, or to the extent that such deeper mappings of the surface forms fail, or are missing, the representations themselves must be judged to be incoherent, flawed, or at least incomplete. They will appear to be symptomatic of disorders. When linguistic representations at the surface are deliberately tampered with and distorted as in the McGurk interactions, as we demonstrated in Chapter 4, meaning dominates and virtually forces the intelligent interpreter to perceive what is expected rather than what is sometimes actually present in the surface forms.

It is for this reason that Bloomfield's recommendation that children be taught to read by using nonsensical strings of letters and sounds is, simply, nonsensical. The exclusive attention to surface forms results in a very high degree of incoherence. And as we showed in Chapter 9, it can produce all of the symptoms of a special kind of instructional dyslexia. To the extent that the pragmatic mapping relations are neglected, inaccessible, or unaccounted for, the theories of disorders likewise will be incomplete. To the same extent, representations at any level are flawed (disordered)—that is, degenerate in the sense of being incomplete—exactly to the extent of their failure to be connected in a coherent way with discoverable meanings (i.e., the real or imagined facts that the surface forms are supposed to represent).

At the Tip of the Mind: Lost in the Minor Hemisphere

Corresponding to the "tip of the tongue" phenomena—where we cannot quite think of a particular word, or name, or a descriptive phrase—there are also what are called the **"tip of the mind"** phenomena (Hostetter & Alibali, 2004). Just as tip of the tongue events are commonly used to get across to nonaphasics the idea about anomic aphasia, we can get an idea of what the agnosias are from the tip of the mind phenomena.

In other instances, we may say or think something like, "I know that I know what that is, or who that person is, but I just can't think where I know them from, or just who or what that thing is." For instance, an object seen in an unfamiliar place or clutter may evoke a certain sense of familiarity but may still fall short of recognition. We know there is something there of interest but do not know what it is. Sometimes, as Hostetter and colleagues have noted, we can help our dominant hemisphere with a little prompting by gestures that seem to suggest what the minor hemisphere was up to. For instance, making a motion like turning a screwdriver may enable recall of a forgotten intention.

In fact, speakers commonly use such seemingly useless, largely redundant gestures to prompt their own thoughts. An example, is the "hurry up, go on" gesture with one or both hands when trying to think of the next sentence to write at the computer. We may do this when no one but us is paying any attention. Are we conveying information to ourselves? Or, as Hostetter and Alibali (2004) noted,

> speakers [for instance on the telephone] often produce representational gestures even when they know that their audience cannot see them, making it unlikely that their intended purpose is solely to help the audience. (2004, p. 589; also see Hostetter, Alibali, & Kita, 2007)

In some of the early split brain experiments as described in lectures by Sperry, Geschwind, Gazzaniga, and others, it became evident that communication between separated hemispheres could be effected by gestures. We will have more to say about that below in the section titled "Associations Between the Hemispheres."

Elaborating the Agnosias:
The Less Studied Hemisphere

At a limit of extreme agnosia the person affected loses the capacity to recognize any familiar objects, persons, spaces, scenes, or contexts. A person with a less extreme **global agnosia** might have the sense that something about a person, place, or thing is familiar and yet they can't quite put their finger on just what it is. The object of thought, the icon that the affected person is trying to think of—say,

The tip of the mind can be thought of as a threshold in the minor hemisphere of the brain where we almost have a complete representation of something, but not quite. We cannot quite think of what a certain actor looks like. We may have the name in front of us and yet be unable to come up with the icon, the facial image, that goes with it.

a person, thing, scene, or context—may be perceivable and may be perceived correctly with respect to properties that can be detected by seeing, hearing, smelling, touching, or tasting and yet the person affected by the agnosia may not be able to recognize it. The key may not connect with the lock that it opens. Likewise, the lock may not trigger the question, "Where is the key?"

The term "agnosia" is loosely and widely applied to any loss of ability to recognize, know, and understand things, their parts, or their properties. The loss may be confined to a particular sense of perception—vision as contrasted with the other senses. For instance, agnosia—or some individual property may be singled out within sensory system or modality of processing.

There is a vast literature on agnosia. With a search on the Web of Knowledge (all databases) for the term "agnosia" we found 1,345 research reports from 1973 to the present. Interestingly, to show just how much more interest and attention is devoted to aphasia, on the same day, April 1, 2009, a search for "aphasia" produced 9,406 hits—seven times as many hits on the same day. It is clear, as we have suggested, that the dominant hemisphere, and language abilities in particular, are getting the lion's share of the research effort.

Meantime, the many articles on agnosias show that they can affect the full range of the iconic, holistic representations involved in sensory, sensory-motor, and sensory-motor-linguistic forms and concepts. The literature describes cases of "agnosia" pertaining to every one of the senses. There are agnosias pertaining to every sensory representations—visual, auditory, **olfactory** (smell), tactile, and **gustatory** (taste). There are also agnosias pertaining to the iconic representation of movements in space and sequence in time (as through coherent gestures), as well as conceptual agnosias where access to knowledge of whole objects, persons, scenes, and contexts is lost or diminished.

The Threshold of Coherence

With agnosias, as we have already suggested, the problem is best understood at the boundary that separates incoherence from what C. S. Peirce [1839–1914] called the **unity of conception**. We proposed to call that boundary the **threshold of coherence**. As Peirce explained, the underlying purpose of representations is to achieve coherence—to make sense of impressions.

Without backing off from the trees, we may not be able to see the forest.

The difference between an incomplete sensory impression—for example, noticing part of a scene or an extreme closeup of a picture that you have not recognized yet—and a whole and meaningful concept is that the partial sensory impression is more or less immediately available as soon as it is noticed. But the holistic concept is not necessarily accessible through the partial impression. The view from inside a boxcar, say, does not enable us to see the whole train, but we may be able to do so from an airplane high above the whole scene. However, once we gain enough information to know what is happening, who is involved, what a statement means, and so on, we have an excess of information. We also gain access to facts and impressions that are not currently part of our sensory impressions. For instance, if we know we are viewing a scene from inside a boxcar on a train, when the protagonist awakens after being knocked out in a previous scene, the noise of the wheels on the tracks is instantly recognized and we know about the tracks though we cannot perceive them.

We have all had an experience of seeing someone somewhere whom we have met before but whom we do not recognize in the new context. We cannot quite put things together. Or we may meet someone whom we know but who does not remember having met us. We may engage in an exchange of information regarding where and when we met, how long ago it was, or what we talked about, and then suddenly, the light goes on. There is an "Aha!" moment where the person says, "Ah yes, I remember, you're the one who . . . " Once that "Aha!" is reached we also gain access to a lot of additional information that is not available in present sensory impressions. For instance, we may remember who else was at the function, another person whom we haven't thought of for years, what we had for dinner that evening, and so on.

Discourse in General Involves the Threshold of Coherence

The same basic coherence threshold is involved in text and discourse processing as well. Take the following example about a "mushy brown peach" as described in the book called *Einstein's Dreams*:

> A mushy, brown peach is lifted from the garbage and placed on the table to turn pink. It turns pink, it gets firm, it is carried in a shopping sack to the grocer's, put on a shelf, removed and crated, returned to the tree with pink blossoms. In this world, time flows backward. (from *Einstein's Dreams* by Alan Lightman, 1993, p. 102)

As Graesser, Millis, and Zwaan (1997) noted, until we get to the last sentence about time flowing backwards, the whole sequence is incoherent because there is no way to understand why anyone would carry a peach from the garbage to the table, and so on. The expected episodic organization depends on the usual directional flow of time. We expect it to flow forward, not backward. But once we are given the key to the mystery, we solve it and it all makes sense.

Dr. Liang Chen, presently on the faculty at the University of Georgia, effectively used the quote from *Einstein's Dreams* to show that we expect events to be reported in the sort of order in which they have occurred, or might occur in experience.

From Surprise to Recognition

Here is how C. S. Peirce (1866/1982b, p. 519) explained our ability to achieve the unity of conception. He said,

> . . . if a conception does not reduce the impressions which it accompanies to unity, it would be a mere arbitrary addition to the latter [those impressions], for there is no other condition for the production of a conception except that it shall make impressions comprehensible.

In other words, if recognition of a person's face added nothing to the face that was not already there, there would be no benefit in the recognition. Nothing would be gained. But there is a huge difference, you will agree, in recognizing yourself in the mirror, or knowing your spouse, and in failing to do either of these simple acts. Both require that we cross the threshold of coherence. The concept of a person's identity is a big step of abstraction away from a mere sensory impression. Peirce takes his argument a step further:

> Now if the impressions could be definitely conceived without the conception, the conception would not reduce them to unity.

The concept of a person's identity is a big step of abstraction away from a mere sensory impression.

That is, nothing would be gained in the recognition of your lover when he or she appears unexpectedly and plants a wet kiss on your lips. But much is gained in such recognition or lost if recognition is missing. Peirce goes on:

> But attention is definite conception; therefore impressions (or more immediate conceptions) cannot be attended to, to the neglect of an elementary conception which reduces them to unity.

That is to say, even paying attention to the person kissing you on the mouth is a conceptual sort of recognition which identifies the event underway as being kissed on the mouth. We could not recognize the person while neglecting to notice that we are being kissed on the mouth. Peirce is not through yet, though:

> On the other hand, when such a conception has once been obtained, there is no reason in general why the premises which have occasioned it

that is, being kissed on the mouth and noticing that it is happening,

> should not be neglected, and therefore the explaining conception may abstract from the more immediate ones and from the impressions. (p. 519)

In other words, if in being kissed on the mouth we happen to notice that the person kissing us is our lover, the kissing itself can take a distant back seat to the importance of the person that we identify as our lover. All the sensory impressions in the world from that one kissing event can be, more or less, set aside in favor of the happy conclusion that goes something like this: "Ah! It's you!" And then, as Richard Gere might have said to Julia Roberts, or vice versa, in *Pretty Woman*, "We kiss 'em right back."

At the boundary that separates the sense that "something seems familiar" and "Aha! I know who (what, when, or how) that is!" We achieve the unity of conception. We know. But in agnosias, some or all of what we have just described cannot happen.

As soon as we cross the threshold of coherence, as Peirce has noted in another context, we have a lot more information than we needed to make the identification of the person—or whatever the logical object of attention may be. We go from a state of some degree of uncertainty, to a state of knowing.

Prosopagnosia

The best known of the agnosias—setting aside the auditory ones which are usually classed with CAPD and/or aphasia and also setting aside the ones associated with literacy which are classed as dyslexia or agraphia—the ones that have been most commonly studied, are in the visual domain. For instance, something like an agnosia occurs when in looking at a photograph, we notice the skin color and yet do not know if we are seeing part of a hand, or face, or leg. Or we may look into a drawer with a tangle of knives and forks, and so forth, and not be able to see, that is, single out and recognize, the particular utensil we are searching for. The object may be right in front of us, "hidden" in plain sight. For persons without any loss, experiences of these "tip of the mind" phenomena are not unknown, though they are uncommon. However, for a person with a genuine agnosia, the type of difficulty just illustrated may be magnified and intensified to a degree that is difficult for persons without the condition to appreciate.

Face Blindness

The special kind of agnosia where a person loses, or perhaps never had, the normal ability to recognize a familiar face is called **prosopagnosia**. The Greek *prosopon* means "face" or "person." If you look at the Greek word from a phonological and semantic point of view, it can be seen and heard that *prosopon* is a cognate of the English word "person." At any rate, Greek and English are known to be derived from a common source language that was spoken over a large part of what is now Europe and India just a few thousands of years ago. Laypersons who find the Greek etymology opaque prefer to call prosopagnosia—"face blindness." It is well described as an inability to recognize, recall, and/or think of faces.

The ability to recognize and recall faces is evidently so specialized that it can be affected when perceptual capacities seem to be intact and other cognitive capacities are evidently unaffected. It can also, it seems, be lost before birth or at any time later on. For an insightful nontechnical description of a single case as viewed from the inside out see the story of Cecilia Burman at her public Web site (2002, retrieved March 7, 2009 at from http://www.prosopagnosia .com/main/cb/index.asp).

Cecilia's Prosopagnosia

Cecilia tells that she has had the condition of "face blindness" as long as she can remember. It was hard to deal with prosopagnosia because people who do not have it cannot easily imagine what it is like. They are apt to suppose that it is merely a problem of trying to remember a long list of unfamiliar names, or to tell similar looking people apart. But prosopagnosia is much more specific than that. Cecelia and other persons with the condition (also see Bill Choisser's book, 2002, retrieved March 7, 2009, from http://www.choisser.com/face blind/) find it difficult to get their friends and even family members to take them seriously, or to understand them, when they explain their situation. Bill Choisser also has had prosopagnosia for as far back as he can remember.

Sorting Through the Research

Although prosopagnosia is a condition that can be "acquired" later in life due to an injury, it may be a prebirth genetic condition. The most recent research with normal brains seeking to discover what is going on when facial recognition succeeds (Bobes et al., 2007) showed that face recognition consistently involves central parietal regions activated about one-half a second after the photo is presented for recognition. When the recognition involves a familiar face expressing emotion, the frontal regions of both hemispheres come into play after only about 350 milliseconds. Carbon (2008) also showed that the context of photos of famous people presented for recognition plays an important role. In disorders involving the loss of ability to recognize faces, according to a recent proposal by Zifan, Gharibzadeh, and Moradi (2007) there appears to be damage to the "medial occipito-temporal region" (p. 146).

Gainotti (2007), consistent with the model suggested in Figure 10–16, examined research on patterns of brain damage associated with prosopagnosia. The cases examined involved right and left hemisphere damage to the front (anterior) temporal lobes. With damage to the left hemisphere deficits generally involved inability to supply the name of a famous pictured person, while damage to the same region in the right hemisphere generally involved inability to store and process the image (i.e., to know that a picture was of a famous person irrespective of the name of that person). This is completely consistent with the pragmatic mapping diagram and the evidence that the dominant hemisphere handles the lexical side

Although prosopagnosia is a condition that can be "acquired" later in life due to an injury, it may be a prebirth genetic condition.

of semantic meaning that must be mapped onto a face, whereas the subordinate hemisphere handles the conceptual aspect of the meaning in a way that is somewhat independent of the lexicon, that is, independent of the name. However, Carbon (2008) has shown that even in the processing of photographs, context is important to the recognition of famous faces showing additional dependence on the transitive relations in narratives—for example, if that is Dallas on November 22, 1963, the picture is of John F. Kennedy, but remove the context and many viewers may not recognize a picture of the familiar famous face.

Consistent with Gainotti's tentative conclusion, and our own amplification of it, but adding some complexity, Anaki, Kaufman, Freedman, and Moscovitch (2007) report a case study of an individual with damage to the left occipital lobe, who "is able to select a famous face from among non-famous distractors" and who is able to demonstrate delayed recognition recall of faces even when certain identifying features have been deleted. He has problems, however, when he has to name the famous person (e.g., "Michael Douglas," "Antonio Banderas," "George Bush," "Tony Blair," "Winston Churchill," "Adolf Hitler," etc.), or when he has to select two faces that share a semantic feature based on the fact that "both are actors," "both are living political leaders," or "both were involved in World War II." On the basis of semantic descriptors he cannot pick the right faces. His deficit seems to be consistent with the differentiation of abilities suggested in Figure 10–16. All of this work on prosopagnosia is consistent with the pragmatic mapping diagram and the hypothesized differentiation of symbolic and iconic functions.

ACROSS THE HEMISPHERES: INDEXING AND MOTOR FUNCTIONS

There are many ways to demonstrate that our two hemispheres normally communicate well with each other. We have already seen that above with reference to the H. Damasio et al. (2004) research showing that for semantic categories of lexical items (words) represented in the dominant hemisphere there are corresponding conceptual representations of the iconic kind (images) in the subordinate hemisphere. Similarly, we see evidence of communication and coordination between the two hemispheres in the theory and research concerning the relation between an anomic aphasia, typically associated with the dominant temporal lobe of the brain, and the corresponding agnosia for facial recognition associated with a lesion in the subordinate occipitotemporal lobe.

There is, in the motor domain, simpler and less abstract evidence of communication between the two hemispheres. We can also demonstrate to ourselves evidence for the dominance of the

There are many ways to demonstrate that our two hemispheres normally communicate well with each other.

major hemisphere (usually the left hemisphere in right-handed individuals) and for the ranking of the major sign systems within each of the two hemispheres: that is, linguistic signs which include motoric and sensory signs are ranked at the top (top and center in the head of the whole body); followed by motoric signs which necessarily include sensory signs in the middle (focused on the face and hands as seen in the motor homunculus of Figures 1–6 and 1–8), and sensory signs at the bottom of the hierarchy (and at the periphery of the body).

Demonstrating Lateralization of Dominance

Here are some illustrations from the motor domain that you can perform to demonstrate the remarkable connectedness and communication between your two hemispheres. If you pat a rhythm with your dominant hand, you can do the same with the subordinate hand. Or you can make the rhythm on either hand hit the off-beats, or a double beat, and so on. However, you will notice, probably, that the main rhythm is easier to maintain with your dominant hand. It is also easier to perform two tasks, for example, rub a circle on your midline with your dominant hand and pat the top of your head with your subordinate hand. With a little practice, it is possible to do the two tasks simultaneously. Then try reversing them. Rub a circle on your midline with your subordinate hand and pat your head with your dominant hand. The task is now more difficult, isn't it? This shows that motor control in the subordinate hemisphere is subject to the dominant hemisphere—that is, the hemisphere that controls your dominant hand also regulates the subordinate hand indirectly by governing the subordinate hemisphere.

> . . . motor control in the subordinate hemisphere is subject to the dominant hemisphere—that is, the hemisphere that controls your dominant hand also regulates the subordinate hand indirectly by governing the subordinate hemisphere.

Coordinating Circular Movements

Here is another series of tasks that show how the two hemispheres typically interact in skilled movements. Pretend you are turning a crank, as in peddling a bicycle—in the **sagittal** plane; Figure 10–17 —with your dominant hand and try imitating the same motion with your left. It is easy to do this. In fact, you can also line up your hands as if the peddles were exactly opposite to one another. In that case, the motion puts you off balance as both hands together move to the front or the the back at the same time. Still, you can easily perform the cranking motion. Or you can pretend you are turning a connected crank shaft, with the peddles as normally arranged, where the left hand is forward when the right hand is to the back, and so on. This motion is easier and more balanced. Now, change the motion. Turn the imaginary crank in your dominant hand in one circular motion and make the crank in the subordinate hand go in the opposite direction. This is harder to do.

However, if you reorient the plane of motion to an *axial* plane (refer again to Figure 10–17)—imagine you are standing with two

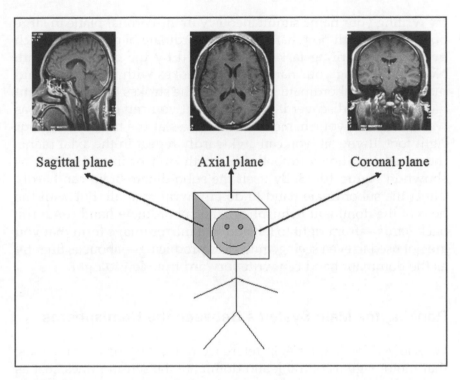

FIGURE 10–17. Differentiating the planes of motion relative to views of the brain created with MRI. Retrieved March 7, 2009, from http://www.med .wayne.edu/diagRadiology/Anatomy_Modules/brain/brain.html. Copyright © 1999 by J. E. Zapawa, A. L. Alcantara, and H. Nguyen. Adapted and reprinted with permission. All rights reserved.

(fixed) bowls of pancake batter on a table and stirring both of them simultaneously, you can stir in the same circular direction with both hands, or you can easily go in opposite directions—where the left hand performs the mirror image motion of the right. The same holds in the **coronal** plane. Imagine you are drawing circles on a wall in large strokes. You can draw two circles, one with each hand going in the same direction, or you can easily reverse the direction with both hands, or you can cause the right hand to go in one direction while the left hand does the mirror image, opposite motion.

If you attempt the same tasks with the subordinate hand operating alone, you will notice that it is more difficult to make a repeated circular motion with the subordinate hand alone than it is to do the motion with your dominant hand while the subordinate hand either follows in the same direction, or does the mirror image motion. Why is this? The answer is simple.

The execution of complex motor movements comes largely under the control of the dominant hemisphere and the subordinate hemisphere is not as good at controlling and producing those movements.

Mirror Writing with the Nondominant Hand

This next demonstration is a clincher. Try writing your name in the air in large bold strokes—as if you were writing on a chalk board or in the dust on a windshield of someone's car. Next try doing it with your subordinate hand. Probably it is difficult. But this time try writing your name simultaneously in the coronal plane in large bold strokes with both hands. The subordinate hand can do much better at the writing task if it is guided by the dominant hand. Next, try writing your name in bold strokes with both hands and make the left subordinate hand mirror the strokes of the dominant hand. You will discover if you try it that you can do just about as well in writing your name in bold strokes at the beach with your right foot. If you sit, you can awkwardly repeat in the axial plane, the parallel writing with both feet, or the mirror image writing as shown in Figure 10–18. By itself the subordinate brain can hardly direct the subordinate hand to do any writing at all. But with the help of the dominant hemisphere, the subordinate hand can write backwards—from right to left and in a mirror image form that you are not used to even seeing, much less producing—about as fluently as the dominant hand can write forward from left to right.

Ranking the Main Systems Between the Hemispheres

We showed in Chapter 4, in reference to the McGurk interactions, that motor signals outrank and dominate the sensory ones, just as visual signals outrank auditory ones in speech perception. Similarly, we also showed in Chapter 4 that meaning functions dependent on linguistic abilities outrank both motor and sensory functions. The relationships involve inclusion. The motor systems encompass sensory ones, and both of them are included within linguistic systems. The higher rank is from more inclusive to less inclusive. Roger W. Sperry (1981) in his Nobel lecture summed up the picture that we diagram in Figure 10–19:

> . . . the two halves of the brain, when connected, work closely together as a functional unit with the leading control being in one or the other. (1981, p. 2; retrieved March 7, 2009, from http://nobelprize.org/nobel_prizes/medicine/laureates/1981/sperry-lecture.html)

Evidently, the subordinate hemisphere normally remains under the control of the dominant hemisphere to such an extent that the subordinate one is helped along and made more efficient than it would be if it were operating by itself. In these simple demonstrations we also see clear evidence of the sign hierarchy where language (meanings especially) outrank movements and both of them outrank sensory representations.

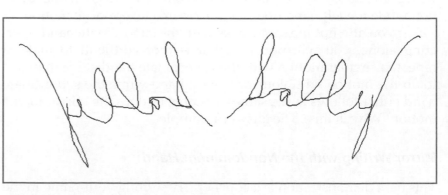

FIGURE 10–18. Mirror writing of the sort that can easily be done with both hands, or even feet, simultaneously.

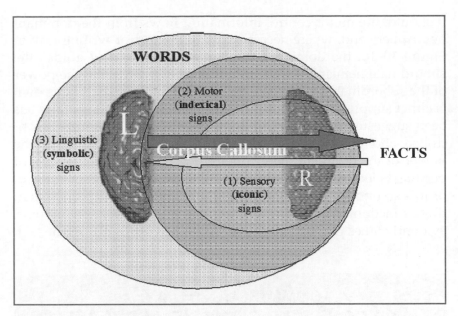

FIGURE 10–19. The pragmatic mapping relation viewed in terms of brain anatomy, known functions, and the major sign systems of the senses, movement, and language.

As shown in our diagram (see Figure 10–19), the control is normally in the dominant (usually left) hemisphere which also specializes in language, and in tasks that, as Sperry described them, are "analytic and sequential." Meantime, the subordinate (usually the right) hemisphere specializes in "spatial and synthetic" functions that require the recognition, comprehension, and holistic management of patterns, faces, designs, and shapes. Sperry continues:

> When this unitary function is rendered defective by a one-sided lesion, the resultant-impaired function prevails with respect to both hemispheres. That is, the two continue to operate as an integral, though defective, functional unit. (p. 2)

When the corpus callosum is intact, the dominant hemisphere handles the motor control of higher learned functions such as speech, writing, signing, producing mathematical equations, writing music, and so forth. It is in charge in producing sequences of abstract symbols or skilled actions and also in interpreting them. Verbal thinking, mathematical reasoning, and essentially all highly abstract analytical functions that require sequences of symbols that can be written in a notational system, for example, musical scores, normally come under the control of the dominant hemisphere. This holds for thinking, speaking, writing, or manual signing.

On the other side of the brain, the subordinate hemisphere specializes in handling iconic signs that are holistic (synthetic)— this includes facial recognition and the recognition of designs, shapes, scenes, and whole contexts. When everything is going along as it should, the motor control information flows from the dominant hemisphere and, where necessary, as in the mirror writing task of Figure 10–18, the dominant hemisphere governs and guides the subordinate hemisphere. The motor control is such that the power of the subordinate hemisphere to generate motor signals of its own is either suppressed (inhibited) by the dominant hemisphere as has been suggested in the work of Reggia et al. (2001) or simply is controlled and guided by the dominant hemisphere. Similarly, the power of the dominant hemisphere to produce holistic images of persons, objects, shapes, scenes, and contexts is normally suppressed, or it is seconded to the subordinate hemisphere that specializes in those functions. Much of this action, though probably not all of it, evidently takes place primarily through the corpus callosum.

COMMISSUROTOMY: DISCONNECTING THE HEMISPHERES

In operations where the callosum is severed, a procedure called **commissurotomy**, some interesting results are observed. We have already discussed effects of lesions in the dominant hemisphere—the main source of the aphasias (loss of language capacities)—and the lesions in the subordinate hemisphere—the main source of the agnosias (loss of capacity to process holistic images)—but we have not said anything yet in this chapter (but see Chapter 6) about the class of disorders known as apraxias—loss of capacity to produce highly articulated skilled movements as in speaking, writing, or manual signing.

The Apraxias

The apraxias can be thought of as varieties of motor aphasia. However, one of the differences is that the various aphasias cannot occur in early childhood, whereas apraxias can. Because "aphasia" involves the loss of a previously acquired language skill it cannot logically occur in an infant that has not yet acquired language skills. By contrast, "apraxias" can occur well before language skills begin to be manifested in infancy. As a result, it is a little strange to refer to **childhood aphasia** though this term is sometimes used and, of course, aphasias are possible in early childhood as a result of brain injuries (see "Childhood Apraxia," 2009, retrieved March 7, 2009, from http://www.apraxia-kids.org/site/c.chKMI0PIIsE/b.700249/k.CC2C/Home/apps/lk/content3.aspx). Generally, however, "motor aphasias" of the "transcortical" variety—also "Broca's aphasia"—are regarded as if they can only occur in adults (e.g., see "Transcortical Motor Aphasia," 2009, retrieved March 7, 2009, from http://en.wikipedia.org/wiki/Transcortical_motor_aphasia).

Setting aside the questions of terminology—whether the apraxias of speech are really types of aphasia, whether agraphia is really a type of apraxia, and so forth—what can we learn from the commissurotomy studies? For one thing, it appears that the subordinate hemisphere can perform tasks that involve linguistic concepts to a much greater extent than was appreciated before. However, there are two motor tasks the subordinate hemisphere is evidently altogether unable to perform at all.

The subordinate hemisphere evidently depends entirely on the dominant (language) hemisphere for the motor production of speech and writing. We see indirect evidence of this finding in the mirror writing demonstration (see Figure 10–18). The subordinate hemisphere cannot produce mirror writing at all fluently without the assistance of the dominant one. Likewise, in commissurotomy patients, the evidence that the dominant hemisphere has charge of motor production of speech and writing is compelling.

> In commissurotomized patients, Sperry and colleagues found that the subordinate hemisphere can neither speak nor write.

The Subordinate Hemisphere Comprehends Language

Although the subordinate half of the brain can recognize and demonstrate comprehension of printed or spoken words and even complex phrases about such abstract concepts as "automobile insurance" or the idea of "providing income for loved ones after a person's death," the subordinate half cannot verbally report this comprehension.

To show that the subordinate hemisphere of commissurotomized patients was able to comprehend words and phrases of considerable complexity and abstractness, investigators, especially Sperry and his colleagues (see Sperry, 1981), set up clever designs where the patient could show comprehension by singling out an object or printed phrase (e.g., by pointing), from an array of possibilities.

> The Commissurotomy patients were also able with the right hemisphere to choose correct written or spoken words to match presented objects or pictures to go correctly from spoken to printed words and vice versa. (Sperry, 1981, pp. 1–2)

Sperry went on to note that the dominant hemisphere of commissurotomized patients also showed the capacity to handle many of the holistic representational tasks that are normally ascribed to the subordinate hemisphere. For instance, they could recognize faces. This was not expected on account of the fact that a person with a lesion in the medial subordinate temporal lobe would normally experience prosopagnosia. However, when communication between the left and right hemispheres was more or less completely cut off by severing the corpus callosum, the dominant half of the brain proved that it had the latent capacity to recognize faces and perform other tasks that were seemingly suppressed by the subordinate hemisphere when the corpus callosum was intact. Sperry proposed that perhaps both hemispheres had the capacity to do all the work of the whole brain.

An opportunity to study that idea, and to test it in an actual case, came in 1967 when Sperry and one of his colleagues learned of an individual who had the congenital condition of never having formed a corpus callosum.

The Agenesis of the Corpus Callosum

In the case of the individual who never formed a corpus callosum —a problem described as **agenesis**—it seems from the reports (Saul & Sperry, 1968; Sperry, 1968) that there were two relatively intact twin brains inside one head. Research with this individual showed that both hemispheres could perform the same tasks about equally well. The individual in question had "an above-average IQ" and motor speech capacities were equally well formed in both of the hemispheres. What was missing were the advantages of a subordinate hemisphere. The individual in question was very good at verbal tasks but performed comparatively less well on tasks requiring the kinds of holistic spatial processing that are normally assigned to the subordinate hemisphere. It seemed that the individual in question had two dominant (language proficient) hemispheres and that this situation had cost him the disadvantage of not developing certain "nonverbal"—holistic and iconic—representational abilities that are normally handled by the subordinate hemisphere. This case, together with the other evidence discussed above, almost completes the picture of the role played by the corpus callosum in communication between the two hemispheres.

We will mention just one other study of an interesting case confirming the theory that sensory information gathered by the subordinate hemisphere (as suggested in Figure 10–19) must be reported to the dominant hemisphere through the corpus callosum. In fact, the case in question suggests that the sensory information communicated from the subordinate hemisphere to the dominant hemisphere critically depends on the region shown in Figure 10–20 known as the **splenium of the corpus callosum**. Suzuki et al. (1998) found evidence in a 14-year-old boy with damage to the back and bottom part of the splenium:

> The only difficulty demonstrated was in reading aloud or copying letters, which were presented tachistoscopically to the left visual field, with his right hand. He could copy letters presented to his left visual field with his left hand, however. . . . Review of 40 reported patients with callosal lesions suggests that the anterior to middle part of the splenium is involved in transferring picture information from the language-nondominant hemisphere to the language-dominant hemisphere and that the ventroposterior part is involved in transferring letter information. (p. 1390)

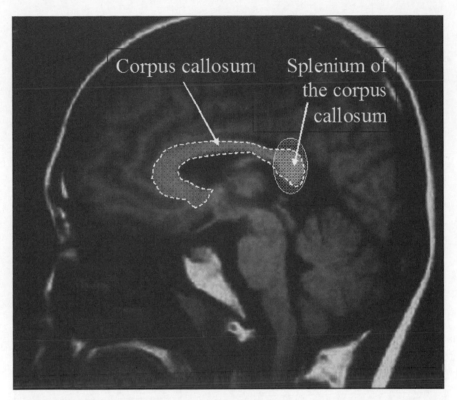

FIGURE 10–20. An MRI of the corpus callosum (dotted outline) and the splenium (in the transparent oval). Retrieved March 7, 2009, from http://www.indiana.edu/~pietsch/callosum.html. Copyright 2008 by Paul A. Pietsch. Adapted and reprinted with permission. All rights reserved.

These findings and their review suggest that the transfer of sensory information from the subordinate to the dominant hemisphere as shown in Figure 10–19 is probably more or less correct, as it is suggested there.

ABRUPT CAUSES OF ADULT NEUROLOGICAL DISORDERS

Some neurological problems—including the aphasias, agnosias, and apraxias—can be traced to a particular event that literally impacted the affected person, for example, a gunshot wound to the head. Although we don't like to call this kind of injury "acquired" it does make sense to call it abrupt, sudden, and shocking. Such events are traumatic. They may involve an encounter with a hard object producing injury or an internal weakness in a blood vessel that suddenly bursts.

The Case of Phineas Gage

In some abrupt injuries we can easily see the *cause*—the steel rod that penetrates the skull as in the case of Mr. Phineas Gage [1823–1860] (Figure 10–21)—and we see the *effect(s)* of the injury.

No Longer the Same Person

In the case of Mr. Gage, who survived for sometime after his accident, there is a record of the cognitive, behavioral, and emotional changes that occurred after the event. Because the changes were abrupt and because they came after the event, a *cause-effect* relation is assumed and warranted. Before the injury, Mr. Gage was gregarious, smart, diligent, and never profane. He worked as a foreman in railroad construction and one day when tamping an explosive it discharged accidentally causing a steel rod of about 2.4 centimeters in diameter to shoot through his head from the jaw line upward penetrating and exiting the skull through the frontal lobes. Subsequently, Dr. J. M. Harlow, who treated and observed Mr. Gage, described him as

> fitful, irreverent, indulging at times in the grossest profanity (which was not previously his custom), manifesting but little deference for his fellows, impatient of restraint or advice when it conflicts with his desires, at times pertinaciously obstinate, yet capricious and vacillating, devising many plans of future operations, which are no sooner arranged than they are abandoned in turn for others appearing more feasible. . . . A child in his intellectual capacity . . . [but with] the animal passions of a strong man. (Phineas Gage, 1860/2008, retrieved March 7, 2009, from http://en.wikipedia.org/wiki/Phineas_Gage)

Traumatic Brain Injury

During and after World War II, aphasias were studied as produced by TBIs from gun shot wounds (Luria, 1947, 1966). Until about the middle of the 20th century, war wounds to the heads of male soldiers were the primary source of information about links between neurological structures and brain functions.

Among the most studied causes of aphasias is **traumatic brain injury** (**TBI**). During and after World War II, aphasias were studied as produced by TBIs from gun shot wounds (Luria, 1947, 1966). Until about the middle of the 20th century, war wounds to the heads of male soldiers were the primary source of information about links between neurological structures and brain functions. However, it is not easy to tell just where the damage is when a projectile pierces the skull and may also enter the brain—rarely does a person survive the sort of injury that occurred to Mr. Phineas Gage. The manifestations of symptoms can vary greatly depending on the severity of the injury, the susceptibility of the individual to damage, age, general health, and so on.

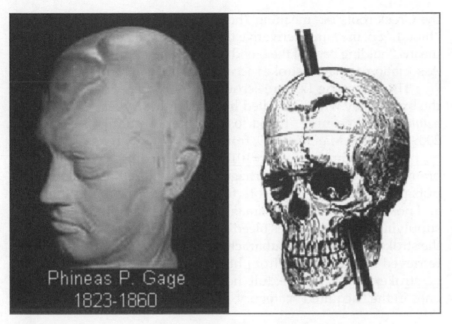

FIGURE 10–21. The death mask of Mr. Phineas Gage (*left*) and reconstruction of his injury (*right*). Retrieved March 7, 2009, from http://en.wiki pedia.org/wiki/Phineas_Gage and http://www.ninds.nih.gov/health_and_medical/pubs/tbi.htm, respectively. Both images are in the public domain —the death mask due to expired copyright and the reconstruction as a publication of the United States National Institute of Neurological Disorders and Stroke (NINDS).

TBI remains one of the most common causes of death and neurological disabilities in children and young adults (Marion, 1999; Brain Injury Recovery Network, 2009, retrieved March 7, 2009, from http://www.tbirecovery.org/Intro.html). TBI can also occur by bruising of the brain, in an automobile accident, or a sports accident, as the brain is slammed against the bony tissue on the inside of the skull. This can happen because of a sudden stop or change in direction of motion. In a forward motion that is stopped suddenly, the brain smashes into the inside front of the skull and then recoils backward into the back side of the skull providing multiple opportunities for bruising and internal bleeding. Shearing (tearing) of the brain tissues is also possible as portions of the brain change velocity at different rates causing additional bleeding and damage.

In a forward motion that is stopped suddenly, the brain smashes into the inside front of the skull and then recoils backward into the back side of the skull providing multiple opportunities for bruising and internal bleeding. Shearing (tearing) of the brain tissues is also possible as portions of the brain change velocity at different rates causing additional bleeding and damage.

Strokes

Aphasias, agnosias, and apraxias of various kinds and of different degrees of severity can also be produced by a **stroke**—or by multiple strokes. The most common kind of stroke involves a blocked blood vessel which causes damage to brain tissue because of deprivation of oxygen. This kind is called an **ischemic stroke**—from the Greek roots *isk-* meaning "holding back" and *-haimos* meaning "blood." So, the Latin derivative that we have borrowed into English means "holding back of the blood." According to the American Heart Association, ischemic strokes account for about 83% of such injuries.

The remaining 17% are accounted for by bleeding in or around the brain or by what are called **hemorrhagic strokes**—from Greek *haimorrhagia* meaning "blood loss" (American Stroke Association, 2009, retrieved March 7, 2009, from http://www.strokeassociation.org/presenter.jhtml?identifier=1014). If the bleeding occurs inside the brain—**intracerebral hemorrhage**—it can cause fluid build up that puts pressure on the brain interfering with normal brain functions and possibly permanently damaging tissues. If a rupture of an artery supplying the brain causes bleeding into the space around the brain the stroke is caused by a **subarachnoid hemorrhage** ("Stroke," 2009, retrieved March 7, 2009, from http://www.ninds.nih.gov/disorders/stroke/stroke.htm). Adult neurological conditions, especially ones in the "acquired" category, can have many different causes.

CUMULATIVE CAUSES OF ADULT NEUROLOGICAL DISORDERS

> There are also injuries that result from cumulative damage where the causes are minute and too numerous to count or observe. They are more like the drops of water in a cloud formation than the projectile that went through Mr. Gage's head.

There are also injuries that result from cumulative damage where the causes are minute and too numerous to count or observe. They are more like the drops of water in a cloud formation than the projectile that went through Mr. Gage's head. Unlike the disorders that follow from observable causal events—a gunshot, getting sprayed by a crop duster, receiving a particular poisonous injection, getting bitten by a snake or spider, and so forth—damage from minute cumulative injuries are difficult to pin down or sort into categories. Although they may involve discrete individual events, they are mixed together with so many other events that it may not even be possible to single them out for attention. Still, we can distinguish relative abrupt, discrete, particular and individual *cause-effect* relations, such as the injury of Mr. Gage, from probabilistic cumulative damage that appears as gradual gains or losses over long periods of time. Such changes can be greatly influenced by minute events at the molecular level.

Pinpointing Cumulative Damage Often Impossible

Many disease conditions that either directly cause or contribute to the severity of neurological and other adult communication disorders are difficult to impossible to pinpoint. Just as multiple systems of great complexity are involved in ordinary human communication, the causes of disorders can be just as diverse and complex. A typical example of cumulative damage can be found in the dementias —of which, Alzheimer's and Parkinson's are the most common and best known. In these disease conditions, extrinsic factors are known to interact in complex ways with body chemistry.

Similarly, neurological disease conditions such as **Lou Gehrig's disease** (also known as *amyotrophic lateral sclerosis*), **multiple sclerosis**, adrenoleukodystrophy, and a great variety of cancers and other undesirable conditions—are directly or indirectly impacted by toxins such as mercury in its various forms (e.g., thimerosal and dental amalgam), and by poisons in general that directly or indirectly damage the nervous system. Contrary to advertisements and sponsored publications of monied interests in the pharmaceutical vaccine lobbies and related medical trade groups—for example, the American Dental Association (see Zentz, 2006, published by the ADA, retrieved March 7, 2009, from http://www.ada.org/public/media/presskits/fillings/testimony_zentz.pdf)—neurotoxins such as mercury are certain to exacerbate neurological diseases and disorders in general.

When mercury, for instance, damages the molecules of the protein **tubulin,** that encases the tiniest of our nerve fibrils. For a demonstration of how this damage occurs with live nerve cells, see the video <u>How Mercury Damages Nerve Fibrils</u> on the DVD (also see Leong, Syed, & Lorscheider, 2001). Diseases and toxins can also impact the nervous system indirectly by damaging the circulatory systems of the blood and lymph, or a particular organ such as the heart.

The impact of some toxins on neurons is direct. The damage, however, may be difficult to detect much less to pinpoint because the fibrils are small and numerous and the damage is at the level of much smaller individual molecules.

The Body's Systems Are Linked

If the heart is unable to supply blood to the brain for a prolonged period of time, three minutes or more—about the length of time you can hold your breath underwater without passing out—the brain can be damaged and the loss can range from mild to severe. If the heart stops long enough, of course, the affected individual dies. Neurotoxins found in pesticides, dental amalgam, industrial products, incinerated wastes, and so on can be indirect causal factors in a heart attack, **arrhythmia**, or any number of related problems. For example, mercury in particular has been singled out as an insidious cause of heart disease (Frustaci et al., 1999; Hagele et al., 2007; R. A. Nash, 2005). Concentrations of mercury along with other trace metals in damaged heart tissue have been shown to be as much as 20,000 times greater than in other muscles. It is supposed that this higher concentration in the heart is partly owed to the intensive neurochemical processes that are necessary to the regulation of heart rhythms (see Frustaci et al., 1999).

Besides the more or less discoverable causes that may leave a trail behind, there are silent kinds of damage being done at the atomic biochemical level that tend to accumulate over time. Deep and mostly silent damage is now known to be major factor in a host of disorders that are lumped together and very loosely described as dementia. The problem of distinguishing them is like the problem of telling just which of many cumulative injuries actually killed the proverbial cat, or which particular straw it was that broke the camel's back.

In the end, as Harman first argued in 1956 (also see Harman, 1972, 1981), it is very difficult to tell the difference between neurological or other damage caused by free radicals from damage caused by related factors. For example, as individual atoms of a heavy metal—like tiny loose cannons bouncing around—impact biologically active molecules and bodily proteins, the damage affects multiple systems. With advancing **nanotechnologies** we are on the brink of not only being able to peer into bodily processes at the molecular level ("Nanotechnology," 2009, retrieved March 7, 2009, from http://en.wikipedia.org/wiki/Nanotechnology), but also to gain control of them (see Bailey et al., 2006).

In the meantime, the debates continue about whether a particular kind of dementia, such as Parkinson's disease, is really caused by direct damage to nerves or by indirect damage owed to inadequate blood supply. Clearly, either sort of event can cause dementia and the research is unequivocal in showing that toxins and oxidative stress play a major role irrespective of whether the precipitating event is owed to oxygen deprivation, nerve damage, or both.

Insidious Genetic Damage

Contrary to some popular theories of genetic mutation, research shows that the vast majority of genetic mutations that are occurring now are harmful.

We know that disorders in general are owed to the accumulation of genetic damage that is inexorably occurring worldwide (Kimura, 1979; Sanford, 2005). As we noted in Chapter 1, there are more than 6,000 known genetic diseases and disorders (Gardner & Snustadt, 1981; also Collins, 2009, retrieved March 7, 2009, from http://www.kumc.edu/gec/geneinfo.html). Also, the fact that the vast majority of mutations are unexpressed in surface form results in the virtual impossibility of selecting "potentially favorable" mutations by either natural or artificial means. The upshot is that mutations are, for practical purposes, universally harmful. The existing research and mathematical models simply do not support the claim that beneficial mutations are likely to occur at all, much less can they accumulate over time as required by standard biological orthodoxy.

As Kimura (1979) showed, the most devastating class of mutations are the relatively mild ("silent") ones. These kinds of mutations are passed from generation to generation without showing up in the surface traits of the organism. Because the cumulative injuries remain **asymptomatic**—without surface effects—they cannot be eliminated by natural selection because they cannot be detected by it. Over time, the silent mutations accumulate and their combined effects are necessarily harmful in the long run (Sanford, 2005). The cumulative damage is analogous in the larger picture and over the long-run in the same way as the minute cumulative injuries to an individual from free radicals are harmful and cumulative (Harman, 1981). The long-term problem of genetic damage is analogous to the problem of individual oxidative stress and mortality as discussed in Chapter 5. However, just as mortality does not cure the problems that cause it, eugenics is no cure for the long-term problem of cumulative genetic damage.

> . . . just as mortality does not cure the problems that cause it, eugenics is no cure for the long-term problem of cumulative genetic damage.

Toxins and Contaminants

Toxins are coming to us through pesticides, preservatives in foods, manufactured products, heavy metals (as in dental amalgam), and vaccines. Some of these can permanently damage the genome. Examples include the thimerosal placed in millions of doses of vaccines administered since the 1980s and still being used in flu vaccines and other medications.

Another harmful substance that was inadvertently introduced into millions of people through polio vaccines was the monkey virus known as **simian virus 40 (SV40)**. It is linked to many varieties of human cancers including brain tumors. It is suspiciously similar to the **human immunodeficiency virus (HIV)** and can lie dormant for years before expressing itself in any symptoms. This particular virus was spread to 98 million Americans and throughout the world through contaminated polio vaccines. It is a known contributing causal agent in **mesothelioma**, a form of lung cancer in humans associated with asbestos exposure. M. Carbone and Bedrossian (2006) showed that this cancer—known to be caused by asbestos—develops more quickly in certain persons exposed to both asbestos and SV40. Feng et al. (2007) showed evidence in research with mice that SV40 interacts with various proteins to promote cancerous tumors (p. 2218). Shi et al. (2007) showed that SV40 promotes malignant growth in surface cells extracted from human prostate glands. M. K. White et al. (2005) found significant concentrations of SV40 in human brain tumors, and Dang, Wuthrich, Axthelm, and Koralnik (2008) showed that SV40 infections would produce encephalitis and meningitis in rhesus monkeys.

More interestingly still, it has been suggested by Dr. Howard B. Urnovitz (1996) that SV40 and the contaminated polio vaccine, which was widely used in central Africa, may have been involved in the genesis of the **human immune virus (HIV)** that causes **acquired immune deficiency syndrome (AIDS)**. In any event, Urnovitz is credited with discovering the **retrotransposons** that are involved in both SV40 and HIV. See a summary of his argument and the science behind it in a paper given at the 8th Annual Houston Conference on AIDS (retrieved April 15, 2009, from http://www.whale.to/vaccines/sweet.html). After SV40 was discovered by B. H. Sweet and Hilleman (1960), it was supposedly killed or removed entirely from vaccines produced after 1961, but it has turned up in later polio vaccines (Carlsen, 2001) and in multiple human cancers in many studies since then. The current research continues to suggest a likeness and a close association between SV40 and the HIV retro viruses (Terpstra et al. 2008). Both are closely linked to human cancers and neuroAIDs, and HIV is the most common cause of dementia in persons under 40 years of age (Comar et al., 2007).

Parkinson's and Alzheimer's

In 2001, Uversky, J. Li, and Fink tentatively suggested that heavy metals were involved in the genesis of Parkinson's disease. Since then, according to the Web of Knowledge on April 1, 2009, their study has been cited 223 times in related research papers and there is no longer any reasonable doubt that metal toxins are factors in the genesis of Parkinson's disease. Liu and Franz (2007) have filled in some of the details concerning the complex biochemistry. Heavy metals are an important part of that picture. They are also implicated in Alzheimer's and neurological disorders.

Kastenholz (2007) has explained how mercury and metal toxicities can cause misfolding (and consequent disfunctionality) of proteins. He cites studies showing that "different high molecular mass metal-containing proteins were isolated in brain samples from Alzheimer's patients" (p. 389). Some of the specific mechanisms at the molecular level have been spelled out by Culotta, M. Yang, and O'Halloran (2006) and by Yokel (2006). Also, Bocca et al. (2006) showed that "imbalances in Alzheimer's disease were found," including higher than expected levels of mercury and significantly decreased antioxidant capacity. Sensible therapies include getting the known toxins out of the brain. Kidd (2005) sums up much of the research as follows:

> Exogenous toxins, such as mercury and other environmental contaminants, exacerbate mitochondrial electron leakage, hastening their demise and that of their host cells. Studies of the brain in Alzheimer's and other dementias, Down syndrome, stroke, Parkinson's disease, multiple sclerosis, amyotrophic lateral sclerosis, . . . aging, and constitutive disorders demonstrate impairments of the mitochondrial citric acid cycle and oxidative phosphorylation . . . enzymes. (p. 268)

Esiri (2007) also notes the incontrovertible evidence that oxidative stress from toxins speeds normal aging and contributes detrimentally to neurological diseases and disorders.

Dantzig (2006) compared 14 individuals with Parkinson disease against 14 control patients. Of the individuals with Parkinson's, 13 of 14 had the red rash around the trunk area, a common symptom associated with mercury poisoning, and mercury in their blood. Charles et al. (2006) studies a large sample of individuals—1,049 men aged 71 through 93 years—who had been exposed to various environmental toxins including mercury. They excluded from their

Conditions of oxidative stress caused by free radicals, heavy metals being among the worst offenders, are linked to neurodegenerative conditions such as Alzheimer's, Parkinson's, and essentially all neurodegenerative conditions (Gaasch et al., 2007; Palomo, Beninger, Kostrzewa, & Archer, 2003; Zahir, Rizwi, Haq, & Khan, 2005).

study any individuals who already had Parkinson's disease and found that "abnormal 'facial expression'" was significantly associated with toxic exposure of all kinds and individuals with high mercury exposure were approximately twice as likely to have abnormal facial movements. There is no reasonable doubt about the involvement of toxins as factors that either trigger or worsen autoimmune diseases and disorders.

> There is no reasonable doubt about the involvement of toxins as factors that either trigger or worsen autoimmune diseases and disorders.

Autoimmunity and Tissue Deterioration

The building up of the body's immune defenses with vaccines is somewhat like preparing for war by engaging in military exercises with live ammunition. There are risks involved. A crash during a war games exercise can be as fatal as a crash in battle.

Similarly, when a vaccine, for example, the polio vaccine, causes polio or inadvertently introduces a formerly unknown latent virus —SV40, for instance—the outcome is a little like a heart transplant that eventually kills both the donor and the patient. With vaccines the theory is that the war games played out under favorable conditions—where the body will prevail against the disease agents in the vaccine—enables full preparation for a real war against disease. Then, when a real threat occurs and a battle ensues, hopefully the body's immune system will win.

However, there is another danger. Just as there can be accidents in war games, in real wars, there is always a danger that the fire intended to destroy enemies will end up killing friends rather than foes. With immune system disorders, in a worst case scenario, the defense system may attack the body that it is supposed to be defending. Among factors that are known to produce **autoimmune disease** is dental amalgam. In particular, where mercury comes in contact with gum tissue, amalgam causes disease. Venclikova et al. (2006) found that 25 of 34 individuals studied showed an immune response to metals including the mercury in the dental amalgam. Of those whose immune system started attacking its own tissues in response to the metals, 20 of 25 had what the authors described as "serious health problems" (p. 61). The study showed "dense particles containing metals" in the gum line of the affected areas.

Pabello and Lawrence (2006) note that the impact of toxins "on the immune system (immunotoxicity) and the nervous system (neurotoxicity)" can result in "the dysregulation of one organ system leading to malfunctions of another" and that these cascading interactions "present a major concern for health" (p. 69). They observe that "substantiated neuroimmunological research" has led to "the multidisciplinary field of neuroimmunotoxicology." Among other things, they focus on:

> mechanisms by which exposure to the prototypic toxicants [toxins], lead, mercury, and PCB's, may directly or indirectly modulate neuroimmune networks [and indirectly] the etiology or progression of diseases and treatments. (p. 69)

With chronic neurotoxicity, the body's defenses become confused, and the body's immune cells attack its own cells, tissues, and organs rather than invaders or disease agents. The number of disorders that are known to have a significant "friendly fire" or autoimmune component is on the rise. Can mercury cause this kind of problem? Research with rats by Day, Reed, and Newland (2005) clearly shows that it can and that it is particularly damaging during gestation. Among the disorders of rising prevalence are many of the most common neurological disorders including autism, Alzheimer's, Parkinsonism, multiple sclerosis, rheumatoid arthritis, and neuroAIDS.

Changing the Medical Paradigm

Koger, Schettler, and B. Weiss (2005) suggest that we have long been engaged in a "vast toxicological experiment" where the guinea pigs are our own children and citizens. They sensibly propose to

> prevent developmental disabilities by mobilizing and affecting public policy, educating and informing consumers, contributing to interdisciplinary research efforts, and taking action within their own homes and communities to reduce the toxic threat to children. (p. 243)

TREATMENT OF ADULT DISEASES AND NEUROLOGICAL DISORDERS

There is excellent empirical evidence that getting toxins out of the mix is beneficial across the board with respect to communication disorders.

There is excellent empirical evidence that getting toxins out of the mix is beneficial across the board with respect to communication disorders. There are also proposals that will not work and that need to be rejected. For example, the history of eugenics shows that it does not work in practice (see Chapters 11 and 12), and for reasons we are about to examine, it cannot logically work at all. After showing why eugenics and cloning cannot solve the problems of cumulative genetic damage, we turn to more hopeful alternatives. It turns out that even the most intractable adult diseases and neurological disorders are treatable.

Eugenics as a Failed Solution

As genetic tests become increasingly available to identify in advance persons carrying defective genes that can lead to neurological disorders, it is certain that the eugenics alternative—one that we encountered in Chapter 1—will gain new interest and support. In

Chapter 11 we show that the idea of eugenics is still lurking in the shadows and in Chapter 12 we consider some of the details of the relevant history showing that eugenics was a major factor in ramping up to major conflicts including World War II. However, eugenics cannot alleviate genetic deterioration on account of the fact that it can only work on the whole genome.

Eugenics in its strongest forms can only prevent certain individuals (and groups) from reproducing. Considering the fact that the genome of every individual is a library of many books—the genes and their components—eugenics in all of its forms basically destroys the whole library while aiming, theoretically, to purge offensive sentences in particular books. The fatal flaw in the plan is that eugenics cannot single out particular books (genes) from the genome library (the so-called "gene pool") one at a time. It is analogous to curing a certain unexpressed tendency by lethal injection—it will prevent overeating as certainly as it will prevent murder, but it cannot single out any genetic tendency whatever.

Perhaps gene splicing or some other genetic intervention can be devised to correct genetic errors directly in individuals, but as yet, the eugenics movements of the past, as a means of ethnic, racial or any other kind of population cleansing—in principle and practice is powerless to reverse the accumulating genetic damage owed to toxins, radiation, and free radical damage. Another idea that has been suggested as a theoretical solution, at least, is **cloning**.

> Preventing reproduction of any individual or group only operates at the level of the whole library of genes associated with that individual or group. It does not single out any one genetic error but operates on all of them.

Why Cloning Also Fails

Over the long haul, cloning cannot solve the problem of cumulative genetic damage. The problem is that clones inherit all of the genetic flaws of their single parent plus any new errors contributed in the cloning process (Sanford, 2005). Therefore, neither cloning, nor eugenics, can provide any way to escape the damage done to the genome before any selection or cloning can take place. On the brighter side, the sources of damage are not altogether unknown to us and many of the causes of cumulative oxidative stress in individuals and of genetic damage to the worldwide population are known to us already. Just as we can reduce our exposure as individuals by avoiding toxic exposures, we can do so by policy and practice.

More Hopeful Alternatives

Tumors, for example, can sometimes be surgically removed with little harm to the individual. The blood vessel that has developed a weak spot that becomes a bubble ready to burst and cause a stroke can sometimes be pinched with a metal clip to prevent or reduce the likelihood of a stroke. The known toxins that attack the nerves directly or indirectly can also be removed from medicines (R. A.

Nash, 2005) and dental practice (Mutter, Naumann, Walach, & Daschner, 2005). As Koger, Schettler, and B. Weiss (2005) noted, we need to seek public policies that will stop the use of neurotoxins, especially in the practice of medicine. If we do that we have reasonable hope of preventing many diseases and disorders, curing some, and making many of them less harmful and less prevalent.

On an individual treatment level, getting toxins out of the picture helps bring disease factors and related disorders under control.

Does it help to get the mercury out of the picture? There is no question that it does. Mutter et al. (2005) showed that removal of mercury in dental amalgam improved symptoms associated with a host of known neurological disorders. The pharmacology literature is also unequivocal in showing that active biochemicals found in certain fruits and vegetables, including traditional herbal medicines, can help to reduce oxidative stress by enabling the body to rid itself of toxins (Nishida et al., 2007). Such procedures are routinely recommended and beneficial in the treatment of neurodegenerative diseases.

SUMMING UP AND LOOKING AHEAD

In this chapter we have dealt with the neurological disorders most commonly associated with adults and with aging processes. We avoid the term "neurogenic" because neurological disorders can arise on the basis of many causes that are outside the nervous system. Causal interactions can involve any and every system of the body. We showed that damage to particular regions and systems of the brain can be diagnostic in helping to reveal the functions that come under the control of the damaged parts. Such evidence led to the discovery of lateralization of brain functions, left brain dominance in right handers (and most left handers as well), and the radical localization hypothesis. Although some claims for localization turned out to be overstated, the basic descriptions of brain anatomy from Brodmann forward have continued to show that different functions tend to be allocated to different anatomical regions of the brain and nervous system.

The research shows that damage to the dominant hemisphere is the primary source of the aphasias. Damage to the subordinate hemisphere likewise is the primary source of the agnosias. The production of articulated movements associated with speech and writing seems to be the sole province of the language hemisphere communicated to the minor hemisphere through the corpus callosum. The minor hemisphere, by the same token, seems to excel at the holistic sensory processing involved in comprehending, recalling, and using whole patterns required for facial recognition and memory, and to understand whole scenes, designs, and patterns.

In this chapter, we developed the idea of pragmatic mapping as a basis for understanding the major losses associated with aphasias, agnosias, and apraxias. We demonstrated brain dominance and the ranking of the main systems of signs through a series of experiments of movements that are easy for the subordinate hand or foot to follow, but that are difficult for the subordinate brain to produce on its own. All of these experimental demonstrations together with results from studies of split-brain patients show that the hierarchy of signs is genuine and that it is reflected in the anatomy of the brain.

Finally, we examined causes and types of common adult neurological disorders such as Alzheimer's and Parkinson's disease and we showed that neurotoxins including mercury and other heavy metals are invariably exacerbating factors. In the next chapter we consider the special problems of assessing and diagnosing communication disorders, especially ones that involve language abilities.

STUDY AND DISCUSSION QUESTIONS

1. Why is it important to keep in mind that genetic and environmental factors can interact especially in the development and expression of adult neurological disorders? What examples can you give of such interactions?

2. In what ways was the radical localization hypothesis too simple? How does the general architecture of the brain figure in this question? What about the integrated brain functions involved in, say, making sense of a story or reporting a sequence of events as in a scientific experiment? What role does "coherence" play?

3. Why is the speed of fMRI crucial to observing language processing? How much faster do the individual frames of slices of brain tissue have to be to depict what is going on in the time it takes to say something like "quicker'n you can say Jack Robinson"?

4. What do the split-brain and hemispherectomy studies show about localization and lateralization theories? For example, what abilities did Roger Sperry and his colleagues find in the subordinate hemisphere of the brain?

5. In what ways did the early brain research emphasize the surface forms of language to the exclusion of its pragmatic connections with the world of experience? How do "tip of the mind" phenomena as well as split-brain studies tend to force attention to the subordinate hemisphere of the brain and its interactions with the dominant hemisphere?

6. What evidence is there that chronological sequencing is a function of the dominant hemisphere while the holistic processing of spatial relations falls to the subordinate hemisphere?

7. How does the "threshold of coherence" involve both hemispheres? Why do we have more information than we needed to identify an acquaintance in a crowd, say, after the recognition

occurs, but before that, we are in a condition of doubt? What happens in the meantime to settle the doubt? What brain components do you suppose are involved when we think to ourselves, "Aha! I know that person! Why that's _____!" where we fill in the blank with the name of the person we suddenly recognize)?

8. Why is it difficult for your subordinate hand to write a mirror image of, say, your own name, without the assistance of the dominant hand? Can you fluently write a mirror image of your name with your dominant hand? If not, assuming you can do so with your subordinate hand when it is literally mirroring the motion of the dominant hand, how is it that you cannot do anything similar with your dominant hand?

9. What are some of the adult neurological disorders that abruptly appear as contrasted with ones that tend to develop gradually over time? Why is it naive to suppose that the gradually appearing disorders, or ones that have been around since before birth, could not have been caused by injuries?

10. What role do neurotoxins play in creating oxidative stress, free radicals, neurodegenerative conditions, and aging?

||||| 11 |||||

Assessment, Diagnosis, and Language/Dialect

OBJECTIVES

In this chapter, we:

1. Discuss the assessment and diagnosis of disorders;

2. Review the special problems presented by language/dialect diversity;

3. Analyze so-called "processing dependent measures"supposed to be independent of knowledge and experience with a particular language/dialect;

4. Examine social Darwinism and eugenics in the United States and connections with IQ testing;

5. Consider the language/dialect factor in assessment of psychological (IQ, competency, aptitude), educational (achievement), personality, and emotional variables;

6. Analyze instructions, reasoning, negation, conjunction, in nonverbal IQ items; and

7. Discuss effects of treatment as distinct from improvement or growth.

KEY TERMS

Here are some key terms of this chapter. Many you may already know, but it may help to review them. These terms are explained in the text and they are defined in the Glossary at the end of the book. They appear in **bold print** on their first appearance in the text.

bias
case studies
ceteris paribus principle
consistency requirement
control group
disproportionate
   representation problem
effect size
innate intelligence
lateral progress
measurement error

monolingual/monodialectal
   assessment
nonverbal/performance
   assessment procedures
nonverbal performance
   assessment procedures
normative expectations
NVPAPs
post hoc ergo propter hoc
   fallacy
principle of consistency

replication requirement
reversion principle
scale of development
standardized IQ tests
theory of the meritocracy
treatment effect
treatment group
universal quantifiers
unreliability
vertical progress

When individuals are assessed in an unfamiliar or foreign language/dialect, or in any representational system that they do not know well, or when they are assessed by persons who do not understand their best language/dialect well or at all, the almost certain outcome will be to underestimate the person's actual abilities.

In this chapter we deal with the essential problems of assessing and diagnosing communication disorders. We see that to do valid assessment and diagnosis it is essential to know the milestones of normal development. The tester/assessor needs to find out just how far along any given individual has already progressed on the road to normal maturity. For any observed level, the question is whether it is at or near what is expected for an individual at the given age. As we will see, it is essential to assess individuals in their strongest and best developed systems of representation when they are performing at or near their best. We need to judge the individual's level of development when that person is wide awake, motivated, and performing at full capacity. Because cognition and social development depend on the shared use of an acquired language/dialect, it is difficult to overestimate the need for the tester/assessor to share the strongest language/dialect of the person being assessed. In fact, it is easy to underestimate the importance of doing so.

As a result, misclassifications are common. Many normal children are misclassified as disabled, disordered, or delayed only because they were tested/assessed in a language/dialect that they either did not know at all or that they did not yet know well. Also, many gifted children who are not yet competent users of the majority language/dialect are commonly overlooked. These two problems taken together can be referred to as the **disproportionate representation problem**.

As we will show, its main cause is the underestimation of abilities by assessment in a language/dialect that the person being assessed either does not know at all or does not know well.

UNDERSTANDING DISPROPORTIONATE REPRESENTATION

There are three possible solutions to the problem of disproportionate representation—classifying language/dialect minority children as disordered, disabled, or delayed when they are not, and failing to recognize them as ahead of the norms when they are gifted.

The Hollywood Rule

The three possible solutions follow the Hollywood film-making rule as put by Jon Shestack. He said that directors aim to make films that are cheap, fast, and good, but you can't have all three. You can have fast and good but it won't be cheap, or you can have good and cheap but it won't be fast, or you can have cheap and fast but the result won't be any good. The solutions to the disproportionate representation problem are like that too.

Three Proposed Solutions

The problem of disproportionate representation can actually be solved in two good ways: One solution that is fast and good (a valid solution) is to hire competent tester/assessors who very well know (read, write, speak, and understand) the foreign language/dialect of the persons to be tested/assessed. This solution is fast and good, but not cheap.

Another solution that is relatively cheap and good (another valid solution) but not fast is to provide ample opportunity for the individual(s) who speak(s) the foreign language/dialect to acquire the language/dialect of the majority. This solution takes time and effort. In nearly ideal settings—ones that are user-friendly and well-planned—for really fast learners it may take only about six months to a year for a child to acquire a new language/dialect, but in most cases two or more years will be needed. This solution is not fast, but it is relatively inexpensive and it can be a very solid and good solution. It requires effective teachers and a friendly accepting social environment where the children who speak the different language/dialect are nurtured, encouraged, and included.

The two good ways to avoid disproportionate representation of language/dialect minorities in categories of disorders and giftedness are: (1) test/assess the student/clients in their own best system of communication; or, (2) enable them to acquire the majority language/dialect.

The cheap and fast way to assess/test children who are not proficient in the language/dialect of the majority of folks in our schools is just to use the majority language/dialect.

Unfortunately, also, in keeping with the Hollywood rule, there is a cheap and fast route that educators can take that is expedient but not a good solution. The cheap and fast way to assess/test children who are not proficient in the language/dialect of the majority of folks in our schools is just to use the majority language/dialect. This is not a good approach, but it is (at least in the short term) fast and cheap. However, like movies that flop at the box office, the practice of testing/assessing individuals in a language/dialect that they do not know well, or in many cases that they do not know at all, is like producing a movie that just won't sell any tickets at the box. Eventually, the time and effort invested in this approach will turn out to have been mostly wasted. Sad to say, it is the most common approach today being used in the schools and even sponsored and recommended by professionals who specialize in communication disorders. By understanding the importance of language/dialect acquisition to the development of cognition and social relations, we will see why the fast and cheap method of just using General American English for assessment, testing, and diagnosis of disorders is a not a good approach. It does not work well and it is, in fact, the cause of the problem of disproportionate representation.

Normal Hills and Valleys Versus Delays, Disorders, and Disabilities

How are teachers, speech-pathologists, pediatricians, and others to distinguish between symptoms of disorders and the normal, sometimes halting fits and starts that commonly occur in the normal development of language and related sign systems? How is it possible to tell the difference between disorders and normal processes of maturation? For instance, if one child seems to devote a large amount of attention and effort to conceptual growth (semantic and pragmatic aspects of language) while another child may concentrate more on perfecting the surface forms of language (phonology and morphology), who is to say which child is more advanced? And on what basis could the judgment be made?

As we have seen in earlier chapters dealing with pervasive developmental disorders (especially, autism, Chapter 5), articulation (Chapter 7), fluency (Chapter 8), and literacy (Chapter 9)—to name just four prominent categories—it is difficult to tell the difference between the normal hills, valleys, and plateaus of development from long-lasting and persistent disorders. When, for instance, is a regression or loss of vocabulary normal? When does a persistently missed articulatory target constitute a language disorder rather than a minor difficulty that will be overcome normally in acquiring a language/dialect? When does hesitation and restarting begin to count as a stuttering disorder? When does a problem in reading count as dyslexia or as an indication of a learning disability?

As we saw in Chapter 1, disorders are defined as unexpectedly long-lasting, persistent, or recurrent difficulties that interfere with

Although normal development does sometimes seem to progress in fits and starts, usually its course is upward through successively broader and higher levels the hierarchy of sign systems.

normal, successful, ordinary communication. Among the most important warning signs that parents, teachers, and other caregivers may become aware of is what many have called a "developmental regression" where the child seems to lose some previous gain. For instance, a child that was speaking in one or two word sentences may suddenly stop doing that and may also stop responding to his or her name. That kind of backward slide is not normal.

Scale of Development

On what may be loosely referred to as the **scale of development** the progress is necessarily **vertical progress** (upward in the hierarchy) if a higher level of abstractness is achieved and **lateral progress** (outward within a given level) if additional elements are added to an existing level. For instance, an example of vertical progress would be discovering the meaning of the first referring term, for example, the child's own name, say, and an example of lateral progress would be the addition of a second, third, and fourth referring term. Both kinds of development come under the control of the learner to a high degree, but the sequence of milestones is quite rigid and in certain respects the sequence cannot be violated at all. For example, there is no way that an infant can progress to noticing mom's bodily actions or states, before noticing mom herself and distinguishing her body from all the other material bodies and persons that come into the child's experience.

Although the marks on the scale of development cannot be measured in interval units such as the standard meter, and though the scale itself is not strictly linear, there is a certain logic to it as we saw especially in Chapters 1 and 4 where we dealt with the hierarchy of sign systems and the ranking of their richly integrated layers. From the theory and research underlying the layering and ranking of sign systems, it becomes obvious that certain systems of signs must be in place before the higher sign systems that depend on them can be developed. So, for instance, a child that has no senses cannot acquire any speech forms or other linguistic signs on account of the fact that sensory signs must first be in place before motor signs can be formed and motor signs must be formed before it will be possible to build up even one single conventional sign of the linguistic kind. Without any senses at all, development of all the higher motor and cognitive representations will be cut off. They will never occur. It was difficult for Laura Bridgman and Helen Keller to acquire language and literacy without sight or hearing. Without any senses at all it would have been quite impossible, just as Aristotle observed long ago.

Success Is Informative

As we saw in Chapter 1, icons must be represented before it will be possible to notice and represent their movements or their relations to each other. Similarly, movements of icons must be noticed and

It was difficult for Laura Bridgman and Helen Keller to acquire language and literacy without sight or hearing. Without any senses at all it would have been quite impossible, just as Aristotle observed long ago.

represented before it will be possible to begin to build up conventional relations such as the kind found in simple referring terms, for example, the name and the person named. Likewise, before it will be possible to refer to an action or state of an object, say, the fact that a certain dog is barking, the child will need to be able to refer to the dog. The barking of the dog can no more occur without the dog than the dancing of a person dancing can occur without the dancer. Noticing and referring to the action, state, or movement of a bodily object requires a higher level of abstraction. And, we can see that some signs have to be in place before certain higher signs that depend on them can be acquired.

As a result, there is a surprisingly strict sequence of signs in normal development with respect to the degree of abstractness of the signs that must be formed. Lower levels have to be acquired first in order to build the higher ones. This is even more certain for complex abstractions than it is for the physical construction, say, of a skyscraper—yet it is more obvious to us in the case of physical constructions. The architects and builders of the Chrysler Building in New York City, or the Empire State Building, or any multistory building, could not just arbitrarily decide to work from the fifth story up. The foundation has to come first and the first floor has to follow that, and so on. It is less obvious but even more certain that very abstract systems, for example, such as the idea of prime numbers, cannot be developed without the idea of numbers and of operations on numbers such as multiplication and division. To know that the number 17 is a prime, for instance, we must not only know that it is divisible by 1 and 17, but that it is not divisible by 2, 3, 4, 5, 6, 7, 8, 9, 10, 11, 12, 13, 14, 15, or 16. Without understanding the idea of what numbers are and the operations of multiplying and dividing, the idea of the underlying factors of a given number and how they are discovered cannot be achieved.

As a result, when a high level of abstraction is displayed linguistically, we may judge with considerable confidence and validity that the lower levels required to achieve the higher abstraction have already been achieved. Success at a high level of performance is diagnostic of the fact that all the required levels below that one have been achieved and surpassed. However, just because we do not see a high level of performance in a given testing or assessment situation does not necessarily mean that the child cannot perform at that level.

> Success is highly indicative of progress and when truly complex sign systems are involved, it cannot be achieved by chance. Failure, on the other hand, is easy to achieve and far less informative.

The Reversion Principle

If we think about it, it is obvious that it would be easier to underestimate an individual's level of development from a poor performance or a lack of success than the reverse. To use the skyscraper analogy, just because we have only taken the stairs from the first floor to the second is no evidence that the third, fourth, and successively higher floors have not been completed. It is always possible that we may have observed a child's behavior at a level well beneath what the child could do in a more interesting or challenging situation. It is possible that we have not observed what the child can do when less shy or inhibited. A child who is already speaking in full sentences can as easily resort to babbling as an adult can when imitating, or conversing with, a babbling infant.

We have all observed conversations, for instance, between normal infants and more mature individuals where the more mature sibling or adult reverts to the level of the infant. Say the baby is at the stage of canonical babbling—where the baby can only create sequences like /bababa/, /dadada/, and /dzadzadza/, and so on, or possibly at the stage of variegated babbling—where the sequences get more complex as in /badzagadzababa/. Suppose further that the older sibling or adult babbles right back to the baby, say, with slight variations on the babbled utterances. Should we diagnose the babbling older sibling or adult as being able to function only at the level demonstrated by the infant? That would not make any sense, but the example serves to show what we call the **reversion principle**. Simply put, it is the fact that any sign user can generally revert to lower levels of abstraction already achieved previously while the reverse is not possible. The child cannot leap up to a floor in the skyscraper that has not yet been built but can easily go down from the highest level that is still under construction to a lower floor.

It is unremarkable when an older sibling, or even an adult, imitates the babbling infants and joins in at their level. Because such phenomena are common—that is, it is common for individuals to adjust their level of signs to that of a less capable interlocutor—we must keep the reversion principle in mind when diagnosing disorders, delays, or any kind of disabilities. The fact is that any individual can usually resort with ease to any lower level of the sign hierarchy that has already been developed. The difficulty comes at the level where construction is underway and, generally speaking, levels above the one under construction are out of reach entirely.

The Zone of Proximal Development

Again, we come to the concept of the "zone of proximal development" (ZPD) that we introduced in Chapter 5. In diagnosing developmental disorders, the ZPD is of paramount importance. It may be useful for us to know just how much learning has taken place within a given system of representation, but it is essential to know just how far up the scale of development a given individual has been able to progress. For diagnosis and for therapeutic intervention it is crucial to find the ZPD of the individual we are assessing.

Because of the logical dependence of higher sign systems on certain lower ones, it is not possible (excepting miracles and

We can easily reach back to a lower level in the sign hierarchy beneath a level we have already achieved, but we cannot easily leap upward to a higher level without going through all the necessary steps in between.

paranormal phenomena) for a person who has never had the opportunity to learn General American English to suddenly start speaking it fluently and carrying on a conversation, say, about the causes of autism. It just cannot happen. Unless you have the right opportunities to develop proficiency in Chinese, Hmong, or Igbo, you will not be able to perform well at all in any of these languages. Similarly, it is not possible for an infant that has just barely achieved the level of variegated babbling to immediately launch into a narrative about why breast milk should be preferred over bottled formula. It just isn't going to happen.

The Highest and Best Level

For all of the foregoing reasons, to assess development validly—that is, to get a true picture of it—it is essential to enable the individual being assessed to perform at that person's highest level of achievement. Otherwise, we will underestimate that person's ability. An underestimation of ability always involves **bias, measurement error**, or what is also called **unreliability**. In fact, we cannot know in cases of underestimation of ability just how far wrong a placement on the scale of ability may be. Say, for instance, that the individual being assessed is observed doing the sort of canonical babble that would be expected of a normal infant sometime between the 5th and 10th month after birth. From such an observation it might be supposed that canonical babbling is the upper limit of that person's linguistic ability. But suppose the observation is an underestimation.

To get a valid idea of how far any individual has advanced on the scale of development we need to find out what is the highest and best performance of which the person assessed is capable.

If so, we do not know whether the individual assessed may be able to produce the two word utterances expected of a normal child at about two years, or whether the person assessed could actually read and discuss this book with perfect comprehension. How are we to know where to place the individual on the scale of development? The answer is that we cannot know how to do that without a reliable and valid measure.

A Poor Showing Is Uninformative

Consider the many ways that unreliable measures or assessments can come about. It might be that the person being assessed was drugged, half-asleep, disinterested, having a bad day, was distracted by internal pain, was suffering from an emotional trauma, and so forth. Or perhaps the person doing the assessment misjudged the data on account of not speaking the language/dialect of the individual tested, or the individual tested may not have understood the task, and so on and on through countless combinations and additional possibilities. The assessment procedures may have been pitched way too high. The tasks may have been too difficult for the individual assessed. Perhaps there was some sort of equipment failure, a recording error, or there may have been a combination of any of the foregoing problems along with others that we have no way of discovering or knowing about after the fact.

A Poor Showing Tells Little

In actuality, there are so many different ways to explain a single poor performance in any given assessment procedure that it is universally agreed by thoughtful professional testers and diagnosticians that *a diagnosis of a disorder should never be based on a single test or assessment procedure* (for example, see Heubert & Hauser, 1999). In fact this rule is so well recognized and accepted that it has been incorporated into law in the United States at least since 1975 in the Education of All Handicapped Children Act which was carried forward at the Individuals with Disabilities Education Act of 2004 (retrieved March 7, 2009, from http://public.findlaw.com/bookshelf-disabil ity-rights-laws/anchor65310.html and at http://frwebgate.ac cess.gpo.gov/cgi-bin/getdoc.cgi?dbname=108_cong_public_ laws&docid=f:publ446.108).

We discuss multiple cases relying on and invoking this principle against schools, municipalities, and states, in courts of law in Chapter 12. The general rule was well put in the case of *Larry P. v. Riles* (1984) in the U.S. Court of Appeals: " . . . no single procedure shall be the sole criterion for determining an appropriate educational program for a child" (793 F.2d, 969, 9th Circuit, p. 8). The same principle was applied by the U.S. Supreme Court in a discrimination case brought against the State of Mississippi in the *United States v. Fordice* (1992). The rule is especially appropriate if performance on a given assessment procedure or test has been unexpectedly weak, low, or judged to be a poor showing.

Single test scores or narrowly defined cutoff scores on a single test are not supposed to be used for exclusionary admission decisions. This is commonly noted in professional manuals for the use of norm-referenced tests. In the *United States v. Fordice* (1992), the U.S. Supreme Court ruled that Mississippi was violating the law of the land (the **Civil Rights Act of 1964** and the equal protection clause of the Fourteenth Amendment) as well as sound measurement standards. Making life-changing decisions on the basis of a single poor performance on a test/assessment procedure is a high-risk gamble. Our argument is that diagnosing a disorder or excluding a child from a gifted program can be such a life-changing decision. It ought never to be made on the basis of a single test or assessment procedure.

But what about the opposite possibility? What if a child or individual does exceptionally well on a single test or assessment

Making life-changing decisions on the basis of a single poor performance on a test/ assessment procedure is a highrisk gamble. Our argument is that diagnosing a disorder or excluding a child from a gifted program can be such a life-changing decision. It ought never to be made on the basis of a single test or assessment procedure.

procedure? Should such an outstanding performance be disregarded? Can it be treated in the same way that we might treat a poor showing?

Repeatedly Strong Performances Are Informative

No one is so lucky that they just happen to succeed on many successive challenging tasks by accident. Repeated successful performances are informative. They do not occur by chance.

For all of the reasons discussed in Chapter 3 concerning the demonstration of Braille writing, successful communication does not come about by accident. It is not the result of unreliable performances. What is more, the higher the level of success in communication, the less likely it is that it could be achieved by chance? A stellar performance or one that shows accelerated development is not apt to occur by accident. It cannot consistently be caused by any of the errors, distractions, and so forth, that cause unreliability in assessments. Individuals do not accidentally just happen to answer many questions successively on a challenging test correctly. A person cannot accidentally get good grades in many courses and on many tests in order to establish a record of a high grade point average. No one is so lucky that they just happen to succeed on many successive challenging tasks by accident. Repeated successful performances are informative. They do not occur by chance.

If a two-year-old is talking in full sentences and expressing abstract ideas, it is reasonable to suppose that the child's success in doing so is because the child is gifted and advanced beyond the expected level for a two-year-old. How do we know this? We know it because the child cannot accidentally leap ahead to such a high level of development without having progressed step by step through all the required pre-requisite stages. No one would suppose that the child's performance could be due to cheating. Even if the child could copy exactly what a more mature sibling was observed to do in the same situation—as if such an unlikely scenario could occur—the capacity of a two-year-old to copy an older sibling in difficult linguistic performances would itself be definitive of a special and unusual giftedness on the part of the younger child. Or take a different example: suppose a college applicant gets a very high score on the *American College Test* or the *Scholastic Aptitude Test* or any similar test. While it might happen by cheating, if that possibility can be ruled out, is there still a reasonable possibility that the high score could be owed to chance? Could it be that the student was just lucky in marking many correct answers?

Or could the high score be owed to unreliability in the test itself? Could the student have just accidentally had a nearly perfect day with a very imperfect test? Could the authors and administrators and the student who took the test all have had an accidentally successful communication experience?

While a bad performance can often be explained as the result of some error factor, a repeatedly successful communication using the advanced representational systems of any language do not come about by accident. The Braille demonstration that we discussed in Chapter 3 succeeded in convincing all concerned that Braille is a suitable writing system for the blind. This was not a crazy accident. It was a valid judgment. Successful performances with even the simplest systems of communication do not result from chance. Logically speaking, they involve all of the desirable qualities of assessment—validity, reliability, and instructional utility. In other words, good testing procedures must contain or illustrate good teaching methods.

To take an analogy that is easy to understand, consider the chance of a golfer hitting a hole in one off the tee. Pretty slim. If we consider the likelihood of someone accidentally hitting two, three, four, or many unlikely shots in a row, we get the idea: A series of very unlikely successes do not come about by chance.

The Low Probability of Multiple Successes

In any multiple choice test, it is easy to miss a large number of items in a row. One way to do it is to get off by one line in marking the answer sheet. All the answers after that one mistake will be incorrect on the answer sheet even if we actually answered all of the questions correctly. A simple distraction can produce a lapse of attention or memory that can prevent communication from succeeding. However, what is the likelihood of answering, say, 100 multiple choice items correctly in a row by accident? Let's say there are 5 choices per item—A, B, C, D, or E. There would be 1 chance in 5 of getting the first item correct by just randomly choosing one of the answers. To answer both items 1 and 2 correctly, by random selection of one of the choices, there would be 1 chance in 25 because we could mark 1A and 2A, or 1A and 2B, and so forth through exactly 25 possible combinations ending with 1E and 2E. We should expect someone to get two items correct in a row 1 time in 25 tries, or 1 in 5^2 chances. So, it follows by simple algebra that the chance of correctly answering all 100 items in a row is 1 in 5 raised to the 100th power, or 5 multiplied by 5, 100 times. The probability of randomly selecting the correct answers to 100 multiple choice items in a row is less than 1 chance in the number 10 followed by 68 zeros. The odds against such a string of good luck are many orders of magnitude greater than a billion to 1 against. By contrast, the probability of answering about 80% of the questions incorrectly by making random selections is nearly 100%.

For all of the above reasons, successful performances are vastly more informative than poor performances. If successful performances accumulate and agree across multiple items, multiple tests, and multiple procedures of assessment, the confidence in the assessment rapidly increases toward a theoretical limit of absolute certainty. Successful communication in even slightly complex situations necessarily contains the properties of validity, reliability,

As the complexity of a communication problem increases, the likelihood of doing it successfully by chance diminishes rapidly toward absolute zero.

If successful performances accumulate and agree across multiple items, multiple tests, and multiple procedures of assessment, the confidence in the assessment rapidly increases toward a theoretical limit of absolute certainty.

and instructional utility. Successful communication intrinsically has these properties. On the other hand, if multiple measures show the same general weaknesses, we must still be cautious in inferring and diagnosing any particular disorder on account of the likelihood that unsuccessful performances can by caused by chance.

One Success Can Trump Countless Failures

Success Counts

Hundreds of failed attempts are less informative than one real success. For this reason, successful experiments—ones that get results or that find what they are searching for—are vastly more informative than experiments where the researchers come up empty handed. Oddly, however, there is a tendency among casual readers of research, and some professionals, to treat unsuccessful attempts to replicate a given outcome as if they were just as informative as the successes. But, failures in communication in any context tell us far less than successes.

When the neurologist, Dr. Roger Bannister (Figure 11–1; also see the video retrieved March 7, 2009, from http://news.bbc.co.uk/onthisday/hi/dates/stories/may/6/newsid_2511000/2511575.stm), broke the four minute mile on May 6, 1954, it counted for a great deal more than all the prior and subsequent failures combined. Until Bannister (2009, retrieved March 7, 2009, from http://en.wikipedia.org/wiki/Roger_Bannister), no one on record had ever run a mile that fast. So how many failures would it take to refute the fact that a human being can run a four-minute mile? The feat was accomplished in front of many witnesses on the first occasion and was repeated by Bannister and by his Australian rival, John Landy, three more times in less than a year. Meantime, many other mile runners failed to break the four minute mile. Does anyone today still remember the failures? Neither should failed experiments be judged as equal to ones that succeed in producing unlikely results. Failures to get results are highly probable, expected, and largely empty of significant information.

By contrast, for anyone who thinks about it, multiple complex measures that produce success in communication and agreement among each other are greatly to be preferred over any single assessment procedure. If Michael Phelps had told his mom when he was just a young boy diagnosed with ADHD that one day he would become one the world's greatest swimmers and possibly the greatest Olympic athlete of all time, it might have seemed unlikely. But by multiple tests and assessments it now appears that this is exactly what he has accomplished (see Michael Phelps, 2009, retrieved

Failures to get results are highly probable, expected, and largely empty of significant information.

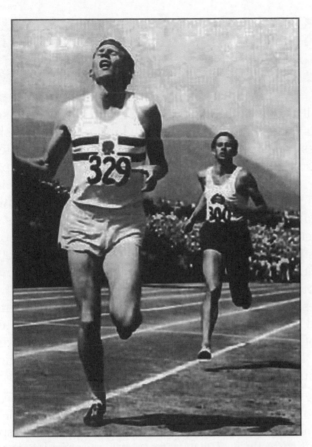

FIGURE 11–1. Dr. Roger Bannister breaking the four-minute mile (http://www.achievement.org /autodoc/page/ban0bio-1). Copyright © 1996–2009 by the American Academy of Achievement. Reprinted with permission. All rights reserved.

March 7, 2009, from http://en.wikipedia.org/wiki/Michael_Phelps). The more observations an assessment is based on, especially when the measures are in agreement, the greater the degree of confidence in its validity. For all of the foregoing reasons, multiple measures from multiple points of view are always preferred and it is essential in all measurement procedures to take care to see to it that the individual being assessed has all the right opportunities and incentives to do the best that is possible for that individual. Failures are virtually meaningless. Successes, on the other hand, are by contrast vastly more informative.

Provided we can determine the most advanced level on the scale of development that an individual can manage, it is reasonable to take that level as diagnostic. If the most advanced sign systems are at the level expected for normal development we should not diagnose any disorder. On the other hand, if the most advanced level is not as expected, or if there has been a regression from a prior attainment, then further assessment is in order.

Provided we can determine the most advanced level on the scale of development that an individual can manage, it is reasonable to take that level as diagnostic.

THE ROLE OF LANGUAGE/DIALECT IN ASSESSMENT

As we will see in this section, research with mental and social tests of all sorts (achievement, intelligence, and personality) shows that for any test that requires instructions that must be understood in some language/dialect, or that involves significant complexities of reasoning, the language/dialect factor is dominant. This is obviously so for any individual who does not already know the language/dialect of the assessment procedure, or who does not know it very well. However, the language/dialect factor has often been treated as if it did not exist. Or, as is the case in the 2000 edition of the *Diagnostic and Statistical Manual of Mental Disorders* in its revised fourth edition, also known as the DSM-IV-TR™, common differences in language/dialect background are apt themselves to be treated as disorders. For instance, the DSM-IV-TR under the heading of "Diagnostic Features" associated with the entire class of disorders lumped under the catch-all term "Phonological Disorder" the authors write:

> Phonological Disorder includes phonological production (i.e., articulation) errors that involve the failure to form speech sounds correctly. . . . The most frequently misarticulated sounds are those acquired later in the developmental sequence (*l, r, s, th, ch*), but in younger or more severely affected individuals, consonants and vowels that develop earlier may also be affected. Lisping (i.e., misarticulation of sibilants) is particularly common. Phonological Disorder may also involve errors of selection and ordering of sounds within syllables and words (e.g., *aks* for *ask*). (p. 65)

Folks in Louisiana are bound to take notice of the choice of examples here on account of the fact that multiple varieties of English—including dialects common to Louisiana and other southern states, not to mention good old England, which Americans commonly refer to as the "mother country"—allow some of the variants that are considered potentially, at least, indicative of phonological disorders. For instance, there are several common dialect variants in the United Kingdom that allow substitutions of [f] for [θ] and [v] for [ð]. To their credit, the authors do mention that "assessments of the developmental communication abilities must take into account the individual's cultural and language contexts, particularly for individuals growing up in bilingual environments" (p. 65), but the terms *dialect*, *language*, and *language variety* do not appear in the index to this 943 page volume. There is an Appendix (pp. 897–903) to assist users "in applying DSM-IV criteria in a multicultural envi-

. . . the language/dialect factor has often been treated as if it did not exist. Or, as is the case in the 2000 edition of the Diagnostic and Statistical Manual of Mental Disorders in its revised fourth edition, also known as the DSM-IV-TR™, common differences in language/dialect background are apt themselves to be treated as disorders.

ronment" (p. 897). There, clinicians are urged to note problems owed to "the individual's first language, in eliciting symptoms or understanding their cultural significance, in negotiating an appropriate relationship or level of intimacy, in determining whether a behavior is normative or pathological" (p. 898)—as if clinicians are generally able to do this for all of the languages of the world. It is a tall order for even a few hundred of those languages, not to mention their many distinct dialect/varieties.

The Predictable Outcome

If the guidelines of the *DSM* are followed, the expected outcome is disproportionate representation of speakers of language/dialect varieties other than General American English in disordered categories. This, in fact, is what we find. Linguistic differences are commonly mistaken for disorders. The mistakes are widespread and have provided a false but popular basis for theories of racial superiority. The problem is not limited to any one language/dialect group or nation, and, just so, America has not been exempted from it. See the section on "The American Eugenics Records Office" later in this chapter.

Monolingual/Monodialectal Assessment

In fact, it is well known that **monolingual/monodialectal assessment** has resulted, especially in the United States, in overdiagnosis of speakers of minority languages/dialects as disordered and their underrepresentation in programs for the gifted (A. A. Ortiz, 1997). Among the proposed solutions to the problem are attempts to get the language and knowledge factors completely out of certain monolingual/monodialectal tests (see the section below titled "Processing Dependent Measures"). The idea in that case has been to try to escape the impact of linguistic and cultural diversity. Another, proposed work-around has been to rely more heavily on so-called **nonverbal/performance assessment procedures (NVPAPs)**. In this chapter we will see why neither of these proposed solutions can work.

The problem is that monolingual/monodialectal assessment tends to diagnose normal individuals who are merely acquiring a new second language/dialect as disordered. It also fails to identify individuals who are advanced on the scale of development but who do not yet know the language/dialect in which they are being assessed. Monolingual/monodialectal assessment is not a reasonable alternative for individuals who happen to have acquired one of 6,911 distinct languages of the world other than General American

As population mobility has accelerated in a world with 6,912 catalogued distinct languages (Ethnologue, 2009, retrieved March 9, 2009, from http://www.ethnologue.com)—not counting distinct dialects of those languages—the problems created by monolingual/monodialectal assessment have greatly intensified.

If we want to communicate well with any individual, we need to use the strongest and best communication systems of the person or persons being evaluated.

English. The more sensible way to deal with language/dialect diversity is to get persons who are competent in the stronger language/dialect of the individual(s) who are to be tested to do the assessments or at least to assist in doing them.

If we want to communicate well with any individual, we need to use the strongest and best communication systems of the person or persons being evaluated. Also, the assessment/diagnosis needs to be done in a variety of settings—as many as are needed to enable the person assessed to perform at optimum efficiency in the highest and best system of communication that person has acquired. We need to use more than one assessment procedure to get the very best performances that the individual being assessed is capable of producing. The assessment needs to take account of the range of contexts of interest and the full range of discourse tasks that the person being assessed is capable of performing or might be called on to perform. *For any school-related task (especially for any test or evaluation procedure) the student needs to be assessed in the language/dialect that he or she understands and is best able to use.*

We are not making an argument against teaching children new languages/dialects. However, we are saying that it is unreasonable to expect any individual to demonstrate their best abilities in a language/dialect that they do not understand well or in some cases at all. It is truly amazing, appalling, and almost unbelievable that many children are commonly tested in our schools on materials and tasks that are presented in a language/dialect that they have had little or no chance to acquire. Yet the fact that this has happened in the past and that it is still happening at the present time is well documented. See the legal cases addressing this point in Chapter 12, especially, *Diana v. the State Board of Education* (1970), *Lau v. Nichols* (1974), *PASE v. Hannon* (1980), *Bonadonna v. Cooperman* (1985), and so forth. The court cases show that the public, parents, and children in schools understand something that seems to be difficult for some educators to grasp: *Testing or teaching children in a language/dialect that they cannot understand, or cannot understand well, does not make any sense.*

However, that practice is not only commonplace (as documented by Cummins, 2003; A. A. Ortiz, 1997; R. Yan & J. W. Oller, 2007), but it is widely defended even by specialists who can easily see that monolingual/monodialectal assessment/testing is not working well at all. Remarkably, to solve the problems created by insisting on monolingual/monodialectal testing/assessment, some researchers have proposed a variation on the theme which, when we examine it critically, actually amounts to more monolingual/monodialectal testing/assessment.

In the next section we deal with a proposal that has gained widespread support in spite of the fact that it claims to remove the natural bias of monolingual/monodialectal assessment by doing more of it.

An Unworkable Proposal: So-Called "Processing Dependent Measures"

It would be truly amazing if it were possible to measure any property of any object of interest by first removing the property to be measured from the objects of interest. However, in 1997, T. Campbell et al. proposed a series of language tests that were designed to remove the language/dialect background factor from those same putative language tests. They said:

> One potential solution to the problem of eliminating bias in language assessment is to identify valid measures that are not affected by subjects' prior knowledge or experience. (p. 519)

Evidently, their proposal sounded sensible to many proponents of monolingual/monodialectal testing because their paper from 1997 has been cited 58 times in the prestige journals tracked on the Web of Knowledge as of March 9, 2009. To our knowledge, only one of the papers published since 1997 that cites T. Campbell and colleagues has also challenged their idea of trying to find or create language tests that would be independent of "prior knowledge or experience" (p. 519). This is the same as saying that it should be possible to find language/dialect tests that could be used with persons who had no prior knowledge of or experience with the language/dialect to be used in those tests. It is, however, just not possible to acquire a language/dialect without any knowledge of that language/dialect or without any experience with it. Nor is there any language/dialect processing task that requires no knowledge or experience to enable the processing. Yet, not only was their idea accepted for publication, it was welcomed by many other researchers as a viable alternative for assessing children in schools who happened not to have any real depth of knowledge or experience in General American English.

In effect, T. Campbell and colleagues proposed to test knowledge of the language/dialect used in the testing—namely, General American English—without requiring the persons tested to have any knowledge or experience whatsoever with that language/dialect. The idea only makes sense if we suppose that it is possible to assess a person's language/dialect proficiency without requiring them to use any acquired proficiency in that language in any way. If the object of measurement were a little less abstract, researchers and clinicians who have attempted to apply the idea of so-called "processing dependent measures" would have been able to see the fallacy they entail. If the original researchers had proposed measuring something more tangible such as height, weight, or momentum without including any reference to actual physical matter, clinicians would have perceived the mistake right away. Imagine trying to measure height with a yardstick that had no length. Or try to think how you could measure the weight of an object with a device from

It would be truly amazing if it were possible to measure any property of any object of interest by first removing the property to be measured from the objects of interest.

. . . removing some of the meaning from language tasks only makes the tasks less meaningful. It does not make them less dependent on knowledge and experience with the particular language/dialect used in the tasks.

which all indications of weight had been removed. Or consider the likelihood that it would ever be possible to measure the velocity and mass of an object from which all trace of mass and movement had been completely removed. If we could imagine how to do any of these things it might make sense to suppose we could develop valid language testing procedures, in a particular language/dialect, that would not require any knowledge or experience with that language/dialect. But, of course none of these things are possible, and the proposal by T. Campbell et al. is logically doomed to fail. It cannot succeed. Yet, evidently because many monolinguals are oblivious to their dependence on a particular variety of a certain language—General American English in the case of most Americans—it does not occur to them that removing some of the meaning from language tasks only makes the tasks less meaningful.

Yet, T. Campbell and colleagues from 1997 forward claimed to have created tasks that were so dependent on "processing" that "background and experience"—presumably meaning and comprehension—could be removed completely or minimized to a point of becoming altogether negligible. To achieve this logical impossibility, T. Campbell et al. proposed three language tasks that were supposed to focus attention so specifically on processing that they would be quite independent of experience and knowledge with the particular dialect of English in which the tasks were presented—namely, General American English.

THREE PROPOSED "PROCESSING DEPENDENT MEASURES"

Details aside, T. Campbell et al. proposed three different tasks that they claimed were measures of linguistic processing that were quite independent of experience with or knowledge of the particular language/dialect in which the tasks were presented. There was a nonsense repetition task, a task requiring recall of words while simultaneously making judgments about the truth or falsehood of a statement or series of statements, and there was a command execution task. Let's first get in mind a brief description of what each of these tasks required of the individuals being tested.

Repetition of Nonsense

First there was a repetition task that required reproducing one, two, three, or four syllables of nonsense that they called the "Nonword Repetition Task." The assessor produces a syllable, such as, "mook" rhyming with "book," or a sequence of syllables, say, "pehfumek" where the vowels rhyme with "left the check," and the person being tested is supposed to repeat the nonsense. To see how dependent this task is on knowledge of the language/dialect used, all we have to do is attempt it in a language with a phonology and syllable structure very different from that of General American English. Any language that we do not already know will serve to demonstrate the point. English speakers find this task difficult if it is presented in Chinese, Korean, or Arabic, for example.

Recalling the Last Word of One to Five True or False Statements

Another task they proposed involved judging the truth or falsity of anywhere from one to five statements such as "trains can fly," and "trees are green," while at the same time remembering the last word of each sentence. They called this the "Competing Language Processing Task." If we try to get the instructions for this task across to anyone in a language/dialect they do not know—for example, try explaining it in Chinese to an English speaking friend (while using all the gestures you like)—we will get the idea that it is decidedly not a language/dialect independent "processing" task. It is not a sensible task, nor is it even vaguely like ordinary communication. The task lacks authenticity.

How often do we have to judge the truth of a sentence such as "trains can fly," or up to five similar sentences in a row while at the same time remembering the last word of each of the five sentences? There are many reasons why this sort of test does not and cannot accomplish the purpose for which T. Campbell et al. supposed it could be used. It certainly cannot be construed as a task that is independent of knowledge and experience with the language/dialect used in presenting the task. Imagine trying to do it in a language that you do not understand at all—say, Turkish or Hottentot. This sort of "processing dependent measure" is clearly not independent of experience and knowledge of the language/dialect used in the task.

If you could not understand the language/dialect, you would not even know what to count as a word, much less would you be able to judge the truth or falsity of statements and also recall their final words.

Contrived Command Execution

A third task that T. Campbell et al. proposed could best be described as a contrived command execution task. Presumably because the task involved changing the arrangement of tangible objects they called it the "Revised Token Test"—a description that is hardly transparent except in its reference to "tokens"? The person being assessed must carry out certain commands related to geometric shapes of different sizes, shapes, and colors (p. 521). For instance, the person being tested is given a series of commands such as, "Touch the green circle," "Pick up the little red square," "Put the big yellow circle on the little green triangle," and so on. Imagine trying to succeed in this sort of task if the commands were all given in Vietnamese. Could you carry them out correctly without translation into a language/dialect that you already understand?

More Monolingual/Dialectal Testing/Assessment

None of the three tasks proposed by T. Campbell et al., nor any pair, nor all of three of them together, could reasonably be construed as tasks that do not require dependence on knowledge and experience with the language/dialect used in the testing. What their proposal amounts to is more monolingual/monodialectal testing.

It is not a solution to the problem of disproportionate representation—it is a caricature, an encapsulation of the source of the problem. The fact that individuals are being assessed in a language/dialect that they do not know at all, or that they do not know well, is the main source of the disproportionate representation problem. The problem is not solved by more of the same.

In Their Favor, Aiming to Reduce Harm

At least the T. Campbell et al. proposal shows some awareness for the difficulty faced by individuals in American schools and clinics who do not already know General American English, and it certainly does not intentionally aim to harm them. On the contrary, the proposal is intended to reduce the harm that is being done by monolingual/monodialectal testing. Also in their favor, T. Campbell et al. have fallen short of the most extreme measures that have both been proposed and used to deal with language/dialect, ethnic, and cultural diversity.

Unfortunately, however, the so-called "processing dependent measures" that have so far been created and/or adapted cannot accomplish their stated objective of getting all the experience and knowledge out of the testing/assessment procedures. Although such procedures are certainly less harmful than the intentional discrimination recommended and practiced less than a century ago by eugenicists and Nazis, relying exclusively on General American English when giving instructions or posing problems in assessment results in subtle but effective discrimination. Even if the discrimination is unintentional, that will not get the schools, municipalities, or state education departments off the hook. The courts have ruled that unintentional discrimination is still discrimination.

Sad to say, the darker side of deliberate discrimination has sometimes reared its ugly head from behind the somewhat naive assumption that our schools are generally unbiased with respect to race and language/dialect differences. They are often factors that are taken for granted—as if neither the language/dialect differences, nor racial differences were issues. But the differences and the resentments against racial discrimination are nonetheless present beneath the surface and sometimes express themselves in violence. When some high school students hung nooses on an "all White" shade tree in Jena, Louisiana just last year, a new wave of racial

> Unintentional discrimination against language/dialect minorities is still discrimination according to the courts (see *Board of Education of New York v. Harris*, 1979).

tensions and violence were grim reminders that there is more work to do in building understanding across linguistic, historical, and ethnic boundaries.

In September 2007, approximately 20,000 people congregated in Jena, Louisiana to protest the racial divide that has persisted nearly a century and a half since the American Civil War. A little history shows why and how the problem of racial discrimination is deeply connected to the way language/dialect differences and disorders of communication are being treated in the schools.

THE AMERICAN EUGENICS RECORDS OFFICE

The American Eugenics Records Office was founded in 1910 at Cold Spring Harbor Laboratory in New York. In 1939, World War II began and the Eugenics Records Office was merged with the Station for Experimental Evolution (Carnegie Institution of Washington, n.d., retrieved March 7, 2009, from http://library.cshl.edu/archives/archives/ciwscope.htm). The latter office still exists today.

Its aim at the beginning was to enable reproduction by individuals judged to be desirable and to suppress the breeding of those judged to be undesirable. At its outset, the director of the American Eugenics Records Office, Charles B. Davenport, authored a basic text with the subtitle: "The Science of Human Improvement by Better Breeding" (Eugenics Archive, n.d., retrieved March 7, 2009, from http://www.eugenicsarchive.org/html/eugenics/static/themes/28.html; also see Allen, 1995; Kamin, 1995; Sedgwick, 1995). When the Eugenics Records Office was transformed into the Station for Experimental Evolution, Davenport stayed on as the first Director of the new organization as well.

It was not until the ideas promoted by American and other eugenicists were applied by Adolf Hitler [1889–1945] in his programs of sterilization, extermination, and experimentation with human beings of ethnicities and races considered inferior, along with disabled persons, that the eugenics movement and social Darwinism (see Chapter 3) began to fall out of public favor in the United States. However, the eugenics movement in America, like Naziism in Europe and elsewhere, did not die out—it went underground. It is well documented that the movement, especially in the United States, was deeply associated from the beginning with racial theories of intelligence and that it is still connected with certain proponents of IQ testing (see Gould, 1981, 1995; Jacoby & Glauberman, 1995; J. W. Oller, 1997; J. W. Oller, S. D. Oller, & Badon, 2006, pp. 325–368). Among its supporters have been certain researchers supported by a group called "The Pioneer Fund" (n.d., retrieved March 7, 2009, from http://www.pioneerfund.org/Grantees.html).

It was not until the ideas promoted by American and other eugenicists were applied by Adolf Hitler [1889–1945] in his programs of sterilization, extermination, and experimentation with human beings of ethnicities and races considered inferior, along with disabled persons, that the eugenics movement and social Darwinism (see Chapter 3) began to fall out of public favor in the United States.

The "Pioneer Fund" and the Meritocracy Theory

The Theory of the Meritocracy

Among the researchers supported by the "Pioneer Fund" was Phillip E. Vernon [1905–1987] who concluded that the observed difference of about 27 points in IQ scores of children born to parents in what he called the "professional class" as contrasted to children born to "unskilled workers" was owed to genetic differences. Vernon did not bother much to consider the fact that there were quite a few immigrant languages represented in the "working class" and that many of them had not yet had sufficient opportunity to fully acquire American English at the time of their testing. Vernon's conclusion was shared later by Richard Herrnstein (1973) in the **theory of the meritocracy**—the idea that genetically superior individuals rise to the top of the social hierarchy while those with less natural ability tend to end up at the bottom (Herrnstein and Murray 1994, pp. 511–512; Sedgwick, 1995).

> Herrnstein and his supporters likewise failed to take language/dialect differences into account.

Herrnstein and his supporters likewise failed to take language/dialect differences into account. They relied on tests in English and argued that they were actually measures of innate abilities. It hardly seems to have occurred to Herrnstein or any of his collaborators and promoters that the tests on which he was relying as measures of innate abilities were mainly measures of acquired language/dialect proficiency. The oversight—failure to consider language/dialect knowledge and experience as factors—was essentially the same as the mistaken supposition by T. Campbell and colleagues in 1997 and subsequently, that they had succeeded in removing all dependence on language/dialect knowledge in their so-called "processing dependent measures."

Of course, differences in abilities do exist across individuals and across social strata. However, the central premise of the meritocracy theory is that IQ tests directly measure innate abilities. But the research shows that IQ tests in general, also tests of achievement, competency, personality, and so forth, mainly measure language/dialect abilities more than anything else. To claim that IQ tests directly measure **innate intelligence** is like insisting that the intelligence of Louis Braille, Laura Bridgman, and Helen Keller could have been validly measured by **standardized IQ tests** before any of the three ever acquired any language or literacy.

It is like claiming that tests in a particular dialect of English applied to children who have not yet learned that language/dialect can directly measure genetically determined abilities rather than acquired language/dialect proficiency. Such claims are false for persons who are tested in a language/dialect that they have not yet had sufficient opportunity to acquire at a high level of proficiency.

An Undercurrent of Racism

An undercurrent of racist eugenics runs through nearly all of the research projects supported by the Pioneer Fund. At their own Web site, their final entry cites Jensen (1998) who claims that "Black-White IQ differences" are valid and that the observed differences show a genetic superiority favoring Whites. Unsurprisingly, Jensen and his collaborators are Whites. But the differences observed in IQ tests are more readily accounted for in terms of the language/dialect factor which is commingled with socioeconomic and educational differences as noted by us and others (Mercer, 1973, 1984; J. W. Oller & K. Perkins, 1978; J. W. Oller, 1997; Stump, 1978). Jensen's conclusions from his research on IQ tests, as supported by the Pioneer Fund, are essentially the same as those of social Darwinism and the American eugenics movement.

They are based on the same flawed arguments that were used to support the institution of slavery. The Pioneer Fund Web site concludes that "IQ tests . . . are not culturally biased against minorities" (retrieved March 7, 2009, from http://www.pioneerfund.org/Grantees.html). But this claim is false. All tests administered in a language/dialect that many of the tested individuals have not yet had an adequate opportunity to acquire are fundamentally biased. The only exceptions would be tests that are interpreted as measures of proficiency in the language/dialect of the test rather than as measures of innate ability, IQ, achievement, aptitude, competency, or anything other than language/dialect proficiency.

The research supported by the Pioneer Fund neglects, the language/dialect factor which is by far the largest component in IQ tests, personality tests, school achievement tests, and all assessment procedures of any kind that depend on the comprehension and/or production of a particular language/dialect. Proficiency in a particular language/dialect is by far the largest factor measured by such tests. In 1998, Arthur Jensen merely updated and reiterated the flawed arguments and conclusions of his 1969 review and his 1980 book.

All three works deny any bias in IQ tests, but Jensen did not take the language/dialect factor into account in any of them. Neither did Hitler, the Nazis, or the slavers of Rhode Island. But it was there all the time and it has not gone away.

The reality of language/dialect differences is especially intense in urban centers where the number of minority language/dialect users, in many places, has become greater than the speakers of the national majority dialect of English. That is, the speakers of General American English are outnumbered by speakers of other languages/dialects (see Finegan & Rickman, 2004). In Providence, Rhode Island, to single out a place of historical interest, the minority language/dialect users are said to outnumber the speakers of General American English by a ratio of about 19 to 1 (personal communication from Pamela Ardizzone, February 21, 2007).

With worldwide population mobility still increasing, in fact, the language/dialect factor in assessment has become more critical than ever before and will continue to grow in importance as the numbers of minority languages/dialects continues to rise in our schools.

Although it tends not to be noticed by educators with a monolingual/ monodialectal background, what IQ tests do measure fairly well, and fairly directly, are acquired language/dialect proficiencies.

WHAT THE IQ TESTS MEASURE BEST

Although it tends not to be noticed by educators with a monolingual/monodialectal background, what IQ tests do measure fairly well, and fairly directly, are acquired language/dialect proficiencies. In fact, all mental and psychological tests depend heavily on the comprehension of some language/dialect. This is obviously true for the instructions to any complex assessment or testing procedure. The first group IQ testers tried to work around the problem of testing/assessing individuals who did not speak General American English, or who were illiterate in any dialect/variety of English, by developing what were called "nonverbal" IQ tests. These were tests that supposedly escaped the need for dependence on instructions provided in English.

The First Group Intelligence Tests

A notorious demonstration of the importance of understanding instructions comes from the manual devised for the first widely used intelligence tests for groups. The nonverbal versions of those tests were created for use with non-English speaking recruits in America during World War I. The objective of the nonverbal tests was to eliminate the need for a common language/dialect between the military recruiters and the persons being tested. Yerkes (1921) said that

> the main burden of the early reports was . . . that the most difficult task was "getting the idea across" . . . [and] a high percentage of zero scores . . . was considered an indication of failure to "get that test across." (p. 379)

Yoakum and Yerkes (1920) said:

> with the exception of the brief introductory statements and a few orders, instructions are to be given throughout by means of gestures instead of words. These gestures accompany the samples and demonstrations and should be animated and emphatic. (p. 80)

Abstract Concepts Depend on Some Language/Dialect

Logical analysis of the sign systems involved in complex reasoning tasks, including the best "nonverbal" IQ tasks that have ever been devised—setting to one side the problem of getting the instructions across, which depends on some shared language/dialect—are nonetheless still dependent on abstract reasoning which can only be done with the assistance of an acquired language/dialect. As we will show below, the so-called "nonverbal" tasks, provided they require reasoning, are deeply dependent on concepts that can only be acquired with the assistance of some language/dialect.

A general theory of signs shows that pictures and gestures without words will utterly fail to express the meanings required. Complex abstractions are needed involving negation (e.g., "do not touch the yellow square when you remove the black circle from beneath it"), disjunction (e.g., "the dot is inside the circle but outside—NOT inside—the triangle"), relations (e.g., "find the figure on the right where the dot can be placed in the same relation to the circle and the triangle that it has in the picture on the left") and **universal quantifiers** (e.g., "all human beings are mortal" or "nothing comes without cost"). Such concepts cannot be demonstrated or learned from pictures or tokens (icons) or pointing (indexes). The acquisition of some language/dialect is required. Therefore, even nonverbal tasks are dependent on a deep language/dialect factor.

Pantomime Does Not Work, But Language Does

As a result, some test authors, notably Ehler and McGhee (2006), have abandoned the idea that instructions to nonverbal tests can be given through vigorous gesturing (pantomime) or that the items in such tests can be constructed or scored without reference to one or more particular languages/dialects. McGhee wrote:

> Our decision to avoid the use of pantomime instructions when administering the *PTONI* (*Performance Test of Nonverbal Intelligence*) was a conscious one . . . nonverbal IQ tests depend on abstract concepts that are only accessible through spoken or written language systems. It is impossible for a child or anyone else to invent a whole language "ad libitum" . . . (see the *PTONI Test Manual*).

Human communities throughout the world rely on acquired abilities in particular languages/dialects. Those acquired abilities are essential to government, law, education, and employment. What is more, research with a vast multitude of mental tests, including educational tests that are supposed to measure achievement, competency, and personality, shows that the majority of variability in the scores is accounted for by acquired language/dialect abilities (see Cummins, 2003; J. W. Oller, Kim, Choe, & Hernandez-Jarvis, 2000).

The language/dialect explanation of differences in IQ scores is simpler, more plausible, and more complete, than the meritocracy theory. Instead of boasting that IQ tests measure innate intelligence the theory of the language/dialect factor simply claims that language tests measure language proficiency. This is not a doubtful or questionable claim. In fact the research shows that we can measure language proficiency with greater accuracy, validity, and reliability, than any other mental construct (J. W. Oller, 1979). Also, the acquisition (or failure to acquire) one or more particular languages/dialects is by a large margin the biggest factor in accounting for differences owed to disabilities.

It follows that the largest factor in explaining the so-called meritocracy is acquired proficiency in one or more languages/dialects.

Race and Disabilities

For all the foregoing reasons, the historical mingling of racial discrimination with the eugenics movement and, in particular, its efforts to prevent "breeding" (reproduction) by persons with disabilities as well as persons of color was as predictable as it was contrary to the principles on which the United States was founded. It was contrary, as we will see in Chapter 12, to every important document dealing with human rights from the American Declaration of Independence forward through the Constitution and the Bill of Rights to all that would follow from them—including the American Revolution, the American Civil War, and especially World War II. But, as we will also see in our final chapter, the struggles for equality under the law and in public education are far from over.

> . . . the historical mingling of racial discrimination with the eugenics movement and, in particular, its efforts to prevent "breeding" (reproduction) by persons with disabilities as well as persons of color was as predictable as it was contrary to the principles on which the United States was founded.

VERBAL REASONING IN NONVERBAL/ PERFORMANCE ASSESSMENT

To solve the special problems presented by the great diversity of languages and dialects to be dealt with in public education, one of the proposed solutions has been to use what are called "nonverbal" or "performance" based tests. All the proposals along this line fall under the umbrella of nonverbal/performance assessment procedures. The "processing dependent measures" as proposed by T. Campbell et al. (1997), as we saw earlier in this chapter, are just a vanilla version of the same thinking. All such efforts claim to remove the language/dialect factor from the tests or assessment procedures used.

In the case of the T. Campbell et al. tasks, the idea was to take the language/dialect factor out of the language/dialect tests. We already showed why this goal is strictly illogical. It involves an underlying self-contradiction on the same level as inventing a yardstick (or any other measure of length) that has no length and yet purports to measure the length of other things. That plan cannot succeed.

But what about the goal of removing all the verbal (linguistic) reasoning—all the language/dialect based thought and concepts—from so-called nonverbal/performance assessment procedures? Is it possible to achieve such a lesser objective? That is, can we devise nonverbal/performance tasks that do not depend at all on the acquired language/dialect proficiency of test takers?

Trying to Remove Experience and Knowledge from Tests?

The idea that it ought to be possible to get all knowledge and experience out of the procedures for assessing intelligence dates to the very beginning of the IQ testing movement. Binet and Simon (1905) wrote:

> It is intelligence alone that we seek to measure, but disregarding insofar as possible, the degree of instruction which the subject [the child tested] possesses. . . . We believe that we have succeeded in completely disregarding the acquired information of the subject. (p. 42)

As a matter of fact, however—except for certain jigsaw puzzles and mazes used by Binet and his successors—every one of the tasks used by Binet and Simon was permeated with the language/dialect factor as would come out in later research.

The kinds of tasks Binet used, and that are still commonly used by intelligence testers, included such performances as: carrying out verbal commands, naming objects, comparing objects, saying how a folded piece of paper will look after a pattern is cut in it and then it is unfolded, arranging objects in a series, repeating a sequence of words or numbers, naming or telling the value of coins or combinations of them, answering questions of fact ("What color is the sky?") or judging the truth or falsity of statements (e.g., "whenever there is a quarrel there is usually a yellow dog standing nearby"), saying what is wrong with a logically strange or false statement (e.g., "in train wrecks the cars at the end are usually damaged the most"), repeating a sentence or summarizing a story or passage of prose, describing a photograph or sequence of pictures, writing from dictation, copying a text, reading a text aloud, describing words or concepts, making change with money, explaining physical, social, legal, or moral problems (e.g., "why is it a bad idea to step off a cliff, hit another person, shoot your neighbor's dog" and so on).

All of the foregoing tasks are obviously dependent on proficiency in the language/dialect used in the procedure. It is interesting, however, that Binet and Simon had already supposed that their tests had succeeded in "completely disregarding the acquired information" of the individuals tested. That conclusion, however, was mistaken. If such tasks, with the possible exceptions of jigsaw puzzles and mazes, are presented in any language/dialect that the persons tested do not already know fairly well, the results will be very disappointing to all concerned and the tests will not be valid.

Nonverbal Performance and Assessment Procedures to the Rescue?

As we have already seen in a prior section of this chapter, it is not possible to get complex instructions across without using words in some language/dialect. But what if NVPAPs were used? Isn't it possible to get the instructions for nonverbal tests across without using any words?

In 1923 Carl C. Brigham was convinced that such tests were possible. He wrote of the first group administered NVPAPs that they consisted of:

> seven different sorts of tests, none of which involved the ability either to read English or to understand spoken English, the tests consisting of pictures, designs, etc., and being given by instructions in pantomime. (1923, p. xxii)

Later, Arthur Jensen (1980) would insist that the best of the modern NVPAPs namely *Cattell's Culture Fair Tests of Intelligence* and *Raven's Progressive Matrices*, could be explained in pantomime. He said that:

> virtually all subjects can catch on to the requirements of the task without verbal instructions, or with pantomimed instructions by the tester. (p. 132)

But Jensen's claim is logically and factually false.

Words and Sentences Are Necessary

It is not possible through gestures and pictures alone to convey the instructions needed to solve a typical nonverbal item of the sort found, for example, in the Cattell test and as illustrated in Figure 11–2. Unless we are already familiar with the instructions to such an item—instructions provided in a language/dialect that we already understand—we cannot see at a glance how to solve it. Nor is it possible by any amount of gesturing—pointing vigorously back and forth between the one illustration on the left to the five alternatives on the right—to explain the instructions that are needed. We have to tell the test-takers in a language/dialect that they can understand that the object of the task is to *find the numbered choice on the right where the small blackened square can be placed in the same relation to one of the several sets of figures at the right that it has to the figures in the illustration at the left*. It is possible for a test-wise person to guess such instructions, but not without relying on verbal concepts that can only be achieved through some particular language/dialect.

The Language/Dialect Factor in Assessment

Once we understand the instructions, we can see that choice 5 is the only one where the blackened square can be placed inside the triangle, but outside the circle. However, consider the verbal con-

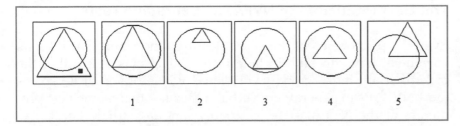

FIGURE 11–2. An NPAP of the type found in *Cattell's Culture Fair Tests of Intelligence*—where the instructions can supposedly, according to proponents of NPAPs, be explained through gestures.

cepts that are in play by the time we get this far. First, there are the concepts differentiating circles, triangles, and squares. These distinct concepts, it is true, can be thought of as visual abstractions from diagramed figures, but are they nonverbal? There are also the concepts of left versus right, and of the "illustration" at the left versus the "choices" at the right. Can each of these conceptual distinctions be made without words?

Perhaps they could be achieved without English, say, by using Chinese, or some other language. But how can such abstractions be known without any vocabulary at all? The test taker requires a vocabulary of abstract meanings that differentiates the concepts and some of their abstract semantic properties. For instance, anyone who can succeed on the task also knows that squares have four sides while triangles have three. The successful test-taker also somehow represents the contrast between the little blackened square and the uncolored circles, triangles, and squares that contain it. There is the contrast between the relation of a figure being inside or outside of another. The little blackened square is inside the triangle but not inside the circle in the illustration. In the choices numbered 1 through 4, the triangle is always contained completely within the circle, so the only place where the small blackened square could be placed outside the circle is in choice 5.

The interesting fact to be noted is that any nonverbal/performance task that involves distinct abstract concepts (circles versus triangles versus squares, etc., for instance), or that involves relations such as inside and outside, or that involves negation (not inside the circle), conjunction (inside one and outside the other), and disjunction (inside one but not inside the other), is so obviously dependent on language that it is remarkable that anyone might ever have supposed that such abstractions were truly "nonverbal" in the first place.

In fact, intensive reviews of the relevant research show that so-called "nonverbal/performance" tasks of a great variety of kinds are deeply permeated by a language/dialect factor (see Cummins, 2003; Carroll, 1993; J. W. Oller, Kim, & Choe, 2001; J. W. Oller, Kim, Choe, & Hernandez-Jarvis, 2000; R. Yan & J. W. Oller, 2007).

The interesting fact to be noted is that any nonverbal/performance task that involves distinct abstract concepts (circles versus triangles versus squares, etc., for instance), or that involves relations such as inside and outside, or that involves negation (not inside the circle), conjunction (inside one and outside the other), and disjunction (inside one but not inside the other), is so obviously dependent on language that it is remarkable that anyone might ever have supposed that such abstractions were truly "nonverbal" in the first place.

The Best Predictors of NVPAPs: Language Tests

Even the proponents of nonverbal testing who claim that IQ tests in general have no built-in language/dialect bias admit that the tasks that are most strongly correlated with nonverbal IQ scores (and NVPAPs in general) are verbal IQ tests—that is, the best predictors of the NVPAPs are invariably language/dialect tests. As Jane Mercer correctly noted in reference to a large scale study in 1984 with groups of more than 600 students in each instance:

> In every case, the verbal factor [i.e., proficiency in General American English] accounts for an overwhelming percentage of the variance. (p. 308)

In fact, the language/dialect factor accounted for 85% of the variance for her White subjects, 87% for Hispanics, and 86% for Blacks. For all three groups (more than 1,800 in all), the best predictor for nonverbal scores was the vocabulary subtest of the verbal kind.

Here is the 411 for IQ testers: The language/dialect factor is the best predictor of NVPAP scores. Proponents of NVPAPs need to ask why. Here is the answer: NVPAPs are *largely dependent on acquired proficiency in some language/dialect*. If this were not so, it would be possible for parrots, dolphins, chimps, and gorillas to do fairly well on NVPAPs—about as well as a human child who has acquired some language/dialect or other. But that never happens. It does not happen because it is not possible to do well on abstract reasoning tasks without acquiring proficiency in some language/dialect. In recent research it has also been shown that in bilingual individuals, the stronger language/dialect is the one that is most correlated with NVPAP scores (see J. W. Oller, Kim, & Choe, 2001).

What is more, on a strictly logical basis, it is evident that the designers of NVPAPs would be entirely unable to devise or agree on scoring procedures for even a single item on any NVPAP without appealing to some particular language/dialect. To determine what answer is to be preferred and why, designers of such tests must use a common language/dialect to discuss the instructions and the reasoning behind the items. NVPAPs are decidedly not independent of language/dialect proficiency.

Basing Diagnosis on the Strongest Communication System

For all of the above reasons, the practice of diagnosing disabilities and disorders for minority language/dialect speakers by using either language tests in General American English or NVPAPs, or both of them combined, comes up short of the goal of valid assessment. It is essential to assess individuals in their own strongest and

. . . the best predictors of the NVPAPs are invariably language/dialect tests.

best system of communication. This is an idea, as we will see in Chapter 12, which has been tested in the U.S. courts of law. Repeatedly, the courts including the U.S. Supreme Court in *Lau v. Nichols* (1974) have concluded that it makes no sense whatever to teach or test children in a language/dialect which they have not yet had a reasonable and sufficient opportunity to acquire.

Invalid Assessment Gives Invalid Results

Assessing individuals in any language/dialect that they do not know, or do not know well, is certain to result in the two most prevalent kinds of diagnostic errors in the schools today—(1) minority language/dialect children will continue to be over-represented as disabled/disordered; and (2) they will also be under-represented in programs for the gifted. In addition to those two errors, children with subtle problems—disorders and disabilities that are difficult to detect—will tend to be overlooked altogether.

DEVELOPMENT VERSUS EFFECTS OF INTERVENTION

Before we close this chapter, there is one more difficult testing and measurement problem to be addressed. How are parents, teachers, therapists, and caregivers in general to know whether a change in performance is owed to ordinary growth that would have taken place without intervention as contrasted with observed changes that can be attributed to some treatment?

As a child gets older, typically more words will be acquired. Phonology can be expected to become more defined—sounds will be more sharply distinguished. Syntax will be advancing. Semantic concepts will be more completely differentiated and enriched. Pragmatic mappings will be clarified and the child will become easier for others to understand while at the same time advancing to the expression of more difficult and challenging ideas. If there is an intervention procedure that has been designed to help the child to acquire more words, for instance, how will it be possible to differentiate the effects of the treatment from the growth in vocabulary that would have occurred normally without the treatment? If the treatment focuses on enriching the conceptual capability of the child to express meanings and ideas, for example, to give a coherent narrative report on a sequence of experienced events, how will improvement owed to the treatment, if there is any, be distinguished from

To validly assess the impact of treatments on developmental disorders, we must have valid information in advance about how development normally proceeds. We must also get valid measurements before and after the treatment at a minimum and valid measurements during the course of the treatment are also desirable.

any improvement that may naturally occur because of maturation and that is quite independent of the treatment.

In other words, how can we be confident that a treatment is the cause of an observed advance in behavior?

Avoiding the *Post Hoc Ergo Propter Hoc* Fallacy

It is difficult in **case studies**—ones that usually involve only a single individual or possibly two or three individuals who receive treatment—to tell the difference between advances owed to the treatment versus advances that might be better attributed to normal development. Just because the improvement occurs after the treatment does not necessarily mean that the treatment caused the improvement. To suppose that is to fall into what is called the *post hoc ergo propter hoc* **fallacy**. This Latin phrase means, "after this fact, therefore, because of this fact." The fallacy lies in assuming that because a certain event B, say, follows another event A, that A caused B to occur. Effects must follow their causes. That is true. So, it is possible that A has caused B if B follows after A. But there may be other factors, call them X, Y, or Z that also preceded B, and that are independent of A, and yet may have caused B. To show that a certain advance was caused by a certain treatment requires more than merely showing that the treatment preceded the advance.

The Essential Role of Normative Expectations

The increased difficulty of assessing or measuring the effects of treatments associated with developmental disorders comes from the fact that development normally advances without any special treatment—that is, without any intervention. If a treatment precedes a noticeable improvement in behavior, because normal development might also produce the same degree of improvement without that treatment, we need to show that the effect observed is greater than what could have been expected without the treatment. Also, if we are going to attribute a particular effect to a given treatment, we need to be sure that the treatment singled out as the cause of that effect was the only factor that could have caused it.

To justify the comparisons needed to assess the effectiveness of any given treatment for a disorder, special care must be taken to ensure that the individuals or groups to be compared are really comparable in all the relevant respects.

The measurements, and whatever theory they may be based on, must enable a reasonable judgment about how any given individual or group was proceeding before the treatment was introduced and how they are doing sometime after the treatment has been introduced. In the end, we must also infer (guess) how things would have proceeded without the treatment and whether or not any particular differences observed can be reasonably attributed to the treatment. To justify a particular inference—that is, to show that it is a reasonable judgment and not just a wild guess or the result of wishful thinking that the treatment has helped any given individual or group—we must make the call depending on whether the advance was greater than would reasonably have been expected without the treatment.

To do this, logically and reasonably, reference *must be* made, in some way or other, to what may be termed **normative expectations**. Such expectations are based on what is known or believed about the development as it usually, typically, and normally proceeds when there are no known disorders or disabilities interfering and where there are no special interventions or treatments to speed things along or slow them down. We must invariably refer to expectations based on the development of communication systems under normal conditions. We have developed this argument especially in Chapter 1 of this book (also in Chapter 4) and we have devoted the whole of the *Milestones* book about *Normal Speech and Language Across the Life Span* to the simplest consistent theory that comprehensively accounts for all of the research that is currently known.

Normative judgments are invariably based on typical cases of development and usually on substantial numbers of individuals. In some experimental studies, a normative **control group**, say, Group N, is used to establish expectations against which the **treatment group** with some disorder of interest, say, Group D, can be compared. If the effect of the treatment dramatically reduces the difference between D and N, provided all other relevant variables have been kept equal, the treatment can be reasonably judged to have been helpful. In an ideal situation, at the end of treatment D will not differ significantly from N in spite of the fact that N and D were very different before the treatment.

The *Ceteris Paribus* Principle: All Else Being Equal

To justify the comparisons needed to assess the effectiveness of any given treatment for a disorder, special care must be taken to ensure that the individuals or groups to be compared are really comparable in all the relevant respects. If we are interested in measuring the contrast between children diagnosed with a particular disorder, Group D, and children who do not have that disorder, Group N, we must assure that Groups D and N are similar in all other respects— that each contains individuals of the same age, gender, language/ dialect, socioeconomic status, educational background, family circumstances, and so forth. This requirement has often been referred to in the research literature in the Latin phrase *ceteris paribus* which means "all else being equal." We refer to this general requirement in assessment and measurement as the *ceteris paribus* **principle**.

If assurances are not provided up front, that is, in the way measurements or observations are obtained before, during, and after treatment, we will not know in the end if differences observed between D and N are because of the treatment or because of differences that may have existed beforehand, or whether any observed

To justify the comparisons needed to assess the effectiveness of any given treatment for a disorder, special care must be taken to ensure that the individuals or groups to be compared are really comparable in all the relevant respects.

differences may have been caused by something other than the treatment of interest. To measure or observe a particular **treatment effect** requires assurance that every necessary and reasonable precaution has been taken to be certain that the only factor that might cause the measure or observation to appear as it does is the treatment itself—the treatment of interest. If the **effect size** attributable to the treatment is large it is possible that no additional control group will be required. That is, if the improvement attributable to the treatment dramatically reduces or removes the contrast between Groups D and N it may be unnecessary to seek a more finely graded comparison.

Suppose the effect size is very small and difficult to detect. In that case it may be necessary to use a less distant reference group. If we think about it, we discover that logically speaking, a perfectly matched individual without the disorder would be the same person if the disorder could be completely removed. Without a complete and sudden cure of the disorder, we cannot get to this ideal situation. However, if we could, Groups D and N would consist of the same persons before and after treatment. But, in the real world, D and N are different persons who differ as little as possible on everything except for the disorder of interest where the difference between D and N is supposedly maximal. The difference at the outset is as large as it can be on account of the disorder.

The maximal difference comparison is the one that is usually of greatest interest. But there are cases where the treatment effect may fall far short of completely removing the disorder and we may want to look at a comparison where the difference between groups is at a minimum.

Zooming In on the Treatment Effect (if any)

To focus on the treatment effect, we need to compare persons who have the disorder and who get the treatment, call them Group $D_{Treatment}$, with a matched group of individuals who also have the disorder but who do not receive the treatment, call them $D_{No\ Treatment}$. In this case, the distance between the comparison groups is minimized. In the ideal case it could be reduced all the way to zero if it were possible to compare each person against him or herself. That could be done only if the treatment did not require any time lapse. However, in the real world treatments require time, so experimenters must settle for groups that are as closely matched as possible to satisfy the *ceteris paribus* principle.

For instance, suppose a team of researchers wants to see if removing known neurotoxins from children diagnosed with neurological disorders will enable them to advance more rapidly than children subject to the same neurotoxins, but who for whatever reason, do not receive the treatment—say, removal of toxins by some form of chelation. In this case, it might be desirable to compare a group of individuals with the disorders in question who receive the treatment, Group $D_{Treatment}$, with matched individuals who also have the disorders in question who do not receive the treatment, Group $D_{No\ Treatment}$. In such a comparison, to make a reasonable judgment in favor of the treatment—to show that it was worth doing—it would be necessary to show that the improvement of Group $D_{Treatment}$ was significantly greater than any change in Group $D_{No\ Treatment}$. Also, it would be important to show that the significant difference was sufficiently great to justify whatever costs, efforts, and possible risks might be have been involved in Group $D_{Treatment}$ undergoing the treatment.

Valid Measurement Required

What is required in all cases where a particular treatment is examined for effectiveness, at a minimum, is valid measurement of the person or group to be treated before the intervention takes place, and afterward as well. A treatment that requires significant effort but that produces no measurable effect cannot be judged to be a good treatment. On the other hand, any poorly designed experiment, like any invalid measurement technique, can fail to find results even if the treatment works very well.

Positive Compared to Null Outcomes (*Ceteris Paribus*)

For all of the reasons we gave earlier, null outcomes in experiments that show no significant effects are like failed efforts of all sorts. They are a lot less informative than ones that show significant effects. One solitary successful attempt at communication is a great deal less likely, and consequently more informative, than any number of failures to communicate under similar circumstances.

Consider the faint communication that resulted in the true life rescue of survivors 18 and 19 from the terrorist attack on the Twin Towers of the World Trade Center in New York after September 11, 2001. If all the failed attempts to get a response from beneath the debris had been weighed equally with the faint tapping by Port Authority Officer, William J. Jimeno, who was buried under the debris, he and John McLoughlin (played by Nicholas Cage in the movie by Oliver Stone, *World Trade Center*, 2006, retrieved March 9, 2009, from http://en.wikipedia.org/wiki/World_Trade_Center_(film)), could not have been rescued at all (see Stone, Berloff, & McLoughlin, 2006). All the failed attempts by Officers McLoughlin and Jimeno to alert rescuers to their presence beneath the rubble were less important to the outcome than their eventual successes. Failures to communicate do not carry the same weight as successes. Millions

. . . null outcomes in experiments that show no significant effects are like failed efforts of all sorts.

. . . if careful and replicable experimental designs—ones that respect the ceteris paribus principle—demonstrate one or many significant treatment effects repeatedly, they must be given more credence than dozens of studies that fail to produce any significant effects.

of failures, all else being equal, count infinitely less than even one success. When two or three other successes are added into the mix, the previous failures have little or no remaining importance.

If the *ceteris paribus* principle is satisfied—that is, if the things that need to be kept equal are kept equal—experiments that get the predicted significant results (for example, the treatment works) are a great deal more informative than failed experiments. Even when all else appears to be equal, failed experiments that do not show treatment effects are still less interesting, less informative, and less apt to be valid, than ones that do show treatment effects. For instance, if careful and replicable experimental designs—ones that respect the *ceteris paribus* principle—demonstrate one or many significant treatment effects repeatedly, they must be given more credence than dozens of studies that fail to produce any significant effects.

The fact that many deaf-blind children before Laura Bridgman and Helen Keller did not acquire language or learn to read is a great deal less informative than the fact that with diligent treatment methods, Bridgman and Keller were able to achieve what seemed to many to be impossible. Similarly, all of the many failed attempts of sighted person's to understand Louis Braille's writing system for the blind were of no consequence in comparison to the successes experimentally demonstrated at the Royal Institution for Blind Youth in February of 1844. When the blind students showed that one of them could write in Braille from dictation and another could read it back, their success counted more than all the prior failures of sighted persons to see the merits of Braille writing.

The Ideal Outcome Versus the Null Outcome

The most dramatic effect that can be shown in the treatment of disorders is for the individual (or group) treated to achieve or surpass what would be expected of the same person (or group) without the disorder(s) in question. Logically this is not only the ideal outcome but it is the most that could be achieved if the treatment were perfectly successful at what it was supposedly designed to do. Of course, the maximal best outcome cannot always be achieved. Still, it is always the implicit ideal goal of treatment. If it cannot be attained, it is still desirable to devise treatments that reduce the negative impacts of the disorder.

The Language/Dialect Factor in Assessment

There are no treatments of disorders that are deliberately devised to achieve null outcomes. Researchers, therefore, who give equal weight to failed experiments attempting to produce positive treatment outcomes as contrasted with experiments that succeed are invariably making a judgment error of a high order. Null outcomes are generally not even worth publishing much less are they worth comparing on any sort of equal basis with demonstrated and desired positive outcomes. If a challenge is to be mounted against some claimed positive outcome, it ought to be on the basis of critical examination of the methods, measures, and procedures of the experiment or experiments that are supposed to have produced it. If fraudulent representations are involved they should be exposed.

However, an attempted replication that fails, or dozens of studies with null outcomes should never be considered as having probative weight. Oftentimes, they only demonstrate ineptness on the part of the experimenters or a flawed design. Successes, or even claimed successes, by contrast, deserve more careful consideration.

Consistency at the Foundation

In all cases, before claims are made for positive effects of a given treatment method, the *ceteris paribus* principle should be satisfied. Observational methods and qualitative approaches that aim to discover patterns must also be subjected to the standard **replication requirement** in the sciences. An experiment that cannot be described well enough to be replicated by a different researcher, or a different team of researchers, is one that cannot be relied on as valid with any reasonable certainty.

In the same way that genuine communication can always be understood by more than one person, it must be possible to describe a successful experiment well enough that other researchers will be able to replicate it. The replication requirement of experimental science is essential, but it is based on the deeper logical expectation that a consistent application of a method ought to give a consistent result. That deeper **principle of consistency** is contained in the *ceteris paribus* principle but does not come from science or empirical investigations of any kind. We do not find complete consistency anywhere in ordinary experience anymore than we count to infinity, find a place where there is absolutely nothing, or where everything is present all at once, or step into the same river twice. Things are always changing in the real world.

Necessary Reasoning Is Necessary

Interestingly, we can only justify the **consistency requirement** on the basis of fully abstract logical and mathematical reasoning. That is, if $A = B$ and if $C = B$, we know that it follows that $A = C$. Or to take a different relation than equality, if A is smaller than B and B is smaller than C, we know that A must also be smaller than C. How do we know this? It is true that we can exemplify all sorts of relations of the kind just described in experience by empirical science. However, the consistency requirement that tells us if A differs in the slightest amount from B it is not quite equal to B, shows why we cannot fully verify or justify the consistency requirement by

We know that things equal to the same thing are equal to each other, but we cannot prove this empirically.

observations based on experience. We can only do so on the basis of purely abstract logic and necessary mathematical reasoning. To carry out such reasoning, as we have already seen above in reference to NVPAPs, requires considerable proficiency in some language/dialect. For a more detailed discussion with proofs showing how all the measurements of science depend on the sorts of transitive relations just described, see J. W. Oller and L. Chen (2007). The claims we are making here have been strictly proved.

Of course, we can approximate the general requirement of consistency in scientific measurements. That is why science can help us to test ideas and show many claims to be false. However, science cannot test the foundations of logic and mathematics. But, by strict logical reasoning of the mathematical kind, we can show that if inconsistencies are permitted anywhere and everywhere—if the *ceteris paribus* principle is abandoned—no meaningful communication of any kind, much less science, is possible. As a result, the consistency requirement is real and valid and for that reason replication of valid experiments must be possible. On the other hand, all sensible mathematical reasoning shows that null results in experiments are infinitely less informative than predicted positive outcomes that can be repeatedly achieved.

... all sensible mathematical reasoning shows that null results in experiments are infinitely less informative than predicted positive outcomes that can be repeatedly achieved.

A Lesson from Lombardi

As Coach Vince Lombardi might well have put it, in the treatment of communication disorders, "Success isn't everything, it's the only thing." People who love individuals with disorders are deeply interested only in studies of disorders that will help those loved ones to succeed as communicators. They don't want their loved ones merely to be treated as objects of study. They want them to be treated as you and I would want to be treated, as human beings, with unalienable rights to life, liberty and the pursuit of happiness. Any lesser goals for therapy and intervention are not sufficiently high. Clinical work may not always achieve the highest possible goals, but that does not make it ethical or desirable to aim for null results even in cases where they are all the therapy may produce. The goal in therapeutic intervention is to make things as much better as possible.

SUMMING UP AND LOOKING AHEAD

In this chapter we have dealt with the essential problems of assessing and diagnosing communication disorders. In measuring and judging developmental communication abilities it is essential to enable the persons assessed to perform at their highest level of competence. Poor performances on tests are as uninformative as failed attempts at communication. Successes by contrast are much more informative. We saw in this chapter that the language/dialect factor is by far the largest and the most important component in assessing communication abilities and in diagnosing disorders. In this chapter we also saw that monolingual/monodialectal assessment of individuals in a language/dialect that they either do not know at all or that they do not know well is the obvious cause of the over-representation of language/dialect minority speakers in disordered/disabled categories and also of their being under-represented in programs for the gifted. Two failed solutions have been proposed: One consisted of "nonverbal/performance assessment procedures" (NVPAPs) and the other involved, so-called "processing dependent measures" (PDMs). Both fail because they require linguistic instructions and concepts and PDMs have the additional flaw of being weak and not very authentic language/dialect tests.

To solve the disproportionate representation problem it is essential to do assessments in the strongest communication system of the individual being tested—their best language/dialect needs to be used. An alternative is to provide adequate opportunity for the acquisition of the language/dialect to be used in assessment. Also, when it comes to the treatment of disorders, assessment and diagnosis are critically involved. In judging the effectiveness of proposed treatments it is essential to focus on claimed and actual validated successes. No treatment ever aimed to achieve a null result. Treatments are supposed to help move the person or group with the disorder toward what would be expected of the same person or group without the disorder. Normative expectations are essential and successful treatments must be validated by replicable demonstrations.

> To solve the disproportionate representation problem it is essential to do assessments in the strongest communication system of the individual being tested—their best language/dialect needs to be used. An alternative is to provide adequate opportunity for the acquisition of the language/dialect to be used in assessment.

STUDY AND DISCUSSION QUESTIONS

1. Why is it essential to understand milestones of normal development in order to diagnose and assess the severity of developmental disorders?
2. Why is successful communication more informative than unsuccessful attempts at communication? How is success in communication similar to correctly answering test questions and to validity in measurement? At the same time, how is unreliability in assessment related to failure to communicate? Why are unreliable procedures also uninformative? Why are successful test performances vastly more informative than unsuccessful ones?
3. What is wrong with assessing all individuals in a single language/dialect or in a single modality of communication? Why not use single test scores for important educational decisions,

for example, such as college admission, diagnosis of disorders, and the like?

4. So-called "processing dependent measures" have included repeating nonsense syllables, judging the truth or falsity of statements and recalling the last word of one or several of them in a row, and carrying out commands that refer to tangible geometric shapes of different sizes and colors. Why can these measures not be judged to be "experience and knowledge independent"? What aspects of acquired knowledge of the language/dialect used in the testing do they rely on?

5. What exactly are the historical relationships between the American Eugenics Records Office, the Pioneer Fund, social Darwinism, and the present day proponents of IQ testing who claim that their tests are completely free, especially the nonverbal/performance IQ tests, of language/dialect bias?

6. What kinds of tests are the best predictors of nonverbal/performance IQ tests? How is it possible to explain the fact that individuals can neither understand the instructions nor even get started on such tests if they have not already acquired some language/dialect? How is it possible to explain the fact that for persons who are becoming bilingual, their stronger language correlates more strongly with their nonverbal/performance IQ as measured by standardized tests?

7. What is the *post hoc ergo propter hoc* fallacy and how does it play into the difficulty of distinguishing a treatment effect from ordinary growth and development?

8. In your view, why is it that caregivers, clinicians, parents, and pediatricians never try to devise interventions that will produce null effects? Why is it, then, that null effects seem to be so highly prized in the research journals pertaining to communication disorders? Why are null outcomes less informative than valid positive outcomes?

9. Why is consistency so critical to measurement in the sciences? Imagine a world in which the exact same experiment would produce a different outcome every time? Would it be possible for a child in such a world to acquire a language? Would science be possible? Why so, or why not?

10. Why is replication of experimental results so highly prized in the sciences? How does experimental replicability relate to our ability to understand different interlocutors or to communicate in different contexts through language?

12

Advocacy, Law, and Ethics

OBJECTIVES

In this chapter, we:

1. Review actions of advocates for persons with communication disorders;
2. Consider the historical links between freedom of the body and the mind;
3. Trace conflicts, precedents, and public laws governing communication disorders;
4. Consider diagnosis and treatment of persons with disabilities under current legislation;
5. Review ongoing litigation and claims concerning vaccine injuries and related issues;
6. Discuss the principle that treatment should benefit and not harm the person treated; and
7. Review the professions that deal with communication disorders.

KEY TERMS

Here are some key terms of this chapter. Many you may already know, but it may help to review them. These terms are explained in the text and they are defined in the Glossary at the end of the book. They appear in **bold print** on their first appearance in the text.

ability tracking system
ADA
adverse impact
Americans with Disabilities Act of 1990
assistive technology
case law
CCC-SLP
Certificate of Clinical Competence in Speech-Language Pathology
civil litigation
Civil Rights Act
Code of Ethics
consent decree
dead-end classes
defendant
Dred Scott decision
EACHA
Education for All Handicapped Children Act of 1975
EHA
Emancipation Proclamation
epenthesis
equal protection clauses
ethical conduct
FAPE
free and appropriate public education

Golden Rule
grade point average
Haemophilus influenzae B
Handicapped Children's Protection Act, 1986
HiB
Hippocratic Oath
Holocaust
IASA
IDEA
IEP
Improving America's Schools Act of 1994
in utero
individualized education program
Individuals with Disabilities Education Act
Individuals with Disabilities Education Act of 1997
Jim Crow laws
jurisprudence
LEA
least restrictive environment
legal discovery
legal injunction
legal precedent
local educational agencies
mainstreaming principle

National Childhood Vaccine Injury Act
National Vaccine Injury Compensation Program
NCLB
No Child Left Behind Act
no-fault
Omnibus Autism Proceeding, 2007
pediatricians
petition for certiorare
petitioner
prima facie evidence
Public Law 88-352
Public Law 94-142
Public Law 99-660
pull-out programs
Rehabilitation Act of 1973
respondent
separate but equal
Special Masters
statute of limitations
Vaccine Adverse Event Reporting System
VAERS
VICP

Historically, advocates for persons with communication disorders have included some interesting persons. In some cases they were individuals who had the difficulty or disorder themselves, as was the case with Helen Keller and Louis Braille. Sometimes they were relatives of the person affected as was the case for Alexander Graham Bell—whose mother and wife were deaf. In other instances, the advocates simply came upon a difficulty and decided to do something about it.

Wars have been waged, the Bill of Rights was written and many legislative acts have been enacted. Court battles are still being slogged through to secure fundamental human rights. Along the way, persons with communication disorders have always been in the background and sometimes they have been brought to the foreground. There is a deep connection between the struggle for equality under the law and modern codes of ethics concerning the treatment of persons with communication disorders and disabilities.

In this chapter, we dig to the foundations of law and ethics to find the principles that motivated current standards of professional organizations that serve persons with communication disorders.

Advocates of individual rights to life, liberty, and the pursuit of happiness have unwaveringly linked the freedom of the mind with that of the body. In the American Revolution, in the American Civil War, and especially in World War II the proposition that "all men are created equal" and entitled by their Creator to "life, liberty, and the pursuit of happiness" has often been challenged.

FREEDOM FROM MENTAL AND PHYSICAL BONDAGE

Freedom of the Mind and Body

Among the heroes enshrined in the stone carvings at New York City's Riverside Church (retrieved March 9, 2009, from http://www.einstein-website.de/images/WestPortal.jpg) we find Valentin Haüy, the early teacher of the blind, along with Abraham Lincoln [1809–1865], the American President who signed the *Emancipation Proclamation* that officially, at least, ended slavery in America. Is it just a coincidence that these two individuals are honored together among at least 14 other humanitarians who pursued freedom of the mind and body?

Was it just curious coincidence that Dr. Samuel Gridley Howe, the great teacher of Laura Bridgman was an advocate for the abolition of slavery? Is it just another coincidence that Julia Ward Howe, whom Samuel Howe married in 1843, was the author of the anthem of abolition known as the "Battle Hymn of the Republic"? You can hear a rendition sung by the St. John's Children's Choir (2009a, retrieved March 9, 2009, from http://www.ez-tracks.com/getsong-songid-267.html and as composed by William Steffe it is performed by the U.S. Army Band, 2009b, retrieved March 9, 2009, from http://lcweb2.loc.gov/diglib/ihas/loc.natlib.ihas.100010422/default.html).

Is it coincidence or thematic appropriateness that the words of the abolition hymn were sung at the funerals of Winston Churchill, Robert F. Kennedy, and Ronald Reagan? Upon reflection all of them were crusaders for freedom along with President Lincoln, Dr. Howe, and Valentin Haüy. All of them also put their lives on the line in the course of public service. Lincoln and Kennedy were actually assassinated and an attempt was made to assassinate Reagan (Lorenz, Lorenz, & Pulte, 1998, retrieved March 9, 2009, from http://www.heptune.com/preslist.html#deaths). Churchill himself—who had a speech impediment of some sort—is remembered as the greatest statesman of World War II and perhaps of the 20th century ("Winston Churchill, 1965/2009, retrieved March 9, 2009, from http://en.wikipedia.org/wiki/Winston_Churchill). His legacy includes the fact that he stood almost alone against Adolf Hitler for several years until the Americans finally entered World War II after the Japanese bombed Pearl Harbor on December 7, 1941.

In similar fashion, the Kennedy brothers—especially, Robert F. Kennedy as the U.S. Attorney General of the 1960s along with his older brother, President John F. Kennedy—are remembered for working to end segregation by race a hundred years after the American Civil War. President Ronald Reagan is remembered by many as the leader who brought down the Berlin Wall marking the end of the long gray period after World War II known as "the Cold War" (see "Berlin Wall," 1989/2009, retrieved March 9, 2009, from http://en.wikipedia.org/wiki/Berlin_Wall). He was also the only president to write a book while in office, and notably his book was a plea to end abortion on demand.

Is it merely a coincidence that Robert F. Kennedy, Jr. has continued in his father's footsteps not only in the pursuit of civil rights but as an advocate for children with autism? In a controversial article about mercury in vaccines (see Kennedy, June 20, 2005, retrieved March 9, 2009, from http://www.rollingstone.com/politics/story/7395411/deadly_immunity/), Robert F. Kennedy, Jr. has argued that many individuals with autism were in fact injured by the mercury in vaccines (see the story and links to extensive documentation on this subject at A-Champ, 2005, retrieved March 9, 2009, from http://www.a-champ.org/cdcmercuryremoval.html). Kennedy also suggested several other known sources of mercury poisoning including dental amalgam. As seen in Chapters 5 and 10, dental amalgam accounts for about 67% of mercury body burden on the average and 55% of the total mercury stored in man-made products. Of course, other sources for mercury are medicines and vaccines that still include thimerosal as a preservative, and other toxins that may be involved in the upsurge in diagnoses of neurological disorders, especially autism (as discussed in Chapter 5). However, the argument brought to the popular press in part by the efforts of Robert F. Kennedy, Jr. has finally reached the U.S. Court of Federal Claims (n.d., retrieved March 9, 2009, from http://www.uscfc.uscourts.gov/). That court, now commonly referred to as the "Vaccine Injury Court," is considering about 5,300 claims that autism was caused by vaccines (*Omnibus Autism Proceeding*, 2008, retrieved March 9, 2009, from http://www.uscfc.uscourts.gov/docket-omnibus-autism-proceeding).

We will return to the issue of toxins and the vaccine story later in this chapter. In the meantime, the question at hand is whether the association between human rights and advocacy for persons with communication disorders is merely coincidental. Putting the punch-line up front, we believe that the association is not a coincidence.

Extreme Eugenics

The historical interest in individuals with disabilities was partly because individuals with severe emotional and mental problems can sometimes threaten the security or peace of mind of others (Bersoff, 1981). According to Boswell (1988), the practice in Greek and Roman times was to exterminate such individuals. In more recent history, from 1939 to 1945 Hitler returned to that practice. The cause of freedom and the rights of the individuals affected by disabilities and by discriminatory treatment are, at their basis, related causes. Laws governing communication disorders are inevitably connected in principle and in fact with those concerned with equal treatment for persons of diversity.

> Historically, in the United States at least, the legal roots of civil rights for persons with disabilities inexorably lead back to the struggles, court cases, and laws concerning slavery and racial discrimination.

Social Darwinism

Although Darwin's ideas have been widely accepted, it is clear from the eugenics movement, also known as social Darwinism, that the rights of individuals in general—and of racial, religious, and ethnic minorities in particular—are inevitably linked to the rights of persons with disabilities and communication disorders. In commenting on the near complete acceptance of the Darwinian perspective, one linguist, Fred Field (2005, p. 50) has asked rhetorically: "Can 50 million Germans be wrong? Absolutely. Can thousands of scientists be wrong? (Your turn to answer.)" In the European **Holocaust**, Hitler and his Nazi followers—many of them supposedly among the best scientists in the world—exterminated 200,000 persons with disabilities. Then they set about to exterminate others that they judged to be genetically or otherwise inferior. Hitler carried eugenics and social Darwinism to its logical limit. The idea was that evolution could be speeded along by human beings taking an active role in killing off all those judged to be unfit. In Nazi Germany, the

> In the European **Holocaust**, Hitler and his Nazi followers many of them supposedly among the best scientists in the world—exterminated 200,000 persons with disabilities.

> "Law for the prevention of Progeny with Hereditary Diseases," proclaimed July 14, 1933, forced the sterilization of all persons who suffered from diseases considered hereditary, such as mental illness (schizophrenia and manic depression), retardation ("congenital feeble-mindedness"), physical deformity, epilepsy, blindness, deafness, and severe alcoholism. . . . In all, between 200,000 and 250,000 mentally and physically handicapped persons were murdered from 1939 to 1945 under the T-4 and other "euthanasia" programs. (see the United States Holocaust Memorial Museum, n.d., retrieved March 9, 2009, from http://www .ushmm.org/education/resource/handic/handicapped.php ?menu=/export/home/www/doc_root/education/foreduca tors/include/menu.txt&bgcolor=CD9544)

In addition, of course, the Hitler regime killed about 6,000,000 Jews—not to mention the Gypsies, Poles, Hungarians, Czechs and others—in its "ethnic cleansing" programs predicated on the misguided theory of eugenics as justified by social Darwinism. The fact is that violations of "unalienable" human rights do not have a logical starting point but they have an end in death. They end in proposing and carrying out the killing of the unfit. It was a fundamental denial of human rights—a plain and complete rejection of the proposition that all human beings are created equal and endowed by their Creator with certain unalienable rights—that led to the holocaust. The same sort of thinking led to the conclusion that some human beings were only suited to be slaves.

The Case of Ota Benga

Recall Darwin's claim about certain races being closer to "the gorilla" (see p. 183 above).

Ota Benga

In 1992, the story of Ota Benga, an African (pigmy) of the Bachichiri tribe (Figure 12–1) was told by Bradford and Blume writing for St. Martin's Press. The book, which won the New York Times book of the year award for 1992, tells the true story of a man who was brought to America supposedly to build an exemplary village here but who ended up in the Bronx zoo with the primates housed there. He was represented as an example of one of their near relatives according to the dictum of Darwin. "Bronx Zoo director William Hornaday saw the exhibit as a valuable spectacle for his visitors, and was encouraged by Madison Grant, a prominent scientific racist and eugenicist" in maintaining the exhibit ("Ota Benga," 1916/ 2009, retrieved March 11, 2009, from http://en.wikipedia .org/wiki/Ota_Benga). After being rescued from captivity by certain opponents to racism and eugenics, Ota Benga, unable to return to Africa, eventually committed suicide in 1916.

The American Civil War and Slavery

It is interesting that from an ethical, legal, and political standpoint, racially based slavery was the central issue in the presidential race of 1860 leading up to the American Civil War [1861-1865]. This can be seen from the writings and speeches of Abraham Lincoln who made slavery the central focus of his debates with Stephen A. Douglas. The word "slavery" was mentioned 84 times in the first debate and 123 times in the last of the seven debates between the two candidates. Douglas opened the seventh of the debates saying:

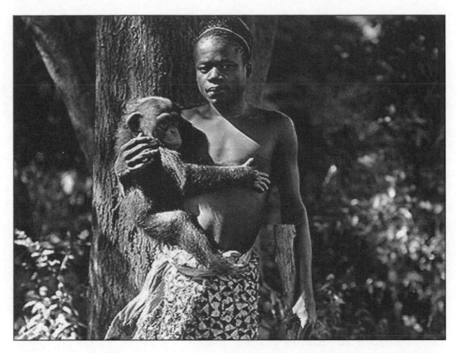

Figure 12–1. Ota Benga in 1906 while living at the Bronx Zoo. Retrieved March 11, 2000, from http://en.wikipedia.org/wiki/Image:Ota_Benga_at_ Bronx_Zoo.jpg. Image in the public domain due to expired copyright.

Mr. Douglas on the Lincoln/Douglas Debates

I confined myself closely to those three positions which he [Lincoln] had taken, controverting his proposition that this Union could not exist as our fathers made it, divided into free and slave States, controverting his proposition of a crusade against the Supreme Court because of the **Dred Scott decision**, and controverting his proposition that the Declaration of Independence included and meant the Negroes as well as the White men, when it declared all men to be created equal (transcripts of all seven Lincoln/Douglas Debates, 1858, retrieved March 11, 2009, from http://www.nps.gov/archive/liho/debate1.htm).

Dred Scott

According to Douglas, slavery led to the question of whether or not the union would survive. It was the focus of the infamous Supreme Court decision against Dred Scott [1795–1858] (Figure 12–2).

Also, slavery was the sole reason for the absurd claim that the phrase "all men" did not include black Africans. Slavery was the central issue of the Lincoln-Douglas debates. Details aside, in the famed Dred Scott decision of 1857, the U.S. Supreme Court ruled 7 to 2 against the Scott family. According to Chief Justice Roger Brooke

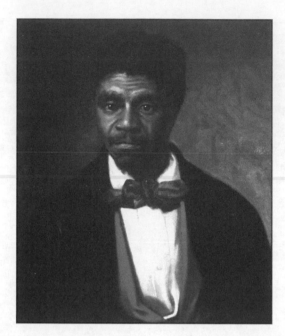

Figure 12–2. Dred Scott circa 1856. Retrieved March 11, 2009, from http://en.wikipedia.org/wiki/Image:DredScott.jpg. Image in the public domain due to expired copyright.

Taney [1777-1864; pronounced "tawney" which rhymes with "brawney" rather than "brainy"], the son of slave-holding tobacco farmers in Maryland (Figure 12–3; Taney, 1864/2007, retrieved March 9, 2009, from http://en.wikipedia.org/wiki/Roger_Taney), ruled that even a

> free Negro of the African race, whose ancestors were brought to this country and sold as slaves, is not a "citizen" within the meaning of the Constitution of the United States. (see the full text of this amazing U.S. Supreme Court decision, Cornell University Law School, 1857/n.d., retrieved March 9, 2009, from http://www.law.cornell.edu/supct/html/historics/USSC_CR_0060_0393_ZS.html)

Interestingly, the record shows that less than a year before the end of the Civil War, Maryland voted to abolish slavery and Taney died the very same day on October 12, 1864.

The Assassination of Lincoln and Slavery

It is also noteworthy that the issue of slavery was, according to the evidence, a principle motive for Booth in Lincoln's assassination (see Norton, 1996, retrieved March 9, 2009, from http://home.att.net/~rjnorton/Lincoln75.html). The historical record shows that John

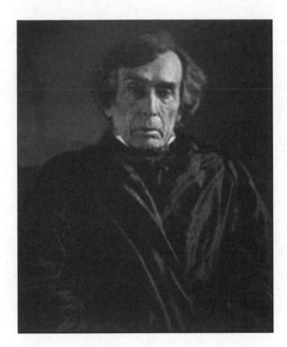

Figure 12–3. Roger B. Taney, Chief Justice of the Supreme Court who wrote the Dred Scott decision. Retrieved March 11, 2009, from http://en.wikipedia.org/w iki/Image:Roger_Taney.jpg. Image in the public domain due to expired copyright.

Wilkes Booth [1838–1865] was present along with one of his conspirators at an impromptu speech Lincoln gave on April 11, 1865. In that speech at the White House, when Lincoln said he wanted African Americans to be granted the right to vote in America, "Booth turned to Lewis Powell and urged him to shoot the President on the spot. Powell refused. Booth (Linder, 2002) said it would be the last speech Lincoln would ever make" (retrieved March 9, 2009, from http://www.law.umkc.edu/faculty/projects/ftrials/linco lnconspiracy/lincolnaccount.html; also see Booth, 1865, retrieved March 9, 2009, from http://en.wikipedia.org/wiki/John_Wilkes_Booth). And so it was. Booth shot and killed Lincoln on April 14, 1865.

It can be argued that advocacy of equal rights for black Africans cost Lincoln his life. Perhaps more importantly from the historical point of view—and because of claims that the American Civil War was mainly about "issues other than slavery" especially the preservation of the Union (e.g., see DiLorenzo, 2003, retrieved March 9, 2009, from http://www.lewrockwell.com/dilorenzo/d ilorenzo37.html)—it is important to bear in mind that Lincoln plainly said in his first inaugural address in 1861 that the impending American Civil War between the seceding states and the Union was caused by slavery. Referring to the Union and the secessionists as different "sections" Lincoln wrote:

One section believes slavery is right, and ought to be extended [to other territories or to non-slave States]; while the other believes it is wrong, and ought not to be extended. This is the only substantial dispute (see Lincoln, 1861b, retrieved March 9, 2009, from http://everything2.com/index.pl?node_id=468294)

Preserving the Union

It is true that Lincoln said that the official purpose of the war was the preservation of the Union and it is also true that he subordinated the slavery issue to the main goal of preserving the Union. He said in a letter to Horace Greeley, editor of the *New York Tribune*, August 22, 1862 (see the entire text of the short letter, parts of which are quoted below, retrieved March 9, 2009, from http://showcase .netins.net/web/creative/lincoln/speeches/greeley.htm):

As to the policy I "seem to be pursuing" as you say, I have not meant to leave any one in doubt.

I would save the Union. If there be those who would not save the Union, unless they could at the same time save slavery, I do not agree with them. If there be those who would not save the Union unless they could at the same time destroy slavery, I do not agree with them. My paramount object in this struggle is to save the Union, and is not either to save or to destroy slavery. . . .

The Less Quoted Statement

In the less often quoted final sentence of his letter to Greeley, however, Lincoln said:

I have here stated my purpose according to my view of official duty; and I intend no modification of my oft-expressed personal wish that all men everywhere could be free.

In fact, according to the same authority and source, at the time the letter was written to Greeley explaining Lincoln's official policy on the war, "a draft of the **Emancipation Proclamation** already lay in his [Lincoln's] desk" (Figure 12–4).

The Threat to the Union: Slavery

Although the official purpose for prosecuting a war is not necessarily the same as the factors leading up to it, the question of restoring the Union would not have come up except for the fact that slavery was supported by a minority of States which were also willing to secede.

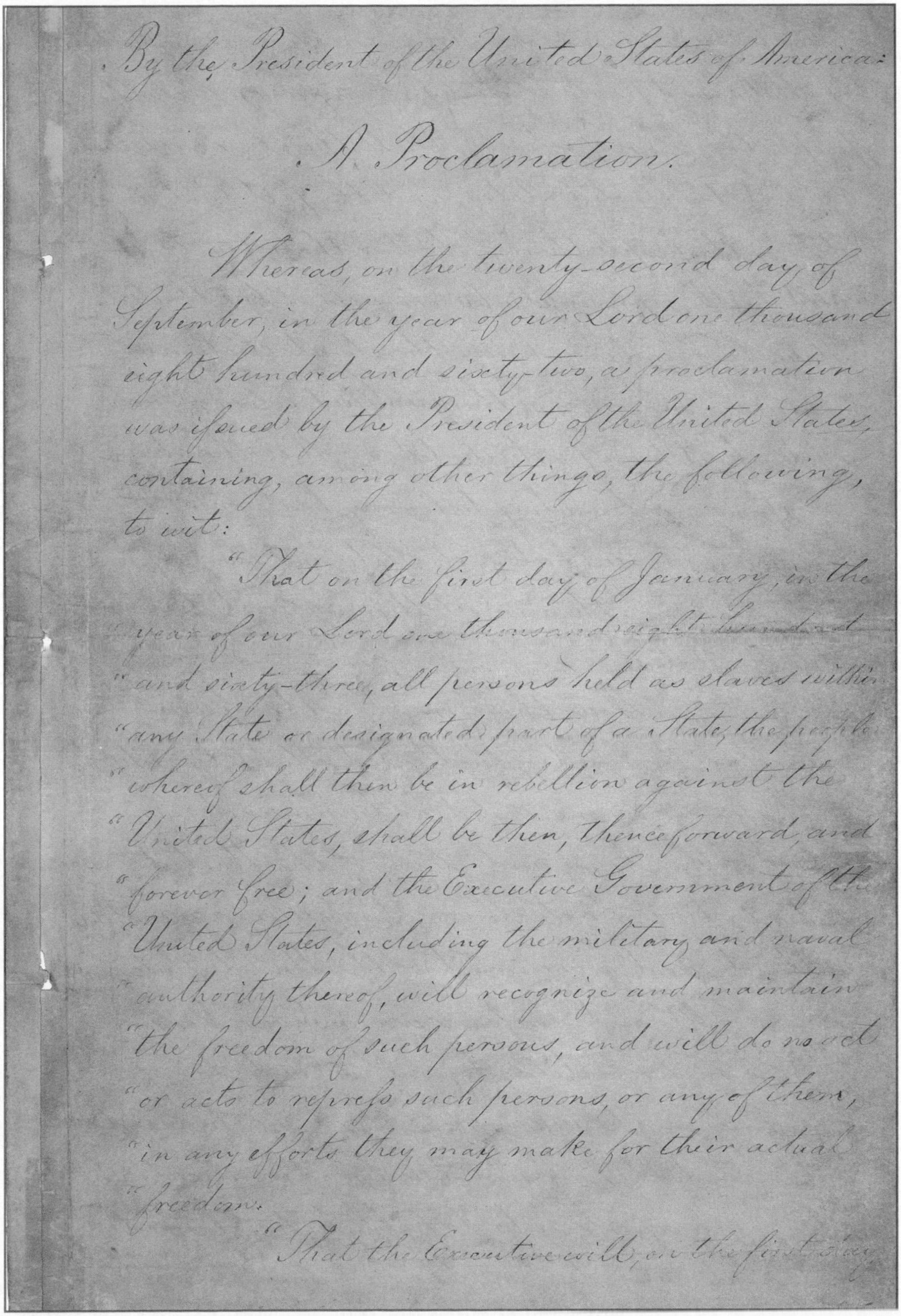

By the President of the United States of America:

A Proclamation.

Whereas, on the twenty-second day of September, in the year of our Lord one thousand eight hundred and sixty-two, a proclamation was issued by the President of the United States, containing, among other things, the following, to wit:

"That on the first day of January, in the year of our Lord one thousand eight hundred and sixty-three, all persons held as slaves within "any State or designated part of a State, the people "whereof shall then be in rebellion against the "United States, shall be then, thenceforward, and "forever free; and the Executive Government of the "United States, including the military and naval "authority thereof, will recognize and maintain "the freedom of such persons, and will do no act "or acts to repress such persons, or any of them, "in any efforts they may make for their actual "freedom.

"That the Executive will, on the first day

Figure 12–4. The first page of the Emancipation Proclamation of January 1, 1863. Public domain image. Retrieved March 11, 2009, from http://www.archives.gov/exhibits/featured_documents/emancipation_proclamation/. United States National Archives and Records Administration photo in the public domain.

With respect to the common claim that the Civil War was mainly about economics, it is necessary to realize that the great plantation industries of tobacco, sugar cane, and cotton were as profitable as they were in large part because of slavery. It must also be remembered that in the Lincoln-Douglas debates, according to Douglas who favored slavery, all of his major points according to his own final summary in the seventh debate were about Lincoln's opposition to slavery. More particularly, Lincoln opposed efforts to extend it. Slavery was the foremost issue in the Lincoln-Douglas debates and the crisis he predicted actually occurred. It was the American Civil War—the costliest conflict in American history. And as Colin Powell noted in an interview on Larry King Live, on June 28, 2007, the struggle for equality isn't over yet. The Union, however, was not lost.

The key outcomes of the American Civil War that ended in 1865 were *the preservation of the Union* and *the abolition of slavery*.

The results of the American Civil War—the preservation of the Union and the abolition of slavery—set the stage for a more humane treatment of all human beings—including individuals with disabilities. It was a decisive but not a final victory in the ongoing struggle for freedom and equality of all human beings. It set the stage for a series of smaller victories and advances in the courts and in the legislatures in favor of the rights of all minorities including those with disabilities. The victory of the free States in the Civil War was a victory for all human beings, and it was crucial to the recognition of the rights of persons with disabilities. The body and the mind really are, so long as a person is alive, intimately connected. To harm one is to damage the other, and the struggle for freedom on both sides—for the body and the mind—was not over yet.

THE LONG ROAD TOWARD EQUALITY UNDER THE LAW

The "War Between the States," as the American Civil War is sometimes referred to, did not end racial discrimination in the United States by a long shot. The famous case of *Plessy v. Ferguson, 163 U.S. 537* (see below) that began in New Orleans and ended in the Supreme Court in 1896 showed that racial injustices stemming from slavery continued long after the Civil War ended.

In some states, segregation was still approved by law, 31 years after the end of the Civil War, and 33 years after the Emancipation Proclamation. In fact, in 1896, almost four decades after the Taney court ruled that Dred Scott and his family—and descendants of slaves in general—were not citizens of the United States and that they had no rights under the Constitution, the U.S. Supreme Court upheld the so-called "separate but equal" provisions allowing segregation by race. It would be 58 years before this landmark case would be overturned. In the meantime, it stood in the way of any real advances on behalf of persons of minority language/dialect background and of persons with communication disorders. Whether by race or by any other perceived limitation, real or not, the segregation laws asserted that some people were inferior and not fit to be included in the "mainstream."

As we will see, the insidious idea that some people are just not suited to be treated as human beings dies hard. The implications of this idea for many persons with disabilities were, in the 20th century, more than just debilitating—the consequences were fatal.

The "Separate But Equal" Jim Crow Laws

The **separate but equal** provision in Louisiana was supposed to mean that the State could provide "separate" accommodations for Blacks and Whites as long as the accommodations were "equal." The whole class of such laws is commonly referred to as **Jim Crow laws** (1876–1965, retrieved March 9, 2009, from http://en.wikipedia .org/wiki/Jim_Crow_laws) after a popular song titled "Jump Jim Crow" performed by a White comedian named Thomas Dartmouth (T. D.) "Daddy" Rice in black face make-up from about 1828 (retrieved March 9, 2009, from http://en.wikipedia.org/wiki/Ju mp_Jim_Crow).

Plessy v. Ferguson (1896)

A few decades after the Civil War, the Jim Crow laws were still firmly in place in some states and Louisiana was one of them.

Separate But Hardly Equal

Homer A. Plessy was a man of mixed race, one-eighth African American, who was not permitted to take a seat in a railroad car reserved for "White" people in Louisiana. He was arrested and fined $300 by the Louisiana Judge John Howard Ferguson. Plessy continued to appeal his case until it was heard in 1896 by the U.S. Supreme Court. In a 7 to 1 decision the court ruled against Plessy and in favor of the racial discrimination permitted by the Jim Crow laws. The lone dissenter was Justice John Marshall Harlan [1833–1911], himself a Kentucky-born son of slave-holders (see Harlan, 1896, retrieved March 11, 2009, from http://www.michaelariens.com/ConLaw/justices/har an.htm). He compared the 1896 decision in *Plessy v. Ferguson* to the *Dred Scott* decision of 1857.

The Dred Scott verdict was never overturned in court but it was reversed on the battlefield and subsequently by the Emancipation Proclamation. However, in 1896 Justice Harlan stood alone against the "separate but equal" law in Louisiana. He wrote:

The thin disguise of "equal" accommodations for passengers in railroad coaches will not mislead any one, nor atone for the wrong this day done [see Harlan, 1896].

> . . . such legislation . . . is inconsistent not only with that equality of rights which pertains to citizenship, national and state, but with the personal liberty enjoyed by every one within the United States. . . .

DISABILITIES IN THE BACKGROUND

Laws throughout history have been the result of conflicts and especially after they were established, there have always been many different ways to violate, interpret, and apply them. For all of these reasons, we have courts to decide disputes. In America, ever since the Civil War, and more recently since World War II, laws and court cases have sought more and more to protect groups and individuals from racial discrimination. As a result, victories won against slavery also enabled advances in the treatment of persons with disabilities.

Although we might wish that laws would be enacted on the basis of high moral considerations, or that they would at least be logically consistent, that is not the way the law commonly works.

Different judges often give different rulings and may seem, on occasion, to reverse their own decisions. In what follows, we review laws and landmark court cases in the United States that have directly or indirectly impacted the treatment of persons with communication problems and disorders.

The Warren Court: *Brown v. Board of Education* (1954)

The *Plessy v. Ferguson* (1896) defense of the "separate but equal" provisions—also known as "the Jim Crow laws"—would stand another 58 years until Chief Justice Earl Warren [1891–1974] delivered the final opinion in the case of *Brown v. Board of Education, 347 U.S. 483* (1954). This time the judgment was unanimous *against* the "separate but equal" laws—especially as they applied in education.

Brown v. Board of Education involved a fifth-grade African American girl, Linda Brown, who was not permitted to enroll in a White elementary school in Topeka, Kansas. The case was argued by Brown's Attorney Thurgood Marshall, who would become the first African American Justice of the U.S. Supreme Court in 1967, 110 years after the *Dred Scott* decision. Although *Brown v. Board of Education* concerned racial discrimination, the case would serve as a foundational precedent with respect to persons with disabilities.

Chief Justice Warren put the unanimous 1954 ruling of the court succinctly:

Jim Crow Laws Finally Overturned

We conclude that, in the field of public education, the doctrine of "separate but equal" has no place. Separate educational facilities are inherently unequal. Therefore, we hold that the plaintiffs and others similarly situated for whom the actions have been brought are, by reason of the segregation complained of, deprived of the equal protection of the laws guaranteed by the Fourteenth Amendment (347 U.S. 483, 496) (retrieved March 11, 2009, from http://www.nationalcenter.org/brown.html).

The "equal protection" guarantee referred to by Justice Warren says "no state shall make or enforce any law which shall abridge the privileges or immunities of citizens of the United States . . . nor deny to any person within its jurisdiction the equal protection of the laws" (Fourteenth Amendment to the U.S. Constitution). The Fourteenth Amendment became part of the Bill of Rights after the Civil War, but the Fifth Amendment supposedly already assured "due process of law" to all citizens.

Reiterating the Fourteenth Amendment

It was only because African Americans had not been treated as citizens prior to the Civil War that "equal protection" clause of the Fourteenth Amendment was deemed necessary. The Warren Court clarified in *Brown v. Board of Education* that "any language in *Plessy v. Ferguson* contrary to this finding is rejected" (see "The National Center for Public Policy Research," n. d., retrieved March 11, 2009, from http://www.nationalcenter.org/brown.html).

One of the inevitable implications, a significant **legal precedent**, of Chief Justice Warren's ruling was that **"pull-out" programs** for persons with disabilities—ones that placed them outside of the mainstream of public education—would end up in conflict with *Brown v. Board of Education* (1954).

Civil Rights Act 1964

After the Warren decision, another decade would pass before the Civil Rights Act of 1964 (**Public Law 88-352**) would effectively generalize the rejection of the "separate but equal" provisions for all possible cases in the United States. The Civil Rights Act of 1964 (retrieved March 11, 2009, from http://en.wikipedia.org/wiki/Civil_Rights_Act_of_1964) was among the first of several broad acts of law impacting the assessment and treatment of persons with communication disorders. In particular its main purposes were to "enforce" the right to vote, to enable District Courts of the United States (Figure 12–5 shows how the districts are organized; retrieved March 11, 2009, from http://www.uscourts.gov/images/Circuit Map.pdf) to enforce the ban against discrimination in public accommodations (the illegal continued practice of segregation), to authorize the Attorney General to institute suits to protect constitutional rights in public facilities and public education, to extend the Commission on Civil Rights, to prevent discrimination in federally assisted programs, to establish a Commission on Equal Employment Opportunity, and for other purposes.

In particular Title VII of that act prohibited tests resulting in the "disparate" treatment of minorities as defined by "race, color,

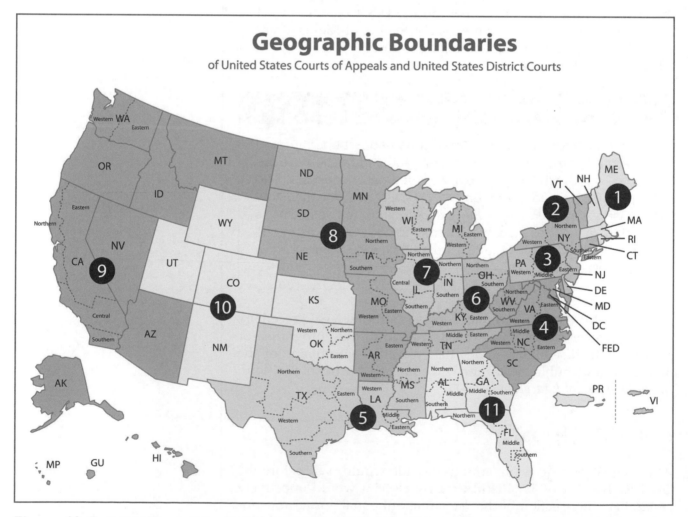

Figure 12–5. Jurisdictions of the United States Courts of Appeals and District Courts. Retrieved March 11, 2009, from http://www.uscourts.gov/courtlinks/. United States Courts publication in the public domain.

religion, sex, or national origin" and especially if those tests could be shown to "adversely affect" an individual's "status as an employee or as an applicant for employment" (section 2000e-2). A common rule for assessing disparate impact came from rules published 14 years later by the Equal Employment Opportunity Commission (1978, 29 C. F. R. Section 1607.4D). According to their so-called "80% rule," a disparate impact is found if the success rate of any protected group is less than four-fifths of the success rate of non-minority individuals (usually White males).

Hobson v. Hansen (1967)

In the case of *Hobson v. Hansen* (1967), Carl Hansen was the Super-intendent of Schools in Washington, D.C. The claim by Hobson and others concerned the **ability tracking system** of the schools. The plaintiff argued that tests used to establish ability groups (also called "tracks") were biased because the tests were normed against White, middle-class data samples.

    The District Court ruled that indeed the tests were inappropri-ate for low socioeconomic groups including African American stu-dents, and the court abolished the tracking system. Circuit Judge J. Skelly Wright ruled in *Hobson v. Hansen* (1967) against using tests to create ability tracking systems (269 F. Supp. 401, District Court of the District of Columbia, 1967). The importance of *Hobson v. Hansen* for special education and communication disorders was that it challenged the classification of children as mentally retarded on the basis of IQ tests normed on children of different linguistic and cultural backgrounds. However, the use of such tests remains the basis for the definition of mental retardation according to the American Psychiatric Association and other professional groups to this day.

The importance of *Hobson v. Hansen* for special education and communication disorders was that it challenged the classification of children as mentally retarded on the basis of IQ tests normed on children of different linguistic and cultural backgrounds.

Diana v. Board of Education (1970)

The case of *Diana v. California State Board of Education* (1970), involved nine families affected by the practice of testing children in English, a language/dialect that they did not know very well, on account of the fact that their native language was in fact Spanish (*Diana v. California State Board of Education*, No. C-70 37 RFP, District Court of Northern California, February, 1970).

Valid Placement Requires Valid Assessment

Diana was just one of the many non-English-speaking children affected by this practice. In fact, she was placed in a program for the mentally retarded on the basis of scores on an IQ test in English. The scores really only showed that Diana hardly knew any English. School personnel did not need an IQ test to discover that she did not speak English, but their conclusion that she was also retarded was the basis for the suit. The question was, how can a valid judgment about mental ability be made in a language the person being tested cannot understand?

Interestingly, the case was decided out of court. It was obvious that no one can perform at peak intellectual capacity in a language they do not know or that they do not know very well. The **consent decree** allowed non-English speaking individuals the prerogative of being tested in their stronger language—which might well not be English. Although the plaintiffs were Spanish speakers, the decree set an important legal precedent for speakers of any one of the 6,911 languages other than English in the world (Ethnologue, 2009). Children from any one of those other languages could conceivably end up in an American classroom. The *Diana* case plainly showed several things:

1. That a diagnosis of mental retardation is not a desirable outcome.
2. That speakers of minority languages are at risk of a false diagnosis of disorder(s).
3. That a false diagnosis of any disorder(s) based on an invalid or inappropriate testing procedure is unjust.

. . . the Diana case forced the California Board of Education representing the most populous state in the United States to acknowledge that a false diagnosis of mental retardation based on an invalid assessment procedure would not stand up in court.

The most important outcome for the future of communication disorders and their diagnosis was the fact that the *Diana* case forced the California Board of Education representing the most populous state in the United States to acknowledge that a false diagnosis of mental retardation based on an invalid assessment procedure would not stand up in court. *Diana* was soon followed by court decisions in Pennsylvania and in Washington, DC.

PARC v. Pennsylvania (1972)

In *PARC v. Pennsylvania* (1972) a class action was undertaken on behalf of all mentally retarded persons in the State of Pennsylvania less than 21 years of age (334 F.Supp. 1257, E.D. PA 1972). The plaintiff was the Pennsylvania Association of Retarded Children (PARC). As a result of this action, certain laws of Pennsylvania were struck down as unconstitutional on account of denying a **free and appropriate public education** (**FAPE**) to all mentally retarded persons in the state (retrieved March 11, 2009, from http://www.faculty.piercelaw.edu/redfield/library/Pdf/case-parc.pennsylvania.pdf). One outcome was the definition of a FAPE—a concept that would be written into subsequent laws by the U.S. Congress. *PARC* also clarified that public education—within reasonable limits of acceptable behavior in schools—is supposed to be not only free and appropriate but also equally available to all students.

Certain laws of Pennsylvania were struck down as unconstitutional on account of not providing a FAPE to all mentally retarded persons in Pennsylvania. The ruling was that mentally retarded persons could not be denied educational opportunities provided by law to other citizens—retarded citizens were equal to nonretarded under the law. Thus, for any child already in a separate program, a pull-out or non-mainstream program, the court required review by Special Masters of the Court of the "educational histories and the educational diagnosis" (Section IV, paragraph 48, p. 14). This review was required for all persons identified as mentally retarded or thought to be mentally retarded between the ages of 4 and 21. It further required "automatic re-evaluation every two years of any educational assignment other than to a regular class" and "an annual re-evaluation at the request of the child's parent or guardian" as well as "an opportunity for a hearing" for anyone not satisfied with the process (Section III, paragraph 12, p. 5).

The State of Pennsylvania was given only 90 days to "identify, locate, [and] evaluate" all persons qualified for relief under the Court Order issued June 18, 1971 (Section IV, paragraph 48, p. 14). The clear intention of the court was to avoid the placing of children who are capable of learning in "dead-end" programs from which no one could be expected to benefit.

The principle in *PARC v. Pennsylvania* was that children should be placed according to the highest level of their abilities to benefit from education and training.

Mills v. Board of Education of the District of Columbia (1972)

In *Mills v. Board of Education*, DC, 348 F.Supp. 866 (D. DC, 1972) a class action was initiated against the District of Columbia schools (retrieved March 11, 2009, from http://www.faculty.piercelaw.edu/redfield/library/Pdf/case-mills.boe.pdf). It directly involved seven "exceptional" children whose parents alleged they had been excluded from the District of Columbia Public Schools and who asked the court to compel the district "to provide them with immediate and adequate education and educational facilities in the public schools or alternative placement [in private schools or tutorial programs] at public expense." The children involved in the suit had been "labeled as behavioral problems, mentally retarded, emotionally disturbed or hyperactive." The presiding judge, District Judge Joseph C. Waddy, generalized the class action to all "exceptional" children in the DC schools:

> The genesis of this case is found (1) in the failure of the District of Columbia to provide publicly supported education and training to plaintiffs and other "exceptional" children, members of their class, and (2) the excluding, suspending, expelling, reassigning and transferring of "exceptional" children from regular public school classes without affording them due process of law.

Quoting from *Brown v. Board of Education* (347 U.S. 483, 493, 1954) Judge Waddy added his own emphasis:

> In these days, it is doubtful that any child may reasonably be expected to succeed in life if he is denied the opportunity of an education. Such an opportunity, where the state has undertaken to provide it, is a right which must be made available to all on equal terms. (348 F. Supp. 866, p. 3)

It is noteworthy that in this and other landmark cases, the deeper issue has always been equality of treatment under the law and the equal opportunity to pursue life, liberty, and happiness—propositions made clear in the American Declaration of Independence of 1776.

As a precedent of **case law**—the kind of law that is created by interpretations of legislation by judges, also known as **jurisprudence** —*Mills v. the Board of Education* argued that public education should prepare individuals for success in life. Judge Waddy's ruling reminds us of Dr. Samuel Howe's aim to provide deaf-blind individuals with access to language and literacy so they could, among other things, be employed.

In Samuel Howe's day the education of exceptional children was considered an act of kindness and philanthropy. By 1972, it had become, in Washington, DC at least, a legal responsibility of public education created more or less, rightly or wrongly, by jurisprudence.

Rehabilitation Act of 1973

The **Rehabilitation Act of 1973** (HR 8070, **Public Law 93-112**), especially in Section 504, explicitly extended certain protections of the Civil Rights Act to persons with a "disability" provided only that they were associated with programs, activities or agencies receiving "Federal financial assistance." Remedies provided in the Civil Rights Act were also made explicitly applicable to cases brought by or on behalf of persons with disabilities. This law supposedly provided teeth to be used against violators. However, there would be certain critical contests where the bite of those teeth left no marks on the offending educational agencies. For instance, in the case of *Smith v. Robinson* (1979, 1984) which is discussed below, the U.S. Supreme Court refused to apply section 504 of the Rehabilitation Act of 1973 to enable the offended party, the Smith family, in that case, to recover the attorneys' fees that were incurred in pursuing the remedies supposedly provided by that section of the law. The Smiths won the court contest but were not awarded the cost of their trouble. But the Rehabilitation Act of 1973 was just the beginning of the laws on the complex issues at stake.

Lau v. Nichols (1974)

In *Lau v. Nichols* (1974) the San Francisco School System was sued for failing to provide comprehensible instruction to about 1,800 Chinese speaking students. Lower courts had twice denied the plaintiffs any relief, but the case eventually found its way to the U.S. Supreme Court. The highest court ruled in 1974:

The failure of the San Francisco school system to provide English language instruction to approximately 1,800 students of Chinese ancestry who do not speak English, or to provide them with other adequate instructional procedures, denies them a meaningful opportunity to participate in the public educational program and thus violates 601 of the Civil Rights Act of 1964 . . . (414 U.S. 563; retrieved March 11, 2009, from http://caselaw.lp .findlaw.com/scripts/getcase.pl?court=US&vol=414 &invol=563)

This was perhaps the most important case up to that time where a public education system felt the bite of the teeth provided to courts under the Civil Rights Act of 1964. It is interesting that this suit was the first to assert plainly in the words of Chief Justice Douglas that language skills are at the heart of learning.

The Core of Public Education

Basic English skills are at the very core of what these public schools teach. Imposition of a requirement that, before a child can effectively participate in the educational program, he must already have acquired those basic skills is to make a mockery of public education. We know that those who do not understand English are certain to find their classroom experiences wholly incomprehensible and in no way meaningful (414 U.S. 563).

Lau v. Nichols established as a principle of law the fact that access to education depends critically on the ability to understand the language of instruction. For that reason, the decision in *Lau v. Nichols* is important to persons and groups whose native language/ dialect, or manner of communication (e.g., manual signed language versus speech) is not the one used in the classroom. It also has the effect of imposing special burdens on public schools. *Lau v. Nichols* clarified that the responsibility for enabling access to a FAPE falls on the public schools rather than on the children who might not understand the language of instruction. The court did not assign the responsibility to the parents of the child, but rather to the schools. It follows by implication that the public schools have the essential responsibility to educate with equity and impartiality those individuals who happen to have some communication disorder.

Lau v. Nichols established as a principle of law the fact that access to education depends critically on the ability to understand the language of instruction.

Education for All Handicapped Children Act, 1975

The **Education for All Handicapped Children Act of 1975** was also known as **Public Law 94-142** (see the full text of the original law retrieved March 11, 2009, from http://users.rcn.com/peregrin.enteract/ add/94-142.txt; also on the DVD). The **EAHCA**, more commonly abbreviated as **EHA**, was an incentive program offering funding to states that already had "in effect a policy that assures all handicapped children the right to a free appropriate public education" (Section 2A). With respect to communication problems it covered:

> specific learning disabilities . . . [of] those children who have a disorder in one or more of the basic psychological processes understanding or in using language, spoken or written, which disorder may manifest itself in imperfect ability to listen, think, speak, read, write, spell, or do mathematical calculations. Such disorders include such conditions as perceptual handicaps, brain injury, minimal brain dysfunction, dyslexia, and developmental aphasia. Such term does not include children who have learning problems which are primarily the result of visual, hearing, or motor handicaps, of mental retardation, of emotional disturbance, or environmental, cultural, or economic disadvantage. (Section 4A)

A Promisory Note

EHA was largely a promisory note from the Federal Government for phased in increasing co-payments from the Federal Government only to the States complying with the eligibility requirements. The allocation of funds was to begin with the Federal Government paying 10% of the costs associated with compliance in 1979 and increasing in 10% increments up to a maximum of 40% of the total costs in 1982. The rest of the funding had to come from State and **local educational agencies (LEAs)**. At the beginning for every 10 cents spent by the U.S. Federal Government the State or LEA would have to come up with 90 cents. The law covered children between ages 3 through 18 until September 1, 1978 and then extended to cover through age 21 by September 1, 1980.

Defined a FAPE

The EHA better known by its number as PL 94-142, formally defined a "free and appropriate public education" (FAPE) as:

> special education and related services which (A) have been provided at public expense, under public supervision and direction, and without charge, (B) meet the standards of the State educational agency, (C) include an appropriate preschool, elementary, or secondary school education in the State involved, and (D) are provided in conformity with the **individualized education program** . . .

The IEP

The mandated "individualized education program" (**IEP**), a concept which would be carried forward in subsequent legislation, especially in the **Americans with Disabilities Act of 1990** (see below), was a written statement for each exceptional child developed in

1. a meeting including
   a. a qualified representative of the school or any other recipient of federal money,
   b. the teacher,
   c. the parents or guardian of the child, and,
   d. if possible the child,
2. and the statement had to include descriptions of
   a. the present levels of educational performance of the child,
   b. annual goals, including short-term instructional objectives,
   c. the specific educational services to be provided, and
   d. the extent to which the child will be included in regular educational programs, and must also include
3. the start-up date for the program and its expected duration (i.e., implying a point of exit from the program), along with
4. appropriate objective criteria, evaluation procedures, and schedules for determining, at least on an annual basis, whether or not the objectives are being achieved.

Least Restrictive Environment

To qualify for federal funds beginning at 10% of costs in 1979, States had to show that children with disabilities had optimal access to the mainstream opportunities and that so-called "pull-out" programs were used only when the nature of the impairment demanded it. The clause stated what we call the **mainstreaming principle**— which, in later versions of this legislation would be referred to as the **least restrictive environment** principle.

In keeping with the principle what are commonly called "pull-out programs"—separate special education classrooms or facilities —were discouraged as follows:

> . . . special classes, separate schooling, or other removal of handicapped children from the regular educational environment occurs only when the nature or severity of the handicap is such that education in regular classes with the use of supplementary aids and services cannot be achieved satisfactorily. (clause 5B under "Eligibility")

Fair Assessment

EHA required "procedures to assure that testing and evaluation materials and procedures utilized for the purposes of evaluation and placement of handicapped children will be selected and administered so as not to be racially or culturally discriminatory" (clause 5C under "Eligibility"). The EHA left two large loopholes: For one, EHA exempted all States where "the application of such requirements would be inconsistent with State law or practice, or the order of any court, respecting public education within such age groups in the State" (PL 94-142, clause 2B under "Eligibility"), and for another it did not cover many categories of communication disorders.

Clause 5B under "Eligibility" states that: to the maximum extent appropriate, handicapped children, including children in public or private institutions or other care facilities, are educated with children who are not handicapped.

The connection between the civil rights of diverse minority groups and those of individuals with disabilities was made more evident than ever before with the passage of Public Law 94-142 in 1975. But that law would eventually be transformed into a much more comprehensive package. In the meantime, some important legal battles would be slugged out in the courts. Those battles would help to shape the development of subsequent laws. In the sections that follow, we concentrate mainly on U.S. Supreme Court cases and a few others that helped to shape national policies and laws impacting the treatment of persons with communication disorders.

University of California Regents v. Bakke (1978)

Reverse Discrimination
An important case showing how conflicted the law and its interpretation can be was the *University of California Regents v. Bakke* (1978). It concerned whether or not a person of majority language and racial status could be discriminated against in favor of less well qualified minority status individuals on account of race (see the entire text of this case retrieved March 11, 2009, from http://caselaw.lp.findlaw.com/scripts/getca se.pl?court=US&vol=438&invol=265).

Mr. Alan Bakke, a White male, sought admission to the School of Medicine at the University of California at Davis in 1973 and 1974 but was denied both times in spite of the fact that his record was stronger than the record of certain minority individuals who were admitted in both of those years.

During that time, the University of California had two admission policies and programs—a relatively lenient one for minority applicants, and a stiffer set of requirements for everyone else (especially White male applicants). Bakke claimed that he was excluded,

> on the basis of his race in violation of the Equal Protection Clause of the Fourteenth Amendment, a provision of the California Constitution, and 601 of Title VI of the Civil Rights Act of 1964. (438 U.S. 265)

When the case was heard by the California Supreme Court, it held that the University of California's "special admissions program violated the Equal Protection Clause" (438 U.S. 265) and it ruled that taking race into consideration was unlawful and ordered the University to admit Mr. Bakke. The State of California then appealed to the U.S. Supreme Court which affirmed the lower California court by ordering the University of California at Davis to admit Mr. Bakke and by invalidating the "special admissions program" for minority applicants (438 U.S. 265, 267). However, in a delicate balancing act, the U.S. Supreme Court reversed the lower California Supreme Court with respect to prohibiting the University of California, and, by implication any other institution of higher education "from taking race into account as a factor in its future admissions decisions" (438 U.S. 265).

In *Bakke*, the U.S. Supreme Court said that excluding a person on account of race is not allowed, but taking race into account in encouraging diversity is allowed. The permission to consider race as a factor was justified for "the purpose of overcoming substantial, chronic minority under representation in the medical profession." In another place the Court justified taking race into account on the basis of prior law which allowed considering race "where there is reason to believe that the evil addressed is a product of past racial discrimination" (retrieved March 11, 2009, from http://caselaw.lp.findlaw.com/scripts/getcase.pl?court=US&vol=438&invol=265).

Board of Education of New York v. Harris (1979)

In the *Board of Education of New York v. Harris* (1979), New York had been sued by Harris, Secretary for the U.S. Department of Health, Education, and Welfare (HEW; later replaced by the Department of Education) for disparate impact under Title VI of the Civil Rights Act of 1964. HEW presented **prima facie evidence**—evidence on its first appearance—of discrimination in hiring and dismissal of minority employees by the Board of Education of New York. The evidence showed racially disproportionate assignment of teachers. The evidence against the Board of Education was not considered sufficient in district court, but the U.S. Department of HEW appealed to the U.S. Supreme Court and won (584 F.2d 576).

The Supreme Court ruled in favor of HEW that the evidence could not be dismissed by New York's claim that there was no intention to discriminate. Rather, the Board of Education of New York had to show either that there was no discrimination or that there was a lawful and compelling reason for the different treatment of racial minority teachers. New York did not do that. Therefore, the Supreme Court affirmed that New York had discriminated under the Civil Rights Act of 1964 (444 U.S. 130, 1979).

The precedent for persons with communication disorders is that States and educational agencies cannot justify discrimination by arguing that it was unintentional.

Parents in Action on Special Education (PASE) v. Hannon (1980)

In *Parents in Action on Special Education (PASE) v. Hannon* (1980) the Chicago Public Schools represented by Hannon et al. were sued in a class action by PASE (506 F. Supp. 831 U.S. District Court for the Northern District of Illinois). The suit concerned the disproportionate number of African American children who were placed in special education classes on the basis of IQ tests. The court examined the three tests relied on by Chicago Public Schools in detail. The tests in question were the *Wechsler Intelligence Scale for Children, Wechsler Intelligence Scale for Children-Revised,* and the *Stanford-Binet IQ Tests.* Although 9 of 488 items were judged to be biased against African American children, according to the judge's evaluation, the IQ tests were fair, and the schools had conformed to the requirements of applicable law, notably the Civil Rights Act of 1964.

We mention this case because it resulted in an outcome opposite to that of *Larry P. v. Riles* which was heard in California in the U.S. Court of Appeals four years later. We are coming to that story, but we note in advance that the placement decisions based on IQ tests in Illinois were allowed to stand in 1980 though they would be disallowed in 1984 in California.

Guardians v. Civil Service Commission of New York City (1983)

In the case of the *Guardians Association v. Civil Service Commission of New York City* (1983) African American and Hispanic police officers protested that New York City Police Department was unfair in using test scores as the basis for hiring and firing on account of disparate impact—discrimination—under the Civil Rights Act of 1964. The District Court under its judgment of violations of Title VI awarded the police officers seniority, back pay, medical and insurance benefits, and the opportunity to take promotional examinations to which their court ordered seniority would entitle them. Under Title VII the City of New York was ordered to use approaches to employment in the future that were nondiscriminatory. Under Title VII any evaluation procedures must be shown to be job-related. The Court of Appeals, on that basis, affirmed under Title VII, but reversed the lower court with respect to the Title VI awards because the Guardians had not provided proof of discriminatory intention as required by Title VI.

The U.S. Supreme Court heard the case on a **petition for certiorare** (463 U.S. 582, 1983)—a request to review the decision of the lower court—and in a carefully argued decision affirmed the decision of the U.S. Court of Appeals for the Second Circuit (No. 81-431). Perhaps the most important outcome of the Supreme Court decision was the notion that compensatory relief would be limited to cases where the offending party could be shown to have intended to discriminate. An example where this requirement was clearly met in a case heard before a lower court is that of *Doe v. Withers* (1992) (see below) where monetary compensation and puni-

> To punish an individual for discrimination, the law requires proof that the individual discriminated intentionally. However, to punish an agency of government intention to discriminate is not required. The agency cannot legally discriminate at all.

tive damages were both awarded to a young man with a learning disability who was subjected to deliberate discriminatory treatment by one of his high school teachers. To demonstrate discrimination by a State, or an organization, proving intention is not necessary as the U.S. Supreme Court ruled in the case of the *Board of Education of New York v. Harris* (1979). However, if punitive damages are sought against an individual, the higher standard of intentional discrimination must be met.

In the next case we will consider, *Larry P. v. Riles*, which went to the U.S. Court of Appeals for the Ninth Circuit in 1984, the standard of intentional discrimination would keep Mr. Riles as State Superintendent of Schools in California from personal liability, but it would not protect the State from liability. The ruling in the U.S. Supreme Court case of *Guardians* (1983), setting a higher standard of intentionality for an individual than for a corporate governing body such as a municipality or a State, would apply again in *Larry P. v. Riles*. Those standards of intentionality would evidently be applied consistently by the courts, but, as we will see, the courts have not been consistent concerning the use of English language IQ tests (normed on mainstream speakers of General American English) to determine whether or not a minority language/dialect child is retarded. Both of these issues are important to persons with disabilities and both came up in *Larry P. v. Riles*.

Larry P. v. Riles (1979, 1984)

In *Larry P. v. Riles* (1979, 1984; retrieved March 11, 2009, from http://wind.uwyo.edu/edec5250/assignments/Larry.pdf) six Black elementary school children petitioned the State of California for relief from being placed in classes for the mentally retarded on the basis of IQ tests. The 1979 decision found Superintendent Wilson C. Riles guilty of intentional discrimination against African American children in California (per 793 F.2d, 969, 9th Circuit, p. 1). The decision, however, was appealed to the U.S. Court of Appeals of the 9th Circuit by Mr. Riles. The Court of Appeals in 1984 handed down its judgment which affirmed the earlier decision in part and reversed it in part. In particular, the higher court reversed the finding that Riles had intentionally discriminated against African American children, but affirmed the ruling against using IQ tests in the placement of African American students. An injunction was issued that blocked California from using IQ tests for any special education placement.

The higher court agreed that Riles, representing the State of California, had violated the Civil Rights Act of 1964, the Education for All Handicapped Children Act (Public Law 94-142), and the Rehabilitation Act of 1973. However, the higher court reversed the claim of the district court that the State of California had violated the **equal protection clauses** of the United States and California

Constitutions. Such clauses are universally required in State Constitutions by the Fourteenth Amendment to the U.S. Constitution which says that "no state shall . . . deny to any person within its jurisdiction the equal protection of the laws." That amendment was passed in 1868 just three years after the end of the Civil War. The same year that the war ended, in 1865, the Thirteenth Amendment dealt the death blow to Justice Taney's decision in the *Dred Scott* case. The Thirteenth Amendment reads as follows:

> Section 1. Neither slavery nor involuntary servitude, except as a punishment for crime whereof the party shall have been duly convicted, shall exist within the United States, or any place subject to their jurisdiction.

> Section 2. Congress shall have the power to enforce this article by appropriate legislation.

It is interesting that perhaps the best precedent for the IQ testing aspect of the 1984 decision in *Larry P. v. Riles*, as well as *PARC v. Pennsylvania* (1972), *Mills v. Board of Education* (1972), and *Lau v. Nichols* (1974), was the case of *Diana v. California State Board of Education* (1970) which was settled out of court. In *Diana*, the court decree clarified that children should be taught and tested in ways they can understand—that it is unfair and unreasonable to test a child in a language/dialect or in a mode of communication that the child does not understand. Just as it would be unreasonable to test the intelligence of English-speaking children in Chinese, or to assess hearing children in a manual signed-language, it hardly makes any sense to assess children in any language or dialect other than the one that they know best (see the discussion in Chapter 11).

It is also noteworthy that the U.S. Court of Appeals generalized the ruling in *Larry P. v. Riles* in 1984 by asserting that the plaintiffs not only represented the six children named in the class action but the *entire population of all*:

> Black children who had been or in the future would be wrongly placed and maintained in special classes for the educable mentally retarded on the bases of IQ test results. (793 F.2d, 969, 9th Circuit, p. 1)

The court ordered the defendants, the State of California and its elected representatives, especially Wilson Riles, to direct each school district to re-evaluate every Black child who had been classified as "educable mentally retarded" (EMR). Also, the schools would have to do so without using standardized intelligence tests (793 F.2d, 969, 9th Circuit, pp. 1–2).

The *Larry P.* case defined the nature of **dead-end classes** by spelling out the fact that under California law the EMR classification is reserved for children considered "incapable of learning in

> It is clear from the arguments in *Larry P. v. Riles* that remedies for injustices done to persons on account of race, if applied consistently, would provide protection for all minorities and for all persons with communication disorders or any other disabilities under American jurisdiction.

the regular classes." The court had also determined that the EMR curriculum "is not designed to help students learn the skills necessary to return to the regular instructional program." In fact, the court argued that the pull-out type of "EMR classes are designed only to teach social adjustment and economic usefulness. The [EMR] classes are conceived of as "dead-end classes",' and a misplacement in EMR causes a stigma and irreparable injury to the student" (793 F.2d, 969, 9th Circuit, p. 3). It was observed by the court that in 1968–1969 while African American children accounted for 9% of the school population, 27% of the EMR population was African American. The court asserted "the only relevant evidence on their cases indicated that they were not retarded" (793 F.2d, 969, 9th Circuit, p. 6).

In addition to pointing to the problem of disproportionality, a problem discussed in Chapter 11, both the District Court (1979) and the U.S. Court of Appeals (1984) involved in hearing *Larry P. v. Riles* agreed that disproportionate representation of minority children in classes for the mentally retarded requires justification. On its face, even in 1984, the over-representation of African American children in EMR classes violated federal laws all the way back to the Fourteenth Amendment. Also, the *Larry P. v. Riles* ruling demonstrated that assessing the innate abilities of any human being in terms of tests administered in a language or dialect that the individual either does not know at all or does not know well, is not valid.

THE LANGUAGE/DIALECT FACTOR IN IQ TESTS

As we saw in Chapter 11, the unfairness pointed to in *Larry P. v. Riles* was owed to failure to take account of differences in language/dialect background. The fact is that communication is paramount to education and learning and communication depends mainly on a common language/dialect system. The courts have generally understood this fact, but they have not been consistent in their rulings about using so-called IQ tests that utterly depend on a language/dialect that, in many instances, the child does not know well or at all. If the common language/dialect requirement for communication is not met, biased and unfair judgments about abilities and disorders are certain to follow.

Intrinsic Bias

Any tests used to define disorders, disabilities, and handicaps that are given in a language/dialect that some students do not under-

The key principle in *Diana v. the State Board of Education* (1970), and in *Lau v. Nichols* (1974), was that children should be tested and taught in a language/dialect that they understand.

stand well or at all are intrinsically biased against those students. In *Larry P.* the U.S. Court of Appeals seems to have understood this in part at least, but in *PASE v. Hannon* (1980) as argued in the U.S. District Court in Illinois, the inappropriateness of diagnosing disorders on the basis of language/dialect based IQ tests that some children could not understand well or at all was, evidently, lost on the court. The U.S. Court of Appeals in California said such so-called IQ tests were invalid while the U.S. District Court in Illinois said they were valid. It cannot logically be both ways. However, neither court connected *Larry P. v. Riles* (1979, 1984) or *PASE v. Hanson* (1980) with the string of prior language-based cases of discrimination leading back to *Lau v. Nichols* (1974) which was the key U.S. Supreme Court case.

> Language/dialect comprehension is essential to education, and, yet, the courts, and some of the key professional organizations in the field, have only partially taken this fact into consideration.

Only intermittently have the courts shown awareness that so-called IQ tests are mainly language/dialect tests (for arguments showing this is so, see Abdesslem, 2002; Cummins, 2003; Gunderson & Siegel, 2001; J. W. Oller, 1997; J. W. Oller, S. D. Oller, & Badon, 2006; A. A. Ortiz, 1997; R. Yan & J. W. Oller, 2007). In *Larry P. v. Riles*, for instance, the U.S. Court of Appeals noted that the California schools had not taken account of "developmental history" or "adaptive behavior" in the placement of children (793 F.2d, 969, 9th Circuit, p. 5). The defendants had failed to show that the IQ tests they used were accurate measures and that "Black elementary school children who scored less than 70 were indeed mentally retarded" (793 F.2d, 969, 9th Circuit, p. 6). The court quoted from EHA the requirement that "no single procedure shall be the sole criterion for determining an appropriate educational program for a child" (793 F.2d, 969, 9th Circuit, p. 8). Likewise, the court quoted from the Senate Report for the EHA where it said "the [Labor and Public Welfare] Committee is deeply concerned about practices and procedures which result in classifying children as having handicapping conditions when, in fact, they do not have such conditions" (793 F.2d, 969, 9th Circuit, p. 8).

Bonadonna v. Cooperman (1985)

Shared Language/Dialect Is Crucial

The parents of Alisa Bonadonna, a hearing impaired child in *Bonadonna v. Cooperman* (1985) sued Cooperman, the Superintendent of New Jersey on behalf of their daughter. The parents won in keeping with the precedents set in *Diana v. Board of Education* (1970), and in *Lau v. Nichols* (1974)—requiring unsurprisingly that children must be evaluated and taught in a language the child can understand.

The court—again, no surprise here—found that evaluations by teachers who were unable to communicate with the child—that is, teachers who did not know manual signed language, signed English, or any other language/dialect system that the child could understand—were invalid. Simply put, people who cannot communicate with a child cannot validly assess that child's abilities or disabilities.

Evaluator Must Be Able to Communicate

The *Bonadonna* case is especially important in interpreting Public Law 94-142 as it would be generalized and later applied to essentially all communication disorders because *Bonadonna* applied precedents for minority languages/dialects to an individual with a hearing disability. It also clarified the constraints on how an IEP can be sensibly designed—educators and teachers have to take the language/dialect of the child into account. For a discussion of this case in particular from the vantage point of parents of children with communication disorders, see P. W. D. Wright and P. D. Wright (2009; retrieved March 11, 2009, from http://www.wrightslaw.com/advoc/articles/iep_guidance.html).

Judge H. Lee Sarokin of the District Court determined that the school's evaluations

> . . . were based almost solely upon observation . . . assessment consisted of primarily non-standardized tasks and procedures . . . no scientific test results seem to have been considered . . . Thus, but one procedure—teacher evaluation—was utilized . . . [which] tended toward discriminatory evaluation, i.e., evaluation that is biased, in this case against deaf children . . . The Court finds that this method of assessment does not meet the requirements of the EAHCA [Public Law 94-142], or its regulations. (EHLR 183, 619 F. Supp. 975, 1985-1986 EHLR DEC. 557:178, D. NJ 1985; P. W. D. Wright & P. D. Wright, 2009, retrieved March 11, 2009, from http://www.wrightslaw.com/advoc/articles/iep_guidance.html)

Solomonic Wisdom

Judge Sarokin, as cited by Aldersley (2002, p. 196) wrote in what Aldersley described as "a Solomonic decision," that:

> . . . the court recognizes, as did the underlying legislation [EHA, Public Law 94-142], the advantages of a handicapped child's participation in a regular school program. Much can be learned from exposure to one's peers and lost if segregation occurs. Social and psychological development are best attained through mainstreaming and may be substantially curtailed if it is denied.

. . . Bonadonna applied precedents for minority languages/dialects to an individual with a hearing disability.

... Although disruption to other class members is a proper consideration, it is significant to note that Alisa's classmates have also benefitted and learned from Alisa's presence in the classroom ... [which] has enhanced ... compassion, understanding and patience ... It is difficult to envision a lesson better worth learning.

The key rule developed in *Bonadonna v. Cooperman* is that segregation deprives everyone.

Shared Language/Dialect Is Crucial

Any separation from the mainstream deprives not only the separated individual or group, but it also deprives the mainstream children by preventing them from having the opportunity to learn from the minority.

Any separation from the mainstream, for this reason, except in cases of imminent danger to either group or to an individual child, has not been favored by the courts (Aldersley, 2002). Such separation from the mainstream seems to create more problems than it solves. For this reason, as in *Bonadonna v. Cooperman*, Judge Sarokin ruled in favor the general principle of the least restrictive environment. EHA (Public Law 94-142) had already established that to the "maximum extent appropriate" exceptional children should be schooled in the same classrooms as nonexceptional children.

Optimizing Communication

The key principle would later be amplified, as pointed out by Aldersley (2002), by emphasizing the term "appropriate" in such a way as to make communication with the child the higher objective. In keeping with this principle, the least restrictive environment is whichever option enables optimal learning and communication from the point of view of the child affected.

Still Pursuing Freedom of the Mind and the Body

The Case Overturned by an Act of Congress

As we continue to trace the history of laws and court precedents leading to the current state of affairs in dealing with communication disorders, we come to the case of that was actually decided in the U.S. Supreme Court but was, in effect, over-

---

The key element is communication and the essential basis for it is a shared language/dialect. For that reason, the language/dialect of the child is a crucial factor. In most cases, it is *by far the most important factor in devising an appropriate IEP*. Of course, in developing an IEP all of the individual's abilities and limits must be taken into consideration as a whole, but those other elements can hardly be determined without establishing communication with the child, as much as it is possible to do so.

turned in the U.S. Congress. The climax would come in 1986, but the story actually began in 1976 with an eight-year old child who had cerebral palsy and related communication disorders. His name was Thomas Smith and he lived in the tiny state of Rhode Island. His case could easily have gone unnoticed except for his mother who stood up for him through an eight year legal battle beginning in 1976 and ending in Congress in 1986. It is a case of interest with respect to the connections between the history of racial discrimination and the treatment of persons with disabilities and communication disorders.

With that case in mind, in the following section, we zoom out to a perspective on history that enables us to connect some of the dots between the freedom of the mind—especially as made possible through socialization and education—and the freedom of the body. To understand the importance of the infamous case of *Smith v. Robinson* (1984) which would, in effect, be reversed in the U.S. Congress in 1986, some background is essential.

JUSTICE AND FREEDOM IN AMERICA

Interestingly, laws are sometimes a reaction to court cases just as court judgments are often used by judges to counteract or sometimes to re-interpret the law. Sometimes the judges take it upon themselves to interpret the law so as to rewrite it—something which legislators generally disapprove. The opposite is also possible and does occur. That is, the legislature can effectively reverse a court decision by changing the law, which is what happened in the case of Tommy Smith. That case illustrates what is meant by the system of "checks and balances" provided by the highest law in the United States, namely, our Constitution.

Interestingly, laws are sometimes a reaction to court cases just as court judgments are often used by judges to counteract or sometimes to re-interpret the law.

Checks and Balances

In 1986, when the U.S. Congress passed the **Handicapped Children's Protection Act**, the legislative branch of government was evidently reacting to the judicial branch. The Congress was in fact reacting to *Smith v. Robinson, 468 U.S. 992 (1984) 468 U.S. 992*, a Supreme Court Case (retrieved March 11, 2009, from http://caselaw.lp.findlaw.com/cgi-bin/getcase.pl?court=US&vol=468&invol=992) where the parents of a child with cerebral palsy were prevented from receiving compensation for attorneys' fees in an action under the EHA (Public Law 94-142). The reasons why the Court did not award the attorney's fees are complex, but they were subsequently decisively reversed, and the law was rewritten and, in this case (believe it or not), simplified by the Congress.

The Supreme Court case, *Smith v. Robinson*, ostensibly, was decided in 1984 in favor of the child with cerebral palsy, but in making the decision supposedly in Tommy Smith's favor, the court refused to award attorneys' fees. This was certainly not a favorable outcome for Tommy's family. They had spent eight years in and out of different courts before getting to the highest court in the land. How could any parent seek relief under Public Law 94-142 or any other law if it was not possible to get their attorneys' fees paid even if they won the final court battle? The case would take another two years before the reaction of Congress would effectively countermand the Supreme Court's call—but it was too late for Tommy Smith to benefit from an "early education" because by the time the Congress reacted in 1986 to the U.S. Supreme Court's decision in *Smith v. Robinson* (1984), Tommy Smith was already 18 years old.

The History of the Rhode Island Connection

Tommy's court battles began in Cumberland, Rhode Island, in November 1976. At that time, Thomas F. Smith, III (Tommy), who had cerebral palsy along with other physical and emotional conditions, was eight years old. The central issue at first was whether or not Tommy would be provided a free and appropriate education, a FAPE under EHA (the 1975 law). The problem came when the Rhode Island school district stopped funding a special program for Tommy and shifted responsibility to "the State's Division of Mental Health, Retardation and Hospitals (MHRH)"—see *Smith v. Robinson*, Section I of the opinion of the Court delivered by Justice Blackmun. The handing off of an exceptional child from one agency to another, as was done in Tommy's case, is a common response to problems that administrators, for any number of reasons, prefer not to have to handle. Tommy's mother took the case all the way to the highest court in the land.

By the time the case was heard in the U.S. Supreme Court in 1984, Tommy was 16 years old, and before the issue would be resolved by the special law passed by Congress in 1986, Tommy would be 18, and the opportunity to provide for his early schooling would be long gone. What the courts all agreed was that Rhode Island violated EHA in Tommy's case by not providing the full hearing required by EHA before passing him off to a different bureaucracy. Because this case, evidently, would literally require the proverbial "Act of Congress" to put things right, what the Rhode Island officials did shows in a remarkable way just how deeply the freedom of the mind is connected throughout history to freedom of the body. In that connection, a brief flashback is in order here.

As we are about to see, the State of Rhode Island has been a focal point of questions about civil rights connecting present day issues concerning language minorities and disabilities with the American slave trade that, oddly enough, provided Rhode Island with its only Ivy League university. The facts to be recounted are well researched and documented: we are not making this up. We are not saying that the history we are about to present caused the situation with Thomas F. Smith, III to develop, but we are saying, however, that the injustices done to Tommy Smith in Rhode Island are part of a much deeper history in that small island State.

Slavery and Justice in Rhode Island

The *Slavery and Justice Report* (2006) is an amazing document commissioned by President Ruth J. Simmons of Brown University, on April 30, 2003 (retrieved March 11, 2009, from http://www.brown.edu/Research/Slavery_Justice/about/charge.html).

The report, which is accessible in its entirety (retrieved March 11, 2009, from http://www.brown.edu/Research/Slavery_Justice/documents/SlaveryAndJustice.pdf), gives a glimpse of the American slave trade and its peculiar connection to the State of Rhode Island and to Brown University in particular. The story begins with Admiral Esek Hopkins whose grand-daughter donated a clock that decorates a corner of the second floor of the oldest building on the Brown University campus known as University Hall. It turns out that the clock came from a slave ship (like the one in Figure 12–6)—a hundred-ton brigantine called the *Sally* owned by Nicholas Brown and Company—"a partnership of four brothers, Nicholas, John, Joseph, and Moses Brown." They were the Providence slavers who provided the original funding for what is now known as Brown University.

The official report (2006, pp. 3-4) says:

> There was nothing unusual about a slave ship departing from Rhode Island. Rhode Islanders dominated the North American share of the African slave trade, mounting over a thousand slaving voyages in the century before the abolition of the trade in 1807 (and scores more of illegal voyages thereafter). . . . The *Sally's* voyage was deadlier than most. At least 109 of the 196 Africans that Hopkins purchased on behalf of the Browns perished, some in a failed insurrection, the balance through disease, suicide, and starvation.

It is estimated that "Rhode Island merchants sponsored at least 934 slaving voyages to the coast of Africa" and that they brought "an estimated 106,544 Africans from their homeland to the New

It is a source of wonder to visitors that Rhode Island—the state where Tommy's plight began—was the state that held a virtual monopoly on the American slave trade during its peak between 1709 and 1807.

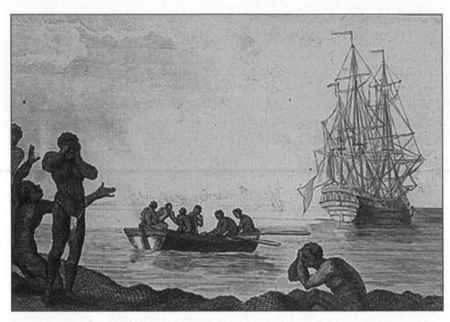

Figure 12–6. One of the slave ships of Rhode Island. A modified portion of a sketch that appeared in Chambon (1783, plate XI). In the public domain because of expired copyright.

World" (Kane, 1998, retrieved March 11, 2009, from http://www.providence.edu/afro/students/kane/slave_trade.htm). After slave-trading was officially outlawed in Rhode Island in 1784, slave ships that formerly off-loaded in Rhode Island just went on down to Charleston, North Carolina. According to a source linked to the official Providence, Rhode Island Web site:

> . . . between 1804 and 1807 of the 202 slave ships which entered the port of Charleston, 59 of the vessels came from Rhode Island, bringing in 8,238 slaves. (retrieved March 11, 2009, from http://www.providenceri.com/NarragansettBay/maritime_commerce.html)

Even today, the history of slavery and the role of Rhode Island as the main off-loading point for Africans brought to America as slaves continues to concern the officials of Rhode Island, the city of Providence, and especially the officials at Brown University. The fact is that Brown's main benefactors were slavers. The slave trade was supposedly banned in Rhode Island in 1807, and almost exactly 200 years later it was officially memorialized in a proclamation on February 24, 2007 by Mayor David N. Cicilline. He wrote the following in response to the *Slavery and Justice Report* (2006):

> I enthusiastically accept my role in joining the University and the Governor in creating a permanent commemoration of the history and role of slavery in Providence and Rhode Island. (Cicilline, 2007, retrieved March 11, 2009, from http://www.providenceri.com/press/article.php?id=191)

Was the purpose to commemorate the role of slavery in helping to build Brown University? From the letter, it seems almost that the mayor was in favor of the slave trade and that in any event he was glad to commemorate its role in Rhode Island history.

In 2009, if Tommy F. Smith is still living, he is about 41 years old. We wonder how he would feel about the role of slavery in Rhode Island. We do not know from the records whether or not he was a descendant of African slaves brought to America through that small state. But many others were and are, and Tommy's experience serves to show that just as certainly as the body is connected to the mind, the injustice of the slavers of Rhode Island is in fact and in principle linked to the case of *Smith v. Robinson* as decided in 1984 by the U.S. Supreme Court.

Although due process and equal protection under the law—regardless of race, religion, or disabilities—were supposedly already among the good objectives sought by honorable people everywhere in 1984, it was clear that the nation still had a long way to go.

In the case of Tommy Smith, the proverbial throwaway remark, "Why, it would take 'an act of Congress' to change this situation!" turned out to be right on the money.

The Handicapped Children's Protection Act, 1986

As Yogi Berra is often quoted as saying—"It ain't over till it's over" (for this and the history of what are affectionately called Yogi-isms by his fans, color us among them, see "Yogi Berra," 2009, Web site retrieved March 11, 2009, from http://www.yogiberra.com/yog i-isms.html). The *Smith v. Robinson* case heard and decided in the U.S. Supreme Court in 1984 was not over yet. The contest was never settled in court. Although Tommy's family, in effect, won the battle over Tommy's right to a FAPE, and they succeeded in showing in court that the Rhode Island officials had violated Tommy's right to a full hearing before they stopped funding his special IEP, the U.S. Supreme Court did not allow Tommy's family to recover the legal fees incurred in pursuing their case.

The majority opinion was that *Smith et al.* had broadened their complaints to include violations, for instance, of due process and equal protection under the Fourteenth Amendment and other laws beyond the ones that Justice Blackmun and the majority of the other Justices saw as applying to the case. In section IV of the Court's split opinion (6 to 3) in *Smith v. Robinson*, Justice Blackmun summed up the gist of the two most relevant laws in the view of the majority—the 1973 Rehabilitation Act and the 1975 EHA (Public Law 94-142):

> While the EHA guarantees a right to a free appropriate public education, 504 [a section of the 1973 Rehabilitation Act] simply prevents discrimination on the basis of handicap. But while the EHA is limited to handicapped children seeking access to public education, [468 U.S. 992, 1017] 504 protects handicapped persons of all ages from discrimination in a variety of programs and activities receiving federal financial assistance.

By asserting violations of due process and equal protection of the Fourteenth Amendment and other laws, according to Justice Blackmun and the majority of the Justices, *Smith et al.* had broadened the case beyond the applicable laws. So, the Supreme Court denied recovery of the legal fees associated with the larger argument. The decision seemed to many to be a transparent miscarriage of justice. How could the U.S. Supreme Court agree that Tommy had been discriminated against because of his disability and yet turn around and not award the fees incurred in getting the case to the Court?

Justices Brennan, Marshall, and Stevens, on this account, registered a dissenting minority opinion. They asserted the following:

An Ironic but True Prediction

Congress will now have to take the time to revisit the matter. And until it does, the handicapped children of this country whose difficulties are compounded by discrimination and by other deprivations of constitutional rights will have to pay the costs. It is at best ironic that the Court has managed to impose this burden on handicapped children in the course of interpreting a statute [namely Public Law 94-142] wholly intended to promote the educational rights of those children.

And, this time, apparently, Congress was evidently listening when the decision in *Smith v. Robinson* was handed down in 1984. It seems also that the Congress sided with the minority of the Justices. Considering how long it usually takes for Congress to act, the **Handicapped Children's Protection Act of 1986** was—on the Congressional clock—an almost lightning quick response aiming to undo the precedent setting decision of the U.S. Supreme Court in *Smith v. Robinson.*

Yell (1990) and Aldersley (2002) have both argued that the Handicapped Children's Protection Act of 1986 was an explicit counter by Congress to the U.S. Supreme Court's decision in *Smith v. Robinson.* The court had denied attorneys' fees for a case of demonstrated discrimination against a disabled child with cerebral palsy. As the minority opinion put it, the decision was "ironic" to say the least—and the Congress evidently considered it just plain wrong.

The Congress reversed the Court's decision by passing a new law to bolster EHA. The 1986 act of Congress provided explicitly for:

1. *the recovery of attorneys' fees in special education lawsuits,* in addition to
2. tuition reimbursement to pay for educational costs incurred on behalf of the exceptional child while the contest was underway, and
3. court intervention—by **legal injunction**—to force an education agency to provide and pay for a FAPE for an exceptional child.

> Yell (1990) and Aldersley (2002) have both argued that the Handicapped Children's Protection Act of 1986 was an explicit counter by Congress to the U.S. Supreme Court's decision in *Smith v. Robinson.*

But, of course, like Yogi said, "It ain't over till it's over" and the struggle to ensure a FAPE for every child with disabilities certainly was not over yet.

Renewal and Extension of EHA, 1986

Another piece of legislation in 1986 was Public Law 99-457 which reauthorized the EHA of 1975 (Public Law 94-142) and extended its applicability to infants and preschool children from birth to the age of 2 years. Although the original EHA applied to the traditional school period of public education—from kindergarten, or in some states from first grade, through grade 12, ages 5 to 18 years—the renewal legislation extended coverage to younger exceptional children. For this reason, as Bloom and Weisskopf (1989) observed, the renewal legislation would require more participation from the medical community. Because it is typically **pediatricians**—doctors who treat infants, toddlers, and preschoolers—Bloom and Weisskopf supposed that doctors would become more involved after the 1986 law. Of course, the renewal legislation of 1986 would also mean that the Federal Government would become more involved in preschool and daycare centers all across the country. In the meantime, the battle continued on various levels and testing remained a key background issue in all the discussions and in some was brought front and center.

In the next section we deal with another 1986 law that impacts every family in America and most of the people in the rest of the world. It is a law that deals with the interface between industry—especially the pharmaceutical companies that manufacture drugs and medicines—and the government that according to President Lincoln's famous Gettysburg Address is "for the people, of the people, and by the people." Unsurprisingly, for that reason the next law also has its own court that was created for the purpose of enabling individuals harmed by the government to be justly compensated for the injury done to them by the government. It is an interesting aspect of the law and it directly comes to bear on many citizens with communication disorders.

NATIONAL CHILDHOOD VACCINE INJURY ACT OF 1986

In 1986, Congress passed the **National Childhood Vaccine Injury Act (Public Law 99-660)**. This act is important to the study of communication disorders because of the fact that as the number of persons being vaccinated increased during the 1980s, the number of injuries also increased—especially the kind associated with neurological communication disorders. The issue reached crisis because of civil suits concerning injuries attributed to the combination shots containing the triple whammy Diphtheria Tetanus Pertussis (DTP) vaccines. According to one story, manufacturers threatened to stop producing the vaccines, shortages supposedly resulted, and Congress enacted the new vaccine law in 1986 (retrieved March 11, 2009, from http://www.answers.com/topic/childhood-vaccine-injury-act?cat=health). There was also, of course, enormous pressure on the vaccine manufacturers by the many civil lawsuits that were being brought against doctors and vaccine manufacturers on account of a rising number of vaccine injuries.

Attorney Tom Powell, speaking in the U.S. Court of Federal Claims on June 11, 2007, asserted that the original purpose of the Vaccine Injury Act was three-fold:

> ## Purposes of the Vaccine Injury Act
>
> The first was to protect manufacturers [of vaccines] from civil liability. The second was to encourage vaccines to be used and administered and developed, and the third was to provide a fair, just, speedy and generous compensation program for those children, hopefully a small number, ideally rare, [with] . . . expected adverse reactions to vaccines (transcript of day 1 in the *Omnibus Autism Proceeding*, p. 10, retrieved March 11, 2009, from ftp://autism.uscfc.uscourts.gov/autism/transcripts/day01.pdf).

In the process of manufacturing or trying to ensure the potency of the disease agents and to try to prevent contamination by other microbes other components are also either deliberately or inadvertently added to the mix.

The 1986 law would turn out to be of special importance to persons with neurological conditions such as autism whose symptoms are known to be caused or exacerbated by toxins, disease agents, and incidental components in vaccines. Such components are what the government has described as "adventitious agents" (FDA/CBER, 2007, retrieved March 11, 2009, from http://www.fda.gov/cber/faq.htm#6). They end up in vaccines and then are placed in the bloodstreams or bodies of human beings in accordance with the federal vaccine schedule as recommended by the CDC. It is, according to standard vaccine theory, necessary for the vaccines to contain agents of the diseases they are supposed to prevent in order to stimulate the immune system to produce antibodies against those agents.

In addition to the disease agents in the vaccines in use in the 1980s, for instance, there was thimerosal, aluminum, formaldehyde, animal proteins, extraneous viruses, and so on. Also in the 1980s, in addition to new vaccines, more so-called "booster" shots were added into the schedule. In the manufacturing process, the vaccines were known to acquire biological proteins, viruses, and other contaminants from the animals—chickens, ducks, rabbits, dogs, and monkeys—used in manufacturing them (Cave, 2001, p. 38). One virus of considerable interest among the 40 plus viruses originating in monkeys, and one that was inadvertently transferred to the human population through the polio vaccines, is the now well-known simian virus 40 (SV40) that we encountered in Chapter 10. That virus is particularly troubling because it can lie dormant in the way the AIDS virus does for a decade or more. Even in mice, SV40 has been shown to last for periods in excess of 6 months (Takeshita et al., 2007). The resemblance of that retrovirus to the human immune virus (HIV) as discovered by Urnovitz (1996) would reinforce many of the concerns that led to the passing of the Vaccine Injury Act of 1986.

Vaccines, Contaminants, and Interactions

In addition to toxins included in the vaccines—mercury, aluminum, and so forth—during the 1980s there was an increasing effort to combine disease agents from several shots into a single one. This was done with the Measles Mumps Rubella (MMR) and Diphtheria Tetanus Pertussis (DTP) vaccines in the 1980s. In these cases, multiple disease agents are introduced simultaneously into a single shot, for the sake of convenience, and for the same reason two or more such shots are commonly administered on the same day. Because of potential interactions, a triple whammy aimed at three different diseases increases the risk for individuals who are vulnerable to injury.

In 1997, as a result of the Vaccine Injury Act, which established two different systems for keeping track of injuries, it was reported that combining the MMR shot with the DTP shot on the same day increased the risk of a seizure within the next 30 days by 210% and administering the DTP a week or two weeks later than the MMR, presumably after the disease agents had time to become active, increased the chance of a seizure by 300% (R. Chen et al., 1997). Also, all of the clinical trials we have consulted for the vaccines containing multiple disease agents show that the interactions increase the associated risks (J. W. Oller & S. D. Oller, 2009). Nevertheless, vaccine combinations for a single shot with up to 20 distinct disease agents have been proposed by manufacturers (for documentation and discussion, see Cave, 2001, and her references), and Paul Offit, a key spokesperson for the CDC on behalf of vaccines has argued, along with some of his colleagues (Offit et al., 2002), that babies should be able to handle up to 10,000 disease agents on a single occasion.

In the case of *Michelle Cedillo v. Secretary of Health and Human Services* (2007; see the section titled "*Omnibus Autism Proceeding*, 2007) the multiple disease agents and toxins in the DTP shot were administered at the same time as the **Haemophilus influenzae B (HiB)** shots—giving her four disease agents plus 25 micrograms

By their method of estimating the relative risk of a seizure within 30 days of a vaccination, R. Chen and colleagues at the CDC, suggested that giving the DTP and the MMR at the same time or giving the DTP a week or two later, resulted in a substantial increase in risk, peaking during the second week after the MMR was given. (We are also grateful to our colleague, Dr. Andrew Wakefield, for his insights into this and related studies.)

Because of the countless ways toxic agents can be combined in different vaccination schedules, there is no way to predict with any reasonable confidence what the results will be for all the many different combinations of vaccines that may be administered.

of mercury to contend with on each occasion from the DTP shots before she was 7 months old. When the DTP vaccines plus the HiB vaccine are combined with thimerosal, the risk is invariably greater. However, it is common practice by pediatricians to administered multiple shots on the same office visit. Logically, if all else were held equal, it is certain that a shorter the time span between shots and a larger number of disease agents and toxins in the mix will increase the risk of injury. For instance, if the order of administration matters, with 8 distinct disease agents or toxins the number of possible permutations is a staggering 40,320 unique combinations $(8! = 8*7*6*5*4*3*2*1)$. No drug company has ever done all the clinical trials needed to show that all those combinations are harmless. Nor is it easy when harm occurs to say just what combination of factors may have caused it. But there is no doubt that combining more and more disease agents and more and more toxins logically increases the associated risks.

Different batches of vaccine and different manufacturing processes make combinations intrinsically unpredictable. The dangers are more acute when the combinations are given within a narrow time frame, but contaminants such as SV40 can have their impact many years after the administration of the vaccine. In any event, as the MMR, Hepatitis B, and HiB shots were added to the recommended United States vaccination schedule during the 1980s there was a corresponding increase in reported neurological disorders. There was also a concomitant increase in known instances of vaccine-caused illness and death. The increase in vaccine injuries during the 1980s was almost certainly the primary cause of the passing of the Vaccine Injury Act by the U.S. Congress in 1986.

Vaccine Adverse Event Reporting System

In 1988, a partial system for monitoring vaccine injuries, the **Vaccine Adverse Event Reporting System (VAERS)**, was set in place. The VAERS national "vaccine safety surveillance program" is administered by the Food and Drug Administration (FDA) and the Centers for Disease Control and Prevention (CDC). It was set up to collect and analyze data from adverse events that occur after a vaccine or some combination of them has been administered to an individual. The official VAERS Web site confirms that adverse effects from vaccines can be severe: "Since 1990, VAERS has received over 123,000 reports" which it assures the public are mostly about "mild side effects such as fever." However, the official site says:

> Very rarely, people experience serious adverse events following immunization. By monitoring such events, VAERS helps to identify any important new safety concerns that otherwise may not come to light before licensure. (retrieved March 11, 2009, from http://www.fda.gov/cber/vaers/faq.htm)

Under-reporting

It is an ongoing matter of concern to the medical community and to everyone involved in vaccine use, that well under 10% of the adverse events are reported (see Cave, 2001, p. xviii). On the positive side, all the data collected under VAERS has been available on-line since 1993; retrieved March 11, 2009, from http://www.medalerts.org/vaersdb/access.html). As parents and thinking professionals commonly notice, the FDA and CDC are in a conflicted position as promoter/marketers of vaccines who are both encouraging universal vaccinations while at the same time they are in charge of monitoring injuries caused by vaccines.

Oversight

The situation of the FDA and CDC as overseers of the vaccine manufacturers is a little like the foxes who joined with a committee of coyotes to protect the chickens. Meanwhile, the chickens were, unknowingly, paying their taxes to the government that appointed the foxes and were one way or another also paying the coyotes to provide them with vaccines. The invariable tendency is for the oversight agencies to report fewer missing chickens than might be reported if there were any chickens on the oversight committees. The fact is that the monitors of vaccines are in charge of marketing them to the public—the CDC wants everyone to be vaccinated—as well as ensuring their safety.

The time frame for the required monitoring of potential vaccine injuries is prescribed by the FDA and CDC in an official "VAERS Table of Reportable Events Following Vaccination" on a vaccine by vaccine basis—each one on its own schedule (retrieved March 11, 2009, from http://www.vaers.hhs.gov/pdf/ReportableEventsTable.pdf). Generally, the timeframes for monitoring adverse vaccine events are about a week, but in some cases they extend to 42 days for the MMR and up to 6 months for Oral Polio Vaccines. Unfortunately, the reporting system time frames are often too short by several country miles. Participants in the recent Adverse Drug Event Reporting Workshop sponsored in 2007 by the National Academies of Sciences commented that:

> studies must be of sufficient duration to detect problems over time. Unfortunately, many postmarketing studies lack these basic characteristics. (retrieved March 11, 2009, from http://books.nap.edu/catalog/11897.html)

The term "postmarketing" is interesting in showing that the FDA and CDC are intentionally participating along with the pharmaceutical companies in marketing vaccines. In the instance of SV40, the virus was spread to millions of people through polio vaccines in the 1960s. In the meantime, the current research shows that the bad effects are still present almost half a century later.

The under-reporting of adverse events along with a host of other problems including drug interactions, educating the public, and the length of monitoring programs, is widely acknowledged along with other problems in the system (see National Academy of Sciences, 2007; also the Institute of Medicine, April 12, 2007, retrieved March 11, 2009, from http://www.iom.edu/CMS/3740/24155/42216.aspx).

It is known that toxic agents introduced by vaccination programs are undoubtedly having effects that are grossly outside the recommended time frames for monitoring.

Inadequate Time Frames for Monitoring

For example, B. Weiss, Clarkson, and Simon (2002) found that the toxic impact of mercury after a single exposure might take five months to show up in behavioral and neurological symptoms. In the Iraq poisoning the symptoms did not show up "until weeks or months after exposure stopped" and in the Minamata, Japan case:

> low chronic doses of methyl mercury may not have produced observable behavioral effects for periods of time measured in years. . . . Parallels are drawn with other diseases that affect the central nervous system, such as Parkinson disease and post-polio syndrome, that also reflect the delayed appearance of central nervous system damage. (p. 851)

Newland and Rasmussen (2003) presented evidence that exposure **in utero**—that is, during gestation—could result in:

> effects [that] extend into adulthood and sometimes accelerate the rate of aging, even when exposure ceases by birth. The neurotoxicant methyl mercury provides an interesting case study that reveals much about how disrupted neural development has lifelong consequences. (p. 212)

VAERS Was About Licensing Vaccines

The VAERS system was actually put in place to help the FDA and CDC continue to license new vaccines. The official Web site (FDA & CDC, 2003) says that VAERS helps:

> to identify any important new safety concerns that otherwise may not come to light before licensure. (retrieved March 11, 2009, from http://www.fda.gov/cber/vaers/faq.htm)

Licensure is the expected outcome even if there are vaccine injuries. However, FDA and CDC have no power or authorization to help the families or individual children who have been injured or even killed by vaccines. That job was given to a special court, as noted above, that is commonly referred to as the Vaccine Injury Court.

The Vaccine Injury Compensation Program

To provide recourse for persons seeking compensation for an injured child, in 1988 Congress established the **National Vaccine Injury Compensation Program (VICP)** which is associated with the U.S. Court of Federal Claims (also known as "the People's Court" and as "the Vaccine Injury Court"; see Lommen Abdo, 2009, retrieved March 11, 2009, from http://www.lommen.com/news_detail.asp

?RecordNumber=149). Under the 1986 law, persons seeking compensation may, if they meet a fairly stringent list of requirements (see the end of this section and in the following section titled "A Special Statute of Limitations for Vaccine Injuries") may be heard in the U.S. Court of Federal Claims—The People's Court. It is the only court in the land where the people can seek reparations for wrongs done to them from the Federal government. It is a special court with distinct procedures and rules. Its original purpose was enunciated by President Lincoln his Annual Message to Congress in 1861 where he said:

> It is as much the duty of Government to render prompt justice against itself, in favor of citizens, as it is to administer the same between private individuals. (Lincoln, 1861a, retrieved March 11, 2009, from http://www.infoplease.com/t/hist/state-of-the-union/73.html)

This sentence is the one that is engraved on the building where the court is housed (Figure 12–7).

In view of its original purpose, it is not surprising that the interests of individuals with disabilities inflicted by government programs would end up there. The U.S. Court of Federal Claims was specifically designed to provide prompt and fair compensation for such injuries. Parenthetically, it is important for parents of vaccine injured children—as well as the speech-language pathologists and others who work with them—to know that filing a report with VAERS does not trigger any action in the Vaccine Injury Court. Rather VAERS is designed to create a permanent data bank of information to track the impact of the nationwide government mandated vaccination programs. To initiate a legal claim under VICP a different report must be filed with a different Federal agency.

In actual fact, the Vaccine Injury Act of 1986 was designed first and foremost to protect the manufacturers of vaccines, and the government agencies that promote their use from suits filed in civil courts by individual citizens. The idea was to provide **no-fault** compensation to the parents or advocates for any child injured by a licensed and/or federally mandated vaccine. In a no-fault system, no person or agency is accused of doing anything wrong that could be punished by law. Instead of a plaintiff, there is a **petitioner**, and instead of a **defendant**, there is a **respondent**. There is no jury and the persons often deciding the case are not judges in the usual sense but **Special Masters** appointed by the court. Individual cases of alleged vaccine injuries can be heard by a single individual acting as the sole arbiter, the whole jury and the judge rolled into one person.

To get on the legal schedule for the Vaccine Injury Court the following requirements must be met:

> (1) . . . the injured person must have received a vaccine manufactured by a vaccine company located in the U.S. and returned

It is interesting that the primary purpose of the U.S. Court of Federal Claims was not to protect the interests of government, pharmaceutical companies, Federal Agencies, large and powerful professional trade associations in medicine, dentistry, and so on, but to protect the rights of individual private citizens against the government.

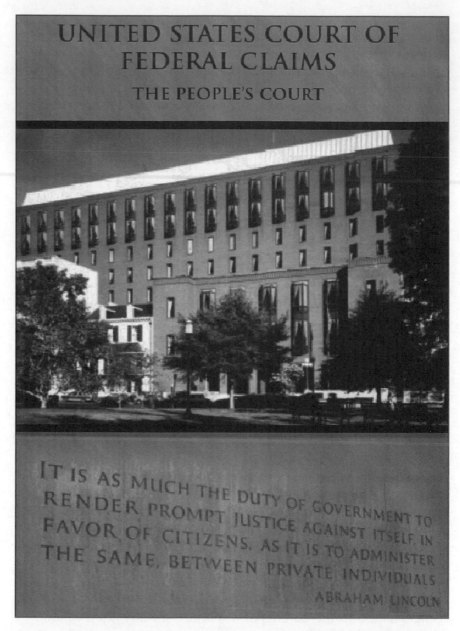

Figure 12–7. Photographs of the building housing United States Court of Federal Claims, also known as the Vaccine Injury Court since 1986. Retrieved March 11, 2009, from http://www.uscfc.uscourts.gov/sites/default/files/court_info/Court_History_Brochure.pdf. United States Court of Federal Claims brochure, in the public domain.

to the U.S. within 6 months after the date of vaccination . . . [and] to be eligible to file a claim, the effects of the person's injury must have lasted for more than 6 months after the vaccine was given; or (2) resulted in a hospital stay and surgery; or (3) resulted in death. (National Vaccine Injury Compensation Program, n.d., retrieved March 11, 2009, from http://www.hrsa.gov/vaccinecompensation/persons_eligible.htm)

A Special Statute of Limitations for Vaccine Injuries

In addition, there is a stringent **statute of limitations** on vaccine injury cases. If they are not filed within three years of the onset of symptoms, the case cannot ever be filed much less can it ever be heard in the U.S. Federal Court of Claims. This statute is "special" because it prevents an injured person, say, who discovers in adulthood that the injury was sustained in infancy from a mandated vaccine, from any kind of compensation. It is also unusual because most statutory limits civil suits concerning injuries that can be shown to have been caused by another individual or by a corporation, say, are not limited in this way (see Sell, 2006, retrieved March 11, 2009, from http://www.autismone.org/download2006.cfm and Included on the DVD by permission).

In neurological disorders, such as autism—which account for the majority of the VICP cases presently being reviewed—throughout the 1980s and 1990s, it was difficult for parents to get a timely diagnosis for their child. In many cases it took years just to get a diagnosis much less to suspect that the onset of symptoms was just after one or several routine vaccinations. Among the children excluded by the statute of limitations were the twin boys of Attorney Jeff Z. Sell. Both boys developed autism after receiving the DTP vaccination with thimerosal but it took just over three years to get a diagnosis and to discover the connection. When seeking to get on the docket for the U.S. Federal Court of Claims, Jeff ran into a wall:

> This rule is inflexible . . . It does not matter that a child's parents did not know about this program, or that they did not know that their child's injuries were related to the vaccine. . . . Most states also have laws which toll (i.e. stop) the running of the statute of limitations while someone is under a disability. . . . In many states a child who is injured does not even have to file a case until sometime after they reach majority [at age 18 or 21 depending on the State] (retrieved March 11, 2009, from http://www.autismone.org/download2006.cfm)

A claim must be filed under the VICP within three (3) years of when the first symptoms occurred.

But in the case of the Federal law governing vaccine injuries, if a diagnosis is delayed, or if a case is not filed within three years of the onset of symptoms, no case can ever be filed even if it should become known that vaccines caused the entire lifelong problems associated with neurological disorders such as autism.

INTO THE NEW MILLENNIUM

When the Vaccine Injury Act was passed by Congress in 1986, no one could have known that a case for more than 5,300 individuals would be heard under the heading of the *Omnibus Autism Proceeding*, which finally got to the People's Court in 2007 after five years of petitioning. Before the case could be heard, however, a number of other additional legal precedents would be set in case law and a great deal of legislation directly or indirectly impacting disabilities and communication disorders would be enacted.

Sharif v. New York State Education Department (1989)

Sharif (a high school student) and her parents, in *Sharif v. New York State Education Department* (1989), sued the New York State Education Department (SED) claiming discrimination against female students in awarding the Regents and Empire Scholarships of New York. It was the policy, at the time, to rely exclusively on the *Scholastic Aptitude Test* (*SAT*) to determine eligibility for those scholarships. District Judge Walker said it was the first case to ask "whether discrimination under Title IX [of the Education Amendments of 1972 (20 U.S.C. 1681 et seq.)] can be established by proof of disparate impact without proof of intent to discriminate" (709 F.Supp. 345, 57 USLW 2491, 53 Ed. Law Rep. 1144, p. 1). The court found that the SED was discriminating and ordered that merit scholarships could no longer be awarded solely based on the *SAT*.

Judge Walker ruled, "The classification of scholarship applicants solely on the basis of *SAT* scores violates the equal protection clause of the Fourteenth Amendment because this method is not rationally related to the state's goal of rewarding students who have demonstrated academic achievement" (709 F.Supp. 345, 57 USLW 2491, 53 Ed. Law Rep. 1144, p. 22). The Court ordered the SED to consider the applicant's **grade point average** in addition to *SAT* scores.

More Than One Measure Required

Sharif affirmed that important educational decisions cannot be made on the basis of any single test score—as had been established long before in EHA 1975. The same principle would be applied later by the U.S. Supreme Court in a discrimination case brought against the State of Mississippi (see the *United States v. Fordice*, 1992, discussed later). Both cases are important in affirming the need for multiple measures especially in high stakes assessments. Such case law is important to the shaping and interpretation of laws governing the diagnosis and treatment of communication disorders.

Americans with Disabilities Act of 1990

The Americans with Disabilities Act of 1990 (**ADA**), **Public Law 101-336**, was signed into law, according to its stated purpose, on

July 26, 1990 (see ADA, 2009 for resources about this act, retrieved March 11, 2009 at http://www.usdoj.gov/crt/ada/adahom1.htm). The succinctly stated purpose of ADA 1990 was supposedly:

> to establish a clear and comprehensive prohibition of discrimination on the basis of disability. (retrieved March 11, 2009, from http://www.usdoj.gov/crt/ada/pubs/ada.htm)

This statement seems to suggest that discrimination against persons with exceptionalities was not already forbidden by prior laws including the Civil Rights Act of 1964, the Rehabilitation Act of 1973, the Education for All Handicapped Children Act of 1975 (Public Law 94-142), the renewals of these laws, and the Handicapped Children's Protection Act of 1986, not to mention the Fourteenth Amendment to the Constitution which dated back to 1868.

The ADA included, in its approximately 61 pages of text, an indirect definition of what is commonly referred to as **adverse impact**. Although the phrase is never used in the document itself, "adverse impact" is defined indirectly as any act of "discrimination":

> that adversely affects the opportunities or status of . . . [any] applicant or employee because of the disability of such applicant or employee. (Section 12112)

According to the ADA the term "disability" was broadly construed to include:

> (A) a physical or mental impairment that substantially limits one or more of the major life activities of such individual;
>
> (B) a record of such an impairment; or
>
> (C) being regarded as having such impairment. (Section 12102, Definitions)

ADA had sweeping implications for the treatment of persons with disabilities in any kind of educational setting in addition to employment and other areas of the law. According to the official introduction to the ADA law at the U.S. Department of Justice Web site (retrieved March 11, 2009, from http://www.usdoj.gov/crt/ada/5yearadarpt/i_introduction.htm), here is the purpose:

The Goal of ADA

"The goal of the ADA is simple—to open up all aspects of American life to people with disabilities. For too long, people with disabilities were held back by old modes of thinking and old methods of building. Prevailing attitudes made it hard for people with disabilities to get an education or to get a job. Barriers in society prevented people with disabilities from getting where they needed to go to build a better life."

ADA regulated building codes for new construction as well as renovations under Title II and Title III which extend to essentially all nonresidential facilities. Enforcement and "technical assistance activities" are estimated to reach 7,000,000 commercial and nonprofit entities, 80,000+ state and local government agencies, 100 federal agencies, and more than "50 million people with disabilities as well as their families and friends." The government Web site for all this, supported by our tax dollars, reads a little like a commercial for utopia. But the law was evidently not yet broad enough. Additional laws would be supplied by the Congress.

EHA Renewal as IDEA in 1990

The act known as **Individuals with Disabilities Education Act (IDEA)** of 1990 (PL 101-476)—also known as the Education of the Handicapped Act Amendments of 1990—was a precursor to a more expansive IDEA law to be enacted in 1997. In the meantime, IDEA 1990 collected prior laws pertaining to persons with disabilities beginning with PL 94-142, the original EHA, and its amendments, especially, PL 99-457, under the new name of IDEA.

In addition to making the abbreviation of the law into a memorable acronym, going from EHA to IDEA, the change from the word "handicapped" to "disabled" reflected an adjustment in the way persons with physical, mental, emotional, or behavioral difficulties were to be viewed and treated. The shift was away from the notion of nameless groups of "*the* handicapped" which could be talked about by Congress and the rest of the world, toward individual human beings. Some might suppose that this was just about "political correctness," but even such a subtle adjustment, from "handicapped" to "disabled," in the larger context of history, seems to represent more than just a change in the words that are publicly acceptable. Today, there is an effort to view problems and symptoms of communication disorders of all kinds as affecting individual persons.

Also, the acronym, IDEA, suggested a more positive and proactive view. The new IDEA law reaffirmed and extended the concepts of the required FAPE and IEP and expanded their reach on both ends. The old EHA laws covered ages 5 to 18 but IDEA 1990 reached down to age 3 and up to 21. Additional coverage and funding were provided for early programs and for **assistive technology**. The technology eventually would provide funding for hardware and software for special keyboards, pointers, joysticks, trackballs, and reading systems to assist individuals with disabilities. IDEA 1990 was also more demanding, in theory at least, by requiring that the IEP for every student by age 16 should include a plan for moving on either to a job or to higher education (Aitken, 2007, retrieved March 11, 2009, from http://onlineacademics.org/IEP.html).

> In addition to making the abbreviation of the law into a memorable acronym, going from EHA to IDEA, the change from the word "handicapped" to "disabled" reflected an adjustment in the way persons with physical, mental, emotional, or behavioral difficulties were to be viewed and treated.

The Vaccine Safety Datalink, 1990

The Vaccine Safety Datalink was established in 1990 "to monitor immunization safety and address the gaps in scientific knowledge about rare and serious side effects following immunization" (retrieved March 11, 2009, from http://www.cdc.gov/od/science/iso/research_activties/vsdp.htm). It is a much larger database than the VAERS. In addition to records of adverse events, the VSD includes data from the large managed care organizations concerning vaccine type, date of vaccination, birth data, and census data, whether there were multiple concurrent vaccinations, and other details.

The Goal of ADA

Curiously, the policy established by law in 1986, that is, in the National Childhood Vaccine Injury Program, put the Vaccine Safety Datalink under the control of the very Federal agencies that it is supposed to be used to monitor—the CDC and FDA.

As we will see below, in reference to the *Omnibus Autism Proceeding 2007*, the federal agencies that are being challenged are the same agencies that are supposed to be protecting the rights of the individuals seeking relief in court. The agencies especially being taken to task are the U.S. Department of Health and Human Services and its subsidiary agency the Centers for Disease Control and Prevention (CDC) that have oversight and control of the Vaccine Safety Datalink. A key item of dispute in the *Omnibus Autism Proceeding 2007* is the refusal of the "respondent" (defendant) to supply access to the data contained there—in the Vaccine Safety Datalink. It may be argued that the VAERS database, which is publicly available, contains everything that is needed but independent researchers and toxicologists interested in the impact of vaccines do not agree (e.g., see documentation in Kirby, 2005; also discussion and data there and in Geier & Geier, 2006a, 2006c).

At the USPHS Web site, the government proudly mentions that it has produced 75 studies based on the Vaccine Safety Datalink. The obvious counter from independent researchers is that many individual researchers can be named who have produced that much work in less time. So the question arises, why does the USPHS not allow access by independent researchers to the Vaccine Safety Datalink? Why does it require expensive litigation to gain access (see Kirby, 2005)? Meantime, in civil courts and in the Congress, the legal battles on behalf of exceptional persons go on.

United States v. Fordice (1992)

In the *United States v. Fordice* (1992; retrieved March 11, 2009, from http://www.law.cornell.edu/supct/html/historics/USSC_CR_05 05_0717_ZS.html), the complaint filed by private citizens, Ayers et al. (case number 90-6588) against Fordice, then Governor of Mississippi, was that the eight public universities of Mississippi remained segregated long after the Mississippi state laws allowing that segregation had been struck down. A key sticking point in maintaining the segregation of the Mississippi universities was the use of the *American College Test* (*ACT*) as the sole basis for some admission exclusions.

By using a certain cutoff score on the *ACT* as the sole basis for refusing to admit certain students, Mississippi was not only violating the universal caveat of professional testers that no high-stakes decision should ever be based on just one test score (Heubert & Hauser, 1999), but according to the U.S. Supreme Court, the way this was being done in Mississippi had a "segregative effect." It was a way of keeping the old Jim Crow laws under the illegal "separate but equal" provisions in effect.

Mississippi Still Discriminating in 1992

In 1992, Mississippi was still operating, in effect, under the defunct Supreme Court ruling of *Plessy v. Ferguson* (1896). That is, Mississippi was doing what the U.S. Supreme Court under Chief Justice Warren in *Brown v. the Board of Education* (1954) had explicitly struck down. The U.S. Supreme Court again in 1992 ruled against the "separate but equal" practice. It also ruled that Mississippi was violating the Civil Rights Act of 1964, the equal protection clause of the Fourteenth Amendment, and sound educational practice. In addition, the Court condemned the use of a single test score in exclusionary judgments about admissions.

In particular, the Court condemned:

> The State's [Mississippi's] refusal to consider high school grade performance along with *ACT* scores . . . since the *ACT*'s administering organization discourages use of *ACT* scores alone . . . (505 U.S. 717, 720)

Again, the principle that multiple measures ought to be used in making important educational decisions was sustained. It would be reiterated in legislation impacting persons with communication disorders (especially see the discussion of IDEA 1997). *Fordice* reminds us again of the fundamental importance of valid assessments especially in high stakes decisions.

By using a certain cutoff score on the ACT as the sole basis for refusing to admit certain students, Mississippi was not only violating the universal caveat of professional testers that no high-stakes decision should ever be based on just one test score (Heubert & Hauser, 1999), but according to the U.S. Supreme Court, the way this was being done in Mississippi had a "segregative effect."

Doe v. Withers (1993)

In _Doe v. Withers_ (1993, on the DVD) an anonymous "learning disabled" student referred to only as "Student D. Doe" sued his high school history teacher, Michael Withers because Withers refused to provide oral testing for Doe. According to the court record, Doe came under the protection of all the legislation covering disabilities including the renewed EHA, that is, IDEA 1990 (Circuit Court of Taylor County, West Virginia, Civil Action No. 92-C-92). Peter Wright has placed the entire case on his Web site (retrieved March 11, 2009, from http://www.wrightslaw.com/law/caselaw/case_Doe_With ers_Complaint.html) and claims there that it "was the first special ed[ucation] jury trial" that awarded damages in a dollar amount to the plaintiff. It also met and affirmed the requirement that Doe had to show Mr. Withers had discriminated intentionally.

Peter Wright points out that Doe's teacher, Michael Withers, was "a prominent member of the General Assembly" and "would not follow the IEP, despite being instructed to" do so by the Superintendent of Schools, his School Principal, the Special Education Director, and the Special Education teacher who worked with Doe. The court awarded the family $50,000 in compensation and $30,000 in punitive damages. The significance of the case for our purposes here is to show the responsibility of individual teachers, and by implication, of clinicians and other professionals for the handling of individuals with disabilities.

> ### Intentionality Counts
>
> It is unlawful to discriminate against any person for race, religion, or disability, and what _Doe v. Withers_ (1993) shows is that punitive damages can be awarded if the discrimination is intentional.

Doe's teacher, Michael Withers, was "a prominent member of the General Assembly" and "would not follow the IEP, despite being instructed to" do so by the Superintendent of Schools, his School Principal, the Special Education Director, and the Special Education teacher who worked with Doe.

Crawford v. Honig (1994)

In _Crawford v. Honig_ (1994), the same judge who sat on _Larry P. v. Riles_ (1979, 1984), Robert Peckham, disregarded his own earlier judgment disallowing the use of IQ tests for African American children (District Court, Northern District of California, C-89-0014 DLJ). This case involved the mixed-race child, Crawford, of an African American mother who was having difficulty at school. His mother wanted to have him tested on standardized IQ tests. However, the school denied the request on the grounds that the child was an African American and that IQ testing was forbidden in such cases by the judgment in _Larry P._—specifically, IQ tests were disallowed for placement in special education in spite of the fact that

Did we mention that the application of the law is not necessarily fair, logical, or consistent? Laws and policies have been exceptionally confused with respect to IQ test uses.

they were allowed, inconsistently, for placement in gifted and talented programs in California.

The mother of the child sued for relief and was eventually advised to identify the child by the race of his father to avoid the problem (37 F.3d 485, 488, United States Court of Appeals of the 9th Circuit, 1994). The upshot of the judgment was to permit the use of IQ tests for placing non-African American minority children (including Crawford himself) in programs for special education, but it left standing the earlier rule against applying the same tests to African American children.

Professional and Legal Inconsistencies

IQ tests couched in a language/dialect that some of the children do not know well or at all have been both required and disallowed. They are required by the latest American Psychiatric Association manual (*DSM-IV-TR*, 2000) in defining mental retardation. Also, according to the American Association for the Mentally Retarded, it is not allowed, under their own published criteria, to define mental retardation *without reference to so-called IQ tests*. Yet two of the tests recommended for use by the American Association for the Mentally Retarded were ones disallowed by the Court of Appeals in *Larry P. v. Riles* (1984) —specifically these were the *Stanford-Binet* and the *Wechsler Intelligence Scale for Children*. These same so-called IQ tests, incidentally, were explicitly pronounced nondiscriminatory in *PASE v. Hannon* (1980) by a different judge (506 F. Supp. 831 U.S. District Court for the Northern District of Illinois).

But in *Crawford v. Honig* (1994), the tests disallowed in *Larry P.* were pronounced perfectly acceptable. Although the rule against using IQ tests was not applied to Crawford himself—who was half African American—that rule was to be left in place for *all other African American children in the entire State of California*. Did we mention that the application of the law is not necessarily fair, logical, or consistent? Laws and policies have been exceptionally confused with respect to IQ test uses. The main problem has been the tendency of courts and educational agencies to disregard or misunderstand the role of language/dialect knowledge in interpreting the tests. The tendency has been to treat all children as if all of them had a single homogeneous language/dialect. But this is not so. Occasionally, the judges and policy-makers recognize that assessments need to be done in the child's best communication system(s)—not in a foreign language or dialect that the child does not know well or at all. The problem is that the widespread assumption that all the children in the American public schools have already had sufficient (ample and approximately equal) opportunity to acquire General

American English—the language/dialect more or less universally used in IQ tests, achievement testing, interviews, observational assessments, diagnosis of disorders, and so forth—is not true. As a result, such assessment procedures are certain to give invalid (unfair, biased, and inaccurate) results in many instances.

With the striking exceptions of *PASE v. Hannon* (1980) and of *Crawford v. Honig* (1994), the other cases we review have generally reached the valid conclusion that it makes no sense to assess any child's capacity to learn in any system(s) of communication other than the one that the child knows best.

Daubert v. Merrell Dow Pharmaceuticals, 509 U.S. 579 (1993)

The case of *Daubert v. Merrell Dow Pharmaceuticals*, 509 U.S. 579 (1993) concerned a child born with a multiple birth defects attributed to a drug manufactured by Merrell Dow (retrieved March 11, 2009, from http://en.wikipedia.org/wiki/Daubert_Standard).

The essential elements of the case were these: In 1974, Jason Daubert was born missing three fingers on his right hand and a lower bone in his right arm. During her pregnancy with Jason, Mrs. Daubert had taken bendectin, an anti-nausea drug, made by Merrell Dow. Tests with lab animals showed that the drug could cause birth defects in rodents. However, the Court held that the evidence from rodents was not relevant and ruled in favor of the pharmaceutical company. Daubert appealed and the case eventually was heard by the U.S. Supreme Court in 1993. The Supreme Court reversed the decision but sent the case back to the Ninth Circuit court, which again ruled in favor of the pharmaceutical company.

The upshot of the case was to refine the idea of what evidence is admissible in court. Succinctly put, the evidence presented by an expert had to be relevant and reliable. The court effectively established in *Daubert* that reliable evidence should have already been subjected to scientific tests that would refute it if it were false, published in peer-reviewed journals or other peer-reviewed venues, and established some measure of its likelihood of being wrong. A still higher standard of being widely accepted as a correct theory or standard knowledge by a relevant community of scientists was considered too high a standard.

It is easy to see why the *Daubert* outcome and the new standards for expert testimony were gladly received by the pharmaceutical companies. As we have already seen, those friends consist not only of their own employees and lawyers but also of the civil servants at the FDA, CDC, and the entire Department of Health and Human Services of the U.S. Federal Government. *Daubert* was not a particularly good result for people with any disabilities that may have been caused by prescribed drugs, medical procedures, or vaccines. But, as Yogi might have added, "It still ain't over till it's over!"

If we test a child in a language/dialect or any system that is foreign to the child's experience, we need to see the test as a measure of language/dialect proficiency and not as a measure of innate ability or intelligence (Cummins, 2003; J. W. Oller, 1997; A. A. Ortiz, 1997).

Daubert made the task of plaintiffs in instances of toxic injury next to impossible and it set a precedent that would later be gleefully introduced in the *Omnibus Autism Proceeding of 2007* by friends of the drug industry.

Alexander et al. v. Sandoval (2001)

In *Alexander, Director, Alabama Department of Public Safety, et al. v. Sandoval* (2001), the State of Alabama sought to defend its English-only policy for driver's license examinations which had been struck down by a lower court. The U.S. Supreme Court reversed the prior judgment on the grounds that the private citizen, Sandoval, who had sued Alabama to challenge the English-only law had no right as a private citizen to claim "disparate-impact" against a law affecting all citizens of Alabama.

The U.S. Supreme Court held that Section 601 of Title VI of the Civil Rights Act of 1964 prohibits *only intentional discrimination* based on race, color, or national origin in covered programs and activities. The question of intentionality in discrimination was dealt with explicitly also in *Guardians Association v. Civil Service Commission of New York City*, 463 U.S. 582. In that case, a majority ruled that compensation for damages could only be provided if the discrimination were demonstrated to be intentional. In *Alexander*, the Court explicitly rejected (5 to 4) the notion that regulations created by subagencies of the federal government could override a state's protection against suits by private citizens. Only Congress can override the state's right to pass its own laws. The Court said:

> Like substantive federal law itself, private rights of action to enforce federal law must be created by Congress. (No. 991908)

Thus, Sandoval had no right under the Supreme Court's interpretation of Title VI of the Civil Rights Act of 1964 to bring the suit in the first place. So, the right of a state to pass English-only laws, and to enforce them over the objection of any single individual who might not happen to speak English was upheld. This decision, however, did not invalidate the right of groups of individuals—as in the cases of *Diana* in 1970, *Lau* in 1974, and *Bonadonna* in 1985— to file and win actions in public education on the basis of attempts to teach or test them in a language/dialect the child had not had a reasonable opportunity to acquire. That issue was not about to go away.

. . . the right of a State to pass English-only laws, and to enforce them over the objection of any single individual who might not happen to speak English was upheld.

Improving America's Schools Act, 1994

The **Improving America's Schools Act of 1994 (IASA)** amended the Elementary and Secondary Education Act of 1965 (20 U.S.C. 2701 et seq.; retrieved March 11, 2009, from http://www.ed.gov/legislation/ESEA/toc.html) and increased funding by $750 million per year with the purpose of serving "all eligible children by fiscal year 2004" (Section 1001a2). The lawmakers asserted that the achievement gap between the "disadvantaged children and other children has been reduced by half over the past two decades" and yet "a sizable gap remains" (Section 1001b1). Further, "educational needs are particularly great for low-achieving children in our nation's highest-poverty schools, children with limited English proficiency, children of migrant workers, children with disabilities, Indian children, children who are neglected or delinquent, and young children and their parents who are in need of family-literacy services" (Section 1001b3).

Individuals with Disabilities Education Act, 1997

Following ADA in 1990, IDEA 1990, and the IASA of 1994, the **Individuals with Disabilities Education Act of 1997**, was really yet another renewal and extension of Public Law 94-142 under the new number Public Law 105-17. This renewal, which extended and refined IDEA 1990, was enacted on June 4, 1997. Justifying the revised legislation of 1997 were specific "Findings" which included the observation that:

> poor African American children are 2.3 times more likely to be identified by their teacher as having mental retardation than their White counterpart. (Section 601, Findings, p. 7)

IDEA 1997 explicitly noted that "the implementation of" the 1975 EHA was.

> impeded by low expectations, and an insufficient focus on applying replicable research on proven methods of teaching and learning for children with disabilities. (Section 601c, Findings, p. 4)

In fact, the 1997 law was about 18 times longer than the 1975 legislation. The 1975 law reads like a rough draft, a mere sketch, of the more explicit and developed 1997 law.

Restricted Educational Agencies

IDEA restricted the power of educational agencies to suspend or expel any disabled child. The IDEA legislation provided that the strongest disciplinary action possible—even if a disabled child carried a "dangerous weapon" and/or used and sold illegal substances (drugs)—was a maximum 45-day suspension (Section 615k1Aii, pp. 65–66). We can only wonder how severely disabled a child might be if that individual were capable of running an illicit drug business on the side and possibly defending it with a lethal weapon, but that was the wisdom of the U.S. Congress, with respect to the most sweeping legislation ever enacted concerning disabilities including essentially all communication disorders.

Assessment Requirements

For such exceptionalities, IDEA required a thorough initial evaluation and periodic re-evaluation (at least every 3 years) using "a variety

IDEA reiterated the 1975 rule that there cannot be any single measure for decision-making and that it is the responsibility of the educational agency to show that the procedures applied "assess the relative contribution of cognitive and behavioral factors, in addition to physical or developmental factors" (p. 52).

of assessment tools and strategies to gather relevant functional and developmental information, including information provided by the parent." All this was to assist in determining disabilities and in shaping the IEP to meet the special needs of that child.

A FAPE under IDEA was defined as:

> special education and related services . . . provided at public expense, under public supervision and direction, and without charge. (Section 602, Definitions, pp. 10–11)

and those services also had to meet all the requirements laid down in IDEA. The term IEP:

> means a written statement for each child with a disability that is developed, reviewed, and revised

in accordance with the seven pages of requirements laid out in Section 614 and in cross-linked parts. It was also necessary under IDEA for the education agency to show that the evaluation procedures are not discriminatory and that they:

> are provided and administered in the child's native language or other mode of communication, unless it is clearly not feasible to do so. (p. 52)

As we saw in Chapter 11, and in many of the cases reviewed in this chapter, the most widespread misuse of assessment and diagnostic procedures are the ones conducted in a language/dialect that the child does not know well or at all. The explicitness of IDEA on this issue—that the child should be evaluated in his or her "native language or other mode of communication" was significant. The evaluation must be complete and must not determine a disability solely on the basis of a "lack of instruction in reading or math or limited English proficiency" (p. 52). The tests and assessment procedures used according to IDEA must cover all suspected areas of disability. IDEA also specified that evaluation involving "assistive technologies"—for example, computers, keyboards, picture boards, or other devices—should be used "in the child's customary environment" (Section 602, 2A, p. 9) and only for the purposes for which they have been "validated." Furthermore, any tests were to be "administered by trained and knowledgeable personnel . . . in accordance with any instructions provided by the producer of such tests" (p. 52).

Defining Disabilities

A key element in the IDEA evaluation process was the determination of disabilities. The IDEA legislation greatly broadened the definition of the covered disabilities in Section 602 from the 1975 EHA. Under the new IDEA, a "child with a disability" was defined as:

a child (i) with mental retardation, hearing impairments (including deafness), speech or language impairments, visual impairments (including blindness), serious emotional disturbance (hereinafter referred to as "emotional disturbance"), orthopedic impairments, autism, traumatic brain injury, other health impairments, or specific learning disabilities; and (ii) who, by reason thereof, needs special education and related services. (p. 9)

IDEA required a team effort for evaluating the child and eventually devising an IEP. The "team" (Section 614d,1, B) had to include the child's parents, one of the regular teachers of the child (provided the child has any), a special education teacher or provider, a representative of the educational agency trained in dealing with disabilities and the general school curriculum, someone who can "interpret the instructional implications of evaluation results" (which may possibly be one of the other persons already mentioned), "at the discretion of the parent or the agency, other individuals who have knowledge or special expertise regarding the child, including related services personnel as appropriate," and if "appropriate, the child" (Section 614, pp. 55–56).

Monitoring Progress

The IEP as specified under IDEA (especially in Section 614d) must be a "written statement" and must include a description of the child's level of performance in the general curriculum and how the child's disability (or disabilities) may affect that performance. It must include a plan for intervention with "measurable annual goals, including benchmarks or short-term objectives" relative to the general curriculum and the special needs of the child relative to any disability. It must also specify accommodations by the educational agency to meet the child's special needs showing how the child will be enabled to participate in the regular activities of the curriculum and in extracurricular activities as well. Explanations are required if the child's participation is limited in any way and especially how the child will be assessed in the curriculum. If the child cannot take part in normal assessment processes, reasons must be given, and an alternative plan set down. The beginning date of any special services, their place, frequency, and duration, must be specified.

The program must consider the strengths of the child, the concerns expressed by the parents, and must be articulated in relation to the most recent evaluation of the child. It must specifically address any noted limitations owing to the child's disability or other special needs, for example, if the child needs accommodations because of not knowing English well, requires Braille, or assistive devices or technologies. The IEP must show the role(s) of the regular education teacher(s) of the child and other school personnel to the extent that their participation may be warranted. It must

The education agency was required to show how the child's progress will be evaluated and how parents (or guardians) will be informed.

include evaluations done at least annually and involving both the regular teacher(s) of the child and any relevant new information provided by the parents or other parties. The frequency of assessment and information provided to parents cannot be less often than for nondisabled children according to IDEA. At the periodic evaluation sessions the education agency must indicate progress toward the annual goals set in the IEP and an assessment of the extent to which the child is going to be able to achieve them.

Transfer of Rights

The law also provides for the transition of very young children with disabilities from programs for preschoolers to programs for school age children and for the eventual transfer of rights formerly accorded to the parents to the child (if not incompetent) when the child reaches the age of majority under state law.

If the child is either judged incompetent or incapable of providing "informed consent" concerning any educational programs covered under IDEA, the state is responsible to appoint either the child's parent or someone else to fill that role on behalf of the child" (Section 615, p. 71). According to IDEA, the burden falls to the education agency to show that the evaluation procedures are not discriminatory.

No Child Left Behind Act, 2001 (NLCB)

The **No Child Left Behind Act** (NCLB) also known as **Public Law 107–110** (retrieved March 11, 2009, from http://www.ed.gov/policy/elsec/leg/esea02/107-110.pdf) was supposed to close the achievement gap between poor and rich schools and to raise standards for teachers across the board. According to IASA 1994, and IDEA 1997, testing was required at least every three years in grades 4, 8, and 12, but under NCLB, testing was required each year of all children in grades 3 through 8 from academic 2005–2006.

Emphasis in NCLB was placed on low achieving schools that get more money initially and additional money during the first two years if they have not shown improvement. However, there is a deadline. If achievement has not advanced in the third and fourth years of NCLB funding, students can get tutoring—even from churches or other organizations—or can be bused to a different public school at federal expense. Where no improvement is observed over a six-year period, changes in staffing are required.

> All schools receiving funding must show that students with limited English skills have attained proficiency in English after three years of school attendance.

Omnibus Autism Proceeding (2007)

On June 11, 2007, the *Omnibus Autism Proceeding*, began with the purpose of hearing the case of *Michelle Cedillo v. Secretary of Health and Human Services* (2007). Michelle's was the first of three test cases on behalf of "nearly 5,000 children [now substantially more than that] diagnosed with autism or similar disorders who have filed claims under the Vaccine Act" (Transcript of Day 1, p. 4). Special Master George L. Hastings, Jr., one of the three assigned to hear and decide the three test cases, was assigned to decide Michelle's case. You can see Michelle herself in an interview with Dr. Sanjay Gupta (April 1, 2008, retrieved March 11, 2009, from http://www.cnn.com/2008/HEALTH/conditions/03/24/autism.vaccines/#cnnSTCVideo). In deciding the disposition of the case of *Michelle Cedillo*, Mr. Hastings, acted alone.

Two other test cases were also heard in the U.S. Court of Federal Claims, also known as the Vaccine Injury Court, and were individually decided by the two other Special Masters, Patricia Campbell-Smith, and Denise Vowell. Each of these test cases, as we saw earlier in Chapter 5, went against the plaintiffs and, in effect, in favor of the CDC and the pharmaceutical companies. The Special Masters, in those three test cases, ruled against the unequivocal findings of toxicological evidence. The complaint that the combined toxins and disease agents in the MMR and thimerosal containing vaccines can cause autism was supposedly laid to rest by Special Master Hastings and colleagues. However, the research evidence, as documented in J. W. Oller and S. D. Oller (2009), contrary to the rulings by the three named Special Masters clearly shows that the measles virus alone, as well as the neurotoxin ethyl mercury as found in thimerosal, all by themselves certainly can and do cause immune dysfunction, brain damage, and autism.

MMR Alone Causes Autism

Although it received less attention in the media, a week after the first test cases went against the petitioning families another test case was decided by Special Master Richard B. Abell concluding that *the MMR shot alone can and did cause the brain damage leading to autism in a boy named Bailey Banks.* What is more, on the heels of that case it was learned that 1,322 other cases complaining that vaccines had caused brain injury, without using the term "autism," had already been decided in favor of the petitioning families. At this point it is safe to say that salvos have been fired by both sides in what appears to be a groundswell of growing public understanding that vaccines and their components are key factors, although not the only ones, in causing epidemic chronic disease conditions including autism. The constituents on one side are relatively less powerful but increasingly numerous individuals affected by the autism epidemic and on the other side there are powerful government agencies (the CDC and FDA) allied with the vast pharmaceutical conglomerates worldwide.

If it were not for the stringent statute of limitations on the filing of vaccine injury cases, as argued by Jeff Z. Sell (2006), a lawyer and parent of two boys with autism, many many more of those cases would already be in the queue for the *Omnibus Autism Proceeding*.

Thimerosal. In addition to hearing each of the remaining test cases, the Court must consider the claims of more than 5,300 other families (Edlich et al., 2007; also Fox, 2009) that as Attorney Tom Powell put it, "thimerosal-containing vaccines caused immune system problems and suppression that makes certain children vulnerable or susceptible to viral infections that can cause neurological injuries, including many of the symptoms of autism, and that the MMR in particular is a viral agent that has caused autism in a number of these children, including in Michelle Cedillo" (transcript for day 1, p. 10, ftp://autism.uscfc.uscourts.gov/autism/transcripts/day01.pdf retrieved March 11, 2009). Michelle Cedillo was almost 13 years old when the proceedings began on her case in the summer of 2007. In the recorded testimony her mother reported that Michelle had been a normally developing toddler, a point conceded by Special Master Hastings in his strangely muddled decision. Michelle had babbled at about 6 months, and had an advancing vocabulary by the time of her MMR shot on December 31, 1995 when she was 15 months of age. Before that time she had received at least 112.5 micrograms of mercury in thimerosal from three shots each for DTP, HiB, and Hepatitis B (same transcript, day 1, p. 34). It is highly probably that the Hastings decision in the Cedillo case will be appealed.

After receiving the MMR, within a week, Michelle developed a high fever that persisted intermittently and was accompanied by about 32 weeks of intense diarrhea. In the summer of 1997, Michelle was seen by a neurologist who wrote that she seemed to be suffering from "post immunization reaction" (p. 37). That July, she was diagnosed with autism. The evidence heard and presented to Special Master Hastings—2917 pages of it in the 14 day transcript ("*Omnibus Autism Proceeding*," 2007, retrieved March 11, 2009 at ftp://autism.uscfc.uscourts.gov/autism/transcripts/day01.pdf) tells a story that is eerily similar to tens of thousands of other cases. Also, as pointed out by R. F. Kennedy, Jr. after the Abell ruling, it is evident that some lawyers urged their clients to sue the government for brain injury and to avoid what he called the "radioactive" term *autism*.

An uneven contest. Most of the available Web sites that deal with the issues at stake have always been on the side of the pharmaceutical companies, the mainstream media (which the pharmaceutical companies largely either own or control), the self-protective federal agencies including the CDC and FDA, and the professional organizations and medical journals that are largely supported by the pharmaceutical industry and that have promoted the offending vaccines and their toxic ingredients. Although the *Omnibus Autism Proceeding* is supposed to be a no-fault judgment, the testimony and arguments presented have all the flavor of the sort of conflict and disagreement usually found in **civil litigation** and even **criminal litigation**. For instance, the petitioners—that is, the parents of children with autism and neurological disorders—have claimed that the government, as the respondent/adversary, is protecting the pharmaceutical companies. The petitioning familes hold that the no-fault system that was supposed to make it easier for injured parties to get reasonable compensation for injuries caused by the government, is actually designed to protect from liability the manufacturers of vaccines and the government promoters of vaccination programs; that the routing of claims of injury to the U.S. Court of Federal Claims, has resulted in cutting off normal access (through what is called **legal discovery**) to critical documents and data such as the Vaccine Safety Datalink (the vast database which extends beyond the 123,000 VAERS, adverse event reporting system).

The problem as well documented by petitioners is that the Vaccine Safety Datalink system has been effectively made secret by the government (e.g., see the publications by the Mark and David Geier and the Web sites maintained by by J. B. Handley and Lisa Handley, 2009, retrieved March 11, 2009, from http://www.putchild renfirst.org/intro.html also http://www.generationrescue.org/). The side of the story pertaining to the thousands of almost anonymous individuals who have complied with the stringent requirements of the Vaccine Injury Act in order to seek redress and compensation is being told almost exclusively by independent researchers, journalists, and by injured parties who have won access to documentation through hard fought legal battles. For example, see the Web sites created by the Handleys' and the documentation presented especially, from http://www.putchildrenfirst .org/intro.html retrieved March 11, 2009.

THE HIGHEST PRINCIPLES OF LAW AND ETHICS

What we call "the law" when we say, "It's the law," loosely includes all levels of government. The law, in that general sense, reflects the attempts of governments, whether successful or not, to resolve disputes, even wars, and to enable communities to survive and hopefully to thrive. Grand examples in U.S. history include several wars beginning with the Revolutionary War leading to the establishment of a new government and the creation of a new nation.

The U.S. Constitution

The law distilled from the Revolutionary War was what we know as the U.S. Constitution and all that flows from it. In arguing our case against the King of England—not to mention his army, navy, and all his loyal subjects—our predecessors wrote:

> We hold these truths to be self-evident, that all men are created equal, that they are endowed by their Creator with certain unalienable Rights, that among these are Life, Liberty and the

Some would say, as the authors of Declaration of Independence did plainly say, that the whole conflict leading to the U.S. Constitution, was about "unalienable rights" of human beings that come from a higher source.

pursuit of Happiness.—That to secure these rights, Governments are instituted among Men, deriving their just powers from the consent of the governed, . . . (Declaration of Independence, 1776, retrieved March 11, 2009, from http://www.ushistory.org/declaration/document/)

The founders evidently believed in, and certainly appealed to, an Almighty Creator, because logically speaking there can be no higher authority than the Creator of the universe.

Unalienable Rights Under the Law

What followed, as they say, is history, but the conflict on behalf of the "unalienable Rights" referred to in the Declaration of Independence certainly did not end in the creation of the U.S. Constitution. The first 10 amendments to the Constitution continued the struggle to codify a workable set of laws that would ensure those basic human rights. Accordingly, that part of the Constitution came to be known as the Bill of Rights (1789, retrieved March 11, 2009, from http://en.wikipedia.org/wiki/United_States_Bill_of_Rights). The rights especially provided for in the Bill of Rights included guarantees in the very first amendment of freedom of religion, of speech, of the press, the right to hold meetings, and to ask for redress of unfair treatment by the government. The last provision of that amendment, it may be argued, implies the right of parents and individuals with disabilities to participate in the construction of an IEP and to ask for changes in it.

The Fifth Amendment to the Constitution, that is the fifth item in the Bill of Rights, provided that none of our other rights to "life, liberty, or property" can be taken from us without "due process of law"—a right that has come up many times in reference to subsequent laws and cases involving the treatment of persons with disabilities. The right to "due process of law" was reiterated and elaborated in the Fourteenth Amendment in the following words:

> All persons born or naturalized in the United States, and subject to the jurisdiction thereof, are citizens of the United States and of the State wherein they reside. No State shall make or enforce any law which shall abridge the privileges or immunities of citizens of the United States; nor shall any State deprive any person of life, liberty, or property, without due process of law; nor deny to any person within its jurisdiction the equal protection of the laws. (Cornell University Law School, n.d.-b, Amendment XIV, retrieved March 11, 2009, from http://www.law.cornell.edu/constitution/constitution.amendmentxiv.html)

This law, along with the Thirteenth Amendment to the Constitution, was largely a result of the most costly dispute over civil rights in the history of the world—namely the U.S. Civil War. The Thirteenth Amendment says:

Neither slavery nor involuntary servitude, except as a punishment for crime whereof the party shall have been duly convicted, shall exist within the United States, or any place subject to their jurisdiction. (Cornell University Law School, n.d.-a, Amendment XIII, retrieved March 11, 2009, from http://www.law.cornell.edu/constitution/constitution.amendmentxiii.html)

Conflicts Anticipated and Balanced

We can see that the law is based on, and to a large extent, derived from the resolution of conflicts. Laws are written acts of government that aim to manage disputes and conflicts and to provide for their resolution. The U.S. Constitution and its amendments provide the most basic laws of the United States. Within that law is the wonderful system of checks and balances between the three branches of government—the Executive, Legislative, and Judicial. Under the Constitution, a law that in the United States establishes the basis for our form of government, the Legislative branch writes new laws, the Judicial branch interprets existing laws, and the Executive branch enforces those laws. As a result of this arrangement, cases argued in the courts, as we have seen in all of the preceding elements of this chapter, provide an important basis for interpreting the law. Similarly, there is a dynamic interaction between all three branches of government with respect to human rights.

However, the story of human conduct does not begin or end with written laws. There are principles that run deeper than the "letter of the law"—deeper than its surface forms of expression, deeper than law enforcement, and deeper than required or forbidden conduct. As we have seen, the story of human rights in U.S. law and history begins with an inheritance that cannot be dated—it cannot be dated to the writing of the Constitution of the United States nor even to the creation of the universe. Those rights, according to the authors of the Declaration of Independence, are "unalienable"—that is, they cannot be separated from human beings because they were granted by the Creator. As the authors of the Constitution wrote the Bill of Rights, the Creator put certain rights in human beings, in the spirit of the genome, that cannot legitimately be abridged or taken away by any government on earth.

Ethical Conduct: A Higher Standard

For all the foregoing reasons, at the earthly end of the human rights spectrum—down here in the schools, clinics, hospitals, courts, and other institutions where day-to-day living takes place—the codified laws of government are universally understood to be incomplete. For this reason, professional organizations—such as the American Speech-Language-Hearing Association, the American Academy of Audiologists, the American Psychological Association, the American

As we saw in the case of *Smith v. Robinson* (1984)—where the U.S. Supreme Court refused to award attorneys' fees to Tommy Smith, to which Congress reacted by establishing a new law, namely, the Handicapped Children's Protection Act of 1986—there is a dynamic interaction between legislatures and the courts.

Counseling Association, the American Psychiatric Association, the American Medical Association, and many others—have all provided additional statements about **ethical conduct**. They provide statements about how the professionals that belong to and that may be certified by these associations should conduct themselves. Those ethical statements invariably refer to principles that are older, deeper, wider, and in all ways more demanding than any that may be codified in specific laws.

Such statements by professional organizations are called **Codes of Ethics**. Organizations such as the American Speech-Language-Hearing Association, ASHA, and the American Academy of Audiologists (AAA) rely on such codes to help define and guide in the setting of standards for the training, practice, and certification of their members. Although laws and authorities may be appealed to in such Codes of Ethics, none of them appeal to a higher authority than the American Declaration of Independence. That document appealed to the highest possible authority—the Creator of the universe—in the act of declaring war on the King of Great Britain. In writing statements of conduct and ethics, however, certainly all the organizations we have mentioned in the previous paragraph have appealed to higher standards than any laws that can be enforced by human governments or institutions.

The Golden Rule

Codes of Ethics for the organizations mentioned all tend to refer, as we will see, to some form of the principle known as the **Golden Rule**—that we ought to treat others the way we ourselves would want to be treated. The translation for communication disorders is to ask: "How would I want to be treated if I had that disorder?"

The Greatest Lesson He Ever Learned

Stephen J. Cannell, the successful screenplay writer, TV producer, and novelist—who was dyslexic and failed three grades in school—in response to a question from one of his fans about the greatest lesson he has ever learned says it was simply, the Golden Rule. In his words, "The greatest lesson . . . is that you should always employ the Golden Rule . . . do unto others as you would have them do unto you. My Dad taught me that lesson early in my life and if you're constantly trying never to do anything that you wouldn't want to have done to you, then, you're gonna be in a good place with people and generally gonna have good relationships . . . " (see and hear Cannell, May 29, 2007, retrieved March 11, 2009, from http://www.cannell.com/videoQA.php?s=9&k=84f011ccbe88f676c6

aeaa73929104fc for the original source see Matthew 7:12 and Luke 6:31).

Doing right by others, as simple as it sounds, is essential to genuine success in communication, business, government, and even in Hollywood. In the book titled *Images that work* J. W. Oller and Giardetti (1999) give both the theory and research in advertising, marketing, and economics showing why Cannell's assessment about Hollywood is correct in a very general way.

Moral Principles

In commenting on the 1992 ethics code of the American Psychological Association, Bersoff (1994) complained that it was "overly long, detailed, and lawyered" and he urged "that those who revise the code in the 21st century" ought to "adhere more closely to fundamental moral principles" (p. 382). Bersoff's main complaint was that the APA Code of 1992 protected the psychologists more than it did the persons they treated. That one-sidedness goes against the Golden Rule which requires equity. The most basic moral principle that Bersoff was talking about was the one that Jesus identified as the basis for the Mosaic law and for the standards of conduct related to it. The most succinct distillation of what is known as the Golden Rule is simply that we should treat others as we want to be treated ourselves.

To meet this almost universally accepted moral obligation (cf. Brooks, 2001), all professional organizations dealing with communication disorders generally ask several things of their members that surpass the requirements and the reach of the codified laws of governments:

1. Genuine acceptance of the worth of persons with communication disorders;
2. Valid up-to-date knowledge about milestones of normal development and how communication disorders arise and how they can be treated successfully; and
3. Respect for, support of, and collaboration with other professionals, parents, individuals with communication disorders, and with the larger community.

In other words, to fulfill the obligation of treating persons with communication disorders, as we (professionals) would want to be treated if the shoe were on the other foot, so to speak, we must make valid assessments based on correct understanding and knowledge. To acquire such valid knowledge necessitates that professionals stay in touch with the larger community of persons, institutions, policy-makers, and especially research and publications concerning normal development and communication disorders.

It also follows from the basic theory of what is true, fair, and right that human beings with disorders and disabilities also have the same rights to life, liberty, and the pursuit of happiness as other human beings do.

Knowledge about how to diagnose, prevent, cure, or treat communication disorders must ultimately be based on empirical evidence—the kind found in the scientific research literature—and all of the foregoing must be tempered with genuine respect for the inalienable rights of all human beings.

Hippocrates

All of the Codes of Ethics referred to above and in the following sections, acknowledge either explicitly or implicitly all three of the numbered principles listed in the previous paragraph. All of them also incorporate the fundamental requirement that Hippocrates codified on the basis of practices already in place in ancient Greece (Figure 12–8).

He wrote down certain commonly accepted principles of physicians nearly half a Millennium before the Christian era. Among the principles was that physicians in particular should above all *do good and not harm to those whom they treat*. This is an idea often generalized to clinicians, speech-language pathologists, special education teachers, and professionals in general who deal with physical, mental, behavioral, and other disorders. Historians who have studied and commented on the **Hippocratic Oath** (Figure 12–9) have universally agreed that its essential elements did not originate with Hippocrates himself, but were widely accepted before he wrote them down.

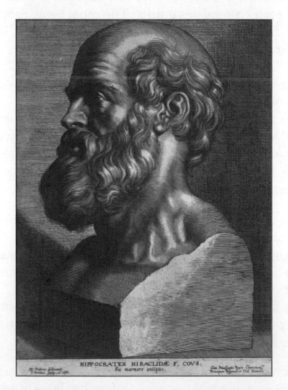

Figure 12–8. Image of a bust of Hippocrates not copyrighted according to *Bridgeman Art Library v. Corel Corporation* (1999)—engraving by Peter Paul Rubens, 1638. Retrieved March 11, 2009, from the National Library of Medicine http://wwwihm.nlm.nih.gov/ihm/images/B/14/555.jpg. Image in the public domain.

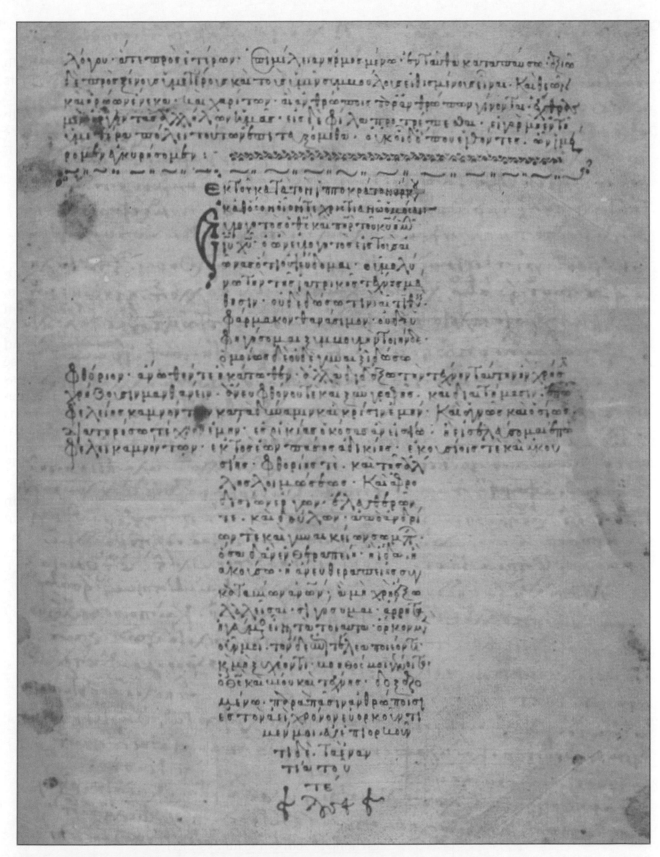

Figure 12–9. A version of the Hippocratic Oath from the Greek-speaking Roman period ca. 1000–1100 AD. Retrieved January 12, 2008, from http://en.wikipedia.org/wiki/Hippocratic_Oath.

Nevertheless, Hippocrates [ca. 460–370 BC] is credited with being "the Father of (Modern) Medicine." However, the oath in its various forms appealed to the highest of authorities. It prohibited euthanasia and induced abortion, and demanded "purity and with holiness" of the physician in how "I will pass my life and practice my Art" (ca, 400 BC, translated by F. Adams, retrieved March 11, 2009, from http://www.cpforlife.org/id19.htm).

Professionals Serving Persons with Communication Disorders

Among the Professional Organizations that serve persons with communication disorders are the ones listed below in this section. We have included the links to their Codes of Ethics and all of them were functional and available on March 11, 2009. Many other organizations could be mentioned that have similar codes of ethics and that in one way or another impact individuals with disabilities. These are singled out for attention mainly because they deal more or less directly with persons known or believed to have communication disorders. They are listed more or less in order with organizations having the widest and most direct impact on communication disorders being listed first. A brief description of what its professional members do is also given:

> Speech-language pathologists are committed to the provision of culturally and linguistically appropriate services and to the consideration of diversity in scientific investigations of human communication and swallowing.

1. The American Speech-Language and Hearing Association (ASHA, 2003, *Code of Ethics*, retrieved March 11, 2009, from http://www.asha.org/docs/html/ET2003-00166.html). The *Code of Ethics* sets the "welfare of persons" served by clinicians as its first ethical principle, and within its *Scope of Practice* document ASHA asserts:

   > The overall objective of speech-language pathology services is to optimize individuals' ability to communicate and swallow, thereby improving quality of life. As the population profile of the United States continues to become increasingly diverse (U.S. Census Bureau, 2005), speech-language pathologists have a responsibility to be knowledgeable about the impact of these changes on clinical services and research needs. For example, one aspect of providing culturally and linguistically appropriate services is to determine whether communication difficulties experienced by English language learners are the result of a communication disorder in the native language or a consequence of learning a new language. (ASHA, 2007, Scope of Practice, retrieved March 11, 2009, from http://www.asha.org/docs/html/SP2001-00193.html#sec1.1)

2. The American Academy of Audiology (2009, *Code of Ethics*, retrieved March 11, 2009, from http://www.audiology.org/publications/documents/ethics/) likewise makes its first principle

also about the persons served, saying: "Members shall provide professional services and conduct research with honesty and compassion, and shall respect the dignity, worth, and rights of those served." In the description of the work and qualifications, the AAA says:

> An audiologist is a professional who diagnoses, treats, and manages individuals with hearing loss or balance problems. Audiologists have received a master's or doctoral degree from an accredited university graduate program. Their academic and clinical training provides the foundation for patient management from birth through adulthood. (2009, What is an audiologist? retrieved March 11, 2009, from http://slhs.sdsu.edu/terms-aud.php)

3. The American Academy of Special Education Professionals (2006a, *Code of Ethics*, retrieved March 11, 2009, from http://aasep.org/about-the-academy/code-of-ethics/index.html).

> . . . for individuals who have dedicated themselves [to] the enhancement of the academic, psychological, physical, and social needs of infants, toddlers, children, adolescents, and young adults receiving services for their special needs. Membership . . . is available to college and university professors, school administrators, educational evaluators, professionals, psychologists, psychiatrists, medical doctors, directors of special education services, directors of early intervention agencies, infant-toddler service coordinators, transition service coordinators, speech and language pathologists, occupational and physical therapists, and all other professionals in the field of special education. (2006b, Overview, retrieved March 11, 2009, from http://aasep.org/about-the-academy/index.html)

4. The American Psychological Association (2002, *Code of Ethics*, retrieved March 11, 2009, from http://www.apa.org/ethics/code2002.html).

> Psychology is the study of the mind and behavior. The discipline embraces all aspects of the human experience—from the functions of the brain to the actions of nations, from child development to care for the aged. In every conceivable setting from scientific research centers to mental health care services, "the understanding of behavior" is the enterprise of psychologists. (2009, Definition of "psychology," retrieved March 11, 2009, from http://www.apa.org/about/)

5. The American Counseling Association (2008, *Code of Ethics*, retrieved March 11, 2009, from http://www.counseling.org/Resources/CodeOfEthics/TP/Home/CT2.aspx) defines the functions of its members as including:

The application of mental health, psychological, or human development principles, through cognitive, affective, behavioral or systematic intervention strategies, that address wellness, personal growth, or career development, as well as pathology. (1997, *The Practice of Professional Counseling*, retrieved March 11, 2009, from http://www.counseling .org/Files/FD.ashx?guid=ea369e1d-0a17-411a-bc08-7a07 fd908711)

6. The American Psychiatric Association (2009, *Principles of Medical Ethics*, retrieved March 11, 2009, from http://www.psych.org/ MainMenu/PsychiatricPractice/Ethics.aspx) advocates the ethical principles laid down by the American Medical Association.

7. The American Medical Association (2001, *Principles of Medical Ethics*, retrieved March 11, 2009, from http://www.ama-assn.or g/ama/pub/category/2512.html).

To promote the art and science of medicine and the betterment of public health. (2009, About AMA, retrieved March 11, 2009, from http://www.ama-assn.org/ama/pub/catego ry/1815.html)

Helping the Person with the Difficulty

The First Principle

All of the Codes of Ethics of the organizations just listed recognize the responsibility of practitioners in these service-oriented professions to place the primary emphasis on the welfare of their clients or patients. According to the American Medical Association in its *Principles of Medical Ethics*, the whole code was "developed primarily for the benefit of the patient" (p. 2). Likewise, ASHA's Code of Ethics requires in its first "Principle of Ethics" that "individuals shall honor their responsibility to hold paramount the welfare of persons they serve professionally" (p. 1). The same idea was clearly expressed by Hippocrates in about 400 BC in the most famous part of what would later come to be known as the "Hippocratic Oath":

I will follow that system of regimen which, according to my ability and judgment, I consider for the benefit of my patients, and abstain from whatever is deleterious and mischievous (as translated and quoted in Sarton, 1952, p. 376).

Judging from his own writings, well before the time of Hippocrates, the essential principles of what would later become known as the

Hippocratic Oath, also the "Law of Hippocrates," were already commonly accepted by prior physicians of that day—about a half a millennium before Christ.

Competence Required

Hippocrates himself also insisted on a "competent knowledge" of the medical arts and deplored "ignorance" and "inexperience as a bad treasure, a bad fund to those who possess it" (see "The Law of Hippocrates," ca. 350 BC/1993, retrieved March 11, 2009, from http://www.cpforlife.org/id19.htm). In fact, the professional codes of ethics in medicine, psychiatry, psychology, counseling, special education, speech-language pathology, and audiology all require competence as a prerequisite to practice. The ASHA Code of Ethics (2003) states in "Principle of Ethics II" that "individuals shall honor their responsibility to achieve and maintain the highest level of professional competence" (retrieved March 11, 2009, from http://www.asha.org/docs/html/ET2003-00166.html#sec1.3). The American Psychological Association (2002) says its members are "committed to increasing scientific and professional knowledge . . . to improve the condition of individuals, organizations, and society" (retrieved March 11, 2009, from http://www.apa.org/ethics/code2002.html).

Educators who deal with communication difficulties and disorders without an adequate grounding in relevant theory and research might be compared to navigators on a stormy sea trying to operate without a compass or pilots flying in bad weather without instruments but with a load of passengers on board. The risks are simply too great and the responsibilities for the lives of other persons are too real to allow for anything less than the utmost diligence.

All of the codes of ethics examined above require adequate documentation of the work performed by practitioners. All of them, along with the Hippocratic Oath, also require respect for the confidentiality of records in order to protect the interests of the clients served. However, there are limits to confidentiality: The professional organizations in medicine, psychiatry, psychology, counseling, and communication disorders put the burden of responsibility on their members to deal with infractions against their respective codes of ethics, and if an individual is a threat to the safety of others there are cases where confidentiality is superseded by moral responsibility.

In cases of ethics violations, the recommended practice by the ACA is first to deal directly with the responsible person(s), and if that fails, to report the violation to the organization. All of the foregoing codes of ethics also make their own members responsible for policing known violations.

The requirements for validity in assessments, diagnosis, testing, and the obligation to examine the practical efficacy of therapies and management programs are especially intense in the codes of ethics of the American Psychological Association and the American Counseling Association. ASHA's Code of Ethics also requires close attention to reliability, validity, and practical consequences of assessments, observations, interviews, measurements, tests, and interventions.

Assessment and Diagnosis as Critical Areas

Speech-pathologists, audiologists, psychologists, and counselors are all required to disclose fully to the persons they treat and their parents (or guardians) all relevant information about assessment, testing, and the efficacy of treatments.

The clear intention in all cases is to provide clients, primary caregivers, and other responsible parties with whatever information they may need to make informed decisions about assessments and interventions. In elaborating on its first principle of ethical conduct, ASHA asserts that its members must "evaluate the effectiveness of services rendered and of products dispensed and shall provide services or dispense products only when benefit can reasonably be expected" (Principle IG). Clinicians as well as researchers and theoreticians are ethically obligated to give attention to the efficacy of proposed and applied therapeutic interventions (ASHA, 2007, p. 3). They must go beyond mere "qualitative description" or honing skills in a particular methodology in order to fulfill requirements for a degree, for instance. Ethical considerations require attention to whether the client/patient/students are benefitting as much as is possible and whether the clinician/teacher/researcher is drawing on the best-known approaches to assessment, diagnosis, and intervention.

Participant observers—who are invariably human beings—also have the obligation, as noted by Guimaraes (2007), to be genuine in their participation. Ethical researcher/clinicians cannot be strictly dispassionate observers who have no prior conception about what our shared purposes as human beings are and of what will work or not work in teaching/therapeutic/clinical interventions. Ethically practitioners are obligated to be informed about the most up-to-date and relevant research and to act according to that knowledge as informed practitioners. Ethical research, intervention, and assessment require concern for whether a given intervention works or not, whether it contributes to recovery or not. Questions of efficacy and the validity of assessment/testing/evaluation are essential to ethical practice.

Validity Is Essential

The ACA (2005) is particularly strict about the use and interpretation of test scores. The aim is not mere description of observed behaviors, but valid description of actual abilities and disabilities based on valid, reliable, and useful tests and assessment procedures. All of this requires, as the ACA noted, that "counselors administer tests under the same conditions that were established in their standardization. . . . In reporting assessment results, counselors indicate any reservations that exist regarding validity or reliability because of the circumstances of the assessment or the inappropriateness of the norms" (see *ACA Code of Ethics*, p. 9, retrieved March 11, 2009, from http://www.counseling.org/Files/FD.ashx?guid=cf94c260-c96a-4c63-9f52-309547d60d0f). Counselors are explicitly forbidden to modify the tests they use.

ASHA (2001), by contrast, formerly encouraged adaptations of assessment procedures with the intention of meeting special needs. The earlier, 2001 "Scope of Practice in Speech-Language Pathology" asserted explicitly "the need to provide and appropriately accommodate diagnostic and treatment services to individuals from diverse cultural backgrounds and adjust treatment and assessment services accordingly" (Ad Hoc Committee on Scope of Practice in Speech-Language Pathology, 2001, pp. I–30). The committee explicitly called for "selection and/or adaptation of materials to ensure ethnic and linguistic sensitivity" and required that clinicians be prepared to "identify, define, and diagnose disorders of human communication and swallowing and assist in localization and diagnosis of diseases and conditions in a wide variety of settings" including schools, clinics, homes, neonatal intensive care units, early intervention settings, preschools, day care centers, and prisons (pp. I–30).

In its more recent statement of the *Scope of Practice in Speech-Language Pathology* (ASHA, 2007), however, the suggestion that speech-language pathologists are qualified to modify tests and assessment procedures in the way suggested in 2001 has been withdrawn, bringing the scope of work more into agreement with the American Counseling Association (2005). ASHA evidently recognizes that assessment and testing cannot just be made up on the spot by unconstrained ethnographers and participant observers as some have urged.

In the 6th edition of *Measurement and Evaluation in Psychology and Education*, Robert M. Thorndike (1997) comments that "the difficulty with individually derived adaptations . . . is that . . . they are often generated *on the spot* by examiners who mean well but do not see enough children with any particular disability to develop a familiarity with appropriate instruments" (p. 404).

Professional Standards

In addition to its Code of Ethics, ASHA also publishes certain standards. For example, for the **Certificate of Clinical Competence in Speech-Language Pathology (CCC-SLP)**, the standards are more explicit than the broad statements in the Code of Ethics. Nevertheless, the standards are also exceedingly broad in describing the range of skills and knowledge required of every certified speech-language pathologist. According to the published *Standards and Implementation for the Certificate of Clinical Competence in Speech-Language Pathology* (ASHA Council on Professional Standards, retrieved March 11, 2009, from http://www.asha.org/about/membership-certification/handbooks/slp/slp_standards.htm) revised July 2008, Standard III-B concerns "basic human communication processes":

The applicant must demonstrate the ability to integrate information pertaining to normal and abnormal human development across the life span, including basic communication processes and the impact of cultural and linguistic diversity on communication. Similar knowledge must also be obtained in swallowing processes and new emerging areas of practice.

In addition, under Standard III-C various areas of knowledge are listed:

articulation;

fluency;

voice and resonance, including respiration and phonation;

receptive and expressive language (phonology, morphology, syntax, semantics, and pragmatics) in speaking, listening, reading, writing, and manual modalities,

hearing, including the impact on speech and language;

swallowing (oral, pharyngeal, esophageal, and related functions, including oral function for feeding; orofacial myofunction);

cognitive aspects of communication (attention, memory, sequencing, problem-solving, executive functioning);

social aspects of communication (including challenging behavior, ineffective social skills, lack of communication opportunities); [and]

communication modalities (including oral, manual, augmentative, and alternative communication techniques and assistive technologies).

In addition, under Standard III-E "the applicant must demonstrate knowledge of, appreciation for, and ability to interpret the ASHA Code of Ethics."

SUMMING UP AND LOOKING BEYOND THIS COURSE

In this chapter we have discussed the historical conflicts, legal contests, precedents, and public laws that provide the social and legal basis for the diagnosis, treatment, and education of persons with communication disorders. We dug down to the foundational principles and crucial documents sustaining the American conception of human rights and the principles that Hippocrates codified.

A basic rule of ethics for serving persons with disabilities is that the person with the least power requires the greatest protection—that would almost always be the student, client, or patient with a disability rather than the professional providing the service. For this reason, the law singles out minorities and persons with disabilities as protected groups. The still deeper underlying principle is that all persons ought to treat others the way they would want

A basic rule of ethics for serving persons with disabilities is that the person with the least power requires the greatest protection—that would almost always be the student, client, or patient with a disability rather than the professional providing the service.

to be treated themselves. It is important to note that without the requisite knowledge, skills, and abilities, it is not possible for educators, diagnosticians, clinicians, doctors, or any professionals that serve persons with disabilities to live up to the standards that their professional organizations routinely demand. For the same reason, laws and regulations governing the treatment of persons with disabilities require competence on the part of the professionals providing treatment. The fact that mainstreaming is preferred over separate or "pull-out" programs for persons with disabilities is consistent with underlying principle that all persons should receive equal treatment under the law. As we look to the future, it will be interesting to see how Congress, the courts, the schools, clinics, hospitals, and so forth, continue to seek equitable solutions to struggles that in the United States, at least, can be dated from the time of the Declaration of Independence forward.

For our part, we subscribe to the proposition that under the law all human beings "are created equal" and have the same fundamental rights to life, liberty, and the pursuit of happiness. We believe that our government needs to remain one that is for, by, and of the people. This includes people of diversity, minority language/dialect backgrounds, as well as individuals with disabilities.

STUDY AND DISCUSSION QUESTIONS

1. What is your view of the relation between freedom of the body and the mind? Was the deafness and blindness of Laura Bridgman and Helen Keller like being imprisoned as Dickens suggested? What about severe autism?
2. What are the similarities and differences between racial segregation and "pull-out" programs for persons with disabilities? Are there any circumstances that you can think of when separate classes are needed, desirable, or beneficial?
3. What costs are associated with separate classes for persons with disabilities? Consider the case of *Bonadonna v. Cooperman* (1985). Explain the principle of the "least restrictive environment" and discuss how it relates to laws against segregation and "pull-out" programs. What about "tracking" or "ability grouping"?
4. What are some examples of inconsistencies and injustices in your view in court cases and laws pertaining to human rights and to disabilities?
5. Why and how are "pull-out" programs inconsistent with *Brown v. the Board of Education* (1954)? What other cases are relevant here?
6. What is the role of IQ tests and language/dialect based assessment procedures and why have they been so controversial in the courts? Why do the courts and laws universally require more than one testing procedure for decisions about disabilities?

7. How could mercury be neurotoxic to animals and not to human beings? Could something have happened during the 1980s and 1990s to make mercury safe during that time frame though after 1999 the FDA, CDC, and pharmaceutical companies decided it was no longer safe and needed to be removed immediately from medicines, especially vaccines?

8. Why are ethical codes invariably more demanding than ordinary laws and court precedents? What do partial birth abortion, slavery, euthanasia, eugenics, social Darwinism, and Nazism have in common? How compatible are they, in your view, with the proposition that all human beings are endowed by their Creator with certain unalienable rights to life, liberty, and the pursuit of happiness?

9. In light of all the cases considered in this chapter what do you think about the role of the U.S. Court of Federal Claims? What do you think the ruling should be in the *Omnibus Autism Proceeding* (2007)?

10. Read the transcript of *Cedillo v. the U.S. Department of Health and Human Services* and then give your own ruling. How would you explain and justify your decision in the case?

Glossary of Terms

The terms in this Glossary are defined with respect to their use in this book. We have tried to use examples that convey the essential meaning of many technical terms, but the reader also may find it useful to consult a specialized dictionary or other on-line resources.

ABA: abbreviation for *applied behavior analysis*.

abducted: pulled apart; the relaxed state of the vocal folds when breathing in or out without voicing.

ability tracking system: a phrase applied with reference to educational systems that claim to differentiate groups by ability and to provide distinct curricula and programs on that basis.

absolute pitch: the ability to detect or produce a particular frequency of a note in singing or other musical performances.

abstractness: the quality of a sign or symbol produced by taking its meaningful content from whatever material objects it may be associated with.

acetylcholine: the main excitatory neurotransmitter of the autonomic nervous system and a key element in the control and regulation of voluntary movements.

acid reflux: the phenomenon commonly referred to as "heartburn" where stomach juices rise into the throat, sometimes as a precursor to vomiting.

acoustic phonetics: the study of the physical aspects of sound waves.

acquired disorder: a type that is not present in the genes of the individual affected by it and that generally occurs owing to some kind of injury after birth.

acquired dyslexia: a disorder where the person affected loses literacy skills owing to something like a *stroke*, head injury, disease, or toxic chemical exposure.

acquired immune deficiency syndrome: a generalized and usually fatal disease caused by a retro virus known as the *human immune virus*.

ADD/ADHD: abbreviation for *attention deficit disorder/attention deficit hyperactivity disorder*.

adducted: drawn together; the dynamic tensional state of the vocal folds when producing voice.

adrenaline: a biochemical consisting of certain amino acids (phenylalanine and tyrosine) that is released by the adrenal gland positioned just above the kidneys; in the bloodstream it acts as a fight or flight hormone and in the nervous system as a neurotransmitter that increases blood flow to the brain and muscles while simultaneously decreasing flow to the skin and the gut—it makes us less sensitive to pain and more capable of movement; also known as epinephrine.

adrenoleukodystrophy: a genetic disorder triggered by long chain fatty acids that build up over time preventing the normal functioning of *myelin*.

adult "neurogenic" disorder: any unexpectedly persistent problem that arises in adulthood and affects the nervous systems of the body; though the term suggests that the disorder originates in the nerves and even is caused by them, in fact, the term "neurogenic" is commonly applied to disorders that merely affect the nervous system in some way.

adverse impact: any effect that discriminates or negatively affects an individual or group, especially, with respect to race, religion, or gender.

afferent nerve fibers: ones ascending to the central nervous system carrying sensory information.

afferent nerves: those that carry sensations and other messages from the periphery to the spinal column and the brain.

agenesis: a complete absence of a system, function, or organ owed to a failure to develop.

agnosias: a class of disorders affecting conceptual understanding, comprehension, or recognition, especially of *icons*.

AIDS: the acronym and abbreviation for *acquired immune deficiency syndrome*.

alexia: technically a condition where literacy is completely lost or fails to develop; also known as *word blindness* or *text blindness*.

alien hand syndrome: a pathological neurological condition where the nondominant hand performs movements that are not under the conscious control of the actor.

allophones: the different surface forms of a given *phoneme* which vary depending on context but which are regarded as manifestations of the same sound by a speaker of the language in question; also see *phones*.

alphabetic principle: the notion or rule that each distinct class of sounds, those that can be used to distinguish the words or surface forms of a given language, should each be represented by just one and only distinct written symbol or *phoneme*; see the *phonemic principle*.

alphabetic writing system: the sort where each written symbol is supposed to represent just one distinct class of sounds; also known as *phonemic writing*.

ALS: abbreviation for *amyotrophic lateral sclerosis*.

alveolar: of or pertaining to the *alveolar ridge*.

alveolar ridge: the hard gum line just behind the upper teeth and in front of the hard palate.

Alzheimer's disease: described by Alois Alzheimer (1906) this condition so commonly affects older persons it has sometimes been referred to as "old-timer's disease" but it is known to be impacted by toxins that damage cortical tissues.

American Signed Language (ASL): the manual language of the Deaf in North America not to be confused with *Signed Exact English*.

amino acids: the basic biochemical building blocks of the proteins that form the essential biochemical systems of plants and living organisms.

amniocentesis: insertion of a needle through the wall of the uterus to withdraw a sample of amniotic fluid to test for genetic defects in a developing fetus.

amodal: a property of concepts that are fully abstract, not involving any of the usual modes of sensory processing.

amplitude: the strength, energy, loudness, magnitude of a signal or waveform.

amyotrophic lateral sclerosis: a progressive neurodegenerative disease of the nerves that control voluntary movements; also known as *Lou Gehrig's disease*.

anosmia: some degree of loss of the sense of smell up to and including no sense of smell at all; technically applicable only to the extreme loss of all sense of smell; also see *dysosmia*.

antioxidants: biomolecules that reduce or prevent the rate of oxidation of other molecules.

anxiety disorder: one characterized by excessive fear or uneasiness.

aphasic jargon: a marginally intelligible string of syllabic speech produced by a person who has lost all or some of the capacity to string words together in discourse in a meaningful way; see *jargon*.

apoplexy: an archaic term for what is commonly known today as a *stroke*.

applied behavior analysis: the systematic application of Skinnerian psychology to the modification and control of behavior in a wide range of situations including the clinical treatment of communication disorders.

apraxia: technically the complete inability to move or coordinate movements but actually used for the full range of disorders of skilled intentional movements.

arcuate fasciculus: the bundle of nerve fibers linking *Broca's area* with *Wernicke's area*.

arrhythmia: an irregular heartbeat that may also be too fast or too slow.

articulation: the result or process of distinct and regular movements of the speech organs, especially the tongue, lips, and jaw, or, in *signed languages*, the distinct movements of the hands in producing meaningful signs; in education, sometimes applied to the coordination of transitions between grades, schools, or educational programs.

articulator: any movable part of the body, especially the mouth or vocal tract (e.g., the tongue, lips, and jaw), or in manual signing, the hands and upper body, that may be involved in speech production or manual signing.

articulatory phonetics: the study of the positions of the moving parts of the mouth, especially the tongue, lips, and jaw in the production of speech sounds.

Asperger syndrome: a condition closely related to classical autism believed by many to be a milder form possibly of high functioning autism which was first described by Hans Asperger (1944); also known as *Asperger's disorder*.

Asperger's disorder: see *Asperger syndrome*.

aspirated: a quality of a sound produced with a puff of air.

aspiration: breathing or sucking air, food, or liquid into the lungs, or, in *articulatory phonetics*, the process of expelling a puff of air in the production of certain plosive consonants such as /p/, /t/, and /k/.

aspiration pneumonia: the type of accumulation of fluid in the lungs that is owed to infections or blockages produce by breathing food or liquid into the lungs (a condition typically produced by swallowing disorders).

assimilation: the process or result of becoming more alike, and in *phonology*, especially, the production of a speech sound in such a way as to make it more like one of its neighboring speech sounds.

assistive technology: any device including special lenses, visual displays, prostheses, chairs, ramps, elevators, and the like, but especially electronic devices such as keyboards and computers that can be used in any way to make communication easier especially for persons with particular communication disorders.

asymmetry: an imbalance or unlikeness in a pattern or arrangement of things.

asymptomatic: without any signs or symptoms of disease or disorder.

ataxic dysarthria: a class of movement disorders where the sequencing of commands to the muscles is specifically disrupted or diminished.

atrophy: deterioration of muscle, tissue, or any bodily function because of disuse.

attention deficit disorder: a condition characterized by inattentiveness, difficulty getting work done, procrastination, and/or organization problems; any unexpectedly persistent difficulty in controlling one's attention and behavior; also see *attention deficit hyperactivity disorder*.

attention deficit hyperactivity disorder: a condition characterized by inattentiveness, difficulty getting work done, procrastination, organization problems, and the additional tendency toward hyperactivity; also see *attention deficit disorder*.

audible electronic text: the output of a program that converts digital text into speech.

audiologists: specialists and clinicians who study and treat disorders of the hearing systems.

audition: the process or result of hearing.

auditory discrimination: the process or result of differentiating sounds.

auditory illusions: phantom sounds that originate in the mind of the person who hears them and may believe that they originate externally.

auditory pattern recognition: the ability, process, or result of categorizing distinct sequences of sounds.

auditory phonetics: the study of the impressions made by sounds, especially the sounds of speech, on the ears.

auditory processing: the ability, process, or result of making sense of a sequence of sounds.

auditory recognition: the process or result of perceiving and knowing the pattern of a sequence of sounds as in a melody or word by comparing the perception whether consciously or subconsciously with one or more memories.

authenticity: the elusive property of discourse in that is naturally produced in the normal contexts of experience; includes such properties as intelligibility, reproducibility, and meaningfulness.

autism: a multiple system metabolic disorder that typically impairs verbal skills, social relations, and ability to take other persons, relations, and attitudes into consideration.

autism spectrum disorders: a growing group of multiple system disorders generally diagnosed on the basis of loss or failure to develop normal verbal abilities, abnormal social interactions, and stereotyped repetitive behaviors such as hand-flapping; a class of disorders now known to be impacted by gut disease, self-immunity, elevated toxicity, and oxidative stress.

autoimmune disease: a condition where the body's defense system attack itself.

autoimmunity: a condition where the body's defense system attacks its own cells.

autonomic nervous system: a normally balanced regulatory system controlling heart rate, glandular secretions, and either the constriction or relaxation of the smooth muscles involved in digestion and other nonvolitional muscle movements; it consists of counterposed components that balance each other—the sympathetic system that increases heart rate and blood pressure and certain glandular secretions and the parasympathetic system that has essentially the opposite functions, reducing heart rate, increasing intestinal and glandular activity, and relaxing sphincter muscles.

autopsy: an examination after the death of an organism, especially a human being, to determine the cause of death.

aversive stimuli: ones that produce a negative reaction or tendency toward avoidance.

axial: the orientation characteristic of any slice or volume that is parallel to the plane that theoretically bisects the brain or body on the horizontal plane in an upright posture.

axon: the bundle of fibrils projecting away from the body of a nerve cell that carries outgoing electrical impulses generated by the cell body.

balanced bilingualism: the ability of an individual whose degree of proficiency in two languages is approximately equal.

basal ganglia: a poorly understood group of nuclei near the center of the brain connecting it with the brain stem.

behaviorism: the materialistic philosophy of psychology that focuses attention on observable acts and their consequences.

Bell's palsy: a type of paralysis of the face owed to damage to or dysfunction of the VIIth cranial nerve (the so-called "facial" nerve) affecting expressions typically on just one side of the face.

Bernoulli effect: the result of the fact that the pressure of a fluid or gas flowing in a contained environment, such as a tube, increases with the velocity of the flow.

beta amyloid: a peptide consisting of many amino acids that are the main constituents of the plaques found in the brains of Alzheimer's patients.

beta-carotene: a form of vitamin A, the main source of the orange color in carrots and sweet potatoes, and a potent *antioxidant*.

bias: an undesirable property of any test, assessment, or measurement procedure which tends to distort and thus increase the error in the process.

bifida: Latin for "cleft" or "split"; see *spina bifida*.

bilabial: produced with both lips.

bimoraic: in *phonology* having two beats as if there were two syllables in a sequence of speech sounds or possibly in a single vocalic element.

binaural hearing: the sort that involves two ears.

Botox: a paralyzing neurotoxin used in cosmetic and other medical procedures to reduce or completely arrest movement of certain muscles.

bottom-up processing: the type that works from surface forms toward meanings and intentions (also see *top-down processing*).

botulinum neurotoxin: the paralyzing neurotoxin produced by the bacterium *Clostridium botulinum* and the primary ingredient in Botox.

botulism: a condition of flaccid (limp muscle) paralysis produced by the neurotoxin botulin.

brain stem: the lower part of the brain connecting it with the spinal cord.

branchial arch syndromes: any one of several conditions that usually appear during the first trimester of a pregnancy when the face is forming; includes *Treacher-Collins syndrome*.

breath group: the length of a sequence of speech sounds or syllables that can be produced on a single exhalation of air.

broadened criteria theory: the notion that the growth in diagnoses of autism and ASDs is owed to the way the criteria for defining ASDs were broadened in 1994.

Broca's aphasia: a loss of speech fluency usually owed to a stroke or brain trauma but that usually leaves the ability to understand speech in tact.

Broca's area: a region in the left frontal lobe of the brain just above and in front of the left ear that is involved in fluent speech production.

bulbar palsy: any paralysis of the types caused by damage to the brain stem and/or the lower cranial nerves.

bulbar region: the brain stem, especially the pons and medulla oblongata.

calligrapher: one who practices the art of decorative writing.

cancellation: in *acoustic phonetics*, a phenomenon where two similar waveforms interact so that each one reduces the effect of the other and in extreme instances may effectively cause each other to be undetectable.

canonical babble: the kind of syllabic repetitive babble that occurs by about the seventh month in normally developing infants.

carcinogenic qualities: cancer-causing.

case law: the sort of legal precedents and interpretive assessments of laws that are created by judges; also known as *jurisprudence*.

case studies: ones which focus attention on actual persons, groups, or instances manifesting the phenomena of interest in real-life contexts.

CAT: abbreviation for *computed axial tomography*.

CCC-SLP: abbreviation for the *Certificate of Clinical Competence in Speech-Language Pathology*.

CDC: abbreviation for the *Centers for Disease Control (and Prevention)*.

Centers for Disease Control (and Prevention): the subagency of the U.S. Public Health Service located outside Atlanta, Georgia, chiefly responsible for monitoring diseases in the interest of public health.

central auditory processes: hearing functions that involve the brain in addition to the ears.

central nervous system (CNS): the brain and spinal cord.

central sulcus: also called the fissure of Rolando, this landmark (see Figure 1–5) separates the motor cortex in the parietal lobes from the sensory cortex in the frontal lobes.

cerebellar ataxia: any one of many disorders resulting in a general lack of coordination of the muscles and limbs; believed to be associated with damage especially to the cerebellum.

cerebellum: a region at the base of the brain on either side of the brain stem just beneath the occipital lobes that is involved in integrating sensory and motor information and in maintaining balance.

cerebral palsy: a disorder of movement and muscular development that involves damage to the cerebrum that can occur before birth, during delivery, afterward up to about age three; some cases are known to be caused by brain trauma, but in most cases the source of the injury is unknown.

cerebrum: the largest part of the brain especially consisting of the outer layer known as the cortex.

Certificate of Clinical Competence in Speech-Language Pathology: one of the professional training requirements to earn a license to be a speech-language pathologist; it can be earned at certain institutions of higher education accredited by the American Speech-Language-Hearing Association by following a prescribed curriculum under the supervision of qualified faculty and by meeting certain other requirements for clinical practice under the guidance of qualified clinical supervisors.

cesarean section: a method of delivering a baby due to lack of cervical dilation or other complications where an incision is made in the mother's abdomen and uterus.

ceteris paribus principle: the essential rule that experimental and observational studies seeking to make valid comparisons between different performances, individuals, groups, or treatments should demonstrate that all other factors have either been eliminated or held equal for the purposes of the comparison at hand.

chelation therapy: removal of toxins by agents that latch on to them and extract them from bodily tissues.

childhood aphasia: a loss of language that in childhood that is caused by brain damage.

chromosome: the part of a sperm or egg cell that consisting of the genetic material which may be passed on to an offspring.

chronological narrative order: a sequence of representations of an event series that is represented to be the same as the sequence in which the events occurred.

civil litigation: any contest in a court of law in which a plaintiff brings a complaint against one or more defendants and the court renders a decision for or against the plaintiff possibly enforcing some right of the plaintiff against the defendant, awarding damages, forbidding a certain act or forcing one, and or making a generalized judgment concerning possible future disputes.

cleft palate: a developmental disorder where the roof of the mouth is not well formed and remains open into the nasal cavities.

clinical neurology: the treatment of disorders and diseases of the nervous system.

cloning: the reproduction of an entire organism through the copying of its *genome*.

Clostridium botulinum: the bacterium that produces botulinum neurotoxin which blocks motor signals to the affected muscles leaving them in a state of flaccid paralysis.

Clostridium tetani: the bacterium that produces tetanus; a spastic paralysis where the affected muscles contract involuntarily as in a muscle cramp.

cluster reduction: the process or result of the tendency to make a single consonant out of two or more consonants; for instance, to convert the final series of consonants in a word such as "jinxed" from /ŋkst/ to /ks/, or in the word "lengths" to make it sound like "links."

cluttering: a theoretically distinct kind of stuttering, according to some authors, where words seem to pile up in a rush like cars simultaneously crashing on a freeway in a heavy fog; see *tachyphemia*.

coarticulation: the simultaneous production to two distinct consonants such as /k/ and /p/, for example—a combination that does not occur in English.

cochlear nuclei: the first level relay stations between the ears connecting them with the muscles of the body and with the higher cortex; where auditory information is integrated and where sensory and motor pathways from the ears to the brain and to the body are connected.

Code of Ethics: any set of rules, usually written down and agreed to by a group of professionals who affirm the rules and promise, in principle, to abide by them.

codon: a sequence of three bases in RNA specifying an amino acid necessary to the construction of a protein (see http://en.wikipedia.org/wiki/Genetic_code visited April 15, 2009).

cognitive momentum: the tendency to complete a thought, inference, or representational process according to expectations; for example, the tendency to expect a certain element to follow on the basis of what has preceded it.

commissure: any bundle of nerves connecting two or more brain systems, but especially large bundles such as the *corpus callosum*, or the *arcuate fasciculus*.

commissurotomy: a severing of major connections between different parts of the brain, but especially the *corpus callosum*.

communication disorder: an unexpectedly long-lasting, persistent, or recurrent difficulty that interferes with normal, successful, ordinary communication.

comorbidity: the condition where two or more diseases, injuries, or disorders exist simultaneously in the same person.

competing acoustic signals: sounds that interfere with each other making it difficult to recognize or understand them.

computed axial tomography: a computational method of converting many x-ray images of the body into a three-dimensional picture where any slice of tissues in any plane or volume of interest can be intensively examined.

concordance rates: the tendency for different individuals to produce the same results or outcomes in a measurement or test.

conduction aphasia: any loss of language ability that affects transfer of information from the sensory systems to the motor systems.

congenital anomalies: deformities that are present at birth—owed to genetic or developmental causes or both.

congenital disorders: ones that are present at birth.

consent decree: an agreement accepted by parties to a lawsuit, usually by the defendant, to stop doing something judged to be illegal in exchange for being released from any further charges or damages under the suit; a kind of voluntary settlement by mutual agreement that comes under the supervision and purview of the court.

consistency requirement: the logical necessity, without which there can be no meaningful signs of any kind, that signs be applied in the same way across individuals and occasions with respect to whatever they signify.

consonant cluster: any systematic, usually consecutive, grouping of two or more consonants in speech production.

consonants: the segments of speech that commonly involve rapid movement at the boundaries of a syllable.

contact ulcer: a sore that forms in the damaged tissue of an injured mucous membrane.

content words: ones that seem to carry a lot of meaning such as nouns, verbs, adjectives, and adverbs seem to do as contrasted with *function words* such as "to" in "He wants to go."

continuous reinforcement: a behavioral training schedule where positive consequences are provided every time a certain behavior occurs.

contralateral: of or pertaining to the opposite side of the brain or body.

contralateral pathways: ones that originate on one side of the body and lead to the opposite side.

control group: in experimental studies, the reference group against which a group receiving some treatment or having some condition of interest is to be compared (assuming that the *ceteris paribus principle* has been followed).

convention: a rule of usage or practice that is implicitly followed in applying symbols in context.

conventional: the primary property of linguistic signs or symbols which arises from their regular use in association with particular objects, persons, relations, or events in experience.

conversation analysis: a particular brand of research tools that are applied in minute detail to the behaviors, gestures, words, phrases, and surface forms used in ordinary conversational discourse.

coronal: the orientation characteristic of any slice or volume that is parallel to the plane that theoretically bisects the front and back of the body down the midline in an upright posture.

corpus callosum: the largest white matter bundle of fibers in the brain connecting the two hemispheres of the cerebrum.

cortex: the surface (outermost layer) of the brain; the thin layer of gray tissue, unmyelinated nerve tissue that covers the surface of the brain and that is involved in complex functions enabling consciousness, memory, reasoning, and language.

cortical deafness: inability to understand words in spite of having otherwise normal hearing.

cortical functions: the essential functions attributed to the cortex, especially the gray matter of the brain.

corticospinal tract: the bundle of nerve fibers connecting the cortex to the motor systems of the body; also known as the *pyramidal tract*.

covert repair hypothesis: the idea that stuttering is the result of trying to some kind of internal breakdown in the process of speech production.

cranial nerves: the sensory and motor nerves that connect the sensory and motor systems with the brain.

craniofacial anomalies: deformities of the face and head.

craniosynostosis: an anomaly of the skull in which distinct bone plates join too early in development.

cranium: the bony part of the skull that contains the brain.

Crohn's disease: an inflammation of the gastrointestinal tract (the tube running from the mouth to the anus) named for the British doctor who described it.

CT: abbreviation for *computed tomography*, a shortened and generalized version of *computed axial tomography*.

cybernetics: the science of purposeful systems that involve feedback and self-control.

cycle of abstraction: the possibly repetitive sequence in which representations are formed first by *discrimination*, then, by *prescission*, and finally, by *hypostasis*.

cystic fibrosis: a progressive disease that mainly impacts the lungs and digestive system.

cytoarchitecture: the systematic structure and arrangement of cells of the body.

DAF: abbreviation for *delayed auditory feedback*.

damp: to reduce the amplitude of a sound.

dead-end classes: ones in which students cannot expect to benefit from at all, that is, where no genuine educational benefits are provided; also called "holding pens."

deceptive representation: one intended to cause someone else to believe, and possibly act on, a false belief.

decoding: the process of figuring out or deciphering a sequence of letters or numbers that represent something other than themselves; commonly applied to the process of "sounding out" a sequence of letters to try to discover the word, phrase, or other sequence of speech units that they may represent; a process that fails with about 50% of the letter sequences in ordinary written English.

decussation of pyramids: the place at the base of the brain stem where the majority of the pyramidal nerve axons descending from the brain cross over to the opposite side of the body.

defendant: the party to a lawsuit who is charged by the *plaintiff* with some wrongdoing that is the basis for the complaint brought to the court.

degenerate: in the logic and grammar, a form that is incomplete or that does not contain all of the parts or elements that are normally expected; in physiology, a form or part that has been damaged and is in a process of progressive deterioration.

degraded acoustic signals: sounds of which the amplitude and/or other qualities have been reduced or distorted.

degrees of freedom: the maximal number of ways in which it is logically (mathematically) possible for contrasted elements in an experimental or empirical study to differ from each other.

delay technique: a behavioral training approach where a reinforcement is withheld momentarily (say for one or two seconds) to allow the actor time to produce an additional, usually more difficult and previously unattained, behavior.

delayed auditory feedback: a condition in which the sound produced by an individual speaker, for instance, is recorded and played back through an amplifier (say a headset) after a lapse of anywhere from 10 to 500 milliseconds; also known as *delayed side-tone*.

delayed side-tone: see *delayed auditory feedback*.

delusional experiences: ones that are internally produced—merely imagined—but that are believed to originate externally by the person having them.

delusional pathology: the sort of disorder where complex imagined events or fantasies are mistaken for real events.

demands and capacities model: the theory that as the complexity of communication increases during early child development, the developing skills and abilities must either keep pace with the increasing complexity or stuttering will be inevitable.

dementia: loss of mental abilities due to deterioration, disease, or cumulative injuries.

dementia pugilistica: deterioration of the brain owed to repeated blows to the head as from a combative sport such as boxing.

dendrites: the fibers of a nerve cell that receive electrochemical signals emanating from other nerves.

dental amalgam: the silverish metal material which is approximately 50% elemental mercury by weight used by many dentists especially in America to fill cavities; the primary source of mercury in human bodies worldwide.

derived signed languages: ones that are based on or derived from the surface forms of a spoken language system, for example, *Signed Exact English*.

detoxification systems: the biochemical systems and organs, especially the gut interacting with the blood, lymph, liver, and kidneys in sequestering and/or transporting poisons out of the body in excrement, urine, mucus, sweat, hair, or nails.

developmental regression: a dramatic loss of previously gained sensory, motor, or, especially, linguistic skills and abilities, as when a child stops responding to his or her name and/or loses vocabulary and verbal skills previously acquired.

developmental stuttering: the kind of abnormal disfluency that begins sometime after the onset of the first meaningful words produced by a child usually sometime after the 18th month and before the fourth birthday.

diabetes mellitus: a disease of metabolism marked by high blood sugar resulting from low production and/or uptake of insulin.

diacritic: a mark added to a letter or string of letters to note some peculiar phonetic quality such as whether a syllable receives contrastive stress or not, or whether the pitch of the voice is rising, falling, level, or some combination of these.

diadochokinesis: the process or ability of rapid and accurate repetitive articulation of markedly distinct nonsense syllables such as "puh," "tuh," and "kuh."

diagnosis: the process of determining the nature and cause(s) of a disease, disorder, or injury.

diagonistic dyspraxia: a condition where the opposite side of the body, for instance, the left hand performs involuntary movements, whereas the other side, say, the right hand, is performing a voluntary movement (also see *alien hand syndrome*).

digital text: a sequence of letters represented in a computer code that can be stored in a computer.

dimercaptuosuccinic acid: an agent used in the chelation of mercury, lead, and other heavy metals.

discourse processing: the production, comprehension, or any use whatever of an intelligible string of representations in one or more languages.

discrepancy approach: a way of defining a disorder or abnormality, especially the notion of *mental retardation* or a *learning disability*, by a difference of a predefined magnitude between verbal and nonverbal scores on some pair of tests aimed at measuring these constructs.

discriminated symbol: the surface form of a word as noticed by a perceiver in contrast to other words or symbols from which the one in question is distinct.

disfluencies: any hesitation, false start, prolongation, interruption, repetition, or any combination of these phenomena during the production of speech or other linguistic signs.

disproportionate representation problem: the fact that language/dialect minorities tend to be over-represented in categories of disabilities and under-represented in gifted categories.

dissimilation: the process or result of making things or behaviors unlike each other and in *phonology*, especially, the production of a speech sound in such a way as to make it unlike one of its neighboring speech sounds.

distributed neural networks: these are generally construed as models of how the brain works with multiple systems of nerves interconnected with each other and working in communication with each other on the same or related processing problems.

distributed processing: different parts of a problem are handled by different systems more or less simultaneously.

dizygotes: identical twins.

dizygotic: the property of fraternal twins (*dizygotes*) who are actually siblings formed from two different unions of distinct egg and sperm cells but happen to be born at the same time.

DMSA: an abbreviation for *dimercaptuosuccinic acid*.

dopamine: a hormone and neurotransmitter that can cross the blood-brain barrier in the medication known as L-dopa used to treat Parkinson's disease.

Down syndrome: a genetic disorder named for John Langdon Down [1828–1896] described in 1866; caused by an extra copy of chromosome 21 (see Lejeune, 1959).

Dred Scott decision: the case argued in the U.S. Supreme Court before Chief Justice Roger Brooke Taney on behalf of a former slave named Dred Scott in which Taney ruled in 1857 that the phrase "all men" in the American Declaration of Independence did not include black Africans.

dual-tasks: ones that involve two distinct sets of complex actions that must be performed more or less simultaneously.

Duchenne-type smile: the universal genuine smile distinguished by cheek raising, spreading, and a friendly and happy squinting of the eyes; the genuine spontaneous kind of smiling named for Guillaume Duchenne who studied its characteristics and identified it as distinct from the professional smile that shows deliberate politeness without spontaneity.

duration: in *phonetics*, the amount of time it takes to produce a particular sound segment or sequence of sounds.

dys-: a Greek prefix applied to terms in English to suggest abnormality or malfunction.

dysarthria: a disorder of movement affecting transmission or reception of motor signals to the muscles.

dysfluencies: the spelling commonly used to signal abnormal *disfluencies* as the intended meaning.

dysgraphia: any disorder or unexpectedly persistent disorder of writing or the ability to string letters or other written symbols together in a meaningful way.

dysosmia: any dysfunction or disorder of the sense of smell.

dysostosis: any condition where the bones are not well formed.

dysphagia: any disorder of swallowing.

dyspraxia: any disorder affecting voluntary skilled movements.

effect size: the relative magnitude of the variability attributable to a predicted outcome—for instance, that persons receiving a certain treatment would recover faster than a control group that did not receive the treatment—which must be judged by taking into consideration the magnitude of variability attributed to errors and to any irrelevant initial differences between the groups.

efferent nerve fibers: ones carrying signals that control movements.

efferent nerves: those that carry messages and commands for movement from the central nervous system and the spinal column to the periphery.

electromyography: a measurement system that involves attaching electrodes to the skin and/or scalp to measure electrical impulses that enervate muscles.

electron: an extremely common basic atomic particle/wave that carries a negative charge.

elicited imitation: an assessment procedure where the person being evaluated is asked to copy or reproduce an action or utterance of another person.

elision: see *ellipsis*.

ellipsis: the omission of a single segment, whole word, phrase, or clause from the surface form of ordinary discourse.

Emancipation Proclamation: the order issued by U.S. President Abraham Lincoln issued on the authority of Article II, section 2 of the United States Constitution in his role as "Commander in Chief of the Army and Navy" during the American Civil War on September 22, 1862; it committed the Union to ending slavery.

embodiment: the association of representations and meanings with actual physically situated bodily objects, persons, and events.

embryological development: in humans, the development from conception to birth; sometimes restricted to that portion of gestation up to the point where the organs and limbs are differentiated sufficiently so that the developing baby resembles an adult in its body parts and extremities.

embryologist: a specialist who studies development from conception to birth.

emphysema: a chronic disease of the lungs typically caused by toxins, for example, an accumulation of nicotine and tar from long-term tobacco smoke inhaled into the lungs.

entrainment: the synchronization in part or in whole of one individual's body rhythms and movements with those of another, as typically seen between speaker and listener when they are fully engaged in conversation.

epenthesis: the phonological process of adding a segment between two others, in order to make the whole consistent with the *phonotactics* of a given language.

epidemic: an incidence of disease at a rate higher than what is expected.

epidemiologists: specialists who study factors contributing to health and disease in populations with a view toward intervention and prevention of disease.

epidemiology: the statistical study of the outbreak and course of diseases that tend to spread in human (or other) populations, including especially the scientific study of epidemics.

epigenetic disorders: ones that are caused by, or that at least involve, some interaction between genes and other factors such as *metabolism* or the *immune system*.

epigenetic systems: all of the bodily systems that are determined in part by genetics and yet interact with the genetic systems so as to produce higher order effects.

epiglottis: the small flap of tissue that normally is open to allow breathing through the mouth and nose but that blocks the opening into the trachea when a swallowing movement is initiated.

epileptic seizures: sudden loss of consciousness accompanied by involuntary spasms of the body associated with abnormal electrochemical hyperactivity in the brain.

epileptics: individuals affected by *epilepsy*.

epinephrine: a biochemical consisting of certain amino acids (phenylalanine and tyrosine) that is released by the adrenal gland positioned just above the kidneys; in the bloodstream it acts as a fight or flight hormone and in the nervous system as a neurotransmitter that increases blood flow to the brain and muscles while simultaneously decreasing flow to the skin and the gut—it makes us less sensitive to pain and more capable of movement; also known as adrenaline.

Equal Protection Clause: the statement in the Fourteenth Amendment to the U.S. Constitution that "no state shall . . . deny to any person within its jurisdiction the equal protection of the laws."

esophagus: the tube leading from the mouth to the stomach.

ethical conduct: actions that conform to understood and sometimes to an explicitly agreed to *Code of Ethics* as of a professional organization.

etiology: the explanation of the cause(s) and/or course of any given disease, injury, or disorder.

eugenics: defined as the "self-direction of human evolution" (Second International Eugenics Conference, 1921); the intentional effort of groups, individuals, or governments to purify the so-called "gene pool" by preventing individuals with deformities or from "undesirable" or "inferior" backgrounds (however they may be defined) from reproducing (and/or surviving); the Nazi extermination programs carried the idea to extreme limits during World War II.

euthanasia movement: a movement advocating "mercy" killing and/or assisted suicide in various forms, for example, to prevent the survival of infants with birth defects, as a means of population control, or as a means of furthering the interest of *eugenics*.

excitatory: tending toward muscular contraction as contrasted with relaxation.

expiratory reserve volume: the amount of air retained in the lungs after breathing out.

expressive aphasia: any loss of language or speech ability affecting the ability to produce speech, writing, or signed language forms.

extinction: in behaviorism, the reduction of the frequency of a behavior until it no longer occurs at all.

extralinguistic elements: aspects of discourse that are not considered by traditional linguists to be part of the language itself, such as the persons involved in creating the discourse.

extrapyramidal tract: the bundle of nerve fibers connecting the cortex to the motor systems of the body; also known as the corticospinal tract.

extrinsic factors: any conditions or contributing elements that influence an organism, person, process, disease, disorder, and so forth, from outside the body and/or the mind.

facilitated communication: an intervention procedure by which the clinician (facilitator) guides or assists the client/patient's hand in typing or otherwise manipulating a keyboard or symbol system.

facilitating context: one that makes something easier or more likely; applied in the literature on stuttering to contexts that make stuttering either more or less likely.

false representation: one that purports to stand for facts that are not as they are represented to be.

FAPE: abbreviation for *free and appropriate public education*.

fasciculation: twitching of a muscle caused by involuntary contraction of one or more muscle cells.

fast speech: the kind produced when reading aloud, for instance, and actually searching for a place in the text, or in rapid recitation of a text that has been memorized.

fetal alcohol syndrome (FAS): a multiple system neurological disorder evident at birth (i.e., *congenital*) believed to be caused by alcohol consumption of the mother during her pregnancy; symptoms include diverse cognitive, motor, and possibly sensory deficits.

fictional representation: one that purports to stand for facts that must be imagined and that are not present in the common physical world of experience.

filtering effects: the results of damping or removing certain frequencies from a sound signal.

fissure of Rolando: this landmark (see Figure 1–5) separates the motor cortex in the parietal lobes from the sensory cortex in the frontal lobes; also known as the central sulcus.

fixed-ratio schedule of reinforcement: a plan for providing positive consequences for a particular behavior on every *n*th occurrence where *n* may be any number greater than 1 and usually less than 7.

flaccid dysarthrias: the type that involve a limp muscle paralysis reduced mobility.

floppy child syndrome: a condition of limp skeletal muscles associated with certain pervasive childhood disorders, for instance, with severe autism in some cases.

fluency shaping: any one of various therapeutic procedures that aim to make distorted fluent speech, such as an extremely slow rate, seem more natural.

fMRI: the common abbreviation for *functional Magnetic Resonance Imaging*.

fontanelles: the soft spots on the neonate's head that allow the skull to flex thus enabling the head to go through the birth canal; there are two such soft spots, one toward the front of the top of the head and one toward the back where bone plates of the skull eventually will join more completely and harden.

foreign accent syndrome: a neurological condition that makes a person sound as if speaking with a foreign accent.

formants: bands of concentrated sound energy in certain frequency ranges produced by resonating cavities, as in speech.

Franceschetti syndrome: another name for *Treacher Collins syndrome*.

free and appropriate public education: defined by law as including services "provided at public expense, under public supervision and direction, and without charge," and meeting certain standards in addition to providing an *individualized education program*.

free radical: a negatively charged atom or molecule that is likely to participate in any possible chemical reactions—a kind of chemical loose cannon looking for a place to lodge.

frequency: the rate at which cycles of a regular sound wave recurs.

fricative sounds: ones that involve noise produced by air molecules rushing between two or more surfaces within the vocal tract.

fricatives: in *phonetics*, sounds that involve significant noise produced by air flowing rapidly between opposed surfaces of the articulators.

frontal lobes: the foremost lobes (divisions) of the brain roughly behind the bony part of the skull known as the forehead and in front of and above the ears.

function words: typically applied (loosely at best) to the so-called "small" words such as "to," "on," "by," and so forth that do not seem to carry easily detectible or consistent content but that work rather as signals about how to take the other meaning laden *content words* that consist mainly of the traditional categories known as nouns, verbs, adjectives, and adverbs.

functional disorders: any unexpectedly persistent problem that affects performance and that has no known physiological or anatomical cause.

functional hemispherectomy: the process or result of producing the effect of removing an entire hemisphere of the brain by isolating that hemisphere from all its connections to the rest of the body and the opposite side of the brain; also see *commissurotomy*.

functional Magnetic Resonance Imaging (fMRI): a method using multiple magnetic fields to measure changes in biochemical systems at a molecular level over time and to transform them into visible images—moving pictures of what is going on inside a living organism.

functional MRI: the process or result of *magnetic resonance imaging* that produces a series of moving pictures of what is going on internally while the person under examination is performing some task.

fundamental frequency: the average rate at which the vocal folds move from a closed position to an open one during speech production.

GABA: an abbreviation for *gamma amino butyric acid*.

gamma amino butyric acid: an amino acid that functions as a neurotransmitter inhibiting the excitation of muscles or nerves.

gas theory of smiling: the absurdly false but popular and widespread notion, propagated by many pediatricians and medical practitioners in the past, and some to this day, that babies smile when they have gas pains.

gastroesophageal reflux disease: persistent heartburn that can damage the delicate tissues of the larynx possibly leading to more serious conditions such as cancer.

gastrointestinal tract: the gut from mouth to anus.

gauss: a unit of measure for the power of a magnet named after the mathematician Johann Carl Friedrich Gauss [1777–1855] (see Gauss, 1855/2007).

gaze: a term applied in speech-language pathology and education to refer loosely to fixations of the eyes, or sometimes, the eye movements involved in *smooth pursuit* or the rapid movements called *saccades*.

gene pool: a misleading term suggesting that there is a collection of genes in a population that can be singled out and selected naturally or artificially for exclusion.

General American English: the variety of English spoken most widely throughout the United States and especially throughout the western half of the country.

generality: the property of abstract signs by which they are enabled to apply to all possible instances of a given kind.

genes plus toxins theory: the idea that ASDs are caused by a combination of genetic susceptibility together with cumulative oxidative stress and toxic injuries.

genetic disorders: ones in which damage to genes plays a role in either causing or enabling the causation of the problem; nearly all diseases have a genetic component.

genetic theory: the idea that ASDs, and many other communication disorders, are caused by genetic factors alone.

geniculate fibers: these are the nerve axons that cross from one side to the other at the brain nuclei forming a shape that is like a knee (Latin: *genu*); literally the "crooked" fibers or "bent ones."

genome: the entire genetic inheritance of any given organism expressed in DNA; the term was created by Professor Hans Winkler (1920), of the University of Hamburg in Germany by combining the word *gene* and *chromosome* (see Lederberg & McCray, 2001, also http://en.wikipedia.org/wiki/Genome visited April 15, 2009) making it a *portmanteau*.

genotoxic: poisoning and thus damaging the genes.

genotoxin: a poison that damages genes or the *genome* of an organism.

GERD: an abbreviation for *gastroesophageal reflux disease*.

germ cells: in reproducing organisms, especially mammals including human beings, these are the cells that contain the chromosomes that will unite with chromosomes from the other parent in the formation of any offspring.

gestational period: the time from conception to birth which in humans is approximately nine months or from 37 to 42 weeks.

give-me-the-money theory: the notion that the number of diagnosed ASDs in recent years has been increasing because more money has been available for ASDs than for other communication disorders; also called the *changing diagnosis theory*.

glial cells: the most numerous cells of the brain outnumbering the rest by a margin of at least 10 to 1 and which are now known to be involved in neural transmissions in addition to their functions in cleaning up and disposing of dead cells, waste products, and reusable pieces of biochemicals in the brain.

glides: speech sounds that are neither considered to be strictly vocalic nor consonantal, but somewhat in between these categories.

gliotransmissions: ones emanating from or originating in the glial cells of the brain.

global agnosia: a generalized inability, usually the loss of ability, to comprehend, or to make use of icons and the abstract concepts associated with them.

global aphasia: a generalized inability, usually the loss of ability, to comprehend, or to make use of symbols but especially language.

glottal plosive: a stop consonant produced by closing the vocal folds completely and then releasing them under pressure.

glottal stop: one produced at the *glottis*.

glottis: another term for the vocal folds.

glutamate: a form of glutamic acid which is involved in inducing the taste known as *umami*.

glutathione: an antioxidant containing glutamate as one of its components that protects cells from toxins.

Golden Rule: the idea from Biblical teaching, especially as put by Jesus of Nazareth, that we should treat others the way we would want to be treated.

GPA: abbreviation for *grade point average*.

Grade 1 Braille: the original form of Braille writing invented by Louis Braille.

Grade 2 Braille: an evolved system of Braille writing that uses various standardized abbreviations and contractions.

Grade 3 Braille: an advanced system of Braille writing adapted by a particular individual complete with multiple shortcuts and abbreviations.

grade point average: the result of a process of assigning a numerical value to letter grades at school, multiplying by the number of credits earned with that grade, and then computing the sum of all points earned and dividing by the number of credits to get the average.

grammar: applied in this book in the linguistic sense to refer to the largely subconscious knowledge that native speakers of a language acquire from childhood—including knowledge of the phonetics, phonology, phonotactics, morphology, lexicon, syntax, semantics, and pragmatics of a language.

granulomas: grain-like nodules seen in many diseases including Crohn's, tuberculosis, and leprosy.

GSH: the chemical abbreviation for glutathione.

Gulf War syndrome: a neurological condition of unidentified causes associated with the vaccinations given to combatants of the 1991 Persian Gulf War; symptoms include immune disorders and birth defects in offspring.

gustatory: of or pertaining to the sense of taste.

Haemophilus influenzae B: a vaccine to immunize recipients against a type of flulike infection caused by a rod-shaped bacterium by the name, *Haemophilus influenzae*.

hallucinations: imagined events that involve fictional elements that are unintentionally and unknowingly being produced by the person experiencing them.

hand-eye coordination: the ability and skill involved in using vision in part to control movements such as reaching and grasping an object, throwing and catching, and the like.

hand-flapping: one of the tell-tale symptoms of Kanner-type autism.

hard glottal attack: the onset of a voiced sound or sequence involving a higher than normal degree of tension in the vocal folds.

hard of hearing: a phrase applied to persons who have difficulty hearing but who are not profoundly deaf.

Helicobacter pylori: a flagellated bacterium found in the gut that is associated with stomach ulcers and cancers.

hemispherectomy: removal of an entire hemisphere of the brain.

hemoglobin: the complex protein that enables red blood cells to carry oxygen from the lungs to other parts of the body.

hemorrhagic strokes: ones involving brain damage attributed to internal bleeding either in the brain or in any part of the tissues and cavities surrounding it.

heritability: the likelihood that a trait will be passed from one generation to the next.

hertz: a basic unit of measure, one cycle per second, applied to repeated cycles as in sound and light waves.

hesitation phenomena: usually applied to the normal processes by which a person maintains the right to speak by gestures and vocalizations such as "uh . . . ummmm" and so forth.

HFA: abbreviation for *high functioning autism*.

HiB: abbreviation for *Haemophilus influenzae B*.

hierarchy: a complex system with layers and ranks where higher elements regulate lower ones.

high functioning autism (HFA): a relatively mild form in which the person affected is highly verbal and able to perform many tasks.

high functioning autism: a relatively mild form of autism where the individuals affected are able to acquire language and perform certain limited tasks.

Hippocratic Oath: a *Code of Ethics* written down in about 380 BC, presumably from existing oral traditions and rules of conduct that were already widely accepted in the medical profession of that time.

HIV: the abbreviation for *human immunodeficiency virus*.

Holocaust: the deliberate extermination between 1939 and 1945 of about six million Jews, many members of certain other ethnic and religious groups, and 200,000 individuals with disabilities by the National Socialists under Hitler.

homeopathic effect: the sort of disputed result where, supposedly, a larger dose of whatever cures a disease may also cause it.

HPV: abbreviation for *human papilloma virus*.

human immunodeficiency virus: the retro virus that can lie dormant for at least 10 to 15 years before activation that causes *AIDS*; also known by its abbreviation, *HIV*.

human papilloma virus: a virus associated with cervical cancer.

Huntington's chorea: a genetic disorder that involves sweeping dance-like movements that are only partially under voluntary control; also known as *Huntington's disease*.

Huntington's disease: a genetic disorder that involves sweeping dance-like movements that are only partially under voluntary control; also known as *Huntington's chorea*.

hydrocephalus: a condition where excessive cerebrospinal fluid builds up in the cavities inside the head.

hyperactivity (ADD/ADHD): the state or result of excessive excitability; a condition of chronic and persistent excitability.

hyperfunction disorders: ones where a performance is accentuated in an extreme way that tends to overshoot the intended actions.

hypernasality: a quality of speech that arises when not only the nasal sounds designated in writing by "m," "n," and "-ng" are *nasalized* but essentially all syllables are nasalized; a common feature of speech associated with a cleft palate; also see *velar insufficiency*.

hypertonia: a spastic condition where the muscle is overstimulated and tends to contract into an almost cramped mode.

hypokinetic dysarthria: a class of movement disorders involving harsh-hoarse voice quality, abnormal speech rhythms, rigidity, and reduced range in the articulators.

hyposmia: reduced sense of smell.

hypostasis: the highest process of nearly complete abstraction by which the content of a representation is completely separated from all the space-time contexts of experience but not from the content of whatever logical object that representation may be used to stand for.

hypostatic symbols: ones that are as abstract as possible; see *hypostasis*.

hypotonia: a flaccid condition where the muscles are understimulated and are limp, tending toward atrophy.

Hz: the abbreviation for *hertz*.

IASA: abbreviation for the *Improving America's Schools Act of 1994.*

icon: any sign that functions as a sign by the property of being like or identical with whatever object, scene, or person that it represents.

IDEA: abbreviation for the *Individuals with Disabilities Education Act of 1997* and later.

ideographic writing: the kind where symbols represent concepts or ideas rather than the surface forms of speech.

IEP: abbreviation for *Individualized Education Program.*

illusion: a regularly produced perceptual error that occurs where a phenomenon seems to be different than it really is, for example, see the *McGurk interactions.*

immune systems: the complex of systems by which an organism protects itself from invaders, such as parasites, bacteria, and viruses.

imperfect: in grammar, this term is applied to actions or states that are ongoing, incomplete, or in progress and the representations that stand for them; for instance, if we say "he was going to town" the action depicted is *imperfect.*

imperforate anus: a malformation of the digestive tract where there is no opening for elimination of solid wastes.

in utero: in the womb.

incipient stuttering: see *persistent developmental stuttering.*

index: any sign that functions as a sign by linking at least two other signs (an *icon* with an *icon*, an *icon* with a *symbol*, a *symbol* with a *symbol*, an *index* with another *index*, and so forth) to each other through the action of one or more sign-users.

individualized education program: under the EHA a required element of a *free and appropriate public education.*

infantile autism: the variety described by Leo Kanner (1943) of which major symptoms included loss of or failure to acquire language, difficulty with social relations, insistence on sameness, repetitive stereotyped movements (e.g., hand-flapping), and gut-related digestive problems; also known as *Kanner-type autism.*

infantile paralysis: the result of having been physically injured in childhood by the disease known as *poliomyelitis,* or simply *polio.*

inflammatory bowel disease: characterized by ulcers in the gut; one of the hallmark symptoms known to affect between 70 and 80% of persons diagnosed with autism.

infrasystems: the subsystems that undergird one or more higher systems in a hierarchy.

inhibitory: tending to prevent or reduce the magnitude or an action, thought, or process.

innate intelligence: the theoretical intellectual capacity that an individual is born with irrespective of whatever experiences and environmental accidents may occur after birth.

inner hair cells: these are very fine hair-like sensors inside the cochlea or inner ear.

inspiratory reserve volume: the additional amount of air that could be inhaled to achieve maximum capacity after drawing a normal breath of air.

instructional dyslexia: the kind that is caused by particular methods of trying to build literacy by teaching rules for associating the distinct surface forms of speech with letters and sequences of letters with minimal or no reference to meaning.

instructional utility: a property of tests, assessment procedures, or measurement approaches that enables persons tested, assessed, or measured to benefit from by learning while participating in the process.

integration training: therapy aimed at enabling the senses and/or sensory-motor systems to work together more efficiently.

inter-rater reliability: the agreement between distinct judges or raters of some performance, activity, quality, or whatever may be the logical object of measurement; usually assessed by some form of statistical correlation.

intermittent schedule of reinforcement: in behaviorism, a plan for providing positive consequences for a given behavior on an unpredictable schedule.

internal capsule: a V-shaped system of axonal fibers connecting the motor cortex with the pyramids just above the medulla oblongata.

International Phonetic Alphabet: a system of writing that aims to full achieve the *phoneme principle* of assigning just one letter to each distinct sound of each of the world's 6,912 known language systems.

interneurons: the kind of nerves within the body that connect sensory, motor, or other interneurons to each other; the main neurons of the gray matter and that also interact with glial cells.

interpretation: the process or result of understanding and translating from one language to another, or paraphrasing the sense of a discourse or segment thereof.

intonation: in speech production, any and all *prosodic elements* that make up the stream of speech and their collective effects.

intracerebral hemorrhage: bleeding that occurs within the *cerebrum* (one of the major hemispheres of the brain).

intrarater reliability: the agreement a single judge or rater with his or her own assessments across different occasions or instances of some performance, activity, quality, or whatever may be the logical object of measurement.

intrinsic factors: any conditions or contributing elements that influence an organism, person, process, disease, or disorder, from within the body and/or the mind.

intubation: the process of putting a tube directly into any opening in the body.

ipsilateral: on the same side.

ipsilateral pathways: ones that originate and terminate on the same side of the body.

ischemic stroke: damage to brain tissue because of deprivation of oxygen; contrasts with *hemorrhagic stroke* where the damage is caused by internal bleeding that may also cause damage by depriving parts of the brain of the normal flow of blood.

isomorphic: having the same form as.

jargon: any special term or collection of terms used in a particular endeavor or profession, for example, the technical language of psychology or of linguistics; in aphasias of certain kinds, especially of the *Wernicke* type, a manner of speaking and the invented vocabulary that is difficult or perhaps impossible for the noninitiated to understand.

Jim Crow laws: state laws that condoned the pretense of providing "separate but equal" facilities in order to continue the practice of racial discrimination after the official abolition of slavery.

jurisprudence: see *case law*.

Kanner-type autism: see *infantile autism*.

kinesics: the study of significant bodily gestures and movements other than linguistic ones.

kinesthetic feedback: sensations within the body informing the actor about actions performed.

lability: the quality of being prone to emotional extremes.

language disorder theory: the notion that stuttering is more than a mere phenomenon of speech and that it involves deeper levels of linguistic processing.

language learning impaired: a disordered quality or state attributed to persons who have unexpectedly persistent difficulty in acquiring a language or some aspect of normal language use, knowledge, or skill.

laryngeal webbing: the pathological formation of web-like connections between the vocal folds.

larynx: the voice box also known as the "Adam's apple."

late-term abortion: any deliberate termination of a pregnancy resulting in the death of the developing baby; also known as *partial birth abortion*.

lateral cerebrospinal fasciculus: the larger bundle of motor nerve fibers extending down the spinal column from each side of the descending corticospinal tract; also known as the *lateral corticospinal tract* and the *crossed pyramidal tract*.

lateral progress: growth in linguistic and cognitive development that involves adding more concepts at the same level of abstraction that a child has already achieved; for instance, adding more words for objects after the first such word has already been attained.

lateralization: the distribution of one or many functions to one side or other of the body and/or brain.

lateralization hypothesis: the notion that certain functions tend to be controlled predominantly or possibly exclusively, as in the production of speech and writing, by only one side of the brain.

LD: an abbreviation for either *learning disability* or *language disorder*; sometimes used deliberately to cover both these terms.

LEA: abbreviation for *Local Education Agency*.

learning disability: any unexpectedly persistent difficulty in acquiring new knowledge, or an additional skill or ability; indistinguishable in common usage and in most aspects of clinical practice from *language disorder*.

least restrictive environment: one that allows the maximal freedom of opportunity to participate in the mainstream and to learn in a school setting.

legal discovery: the process or result of gaining access to the documentary evidence and data to be presented by the opposition in a lawsuit.

legal injunction: an order issued by a court to stop an illegal practice.

legal precedent: any principle of law that is established by the interpretive role of a court.

legal sanity: the state of being responsible under the law for one's intentional actions; in general, construed as the ability to represent and understand the potential or actual consequences of one's actions.

Lidcombe Program: a positive behavioral therapy for stuttering named for the suburb of Sydney, Australia where it originated; it rewards fluent stretches of speech in order to increase their likelihood.

linear processing: the kind that occurs in sequence where event A is produced or perceived ahead of B which is produced or perceived ahead of C and so forth.

linguistic expectations: forward looking inferences based on knowledge of language and how it is normally arranged with respect to meanings and surface forms.

lip reading: the result, ability, or process of comprehending speech by attending wholly or in part to movements of the visible articulators.

liquids: the peculiar class of speech sounds that function both as consonants and vowels.

literacy modality: the capacity, ability, or manner of processing written material as in reading versus writing, or in reading silently as contrasted with reading aloud.

LLI: an abbreviation for *language learning impaired*.

LMN: abbreviation for *lower motor neuron* (system).

local educational agencies: ones that come under the control of local authorities rather than the state or federal government.

localization hypothesis: the notion that certain sensory, motor, representational acts, or mental functions are controlled by a particular isolable portion of brain tissue which, if damaged will impair the function in question up to a limit of complete obliteration if the region in question is completely destroyed.

localization: the tendency for certain neurological functions to be associated with certain regions of the nervous system, especially the brain.

logographic writing: the type that directly represents words rather than sounds, syllables, or other surface forms of speech.

Lou Gehrig's disease: see *amyotrophic lateral sclerosis.*

lower motor neurons: the descending nerve fibers from the brain stem to the spinal cord reaching out to the muscles.

macrophages: these are immune system cells within tissues that originate from white blood cells whose role is to engulf and digest cellular debris and disease agents.

magnetic resonance imaging: the process or result of creating an image of a slice or volume of a three-dimensional material, commonly the insides of a living person; a process that relies on a powerful magnet augmented by three smaller magnets arranged at right angles to each other generating a highly homogeneous magnetic field through which radio waves are propagated; the molecular systems within the magnetic field distort the radio waves somewhat in the manner that the shape of the oral and nasal cavities shape the spectrum of speech sounds passing through them; subsequently the density, dimensions, and other molecular qualities of the material within the magnetic field can be converted into visible images showing the inside of the material (or body) in great detail—theoretically down to the level of molecules.

mainstreaming principle: the idea the children with disabilities should be educated alongside normally developing children as much as possible.

mandibulofacial dysostosis: any one of many deformities of the bones and tissues of the jaw and face; see the case of Joanna Jepson discussed in Chapter 2.

manner of articulation: the way a speech segment is articulated, for instance, whether or not it involves friction, *aspiration* (in the *phonetic* sense), *nasality*, and so on.

manual babbling: the type of repetitive hand movements made by deaf infants in experimenting with the surface forms of manual signed languages; parallels ordinary babble.

manual modality: the avenue for producing language commonly used by Deaf communities worldwide.

manual signs: the kinds of linguistic signs produced by individuals and communities that share a manually signed language; the words, phrases, and sequences of such a language.

Manually Signed English (MSE): a form of signed language derived from the surface forms of spoken English.

masking effects: processes or results of processes where certain sensory signs (possibly linguistic surface forms or gestures) tend to be covered up by other signs that interfere with processing.

McGurk effect: any one of several sensory, sensory-motor, or sensory-motor linguistic phenomena where signs at a higher level tend to mask or override signs at a lower level; see *McGurk interactions*.

McGurk interactions: the process or result of cross-modal transfer or interference where signs at a higher level tend to mask or override signs at a lower level.

meaningful sequence: any arrangement of a series of words, phrases, and higher units of discourse so that they make sense and involve conformity to ordinary expectations about how things work in ordinary experience; for instance, a story reported in a chronological order which begins with the first event in a series and ends with the resolution of some conflict telling how things came out.

measurement error: any variability in a measure or assessment that can be attributed to chance or any biasing factor rather than to the particular object or attribute that the procedure is supposed to measure or assess; also known as *unreliability*.

mechanical injuries: ones caused by collisions between moving material bodies, for instance, see *traumatic brain injury*, also *dementia pugilistica*.

median canal: the tube inside the cochlea beneath the vestibular canal, above the tympanic canal, and to the outside of the tiny tube known as the organ of Corti.

medulla oblongata: the lower part of the brain stem which is chiefly responsible for autonomic systems.

mercury: the most potent xenobiotic toxin among the naturally occurring heavy metals.

merthiolate: a brand name for *thimerosal*.

mesothelioma: a form of cancer usually of the lungs that develops in any one (or more) of the sacks—called "mesothelia"—that enclose the internal organs of the body, especially those within the chest cavity enclosing the lungs, heart, and so forth; usually associated with asbestos exposure.

metabolism: the biochemical processes that enable survival of living organisms and the processes that convert matter into energy.

metathesis: the process by which neighboring sounds in a string of sound segments of speech may sometimes exchange positions, for instance, as happened in the Spanish word "milagro" derived from the Latin "miraculum."

microglia: immune defense cells unique to the brain and spinal cord.

minimal pair: two words that differ in just one sound segment but have distinct meanings, such as, "pat" and "cat."

mixed dysarthrias: a catch-all term for movement disorders of the lower motor neuron system that do not neatly fit any of the other categories.

modular: the kind of processing that is, at least theoretically, distributed to distinct components or "modules."

modules: the distinct and somewhat independent components dedicated (theoretically at least) to the processing of distinct aspects of knowledge, skills, or abilities, and especially, language.

monitoring functions: ones by which feedback is used to assess how an ongoing process is working.

monolingual/monodialectal assessment: any testing or evaluative procedure that is exclusively dependent on instructions, explanations, and communications the rely on shared proficiency in just one language by the persons doing the assessment and the persons being assessed.

monomoraic: receiving only a single beat or having the duration of a short, unaccented syllable.

monosyllabic word: one with a single syllable, such as *dog, cat, come, go*, and so on.

monotone: in speaking, a level pitch that changes little or not at all throughout its duration.

monozygotes: fraternal twins, that is, ones that are merely siblings born of the same mother at the end of the one pregnancy.

monozygotic: a unique quality of identical twins (*monozygotes*) formed from the union of a single egg and sperm cell.

mora: a beat representing the shortest duration of a syllable in a language.

mora timed: a language where the length of a given syllable is determined not by stress, nor by the average length of syllables, but by a deeper underlying phonological convention that arbitrarily assigns a length of one, two, or three beats to a given syllable.

mortality: the inevitable process and result of biological decay owed to cumulative injuries from disease, trauma, and so forth.

motor cortex: also called the "primary" motor cortex which consists of the strip of brain tissue just in front of the fissure of Rolando (the central sulcus) in the frontal lobes which maps onto the parts of the movable body that come under volitional control.

motor phonetics: the study of the production of speech.

motor strip: see *motor cortex*.

MRI: abbreviation for *magnetic resonance imaging*.

multimodal: affecting or involving more than one modality of sense, movement, or language.

multimodal integration: the process or result of the working together and mutual influence on distinct modalities of sensory, sensory-motor, and sensory-motor linguistic processing.

multiple sclerosis: a persistent, inflammatory disease that destroys the demyelinates nerve cells of the brain and spinal cord.

myasthenia gravis: a disease of the nerves and muscle characterized by intermittent weakness and quick tiring during mild exertion; an autoimmune disorder where the body's defense system blocks the uptake of acetylcholine and prevents its normal stimulative effect.

myelin: the protein that forms the insulating sheath covering and enabling nerve fibers to carry electrical impulses.

myoelastic aerodynamic theory of phonation: a theory explaining voicing of speech sounds from van den Berg (1958) by applying Bernoulli's theory of the dynamics of fluid motion.

mythomania: a delusional disorder where the liar at the point of inception of the pathology becomes entrapped into believing his or her constructed falsehoods—the liar becomes deluded by the lies of his or her own creation; also known as pathological lying and pseudologia fantastica.

nanotechnologies: those that enable the examination and manipulation of very tiny systems at the level of individual atoms and molecules; ones that depend on models, machines, and processes that must be measured in units of 1 to 100 billionths of a millimeter.

nasal: a quality of sound segments accompanied by resonance caused by air passing through the nose, or, when used as a noun, any such segment.

nasalized: a quality of sounds produced by resonance of sound pressure waves resonating in air passing through the nasal cavities.

National Vaccine Injury Compensation Program: one established by law in 1986 designating the U.S. Court of Federal Claims as "the Vaccine Injury Court" to provide legal recourse and possible compensation for injuries if certain stringent requirements for filing, and so forth, were met.

native models: persons who have acquired a particular language from birth and use it as their so-called "mother tongue."

natural signed languages: ones that are not derived from any particular spoken language and that are common to Deaf communities.

negative inertia: a momentum propelling a person, object, or thought in the wrong direction; in other words, a momentum that is contrary to the purpose or intention at hand.

negative reinforcement: the provision of negative consequences for behavior, also known as punishment.

neologisms: new words.

neuroAIDS: a new form of acquired immune deficiency syndrome that attacks the central nervous system.

neurofibrillary tangles: pathologically twisted nerve fibrils found in the brain tissue of persons affected by Alzheimer's disease.

neurogenic disorders: strictly speaking, ones that have a neurological point of origin; often extended to all those that are believed primarily to impact the nervous system.

neurogenic stuttering: a condition of persistent abnormal disfluency that is attributed to an injury or disorder of a neurological kind.

neurolinguistics: the study of the ways in which the nervous system, especially the brain, is involved in and essential to the comprehension, acquisition, and use of language.

neurological disorders: any of those affecting the nerves or nervous system, especially the brain.

neurons: nerve cells, central units of the entire brain and nervous system.

neurotoxicity: a state of poisoning that affects the nerves and nervous system.

neurotransmitter: any one of a relatively small number of biochemicals, more than 10 but probably fewer than 100, that are involved in promoting and/or inhibiting neural signals; among the most important are glutamate, with an excitatory function, and gamma amino butyric acid (GABA) which has an inhibitory role.

nonverbal/performance assessment procedures: those that purport to rely on sensory and motor systems that do not require any comprehension or production of one or more languages; a hypothetical kind of testing or assessment that exists only in theory on account of the fact that all assessment procedures that involve abstract reasoning require the use of concepts that are only accessible through some particular language.

normal speech: this phrase has reference to the rate and manner in which users of a particular language commonly speak—as contrasted with *fast speech* and *slow speech*.

normative expectations: the kind that depend on what is known or believed about the development as it usually proceeds when there are no known disorders or disabilities interfering and where there are no special interventions or treatments to speed things along or slow them down.

nuclei of the cranial nerves: the places where the major nerve bundles of the two hemispheres of the brain and its various parts converge ostensibly to enable communication between the two sides of the body.

NVPAPs: abbreviation for *nonverbal/performance assessment procedures.*

olfactory: of or pertaining to the sense of smell.

onset: in *phonetics,* the beginning of a sound segment, syllable, or higher unit.

operant: a behavior that is conditioned by contingent consequences.

operant conditioning: the process or result of using contingent consequences to shape, establish, or extinguish some behavior or set of behaviors.

oral babbling: the repetitive production of syllabic vocalizations by normal infants as they acquire speech and language.

organ of Corti: the neurological center of hearing; sometimes compared to an electronic microphone and/or amplifier but vastly more complex than any existing complex of such manufactured electronic devices presently in existence.

ossification: the hardening of pliable tissue into bone.

otitis media: an inflammation of the middle ear.

otoacoustic emission (OAE): sounds produced by the inner ear that are associated with its function as an amplifier/interpreter of sounds.

outer hair cells: sensitive cilia in the organ of Corti that amplify certain frequencies of sounds impacting the fluid in the cochlea.

oxidation: the loss of one or more electrons by an atom or molecule.

oxidative stress: a condition of biochemical instability where many biomolecules have been oxidized and are seeking to regain equilibrium by borrowing one or more electrons from some other donor atom or molecule.

pancreas: the organ that produces insulin enabling the burning of bodily sugars.

paralinguistic devices: any of the actions and changes in the surface forms of discourse, such as raising the voice, gesturing, or any combination of such actions that may influence the way the discourse is understood.

parallel neural networks: ones that operate simultaneously, possibly on very different tasks.

parallel processing: the sort that occurs in multiple systems simultaneously.

parallel universes: the ones that we cannot perceive but that some theoreticians seem to think may exist contemporaneously with the one can perceive.

paranormal phenomena: any events that cannot be explained by ordinary normal processes of the body or mind.

parietal lobes: the lobes of the brain that lie just behind the central sulcus, thus, behind the frontal lobes, and just in front of the occipital lobes at the very back of the head; they extend roughly along the top of the skull above the ears and ending at about the base of the skull cap.

Parkinson's disease: a degenerative condition described by James Parkinson (1817) as "the shaking palsy" because it is characterized by tremors among other symptoms such as rigidity, jerky movements, and so on.

parosmia: a disorder of smell in which phantom odors occur.

parotid salivary gland: the largest of the salivary glands located in front of the ear and at the back of the jaw on both sides of the head.

parsing: dividing up.

partial birth abortion: a procedure during which a live infant is killed during its delivery by a physician; also see *late term abortion*.

pathological lying: see mythomania.

PD: abbreviation for *Parkinson's disease*.

PDD: abbreviation for *pervasive developmental disorder*.

PDD-NOS: abbreviation for *pervasive developmental disorder not otherwise specified*.

pediatric surgeon: a physician who performs surgical procedures mainly on infants and young children.

pediatricians: doctors whose main patients are children rather than adults.

peptic ulcers: the most common type of sores inside the gut, especially the small intestine and stomach.

perceptual defense: the process or result of a negative anticipatory reaction to undesirable stimuli, for example, the filtering out of an undesirable stimulus or message.

perceptual vigilance: the process or result of a positive anticipatory reaction to a desirable stimulus, for example, the amplification of a desirable stimulus or message as when hearing one's name spoken in a conversation.

period: in physics, the time from the greatest height of a wave to its deepest trough, or the time required to complete a single cycle.

peritoneum: the sack that contains the intestines.

peritonitis: inflammation of the *peritoneum*.

persistent developmental stuttering: the kind that seems to gradually develop into the performance of an individual and then remain indefinitely; also known as *incipient stuttering*.

pervasive developmental disorders not otherwise specified: ones that affect multiple systems but that have not been specifically named, diagnosed, or identified (a catch-all especially for autism-like conditions).

pervasive developmental disorders: ones that affect many systems simultaneously, for example, *autism*, *Asperger syndrome*, *Rett syndrome*, and so forth.

pervasive developmental disorders: ones that tend to affect multiple systems of development.

PET: abbreviation for *positron emission tomography*.

petition for certiorare: a formal request for a higher court, for instance, the U.S. Supreme Court, to review a decision of a lower court and possibly overturn it.

petitioner: the person making a legal request of the court.

pharyngeal cavity: the region above the larynx and beneath the back of the tongue; also known as the *pharynx*.

pharynx: the region above the larynx and beneath the back of the tongue; also known as the *pharyngeal cavity*.

philtrum: the indentation of facial tissue just above the upper lip and under the nose.

phonation: the process of producing voice or sounds by voluntary vocalization.

phoneme: in traditional linguistics a class—but, better, a system—of speech sounds that can be used by speakers of a given language to distinguish meanings in that language.

phonemic awareness: the linguistic ability to understand explicit references to the sounds of speech and to manipulate them overtly on command; for instance, to produce a series of words that have the same initial sound, or to produce a new word by moving the initial sound to the end of the word, and so forth; a concept based on a superficial theory of language whose proponents represent themselves as expert teacher/clinicians able to explain the causes and remedies for disorders described variously under the vaguely defined terms *LD*, *dyslexia*, *LLI*, and the like; synonymous with *phonological awareness*, a closely related concept that also tends to emphasize knowledge of the surface forms of speech so much that the concepts themselves (and the theories on which they are based) tend toward nonsense—a commonly recommended approach for teaching and testing of literacy skills by proponents of these superficial notions.

phonemic segments: see *phoneme*.

phones: the different surface forms of a given *phoneme* which are regarded as manifestations of the same sound by a speaker of the language in question.

phonetic code: a system of writing or representation based on the distinctive sounds or classes of sounds that constitute the syllables of a spoken language.

phonetic features: the distinguishable qualities of a *phonemic segment* that enable users of such segments in some particular language to recognize it as a *phonemic segment* in that particular language.

phonetic segments: in the traditional phonemic theory, the actual sounds that constitute the actual spoken surface forms of *normal speech* in any particular language.

phonetic transcription: a system of transforming speech into a written form that purports to represent the individual sound segments of which the speech is supposed to consist.

phonetician: a specialist who studies the sounds of speech.

phonics: the class of approaches to the teaching of literacy skills that emphasizes rules of sound-to-letter correspondences and the sounding out of letter sequences in the process of reading along with the reverse process in writing as the essential foundation; also see the *phonemic principle, phonemic awareness,* and *phonological awareness.*

phonological awareness: see *phonemic awareness* which is virtually the same theoretical construct; also, note that the supposed differences between the two phrases in question are equally impoverished on account of the fact that language—whether spoken, written, or signed—cannot be reduced entirely to the surface forms of writing, speaking, signing, or correspondences between them. Meaning also must be taken into consideration to complete such theories.

phonotactics: the rule system governing the way sounds are to be strung together in any forming the syllables, words, phrases, and higher surface forms of any spoken language system—sometimes generalized to include the analogous constraints on manually signed language systems.

phylogenetic speculation: a phrase invented by Chomsky and colleagues to disparage the tendency of Darwinian enthusiasts to invent fanciful (unverifiable) stories about how men could have descended from apes while at the same time developing the entire design for the human language capacity and all that comes with it.

pinna: the outer ear (the visible part).

pitch: the basic frequency of a sound, note, or complex waveform.

place of articulation: in *phonetics* the primary articulatory target of consonantal speech segments; also known as *point of articulation.*

plagiarism: the process of deliberately copying verbatim the words of someone else without giving credit to the source.

plaintiff: the person bringing the complaint against a *defendant* in a lawsuit.

planum temporale: a cortical area just behind the auditory cortex in both hemispheres that has been associated with in such phenomena as stuttering and with *absolute pitch.*

plaques: an accumulation of undesirable protein debris that forms an obstructive covering of some tissue.

plosive: any sound of speech that involves a rapid release of air under pressure; also known in traditional linguistics as *stop consonants.*

point of articulation: see *place of articulation.*

polio: see *poliomyelitis.*

poliomyelitis: a disease caused by the polio virus that infects and causes inflammation and possibly destruction of motor neurons leading potentially to paralysis followed by extreme atrophy or stunting of body parts especially the limbs.

polyp: a fleshy growth on a mucosal membrane, usually benign.

portmanteau: a word formed by combining two or more others by "smushing" them together to use a popular example from *smash* and *crush*; the term is a combination of French *porter* meaning "to carry" and *manteau* meaning "overcoat, mantel, or covering"—in French it means a bag suitable for carrying an overcoat; it was introduced into English by Charles Lutwidge Dodgson also known as Lewis Carroll in the famous Jabberwocky poem of *Alice in Wonderland* (http://en.wikipedia.org/wiki/Portmanteau visited April 15, 2009).

positions of discourse: those occupied by producer, consumer, and the surface forms of the discourse itself; also commonly referred to as the "persons" of grammar—first, second, and third.

positive reinforcement: in behaviorism, a consequence of a behavior that tends to increase the likelihood of its recurrence.

positron: the relatively rare antimatter particle (or wave) that is the positive counterpart of its more common negative opposite which is the *electron.*

positron emission tomography: a computer-dependent imaging technique for looking at the inside of a living body that takes advantage of the physical destruction that takes place when a negatively charged electron collides with a positively charged particle call a *positron*.

possible worlds: any imaginary setting that has even a vague resemblance to the common world of ordinary experience.

post hoc ergo propter hoc fallacy: the often false idea that because a certain event B happens after some other event A, that A caused B; an inference that is sometimes true but often false; for instance, just because a yellow dog came into the alley just before the robbery occurred, we cannot reasonably infer that the dog caused the robbery.

post-traumatic stress syndrome: a generalized complex of neurological, psychological, and possibly physical and/or behavioral symptoms attributed to a prior ordeal or fear producing event or series of events, for example, the terror produced by battle.

postmodernism: a naive "critical" philosophy of the 20th century (and later) pretending to be so enlightened as to transcend the term "modern"; a mixed bag of self-contradictions claiming that meaning is always uncertain and that it is itself, therefore, indefinable.

pragmatic isomorphism: a complete similarity of abstract form.

pragmatic mapping: the association of one or more signs with its intended content in some actual context of experience.

precipitating factors: ones that are believed to bring about or cause a certain phenomenon such as a severe stuttering episode.

preparatory set: the cognitive and/or emotional readiness that makes it easier (or possibly harder) to process a certain signal; for instance, see *perceptual defense* and *perceptual vigilance*.

prescinded symbol: one that is abstracted sufficiently from the contexts of its occurrence that it can be and is independently produced on a new occasion.

prescinding: the process of abstracting a representation from the context in which its object can actually be perceived; for instance, a moving object *prescinds* itself from its former location so that to represent the object where it was before it moved, or where it will end up after it moves some more requires the representer to *prescind* a representa-

tion from the percept of the moving object by imagining it where it was or will be.

prestin: the protein enabling the motor functions of the outer hair cells in the organ of Corti.

prevalence: the total number of cases of a disease, condition, injury, or whatever, in a particular population at a given time.

prima facie evidence: that which seems to prove a particular claim with little or no interpretation, for instance, a written promise to perform a certain action shows by its very existence that a written promise was made.

principle of consistency: the notion that meaningful reports of experiments must be sufficiently interpretable that the same results can, in principle, at least be achieved by someone else using similar methods; see the *consistency requirement* and also the *replication requirement*.

processing malfunction models: theories of stuttering that involve the breakdown of any of the systems by which speakers check the accuracy of the surface forms and meanings of their own productions.

profound deafness: total loss or failure to develop the sense of hearing.

prognosis: the likely course an undesirable condition, disorder, or disease is expected to follow.

progressive palsy: a degenerative form of paralysis the is expected to worsen over time.

proposition: the idea underlying a complete and intelligible declarative sentence, for example, the idea that all human beings are mortal can be expressed in countless distinct surface forms in any language system in the world and yet it is essentially the same abstract idea.

prosodic elements: the subtle qualities including tone of voice, facial expression, and intonation that impact the manner in which the surface forms of speech—but of writing too by analogy—may be intended, understood, or interpreted; of or pertaining to *prosody*.

prosody: the variation in sequences of syllables involving rate, loudness, and pitch.

prosopagnosia: the loss of, or possibly the failure to develop, the ability to recognize faces.

prospective study: one that selects a sample of persons fitting a particular description and then asks if they have some other predicted or expected condition as well.

proton: a subatomic particle with a positive charge and a mass about 1836 times greater than an electron.

pseudobulbar palsy: paralysis on both sides owed to damage of the lower cranial nerves, 9, 10, 11, and 12.

pseudologia fantastica: see *mythomania*.

pseudologue: a technical term used to refer to a pathological liar.

psychogenic stuttering: a condition of persistent abnormal disfluency that is attributed to a psychological, mental, or emotional trauma or disorder.

psycholinguistics: the study of the psychology of language comprehension, acquisition, and use.

psychosis: a term applied loosely to almost any persistent psychological condition that interferes with normal life and experience; for instance, see *schizophrenia*.

psychotics: individuals persistently manifesting behavioral symptoms of *psychosis*.

PT: abbreviation for the *planum temporale*.

public awareness theory: the idea that the increasing number of cases diagnosed with ASDs in recent years can be explained by greater public awareness about ASDs.

pull-out: in the stuttering literature this term is applied to the intentional self-interruption that occurs when we stop talking; in educational settings, this term is generally applied to programs where children are taken out of their regular classroom for special tutoring or therapy.

pull-out programs: ones in which the persons undergoing treatment for whatever reason are taken out of the mainstream classroom and placed in a separate location for treatment.

punishment: see *negative reinforcement*.

pyramidal tract: the bundle of nerve fibers connecting the cortex to the motor systems of the body; also known as the corticospinal tract.

radioactive tracers: elements injected into the body consisting of atoms with unstable nuclei that predictably emit particles or electromagnetic waves that can register on a photographic plate or other device to form a picture or image of the inside of the body.

raised print: a now archaic system of writing invented by Valentin Haüy for the Blind, replaced almost completely by *Braille*.

reading readiness: the time at which, in theory, a child is well-prepared or able to undertake the acquisition of skills in reading and writing.

real-time processing: the recording, imaging, copying, comprehension, production, or other use of rapidly occurring events—such as conversational exchanges, reading, signing, calculation, perception, thinking, or some combination of these—as they are actually occurring.

receptive aphasia: the type of language loss that affects the ability to process or understand verbal productions or discourse produced by someone other than the person affected by the loss.

receptive repertoire: the inventory of sounds, syllables, words, or other representations that an individual is able to comprehend (but not necessarily produce).

recurrence risk: in related persons such as siblings or twins, the likelihood that a disease condition observed in one sibling will also be found in a twin, or in a younger sister or brother, or the likelihood that a disease condition of one or both parents will be passed on to their children.

redox: the combined processes of *oxidation* and *reduction* whereby an atom or molecule may either lose or gain (respectively) one or more electrons.

reduction: the process by which an atom or molecule gains an electron.

referential content: the things, persons, events, or sequences of events that are signified and pointed to in discourse; in other words, its pragmatic content, for example, the referential content of the assertion that *the dog bit the postman* would include the dog, the postman, and the biting of the postman by the dog.

referring term: any word, phrase, or symbol that is used to point out or signify something other than itself, possibly another symbol.

reflex: a movement that occurs in response to an external stimulus but that does not come under conscious volitional control.

reflex arc: a term applied, somewhat misleadingly by German neurologist, Ludwig Lichtheim [1845–1928] to refer to the neurological basis for the comprehension and production of spoken discourse; what is misleading in this usage is the implication that language use is fundamentally like the well known knee jerk reflex, for instance, which does not involve intentionality, volition, or higher cortical functions.

reinforcing stimuli: ones which increase the likelihood that a given behavior will recur.

reliability: a property of a measure or test consisting of that portion of its variance that can be repeatedly obtained by applying the procedure under the same conditions.

replication: the process of reproducing or copying especially as applied to genetic material.

replication requirement: in the sciences, the universal demand that valid experimental results should be attainable repeatedly by applying the same methods of experimentation, measurement, and so forth.

residual volume: the air remaining in the lungs after breathing out.

resin composite: any of several materials used as alternatives to the so-called "silver" metal fillings that are actually about 50% mercury.

resonance: in acoustic phonetics, the quality of a complex sound wave produced by its reflection within a cavity or chamber where the distance between the reflecting walls is approximately equal to or an even multiple of the wavelength of the sound source.

respondent: someone who answers a charge, question, or complaint.

retrotransposons: genetic elements that can increase their own numbers by looking back to an earlier state to copy themselves either forward or backwards into a new location in the genome or in one of its RNA products involved in biochemical processes of the body; *retroviruses* such as *HIV* and the *neuroAIDS* viruses seem to imitate *retrotransposons*.

Rett syndrome: a genetic disorder that almost exclusively affects girls and that is included as one of the PDDs by the American Psychiatric Association (1994).

reversion principle: the logical expectation that sign users will generally be able to revert to a simpler system of signs than the more complex ones at hand, but that leaping ahead to a much higher and more complex system that has not yet been achieved is virtually impossible.

rigid transliteration: the sort of translation that works from minute forms such as letters or parts of words

and phrases and translates them one by one into a new sequence of letters, words, or signs.

rime: the British spelling for "rhyme" that is commonly applied in *phonology* to the vowel center and whatever terminal consonants may be associated with a syllable that are also associated with one or more distinct syllables; for instance, the *rime* of the word "rhyme"—as well as "mime," "time," "climb," "dime," "I'm," and so on—is the portion that follows the initial consonant if there is one—the phrase "I'm" as in "I'm rhyming and miming all the time" has no initial consonant but has the same *rime* as "rime" does.

rounded: in speech sounds, the quality of being produced with the lips in the position required to produce the vowels /u/ and /o/.

saccades: rapid movements of the eyes from one point of fixation to another; contrasted with *smooth pursuit* or *gaze*.

sagittal: the orientation characteristic of any slice or volume that is parallel to the plane that theoretically bisects the left and right sides of the body in a vertical upright orientation.

sandhi: the processes especially of assimilation and dissimilation involved in normal speech production—extending to epenthesis, metathesis, and so forth.

scale of development: a systematic definition, differentiation, and/or demarcation of distinct milestones and the order in which they usually are (or logically must be) achieved as a child grows from conception to maturity.

schedule of reinforcement: in behaviorism, the planned rate at which positive or negative consequences are provided when a given behavior occurs.

schizophrenia: a little understood class of disorders involving persistent recurrent hallucinations or delusions as their primary defining trait.

schizophrenics: individuals affected by *schizophrenia*.

secondaries: see *secondary behaviors*.

secondary behaviors: a phrase from the stuttering literature referring to behaviors such as foot-stomping, teeth grinding, or tongue protrusion, or other distracting acts that tend to become associated with severe stuttering in many cases; also known merely as *secondaries*.

secondary injury: the sort of tissue damage caused by the toxins and disease agents contained within cells or their parts that are released when the containing membranes are broken by a primary injury such as a bruise or puncture wound.

segmental sounds: see *phonetic segments*.

self-contradiction: the process or result of producing an argument that refutes itself; a necessarily false form of argumentation.

semantic aphasia: a loss of language ability particularly affecting comprehension of words and linguistic concepts; also known as *Wernicke's aphasia* and *receptive aphasia*.

semantic function: any function having to do with the abstract and general meaning of a sign; for example, the constraints on other signs that arise from the meaning associated with a different sign is a semantic function—for instance, a phrase such as "silent paint" is odd because "paint" is not the sort of thing that can ordinarily make any noise.

semiconsonants: sounds such as the first segment of "yet" and "wet" or the final segments of "sigh" and "sew" that seem to have some consonantal qualities and yet do not quite achieve the full status of a consonant according to some phonologists; also see *glides*.

semiotics: the general study of signs and representations which includes linguistics as a central element.

semivowels: sounds such as the first segment of "yet" and "wet" or the final segments of "sigh" and "sew" that seem to have some vocalic qualities and yet do not quite achieve the full status of a vowel according to some phonologists; also see *glides*.

senile dementia: see *Alzheimer's disease*.

sensorineural hearing loss: the type of loss in either or both ears that involve the functions of the inner ear (especially the cochlea) and connections to the brain.

sensory alexia: the hypothetical peculiar, and relatively complete loss of ability to sense and/or perceive written words while perceptions of other nonlinguistic phenomena, and the speech modality, remain relatively unaffected.

sensory aphasia: any loss of the ability to notice and recognize surface forms of one or more languages; see *alexia* as well as *subcortical* and *transcortical sensory aphasia*.

sensory asignia: the hypothetical generalized loss of ability to sense and/or perceive signs of any

kind while the ability to conjure up signs internally or to think in signs remains intact.

sensory cortex: the portion of the brain, especially the strip of tissue in the parietal lobes on each side just behind the central sulcus, that maps onto the sensory functions of the opposite side of the body; also called the *somatosensory cortex*.

sensory dyslexia: the hypothetical peculiar loss of ability to sense and/or perceive words while perceptions of other nonlinguistic phenomena, or the speech modality, remain relatively unaffected.

sensory prejudices: false judgments made in advance about the senses and information available to a person lacking one or more avenues of sense.

sensory strip: see *sensory cortex*.

sensory systems: all of the systems of the body involved in sensation but especially the senses of seeing, hearing, smelling, touching, and tasting.

separate but equal: a legal term applied to the pretentious claims of certain state legislatures that intentionally permitted racial discrimination against Blacks long after the American Civil War, but that were effectively struck down in *Brown v. the Board of Education* in 1954.

sequential (episodic) organization: see *meaningful sequence*.

Sequoia: the American, a Cherokee Indian, who invented a *syllabary* for what was beforehand an unwritten American language.

serial neural networks: ones that fire or communicate with each other in a certain sequence.

serial processing: the types where signals are handled in sequence one after another; for example, as in many aspects of speech perception.

short-term memory: the process of recording and/or recalling or the normal ability to recall a conversation or event that has occurred within the previous three or four seconds up to a three or four-minute time frame.

sibilant: a speech sound accompanied by a hissing fricative quality such as found in the first segment of the word "sit" and the final segment of "hush."

sickle cell anemia: a genetic disease where red blood cells tend to be deformed into an oblong sometimes taking the shape of a sickle.

signal detection: the process or result of noticing a sound or other sensory stimulus.

Signed Exact English (SEE): a manual language derived from the surface forms of spoken English.

simian virus 40: a *retrovirus* from monkeys and/or other nonhuman primates that was inadvertently transferred to millions of humans through polio vaccines and that has been associated with many cancers, diseases, and disorders; the 40th simian virus identified in serums used in the manufacture of vaccines and medicines.

simple frequency theory: the idea that differences in our ability to process patterns of distinct signals—such as words or sequences of them, for instance—depends almost exclusively on how often those signals or patterns are experienced.

simultaneous interpretation: usually a sentence by sentence translation from one language to another that is provided at the same time that someone else is speaking; for example, translation from speech to manual signs while someone else is doing the speaking.

singer's nodes: hard nonpliable tissue formations in the vocal folds.

single nucleotide polymorphism (sn): a variation in a gene sequence in DNA where one of the pairs of four bases (A, T, C, G) is different than expected or required for the construction of a particular protein (see http://en.wikipedia.org/wiki/Single_nucleotide_polymorphism visited April 15, 2009); for example, see *sickle cell anemia*.

situation based: a defining quality of certain theories of language and discourse that emphasize the importance of the material and social contexts in which linguistic discourse is produced.

slow speech: carefully articulated speech where each segment is deliberately contrasted with each other.

Smith-Magenis syndrome: a complex of genetic abnormalities that result in multiple system disorders evident from infancy involving facial appearance, feeding problems, low muscle tone, developmental delays, mental retardation, skeletal anomalies, and decreased sensitivity to pain.

smooth pursuit: the process of focusing on a moving object and following it with the eyes as it moves on a trajectory through the visual field.

social Darwinism: the consequences in society and public policy that flow naturally from Darwin's theory of evolution as applied to his false views about race; for example the claim that Black Africans were closer to apes than White Caucasians like himself.

sociolinguistics: the study of the sociology of language comprehension, acquisition, and use.

solar plexus: the indentation just below the rib cage centered on the diaphragm behind which a nexus of nerve systems controlling breathing and digestion is located; also known as the *celiac plexus*.

somatic (bodily) systems: see *sensory systems*.

somatosensory cortex: see *sensory cortex*.

somnambulism: sleep walking, or the tendency to physically perform actions while in a dream state that normally would be suppressed.

spastic dysarthrias: any one of the pathological conditions where the vocal folds are hypertonic (too tense).

spastic dysphonia: a condition where the vocal folds are too tight during speech production resulting in strained, harsh, and gruff-sounding speech.

special education: instruction that is modified to address the special needs, including communication disorders or special gifts, of individual children in schools.

Special Masters: the individuals who decide cases presented to the Vaccine Injury Court.

spectral properties: the qualities of a complex wave form by which distinct frequencies and ranges or bands of them are activated at distinct intensities.

spectrogram: a visible representation of a complex wave form showing distinct levels of energy at different frequencies over time.

spectrum: the range of frequencies across which distinct levels of wave energy may be expressed.

speech-language pathology: the study of speech and language related communication disorders and the clinical practice of therapies and interventions designed to treat such disorders.

speech to text: a phrase applied to the automated process or result of converting (or attempting to convert) spoken forms into written ones by an algorithmic (computerized) system.

sphere of reference: the logical domain within which distinctions between things, events, persons, or sequences of them are or can be distinguished.

spina bifida: a Latin term meaning cleft spine and referring to any one of several conditions where the spine is exposed at birth.

spinal cord: the bundle of nerve fibers in mammals that is encased within the back bone leading from the nerves at the periphery to and from the brain.

splenium of the corpus callosum: in a sagittal section of the brain, the bulbar-shaped posterior end of the central *commissure* connecting the two hemispheres of the brain.

split-brain experiments: ones in which the two hemispheres of the brains of patients, usually suffering from *epileptic seizures*, are prevented from communicating with each other by either the removal of an entire hemisphere or a *commissurotomy*.

spondee: a two syllable word that has the same stress pattern and rhythm as this word, that is, as spondee.

standardized IQ tests: tests administered according to set procedures that are supposed to measure innate intelligence but that depend directly and predominantly on acquired language proficiency.

startle response: a reaction of the body that involves contraction of peripheral muscles of the arms and legs, as well as eye closure, sudden increase in blood pressure, and more rapid breathing.

statute of limitations: a rule of law preventing the filing of a claim when a certain lapse of time has occurred after the injury.

stereotyped movements: ones that tend to recur especially in ASDs.

stop consonant: see *plosive*.

stress pattern: see *stress*.

stress: the quality of a syllable consisting of its amplitude, pitch, and length relative to other syllables in a stream of speech.

stress timed language: one in which the rhythm of sequences of syllables and their length in particular is determined by the relative *stress* placed on distinct syllables.

stridor: the high-pitched croaky sound produced by forcing air through a blocked or hypotonic larynx.

stroke: damage to the brain owed to deprivation of oxygen which may be caused by loss of blood flow owed to heart stoppage, blocked blood vessels, buildup of fluid in or around the brain, or by bleeding in or around the brain or loss of blood in another part of the body.

structural linguistics: the traditional variety of American linguistics advocated by Bloomfield and his successors that placed emphasis on surface forms of speech almost to the exclusion of all else, but especially de-emphasizing meanings, intentions, and interpretive processes.

stuttering block: an occasion where speech is interrupted that may often be accompanied by distracting *secondary behaviors*.

stuttering events: occasions in speech during which abnormal disfluencies occur or abnormal adjustments are made by the speaker, such as using a circumlocution, or momentary silence, to try to avoid their occurrence.

stuttering modification: any change in the manner of producing speech, possibly highly disfluent speech, that may be employed to try to reduce or reshape disfluencies so as to enable more fluent speech production on the part of a person who stutters.

stuttering severity index: any one of various subjective measures that have been applied to try to assess the degree to which an individual's tendency toward disfluencies will interfere with communication.

stylopharyngeus: the long thin muscle (on both sides of the cheek extending down to the pharynx) shaped roughly like an old time writing quill or stylus that enlarges the pharynx to enable swallowing of a large mouthful of food or liquid.

subarachnoid hemorrhage: bleeding in the space around the brain.

subcortical motor aphasia: loss of capacity to produce fluent speech but without significant impairment of linguistic comprehension, reading and/or writing; owing, presumably, to damage to regions of tissue beneath the *cortex* including the *thalamus*, *internal capsule*, and *basal ganglia*; a disorder that incidentally affects speech and that some specialists would prefer to class as an *apraxia* or even *dysarthria*.

subcortical sensory aphasia: a peculiar loss of ability in which sounds, syllables, words, and phrases can be heard and sometimes repeated, but no longer make sense to the person affected; also known as *word deafness* and *central auditory processing disorder*; with respect to literacy also see *alexia* also known as *word blindness*, which, if it occurs in a pure form (where the loss does not impact auditory or other sensory modalities, and where the ability to speak, think, and write remain unaffected) would also qualify as a *subcortical sensory aphasia*.

subliminal messages: ones that are too faint or too fast to be noticed consciously and yet that are present nonetheless and have an effect at a sub-conscious level.

substantia nigra: the dark colored tissue deep within the basal ganglia involved in the production of *dopamine*.

supplementary motor area: the regions neighboring *Broca's area* that seem to be involved in complex volitional motor planning; especially in Brodmann's area 6.

suprasegmental elements: usually limited to stress and intonation as these are associated with the surface forms of speech represented as a string of phonetic segments (usually excluding gestures and facial expressions).

surface forms: the parts or aspects of signs of any kind that are perceivable.

suture: the juncture at which plates of tissue, especially the bones of the skull, are joined or sewed together.

SV40: abbreviation for *simian virus 40*.

syllabary: a writing system in which the symbols represent whole syllables rather than other sound segments or higher units.

syllabic writing: see *syllabary*.

syllable: the smallest pronounceable unit of speech containing at least a vocalic nucleus possibly bounded before and after by consonants at the margins; the basic building block of every sequence of spoken words; for example, the word *caught* consists of one syllable.

syllable timed: a language in which the length of a syllable is relatively constant and in which the rhythms of speech are governed more or less by the average length of a syllable in that language.

symbol: any sign that functions as a sign by virtue of its conventional associations or its representational value; in other words, a sign that arbitrarily by conventional use stands for something other than itself is a symbol; for example, a name.

symptomology: the scientific study of the signs (symptoms) of a disease, disorder, or condition.

synapses: the junctions at which nerve cells connect with each other and across which they express electrical impulses and electrochemical exchanges.

synostosis: a condition where the bones merge abnormally forming either a premature or malformed union.

syntax: that aspect of grammar pertaining to the sequence of units at any level, but especially within phrases consisting of words or higher units.

synthesized speech: the kind produced by a computer as from a series of acoustic, digital, or other nonspeech signals.

syphilis: a sexually transmitted disease involving infection by the bacterium, *Treponema pallidum spirochete*; see "Treponema pallidum" retrieved April 15, 2009, from http://en.wikipedia.org/wiki/Treponema_pallidum .

syphilis lesion: a sore attributed to the venereal disease of *syphilis*.

tachyphemia: an abnormally persistent form of excessively fast speech where words seem to pile up in unintelligible batches; see *cluttering*.

TBI: abbreviation for *traumatic brain injury*.

telegraphic: the kind of speech that tends to consist almost exclusively of crucial *content words* without normal grammatical marking, or morphological completeness, and with reduced use of or absence of *function words*.

temporal integration: the working together of distinct systems in processing of signals that occur across time; for instance, in understanding a sequence of spoken words, written signs, or moving pictures.

temporal integration threshold: the length of time necessary for a perceiver to notice a silent space between two distinct beeps or tones.

temporal lobes: the portions of the brain that are behind the frontal lobes, beneath the parietal, and in front of the occipital.

temporal masking: a phenomenon where the occurrence of a signal (possibly a sound) makes it difficult or impossible to detect another distinct signal that occurs just before or afterward.

temporal ordering: the arrangement of distinct signs that is produced or noticed in a certain sequence; for instance, where sign A precedes sign B, which precedes sign C, and so on.

temporal resolution: the accuracy or degree of precision attainable in distinguishing and recognizing signs produced in a sequentially organized complex waveform where distinct elements run together and overlap as in speech.

teratology: the study of deformities, from the Greek roots *tera-* meaning "monster" and *logo-* meaning "word or concept."

testosterone: a male hormone of which human males produce in significantly greater quantity than females, by 50 times, and that is known to be associated with an increase in oxidative stress.

tetanospasmin: the neurotoxin produced by clostridium tetani that causes the disease known as tetanus by blocking GABA and thus upsetting the balanced control of muscles which causes *tetanic spasms* that are irreversible.

text to speech: the computerized process of converting a sequence of written symbols into a stream of audible speech.

theory of abstraction: a particular proposal about how signs are formed by intelligent agents by transforming concrete things, relations between them, and events into abstract concepts or signs.

theory of the meritocracy: the notion (from proponents of IQ tests) that brighter people end up at the top of the social hierarchy and receive educational and economic benefits commensurate with their ability, whereas individuals with less ability end up at the bottom.

thimerosal: the technical name for the preservative used in many vaccines and other medications from the 1930s forward, as produced by the Eli Lilly company; also known as *thiomersal* and *merthiolate*.

threshold of coherence: the theoretical boundary between comprehension, say, of discourse or a complex sequence of events and the failure to comprehend.

threshold of insanity: the theoretical level beyond which a merely odd behavior is regarded, under the law, as showing that the actor is incapable of deliberate volitional control and therefore legal responsibility for his or her actions.

tinnitus: a ringing in one or both ears that may be intermittent or persistent and may be caused by internal neurological events or by damage to the inner ear; it is generally considered to be a pathological condition.

tip of the mind: by analogy with the *tip of the tongue* phenomenon where a known word seems to be just out of reach and cannot be called to consciousness; in this case, it is the concept, person, object, event, or referent itself that cannot be called up for conscious thought; for instance, the idea, thought, or concept that occurred to us that we cannot quite recall.

tip of the tongue: the phenomenon where we try to think of a word or name and yet cannot quite bring it to consciousness in spite of the fact that it is a familiar form that we know very well and commonly use.

tip of the tongue phenomenon: the instance where a known word, name, phrase, lyric, or line of poetry seems to be just out of reach and cannot be called to consciousness; a phenomenon that can also occur with tunes, melodies, or jingles which might be called "edge of the voice phenomena."

top-down processing: the type where prior knowledge of abstract ideas, subject matter, intentions, and the like, guide perception and understanding of discourse to correct inferences about its content and meaning.

toxicology: the study of poisons.

toxin: any substance capable of injuring the body and its organs at the atomic and/or molecular levels.

trachea: the windpipe or tube leading into the brachii that lead to the lungs.

tracheostomy: the opening of a hole in the throat and windpipe to enable breathing directly through the trachea.

transcortical motor aphasia: loss of the linguistic ability to perform complex sequencing and planning of discourse while comprehension and ability to repeat verbal material, read aloud, and write from dictation remain relatively unimpaired (Brookshire, 1997, pp. 141–142).

transcortical sensory aphasia: the loss of capacity to make sense of discourse sequences though the ability with prompting to recite complex sequences such as a prayer or poem remains relatively intact (see Goodglass & Kaplan, 1983; and McCaffrey, 2001).

transcribe: to represent surface forms in writing.

transitive relations: the kind where the presence of a certain element in a connected sequence of elements enables us to correctly infer other elements.

translation: the process or result of interpreting a string of symbols in one form (usually a distinct language) into another.

trauma: the process or result of sudden injury, for example, as by a collision between a person and some other bodily object.

traumatic brain injury: any damage to the brain that is caused by a sudden blow or collision that produces bruising or internal bleeding.

traumatic injury: the sort of sudden injury produced by a collision or trauma.

treatment effect: an observed difference between performances, persons, or groups that can be reasonably—reliably and validly—attributed to a particular therapy, medicine, method, and so forth (the "treatment"), that some received while others did not.

treatment group: the cases receiving a certain therapy, medicine, method, and so forth (the "treatment"), that other cases—the *control group*—did not receive.

triangulate: to measure or infer the time or distance to a certain object (or event) from the known time or distance to two other locations distinct from the first.

trigeminal neuralgia: a painful facial pathological condition involving the Vth cranial nerve; a disorder also referred to as the "suicide disease" because persons with this condition commonly take their own lives if they cannot find successful treatment.

trilingualism: the state of proficiency attributed to a person who knows and uses three languages.

trimoraic: a sequence of sounds, especially a single syllable, consisting of or containing three *moras*.

trochee: a two-syllable word that has the same *stress pattern* as the word "trochee" pronounced like "croaky."

true narrative representation: the report, perception, or experience of a sequence of events or facts that have really occurred as they are represented to have occurred.

TTS: abbreviation for *text to speech*.

tubulin: a protein that forms the sheath around the tiniest nerve fibers of both snails and other organisms including human beings and one of the principle components of *myelin*.

tympanic canal: the larger and lower fluid-filled tube of the cochlea that is most directly connected to the ear "drum" (the latter also being known as the *tympanic membrane*).

UMN: abbreviation for the *upper motor neuron* (system).

unilateral motor neuron dysarthria: the kind that only affects movements on one side of the body.

unity of conception: the point at which comprehension is achieved such that all the elements of a problem, event sequence, a coherent discourse, or especially a *true narrative representation* makes sense so that all of the important elements of the whole are accounted for.

universal quantifiers: elements of language, logic, and conception that apply to all possible cases of a given kind or to none of them; for instance, the meanings underlying the words "all," "no," and "every."

unreliability: the variability in a measure or assessment procedure that is attributable to error; see *measurement error*.

unrounded: in *phonetics*, any sound segment that is produced without the rounding of the lips, for instance, the vowels /i/ and /a/ are *unrounded*.

unvoiced: in speech production, the quality of sound segments in which the vocal folds are not vibrating; also known as *voiceless*.

upper motor neuron (system): the system of motor neurons contained in the brain and extending downward to the brain stem and ending at the decussation of the pyramids.

Vaccine Adverse Event Reporting System: a system established in 1988 for the supposed purpose of monitoring injuries from vaccines administered according to federal mandates.

VAERS: abbreviation for the *Vaccine Adverse Event Reporting System*.

validity: the extent to which variability in a measure, test, or assessment procedure can be attributed truly to whatever object, property, or phenomenon that procedure is supposed to assess.

variegated babble: the speechlike stage just beyond *canonical babble* at which distinct syllables can be produced in rapid succession.

vegetative: a state or property of a sign act or sign producer which cannot be attributed to intentional and/or volitional action.

vegetative movements: those involved in chewing, swallowing, and digestion.

velar: the place or *point of articulation* of speech sounds that are formed by contact between the back of the tongue and the *velum*.

velopharyngeal insufficiency: a condition in which the velum does not flex or reach far enough to close the pharyngeal airway leading to and from the nasal cavities, especially in speech production.

verbal behavior: often construed as a term only applying to speech, but also sometimes extended to other kinds of linguistic and discursive behaviors including writing, signing, and linguistic thought.

vertical progress: development or growth of the intellectual and linguistic kind that involves the attainment of a higher level of abstraction in a sign system; contrasts with *lateral development*.

vestibular canal: the upper tube of the cochlea that is involved in maintaining balance and the sense of positional orientation and posture, that is, whether we are upright, lying down, and so on.

vestibular system: the representational basis for our sense of balance, posture, and movement.

VICP: abbreviation for the *Vaccine Injury Compensation Program*.

visible speech: a phrase used by Alexander Graham Bell in advocating that deaf persons should learn to speak by looking closely at the articulatory movements of speaking models.

visuocentricity: the prejudice of seeing persons against those who are blind or visually impaired.

vital capacity: the entire capacity of the lungs to contain air consisting of the maximal inhalation plus the residual volume left after a maximal exhalation.

vitamin C: a well-known antioxidant and the vitamin that prevents "scurvy" or "Rickets disease."

vitamin E: an antioxidant that reduces tissue scarring in certain injuries.

vocal folds: referred to popularly as the "vocal cords" these strands of mucous membrane are normally open during breathing and close together during voiced speech producing the oscillating vibrations that we call the "voice."

vocal hygiene: the care and maintenance of the voice.

vocal nodules: growths that form on the vocal folds.

vocal timbre: all of the qualities of the voice other than pitch and volume.

vocal tract: the mouth and the tubes that connect it to the voice box (the larynx), the lungs, and the stomach.

vocalic center: in any syllabic production this is the approximate center of the vowel or what is called the "vocalic" part of the syllable.

voice disorder: any abnormal condition of the larynx or related systems involved in the production of voicing in speech or speech-like vocalizations.

voiced: in speech production, the quality of sound segments in which the vocal folds are vibrating.

voiceless: see *unvoiced*.

voicing: the action that is necessary in speech to produce *voiced* sound segments.

volitional control: the kind that can be attributed to the intentional, free will of the actor.

vowels: the kind of sound segments that can form the center of a syllable and that can be lengthened in such a way that they occupy the full length of an entire *breath group*.

wavelength: the distance from the highest peak to the lowest rough of a repeating wave form.

Wernicke's aphasia: a loss of the ability to comprehend language, especially speech.

Wernicke's area: a region in the left hemisphere which Carl Wernicke (1874/1977) associated with the ability to comprehend speech; also sometimes referred to as *receptive aphasia* or *semantic aphasia*.

white noise: noise that tends to be spread randomly over the whole spectrum of sound.

word deafness: *subcortical sensory aphasia* especially of the auditory kind.

word recognition: the process or result of exercising the ability to read words aloud one at a time as in a list, or in the sounding out of letters in sequence that is advocated by proponents of *phonics*.

xenobiotic: any substance that is foreign to the body, especially, any manufactured toxin such as those found in pesticides, preservatives, and the like.

zone of proximal development: on a scale of development, the next step upward that an individual is prepared to take with some assistance.

ZPD: abbreviation for *zone of proximal development*.

References

Abdesslem, H. (2002). Redefining motivation in FLA and SLA. *Cahiers linguistiques d'Ottawa, 30,* 1–28.

Abe, N., Suzuki, M., Mori, E., Itoh, M., & Fujii, T. (2007). Deceiving others: Distinct neural responses of the prefrontal cortex and amygdala in simple fabrication and deception with social interactions. *Journal of Cognitive Neuroscience, 19*(2), 287–295.

Abell, R. B. (n.d.). Bailey Banks v. Secretary of the Department of Health and Human Services, United States Court of Federal Claims, Office of Special Masters, No. 02-0738V, Filed: 20 July 2007. Retrieved April 17, 2009, from http://www.uscfc.uscourts.gov/sites/default/files/Abell.BANKS.02-0738V.pdf

Abortion at 24 weeks for a cleft palate. (2003, November 25). Retrieved April 17, 2009, from http://web.archive.org/web/20050101061713/www.bbc.co.uk/radio4/womanshour/24_11_03/tuesday/info4.shtml

Ad Hoc Committee on Scope of Practice in Speech-Language Pathology. (2001). *Scope of practice in speech-language pathology.* Rockport, MD: American Speech-Language-Hearing Association. Retrieved April 17, 2009, from http://www.asha.org/NR/rdonlyres/4FDEE27B-BAF5-4D06-AC4D-8D1F311C1B06/0/19446_1.pdf

ADA (2009). *U.S. Department of Justice, Americans with Disabilities Act.* Retrieved April 17, 2009, from http://www.usdoj.gov/crt/ada/adahom1.htm

Adverse Drug Event Reporting Workshop. (2007). *Adverse drug event reporting: The Roles of consumers and health-care professionals: Workshop summary.* Retrieved April 17, 2009, from http://books.nap.edu/catalog/11897.html

Advocates for Children's Health Affected by Mercury Poisoning (A-CHAMP). (2005). *Centers for Disease Control failure to remove mercury from vaccines.* Retrieved April 17, 2009, from http://www.a-champ.org/cdcmercuryremoval.html

Ainswort, W. A. (1973). System for converting English text into speech. *IEEE Transactions on Audio and Electroacoustics AU21*(3), 288–290.

Aitken, J. E. (2007). *IDEA-2004, IEP, transition, and the law.* Kansas City, Missouri. Retrieved April 17, 2009, from http://onlineacademics.org/IEP.html

Aldersley, S. (2002). Least restrictive environment and the courts. *Journal of Deaf Studies and Deaf Education, 7*(3), 189–199.

Aldridge, M. A., Stillman, R. D., & Bower, T. G. R. (2001). Newborn categorization of vowel-like sounds. *Developmental Science, 4* (2), 220–232.

Aleka Titzer. (2009). "Aleka Titzer," and "Aleka and Friends." On the DVD.

Alexander, L. (1947, July 14). *Military tribunal, Nuremberg: Closing argument for the United States of America.* Harvard Law School Library Item No. 2. Retrieved April 17, 2009, from http://nuremberg.law.harvard.edu/php/pflip.php?caseid=HLSL_NMT01&docnum=2&numpages=78&startpage=1&title=Closing+argument+for+the+United+States+of+America.&color_setting=C, (p. 76).

Alexander, L. (1949, July 14). Medical science under dictatorship. *New England Journal of Medicine,* pp. 39–47.

Allen, G. E. (1995). Eugenics comes to America. In R. Jacoby & N. Glauberman (Eds.), *The bell curve debate: History, documents, opinions* (pp. 441-475). New York: Random House.

Alzheimer's disease. (2009). Retrieved April 17, 2009, from http://en.wikipedia.org/wiki/Alzheimer's_disease

Ambidextrous pitcher. (2009). Retrieved April 17, 2009, from http://www.youtube.com/watch?v=8U2xkHOTvvw

Ambrose, N. G., & Yairi, E. (1999). Normative disfluency data for early childhood stuttering. *Journal of Speech, Language, and Hearing Research, 42,* 895–909.

American Academy of Audiology. (2009). *What is an audiologist?* Retrieved April 17, 2009, from http://www.audiology.org/resources/consumer/Documents/FSAudiologist08.pdf

American Academy of Audiology. (2009). *Code of ethics.* Retrieved April 17, 2009, from http://www.audiology.org/publications/documents/ethics/

American Academy of Pediatrics. (1998, August). Auditory integration training and facilitated communication for autism (reaffirmed in 2006). *Pediatrics, 102*(2), 431–433.

American Academy of Special Education Professionals. (2006a). *Code of ethics.* Retrieved April 17, 2009, from http://aasep.org/about-the-academy/code-of-ethics/index.html

American Academy of Special Education Professionals. (2006b). *Overview.* Retrieved April 17, 2009, from http://aasep.org/about-the-academy/index.html

American Counseling Association. (1997). *The practice of professional counseling.* Retrieved April 17, 2009, from http://www.counseling.org/Files/FD.ashx?guid=ea369e1d-0a17-411a-bc08-7a07fd908711

American Counseling Association. (2005). *Code of ethics.* Retrieved April 17, 2009, from http://www.counseling.org/Resources/CodeOfEthics/TP/Home/CT2.aspx

American Dental Association. (2005, August 5). *Summary of recent study of dental amalgam in wastewater.* Retrieved April 17, 2009, from http://www.ada.org/prof/resources/topics/topics_amalgamwaste_summary.pdf

American Dental Association. (2007, June). *Amalgam (silver-colored) fillings.* Retrieved April 17, 2009, from http://www.ada.org/public/topics/fillings_faq.asp

American Dental Association. (2007, December). *Amalgam.* Retrieved April 17, 2009, from http://www.ada.org/prof/resources/topics/amalgam.asp

American Dental Association. (2007a). *Best management practices for amalgam waste.* Retrieved April 17, 2009, from http://www.ada.org/prof/resources/topics/amalgam_bmp.asp

American Dental Association. (2007b). *Dental amalgam.* Retrieved April 17, 2009, from http://www.ada.org/public/topics/fillings.asp

American Diabetes Association. (n.d.). *All about diabetes.* Retrieved April 17, 2009, from http://www.diabetes.org/about-diabetes.jsp

American Medical Association. (2001). *Principles of medical ethics.* Retrieved April 17, 2009, from http://www.ama-assn.org/ama/pub/category/2512.html

American Medical Association. (2009). *About AMA.* Retrieved April 17, 2009, from http://www.ama-assn.org/ama/pub/category/1815.html

American Psychiatric Association. (1994). *Diagnostic and statistical manual of mental disorders* (4th ed.). Washington, DC: Author.

American Psychiatric Association. (2000). *Diagnostic and statistical manual of mental disorders* (4th ed., Text Revision). Washington, DC: Author. Retrieved April 17, 2009, from http://www.psychiatryonline.com/referral.aspx?gclid=CNvV_Lvn05ACFQUllgodIXM5WQ

American Psychiatric Association. (2009). *Principles of medical ethics.* Retrieved April 17, 2009 from http://www.psych.org/MainMenu/PsychiatricPractice/Ethics.aspx

American Psychological Association. (2002). *Code of ethics.* Retrieved April 17, 2009, from http://www.apa.org/ethics/code2002.html

American Psychological Association. (2009). *Definition of "psychology."* Retrieved April 17, 2009, from http://www.apa.org/about/.

American School for the Deaf. (2005). *A turning point in American history.* Retrieved April 17, 2009, from http://www.asd-1817.org/history/index.html

American Signed Language (ASL) Dictionary. (n.d.). Retrieved April 17, 2009, from http://www.lifeprint.com/asl101/pages-layout/signs.htm

American Speech-Language-Hearing Association. (1996). Central auditory processing: Current status of research and implications for clinical practice. *American Journal of Audiology, 5*(2), 41–54.

American Speech-Language-Hearing Association. (2003). *Code of ethics.* Retrieved April 17, 2009, from http://www.asha.org/docs/html/ET2003-00166.html.

American Speech-Language-Hearing Association, Ad Hoc Committee on Scope of Practice in Speech-Language Pathology. (2008). *Scope of practice in speech-language pathology.* Rockport, MD: Author.

American Speech-Language-Hearing Association, Council on Professional Standards. (2000). *Speech-language pathology standards (effective 1/1/05): Standards and implementation for the Certificate of Clinical Competence in Speech-Language Pathology.* Rockville, MD: Author.

American Speech-Language-Hearing Association, Council on Professional Standards. (2008). *Standards and Implementation for the Certificate of Clinical Competence in Speech-Language Pathology.* Retrieved April 17, 2009, from http://www.asha.org/about/membership-certification/handbooks/slp/slp_standards.htm

American Stroke Association. (2009). *What are the types of stroke?* Retrieved April 14, 2009, from http://www.strokeassociation.org/presenter.jhtml?identifier=1014

Americans with Disabilities Act of 1990, Pub. L. No. 101-336, §2, 104 Stat. 328. (1991). Retrieved April 14, 2009, from http://www.usdoj.gov/crt/ada/pubs/ada.htm

Amyloid plaques and neurofibrillary tangles. (2008). Retrieved April 14, 2009, from http://www.ahaf.org/alzdis/about/AmyloidPlaques.htm

Anaki, D., Kaufman, Y., Freedman, M., & Moscovitch, M. (2007). Associative (prosop)agnosia without (apparent) perceptual deficits: A case-study. *Neuropsychologia, 45*(8), 1658–1671.

Andersen, D. H. (1938). Cystic fibrosis of the pancreas and its relation to celiac disease: A clinical and pathological study. *American Journal of Diseases of Children, 56,* 344–399.

Annie Sullivan. (1936/2009). Retrieved April 14, 2009, from http://www.lkwdpl.org/wihohio/sull-ann.htm

Answers.com. (2009). *Autism.* Retrieved April 14, 2009, from http://www.answers.com/autism&r=67

Aposhian, H. V., Bruce, D. C., Alter, W., Dart, R. C., Hurlbut, K. M., & Aposhian, M. M. (1992). Urinary mercury after administration of 2,3-dimercaptopropane-1-sulfonic acid—correlation with Dental Amalgam Score. *FASEB Journal, 6*(7), 2472–2476.

Aristotle. (ca. 350 BC). *Posterior analytics* (G. R. G. Mure, Trans.). Retrieved April 14, 2009, from http://classics.mit.edu/Aristotle/posterior.1.i.html

Armstrong, D. F., Stokoe, W. C., & Wilcox, S. E. (1995). *Gesture and the nature of language.* New York: Cambridge University Press.

Arons, B. (1992, September). *Techniques, perception, and applications of time-compressed speech.* Paper presented at the 1992 Conference, American Voice I/O Society. Retrieved March 6, 2009, from http://www.dcc.uchile.cl/~abassi/WWW/Voz/avios92.html

Atianjoh, F. E., Ladenheim, B., Krasnova, I. N., & Cadet, J. L. (2008). Amphetamine causes dopamine depletion and cell death in the mouse olfactory bulb. *European Journal of Pharmacology, 589*(1–3), 94–97.

Auditory integration training. (2004). Retrieved April 14, 2009, from http://www.aitresources.com/

Auditory nerve. (n.d.). Retrieved April 14, 2009, from http://www.uni-tuebingen.de/uni/khh/glossary.htm

Autism Developmental Disabilities Monitoring Network. (2007). *Prevalence of the Autism Spectrum Disorders (ASDs) in multiple areas of the United States, 2000 and 2002.* Retrieved April 14, 2009, from http://www.cdc.gov/ncbddd/autism/documents/AutismCommunityReport.pdf

Autism Society of America. (n.d.). *Defining autism.* Retrieved April 14, 2009, from http://www.autism-society.org/site/PageServer?pagename=about_whatis_characteristics

Autism Speaks. (2009). Retrieved April 14, 2009, from http://www.autismspeaks.org/

Autism Speaks. (July 16, 2008). *Autism speaks applauds Louisiana Governor Bobby Jindal for signing autism insurance reform legislation into law.* Retrieved September 7, 2008, from http://www.autismspeaks.org/press/governor_signs_louisiana_insurance_law.php

Autism07. (2007, April 12–14). *The Sertoma International Conference on Autism Spectrum Disorders.* Retrieved September 24, 2008, from http://www.autism07.com/index.html

Azar, B. (1998, June). Why can't this man feel whether or not he's standing up? *APA Monitor, 29*(6). Retrieved April 14, 2009, from http://www.apa.org/monitor/jun98/touch.html

Backlund, H., Morin, C., Ptito, A., Bushnell, M. C., & Olausson, H. (2005). Tactile functions after cerebral hemispherectomy. *Neuropsychologia, 43*(3), 332–339.

Badon, L. C. (1993). *Comparison of word recognition and story-retelling under the conditions of contextualized versus decontextualized reading events in at-risk poor readers.* Unpublished doctoral dissertation, Louisiana State University, Baton Rouge.

Badon, L. C., Oller, J. W., Jr., & Oller, S. D. (2005). Enabling literacy in at-risk learners: Decoding surface form versus attending to meaning and narrative structure. *Psychology of Language and Communication, 9*(1), 5–27.

Bailey, D. M., Roukens, R., Knauth, M., Kallenberg, K., Christ, S., Mohr, A., et al. (2006). Free radical-mediated damage to barrier function is not associated with altered brain morphology in high-altitude headache. *Journal of Cerebral Blood Flow and Metabolism, 26*(1), 99–111.

Bajaj, A. (2007). Analysis of oral narratives of children who stutter and their fluent peers: Kindergarten through second grade. *Clinical Linguistics and Phonetics, 21*(3), 227–245.

Bajaj, A., Hodson, B., & Westby, C. (2005). Communicative ability conceptions among children who stutter and their fluent peers: A qualitative exploration. *Journal of Fluency Disorders, 30*(1), 41–64.

Baker, J. (2003). Psychogenic voice disorders and traumatic stress experience: A discussion paper with two case reports. *Journal of Voice, 17*(3), 308–318.

Balasubramanian, V., Max, L., Van Borsel, J., Rayca, K. O., & Richardson, D. (2003). Acquired stuttering following right frontal and bilateral pontine lesion: A case study. *Brain and Cognition 53*(2), 185–189.

Baler, R. D., Volkow, N. D., Fowler, J. S., & Benveniste, H. (2008). Is fetal brain monoamine oxidase inhibition the missing link between maternal smoking and conduct disorders? *Journal of Psychiatry and Neuroscience, 33*(3), 187–195.

Ball, M. J., & Muller, N. (2005). *Phonetics for communication disorders.* Mahwah, NJ: Lawrence Erlbaum.

Ballard, D. H., Hayhoe, M. M., Pook, P. K., & Rao, R. P. N. (1997). Deictic codes for the embodiment of cognition. *Behavioral and Brain Sciences, 20,* 723–767.

Banerjee, S., & Bhat, M. A. (2008). Glial ensheathment of peripheral axons in Drosophila. *Journal of Neuroscience Research, 86*(6), 1189–1198.

Bannister, R. (1954). *Bannister breaks four-minute mile.* Retrieved April 14, 2009, from http://news.bbc.co.uk/onthisday/hi/dates/stories/may/6/newsid_2511000/2511575.stm

Bannister, R. (2009). Retrieved April 14, 2009, from http://en.wikipedia.org/wiki/Roger_Bannister

Baratz, J. (1969). A bidialectal task for determining language proficiency in economically disadvantaged Negro children. *Child Development, 40,* 889–901.

Barbeau, E., & Poncet, M. (2001). Diagonistic dyspraxia in anterior and posterior corpus callosum lesions. *Revue de Neuropsychologie, 11*(2), 241–255.

Barlow, B. K., Cory-Slechta, D. A., Richfield, E. K., & Thiruchelvam, M. (2007). The gestational environment and Parkinson's disease: Evidence for neurodevelopmental origins of a neurodegenerative disorder. *Reproductive Toxicology, 23*(3), 457–470.

Barr, L. (2004). *EPA's draft use reduction program.* Retrieved September 24, 2008, from http://www.epa.gov/region5/air/mercury/meetings/Nov04/barr.pdf

Barsalou, L. W. (1999). Language comprehension: Archival memory or preparation for situated action? *Discourse Processes, 28,* 61–80.

Barwise, J., & Perry, J. (1983). *Situations and attitudes.* Cambridge, MA: MIT Press.

Battle Hymn of the Republic. (2009a). [Sung by the St. John's Children's Choir.] Retrieved April 14, 2009, from http://www.ez-tracks.com/getsong-songid267.html

Battle Hymn of the Republic. (2009b). [U.S. Army Band performs composition by William Steffe.] Retrieved April 14, 2009, from http://lcweb2.loc.gov/diglib/ihas/loc.natlib.ihas.100010422/default.html

Bauer, A. (2005). *A wild ride up the cupboards.* New York: Scribner.

Bellinger, D. C., Trachtenberg, F., Barregard, L., Tavares, M., Cernichiari, E., Daniel, D., et al. (2006). Neuropsychological and renal effects of dental amalgam in children: A randomized clinical trial. *Journal of the American Medical Association, 295,* 1775–1783.

Benson, J. D., Debashish, M., Greaves, W. S., Lukas, J., Savage-Rumbaugh, S., & Taglialatela, J. (2004). Mind and brain in apes: A methodology for phonemic analysis of vocalizations of language competent bonobos. *Language Sciences, 26*(6), 643–660.

Bentivoglio, M. (1998, April 20). *Life and discoveries of Santiago Ramón y Cajal.* Retrieved April 14, 2009, from http://nobelprize.org/nobel_prizes/medicine/articles/cajal/index.html

Bergmann, C., Morlot, S., & Ptok, M. (2007). Speech impairment and the Smith-Magenis syndrome [in German]. *HNO, 55*(8), 644–646.

Berlin Wall. (1989/2009). Retrieved April 14, 2009, from http://en.wikipedia.org/wiki/Berlin_Wall

Bermpohl, F., Pascual-Leone, A., Amedi, A., Merabet, L. B., Fregni, F., Gaab, N., et al. (2006). Attentional modulation of emotional stimulus processing: An fMRl study using emotional expectancy. *Human Brain Mapping, 27*(8), 662–677.

Bernard, S. (2004). Association between thimerosal-containing vaccine and autism *Journal of the American Medical Association, 291,* 180.

Bernard, S., Enayati, A., Redwood, L., Roger, H., & Binstock, T. (2001). Autism: A novel form of mercury poisoning. *Medical Hypotheses, 56,* 462–471.

Bernard, S., Enayati, A., Roger, H., Binstock, T., & Redwood, L. (2002). The role of mercury in the pathogenesis of autism. *Molecular Psychiatry, 7*(Suppl. 2), S42–S43.

Bernard, S., Redwood, L., & Blaxill, M. (2004). Thimerosal, mercury, and autism: Case study in the failure of the risk assessment paradigm. *Neurotoxicology, 25*(4), 710–710.

Bernstein-Ratner, N., & Tetnowksi, J. (Eds.). (2006). *Current issues in stuttering research and practice.* Mahwah, NJ: Lawrence Erlbaum.

Bersoff, D. N. (1981). Testing and the law. *American Psychologist, 36*(10), 1047–1056.

Bersoff, D. N. (1994). Explicit ambiguity—the 1992 Ethics Code as an oxymoron. *Professional Psychology-Research and Practice, 25*(4), 382–387.

Bickerton, D. (1981). *Roots of language.* Ann Arbor, MI: Karoma.

Biklen, D. (1990). Communication unbound—Autism and praxis. *Harvard Educational Review, 60*(3), 291–314.

Bill of Rights. (1789). Retrieved April 14, 2009, from http://en.wikipedia.org/wiki/United_States_Bill_of_Rights.

Binet, A., & Simon, T. (1905). New methods for the diagnosis of the intellectual level of subnormals. *L'Année Psychologique, 5,* 191–244.

Biran, I., Giovannetti, T., Buxbaum, L., & Chatterjee, A. (2006). The alien hand syndrome: What makes the alien hand alien? *Cognitive Neuropsychology, 23*(4), 563–582.

Birdwhistell, R. (1970). *Kinesics in context*. Philadelphia: University of Pennsylvania Press.

Birnholz, J., Stephens, J. C., & Faria, M. (1978). Fetal movement patterns: A possible means of defining neurologic developmental milestones in utero. *American Journal of Roentology, 130,* 537–540.

Björk, E. A. (1999). Startle, annoyance and psychophysical responses to repeated sound bursts. *Acustica (Acta Acustica), 85,* 575–578.

Black, J. W. (1951). The effect of delayed side-tone upon vocal rate and intensity. *Journal of Speech and Hearing Disorders, 16,* 56–60.

Blass, E. M., & Camp, C. A. (2001). The ontogeny of face recognition: Eye contact and sweet taste induce face preference in 9- and 12-week-old human infants. *Developmental Psychology, 37,* 762–774.

Blind Children's Learning Center. (2007). Retrieved April 14, 2009, from http://www.blindkids.org/speech.html

Bloodstein, O. (1950). A rating scale study of conditions under which stuttering is reduced or absent. *Journal of Speech and Hearing Disorders, 15,* 33.

Bloodstein, O. (1959). *The nature of stuttering*. From the 1959 Symposium on Stuttering sponsored by the University of Wisconsin, Madison. Retrieved April 14, 2009, from http://www.mnsu.edu/comdis/voices/voices.html

Bloodstein, O. (1960). The development of stuttering. II. Developmental phases. *Journal of Speech and Hearing Disorders, 25,* 366–376.

Bloodstein, O. (1974). The rules of early stuttering. *Journal of Speech and Hearing Disorders, 39,* 379–394.

Bloodstein, O. (1995). *A handbook on stuttering* (5th ed.). San Diego, CA: Singular.

Bloodstein, O. (2006). Some empirical observations about early stuttering: A possible link to language development. *Journal of Communication Disorders, 39*(3), 185–191.

Bloodstein, O., & Gantwerk, B. F. (1967). Grammatical function in relation to stuttering in young children. *Journal of Speech and Hearing Research, 10,* 786–789.

Bloodstein, O., & Grossman, M. (1981). Early stutterings: Some aspects of their form and distribution. *Journal of Speech and Hearing Research, 24,* 298–302.

Bloom, A. S., & Weisskopf, B. (1989). The physician under Public Law 99–457. *Journal of the Kentucky Medical Association, 87*(6), 275–279.

Bloomfield, L. (1933). *Language*. New York: Holt, Rinehart, and Winston.

Bloomfield, L., & Barnhart, C. L. (1961). *Let's read: A linguistic approach*. Detroit, MI: Wayne State University Press.

Blotcky, A. J., Claassen, J. P., Fung, Y. K., Meade, A. G., & Rack, E. P. (1995). Optimization of procedures for Hg-203 instrumental neutron-activation analysis in human urine. *Journal of Radioanalytical and Nuclear Chemistry—Articles, 195*(1), 109–116.

Blumstein, S. E., & Kurowski, K. (2006). The foreign accent syndrome: A perspective. *Journal of Neurolinguistics, 19*(5), 346–355.

Board of Education of the City of New York v. Harris, 622 F.2d 599. (1979). Retrieved April 14, 2009, from http://caselaw.lp.findlaw.com/scripts/getcase.pl?court=us&vol=444&invol=130

Bobes, M. A., Quiñonez, I., Perez, J., Leon, I., & Valdes-Sosa, M. (2007). Brain potentials reflect access to visual and emotional memories for faces. *Biological Psychology, 75*(2), 146–153.

Bocca, B., Alimonti, A., Bomboi, G., Giubilei, F., & Forte, G. (2006). Alterations in the level of trace metals in Alzheimer's disease. *Trace Elements and Electrolytes, 23*(4), 270–276.

Bocca, E. (1958). Clinical aspects of cortical deafness. *Laryngoscope, 68,* 301–309.

Bocca, E., Calearo, C., & Cassinari, V. (1954). A new method for testing hearing in temporal lobe tumor. *Acta Otolaryngologica, 44,* 219–221.

Bocca, E., Calearo, C., Cassinari, V., & Migliavacca, F. (1955). Testing cortical hearing in temporal lobe tumors. *Acta Otolaryngologica, 42,* 289–304.

Bodaghi, B., Weber, M. E., Arnoux, Y. V., Jaulerry, S. D., Le Hoang, P., & Colin, J. (2005). Comparison of the efficacy and safety of two formulations of diclofenac sodium 0.1% eyedrops in controlling postoperative inflammation after cataract surgery. *European Journal of Ophthalmology, 15*(6), 702–711.

Boeing. (2007). *Statistical summary of jet airplane accidents worldwide operations 1959–2007*. Retrieved September 24, 2008, from http://www.boeing.com/news/techissues/pdf/statsum.pdf

Bohland, J. W., & Guenther, F. H. (2006). An fMRI investigation of syllable sequence production. *Neuroimage, 32*(2), 821–841.

Bolhuis, J. J., & Gahr, M. (2006). Neural mechanisms of birdsong memory. *Nature Reviews Neuroscience, 7*(5), 347–357.

Boorstin, J. (1990). *The Hollywood eye: What makes movies work*. New York: Harper Collins.

Booth, J. W. (1865). Retrieved April 14, 2009, from http://en.wikipedia.org/wiki/John_Wilkes_Booth

Borgeat, F., David, H., Saucier, J. F., & Dumont, M. (1994). Perceptual defense and vulnerability to postpartum depression. *Acta Psychiatrica Scandinavica, 90,* 455.

Borgeat, F., Sauvageau, I., David, H., & Saucier, J. F. (1997). Perceptual defense and vigilance to perinatal stimuli. *Perceptual and Motor Skills, 85* (3, Pt. 1), 1136–1138.

Bornstein, H. (1973). A description of some current sign systems designed to represent English. *American Annals of the Deaf, 118*(3), 454–463.

Bornstein, H. (1979). Systems of sign. In L. Bradford & W. Harly (Eds.), *Hearing and hearing impairment* (pp. 333–361). New York: Grune & Stratton.

Bosshardt, H. (2006). Cognitive processing load as a determinant of stuttering: Summary of a research programme. *Clinical Linguistics and Phonetics, 20*(5), 371–385.

Boswell, J. (1988). *The kindness of strangers: The abandonment of children in Western Europe from late antiquity to the Renaissance.* New York: Pantheon Books.

Botox. (2009). Retrieved April 14, 2009, from http://www.botoxcosmetic.com/

Bower, T. G. R. (1997). Contingencies, logic, and learning. *The Behavior Analyst, 20,* 141–148.

Bradford, P. V., & Blume, H. (1992). *Ota Benga—The pygmy in the zoo.* New York: St. Martin's Press.

Braille. (1852/2009). Retrieved April 14, 2009, from http://en.wikipedia.org/wiki/Braille

Braille, L. (1809–1852). Retrieved April 14, 2009, from http://en.wikipedia.org/wiki/Louis_Braille

Brain Injury Recovery Network. (2009). Retrieved April 14, 2009, from http://www.tbirecovery.org/Intro.html

Branigan, E. (1992). *Narrative comprehension and film.* London: Routledge.

Bransfield, R. C., Wulfman, J. S., Harvey, W. T., & Usman, A. I. (2008). The association between tick-borne infections. Lyme borreliosis and autism spectrum disorders. *Medical Hypotheses, 70*(5), 967–974.

Bridgeman Art Library v. Corel Corp., 36 F. Supp. 2d 191 (S.D.N.Y. 1999).

Brigham, C. C. (1923). *A study of American intelligence.* Princeton, NJ: Princeton University Press.

British Broadcasting Company. (2003, December). *Curate wins abortion challenge.* Retrieved April 14, 2009, from http://news.bbc.co.uk/1/hi/health/3247916.stm

British Dyslexia Association. (2009). *About dyslexia.* Retrieved April 14, 2009, from http://www.bdadyslexia.org.uk/aboutdyslexia.html

Broca, P. P. (1861). Perte de la parole; ramolissement chronique et destruction partielle du lobe antérieur gauche de cerveau (Loss of speech: Chronic softening and partial destruction of the left frontal lobe of the brain). *Bulletins de la Société d'Anthropologie de Paris, 2,* 235–238.

Broca's aphasia. (2009). Retrieved April 14, 2009, from http://en.wikipedia.org/wiki/Paul_Broca

Brodman, K. (1909/1999). *Localization in the cerebral cortex* (L. Garey, Trans.). London: Imperial College Press. (Original work published in 1909).

Brodmann's areas. (2009). Retrieved April 14, 2009, from http://en.wikipedia.org/wiki/Brodmann_area

Brooks, R. B. (2001). Fostering motivation, hope, and resilience in children with learning disorders. *Annals of Dyslexia, 51,* 9–20.

Brookshire, R. H. (1997). *Introduction to neurogenic communication disorders* (5th ed.). St. Louis, MO: Mosby.

Brown v. Board of Education, 347 U.S. 483. (1954).

Brown, A. M., Kenwell, Z. R., Maraj, B. K.V., & Collins, D. F. (2008). "Go" signal intensity influences the sprint start. *Medicine and Science in Sports and Exercise, 40*(6), 1142–1148.

Bruce Willis. (2002). Retrieved April 14, 2009, from http://www.rd.com/images/content/021102/bruce_willis_interview.pdf

Bruner, J. (n.d.). *Best image depicting science or technology.* Retrieved September 24, 2008, from http://www.life.com/Life/eisies/eisies2000/scienceSingle_blowup.html

Bruner, J. S. (1975). From communication to language: A psychological perspective. *Cognition, 3,* 255–287.

Bruner, J. S. (1983). *Child's talk: Learning to use language.* New York: Norton.

Brunotto, M., Frede, S., De Gelfo, A. M. Z., Cismondi, I. A., Hliba, E., & De Halac, R. I. N. (2003, December). Study of human papiloma virus infection on mouth and genital epithelium. *Journal of Dental Research, 82*(Special Issue C), 32–32.

Bullock, T. H., Bennett, M. V. L., Johnston, D., Josephson, R., Marder, E., & Fields R. D. (2005). The neuron doctrine, redux. *Science, 310*(5749), 791–793.

Burbacher, T. M., Shen, D. D., Liberato, N., Grant, K. S., Cernichiari, E., & Clarkson, T. (2005). Comparison of blood and brain mercury levels in infant monkeys exposed to methyl mercury or vaccines containing thimerosal. *Environmental Health Perspectives, 113*(8), 1015–1021.

Burghaus L., Hilker, R., Thiel, A., Galldiks, N., Lehnhardt, F. G., Zaro-Weber, O., et al. (2006). Deep brain stimulation of the subthalamic nucleus reversibly deteriorates stuttering in advanced Parkinson's disease. *Journal of Neural Transmission, 113*(5), 625–631.

Burman, C. (2002). *Hello fellow face-blind friend.* Retrieved April 14, 2009, from http://www.prosopagnosia.com/main/cb/index.asp

Burr, C. W. (1905). *Report of an adult signer.* Presented at the Seventeenth Meeting of the Annual Convention of Instructors of the Deaf. Morgantown, PA.

Bushnell, I. W. R., Sai, F., & Mullin, J. T. (1989). Neonatal recognition of the mother's face. *British Journal of Developmental Psychology, 7,* 3–15.

Butler, S. R. (1997). Hemispheric specialization and neuronal plasticity. *Developmental Brain Dysfunction 10*(4), 187–202.

Butovskaya, M. L. (2005). Man and apes: Linguistic abilities and dialogue potentialities. *Zoologichesky Zhurnal*, *84*(1), 149–157.

Buyske S., Williams, T. A., Mars, A. E., Stenroos, E. S., Ming, S. X., Wang, R., et al. (2006, February 10). Analysis of case-parent trios at a locus with a deletion allele: Association of GSTM1 with autism. *BMC Genetics, 7*, Art. 8.

C. Everett Koop (2009). Retrieved April 14, 2009, from http://en.wikipedia.org/wiki/C._Everett_Koop

Cabrera, S., Barden, D., Wolf, M., & Lobner, D. (2007, October). Effects of growth factors on dental pulp cell sensitivity to amalgam toxicity. *Dental Materials, 23*(10), 1205–1210.

Campbell, D. B., Sutcliffe J. S., Ebert, P. J., Militerni, R., Bravaccio, C., Trillo, S., et al. (2006). A genetic variant that disrupts MET transcription is associated with autism. *Proceedings of the National Academy of Sciences of the United States of America, 103*(45), 16834–16839.

Campbell, S. (2004). *Scans uncover secrets of the womb.* Video and Audio News (Interview) with the BBC's Vicki Young. Retrieved September 24, 2008, from http://news.bbc.co.uk/2/hi/health/3846525.stm.

Campbell, T., Dollaghan, C., Needleman, H., & Janosky, J. (1997). Reducing bias in language assessment: Processing-dependent measures. *Journal of Speech, Language, and Hearing Research, 40*(3), 519–525.

Cannell, S. J. (2006). *Dyslexia videos, article and resources.* Retrieved September 24, 2008, from http://www.cannell.com/dyslexia.php

Cannell, S. J. (May 29, 2007). *The greatest lesson I've learned.* Retrieved September 24, 2008, from http://www.cannell.com/videoQA.php?s=9&k=84f011ccbe88f676c6aeaa73929104fc

Capo, F. (2008, May 7). *World's fastest talker.* Retrieved March 6, 2009 from http://www.youtube.com/watch?v=aZb6iBmHqkY

Caputi, F., Spaziante, R., de Divitiis, E., & Nashold, B. S. (1995). Luigi Rolando and his pioneering efforts to relate structure to function in the nervous system. *Journal of Neurosurgery, 83*(5), 933–937.

Carbon, C. C. (2008). Famous faces as icons. The illusion of being an expert in the recognition of famous faces. *Perception, 37*(5), 801–806.

Carbone, M., & Bedrossian, C. W. M. (2006). The pathogenesis of mesothelioma. *Seminars in Diagnostic Pathology, 23*(1), 56–60.

Carlsen, W. (2001, July 22). New documents show the monkey virus is present in more recent polio vaccine. *San Francisco Chronicle*, p. A6.

Carnegie Institution of Washington. (2005). *Brief historical time line for Carnegie Institution of Washington (CIW) at Cold Spring Harbor.* Retrieved September 24, 2008, from http://library.cshl.edu/archives/archives/ciwscope.htm

Carpi, A. (1999). *Atomic structure.* Retrieved September 24, 2008, from http://web.jjay.cuny.edu/~acarpi/NSC/3-atoms.htm

Carroll, J. B. (1993). *Human cognitive abilities: A survey of factor analytic studies.* Cambridge: Cambridge University Press.

Carroll, L. (1871). *Through the looking-glass, and what Alice found there.* London: Macmillan.

Carvey, P. M., Punati, A., & Newman, M. B. (2006). Progressive dopamine neuron loss in Parkinson's disease: The multiple hit hypothesis. *Cell Transplantation, 15*(3), 239–250.

Cave, S. (2001). *What your doctor may not tell you about children's vaccinations.* New York: Time Warner Books.

Cedrola, S., Guzzi, G., Ferrari, D., Gritti, A., Vescovi, A. L., Pendergrass, J. C., et al. (2003, March). Inorganic mercury changes the fate of murine CNS stem cells. *FASEB Journal, 17*(3), 869.

Centers for Disease Control. (n.d.-a). *Autism: Learn the signs act early.* Retrieved September 24, 2008, from http://www.cdcfoundation.org/healththreats/autism.aspx

Centers for Disease Control. (n.d.-b). *Increase in autism.* Retrieved September 16, 2006 from http://www.cdc.gov/od/ads/autism/autism.htm

Centers for Disease Control. (1986, June 6). Perspectives in disease prevention and health promotion premature mortality due to unintentional injuries—United States, 1983. *MMWR Weekly, 35*(22), 353–356. Retrieved September 24, 2008, from http://www.cdc.gov/mmwr/preview/mmwrhtml/00000741.htm

Centers for Disease Control. (2006). *Prevention and Control of Influenza: Recommendations of the Advisory Committee on Immunization Practices (ACIP).* Retrieved September 24, 2008, from http://www.cdc.gov/mmwr/preview/mmwrhtml/rr5510a1.htm

Centers for Disease Control. (2006, October 31). *Measles, mumps, and rubella (MMR) vaccine and autism fact sheet.* Retrieved September 24, 2008, from http://www.cdc.gov/nip/vacsafe/concerns/autism/autism-mmr.htm

Centers for Disease Control. (2007, February 9). Surveillance summaries. *Morbidity and Mortality Weekly Report (MMWR), 56*, No. SS-1. Retrieved September 24, 2008, from http://www.cdc.gov/mmwr/PDF/ss/ss5601.pdf

Centers for Disease Control/Vaccine Safety Datalink. (1990). *Vaccine Safety Datalink (VSD) Project.* Retrieved September 24, 2008, from http://www.cdc.gov/od/science/iso/research_activties/vsdp.htm

Chadwick, R. S. (1998, December 8). Compression, gain, and nonlinear distortion in an active cochlear model with subpartitions. *Proceedings of the National Academy of Sciences, USA, 95*(25), 14594–14599.

Chamberlain, D. (2009). *Life before birth.* Retrieved March 20, 2009, from http://www.birthpsychology .com/lifebefore/

Chambon, M. (1783). *Traité général du commerce de l'Amérique.* Amsterdam: Librairie Portal.

Chandrashekar, J., Hoon, M. A., Ryba, N. J. P., & Zuker, C. S. (2006). The receptors and cells for mammalian taste. *Nature, 444*(7117), 288–294.

Chard, D. J., & Dickson, S. V. (1999). *Phonological awareness.* Retrieved April 14, 2009, from http://www.ld online.org/article/6254

Charles, L. E., Burchfiel, C. M., Fekedulegn, D., Kashon, M. L., Ross, G. W., Petrovitch, H., et al. (2006). Occupational exposures and movement abnormalities among Japanese-American men: The Honolulu-Asia Aging Study. *Neuroepidemiology, 26*(3), 130–139.

Charles Macklin. (ca. 1797). Retrieved April 14, 2009, from http://en.wikipedia.org/wiki/Charles_Macklin

Chartrand, T. L., & Bargh, J. A. (1999). The Chameleon effect: The perception-behavior link and social interaction. *Journal of Personality and Social Psychology, 76*(6), 893–910.

Chauhan, A., Chauhan, V., Brown, W. T., & Cohen, I. (2004). Oxidative stress in autism: Increased lipid peroxidation and reduced serum levels of ceruloplasmin and transferrin—The antioxidant proteins. *Life Sciences, 75*(21), 2539–2549.

Chauhan, A., Chauhan, V., Cohen, I. L., Mehta, P., Brown, W. T., & Barshatzky, M. (2006, July). Increased oxidative stress and inflammation in autism. *Journal of Neurochemistry, 98*(Suppl. 1), 29.

Chauhan, A., Essa, M. M., Muthaiyah, B., Brown, W. T., & Chauhan, V. (2008). Increased oxidative damage and free radical generation in lymphoblasts from autism. *Journal of Neurochemistry, 106*(Suppl. 1), 44.

Chen, C. S., & Miller, N. R. (2007). Botulinum toxin injection causing lateral rectus palsy. *British Journal of Ophthalmology, 91*(6), 843–843.

Chen, R. T., Glasser, J. W., Rhodes, P. H., Davis, R. L., Barlow, W. E., Thompson, R. S., et al. (1997). Vaccine Safety Datalink project: A new tool for improving vaccine safety monitoring in the United States. *Pediatrics, 99*(6), 765-773.

Chermak, G. D., & Musiek, F. E. (1997). *Central auditory processing disorders.* San Diego, CA: Singular.

Cherokee. (2005). Retrieved April 14, 2009, from http://www.ethnologue.com/14/show_language.asp?c ode=CER

Cherry, S. R., Sorenson, J. A., & Phelps, M. E. (2003). *Physics in nuclear medicine* (3rd ed.). Philadelphia: Saunders/Elsevier Science.

Chiat, S. & Roy, P. (2007). The preschool repetition test: An evaluation of performance in typically developing and clinically referred children. *Journal of Speech Language and Hearing Research, 50*(2), 429–443.

Childhood apraxia. (2009). The Childhood Apraxia of Speech Association of North America (CASANA). Retrieved April 14, 2009, from http://www.apraxi a-kids.org/site/c.chKMI0PIIsE/b.700249/k.CC 2C/Home/apps/lk/content3.aspx

Children's corner. (n.d.). *Bio of Stan Kurtz.* Retrieved April 14, 2009, from http://www.childrenscorn erschool.com/stankurtz.htm

Choisser, B. (2002). *Face blind!* Retrieved September 24, 2008, from http://www.choisser.com/faceblind/

Chomsky, N. A. (1957). *Syntactic structures.* The Hague: Mouton.

Chomsky, N. A. (1959). A review of B. F. Skinner's *Verbal Behavior. Language, 35*(1), 26–58.

Chomsky, N. A. (1965). *Aspects of the theory of syntax.* Cambridge, MA: MIT Press.

Chomsky, N. A. (1972). *Language and mind.* New York: Harcourt, Brace, & World.

Chomsky, N. A. (1980). On cognitive structures and their development: A reply to Piaget. In M. Piatelli-Palmarini (Ed.), *Language and learning: The debate between Jean Piaget and Noam Chomsky* (pp. 35–54). Cambridge, MA: Harvard University Press.

Chomsky, N. A. (1988). *Language and problems of knowledge: The Managua lectures.* Cambridge, MA: MIT Press.

Chomsky, N. A. (1995). Language and nature. *Mind, 104*, 1–61.

Chomsky, N. A. (2002). *On nature and language.* New York: Cambridge University Press.

Chomsky, N. A., & Hornstein, N. (2005). *Rules and representations.* New York: Columbia University Press.

Chomsky, N. A., & Fodor, J. A. (1980). The inductivist fallacy. In M. Piatelli-Palmarini (Ed.), *Language and learning: The debate between Jean Piaget and Noam Chomsky* (pp. 259–275). Cambridge, MA: Harvard University Press.

Chomsky, N. A., & Halle, M. (1968). *The sound pattern of English.* New York: Harper and Row.

Christopher Burke. (2009). Retrieved April 14, 2009, from http://www.nndb.com/people/380/000086122/

Cicilline, D. N. (2007). *Statement from Mayor David N. Cicilline regarding Brown University's commitment in response to the Slavery & Justice Report.* Retrieved April 14, 2009, from http://www.providenceri.com /press/article.php?id=191

Civil Rights Act of 1964, Pub. L. 88-352, 78 Stat. 241. (July 2, 1964). Retrieved April 14, 2009, from http:// en.wikipedia.org/wiki/Civil_Rights_Act_of_ 1964

Clancy, M. (2001). *Story of the "fetal hand grasp" photograph*. Retrieved April 17, 2009, from http://www.michaelclancy.com/story.html

Clarkson, T. W., & Magos, L. (2006). The toxicology of mercury and its chemical compounds. *Critical Reviews in Toxicology, 36*, 609–662.

Claus, B., & Kelter, S. (2006). Comprehending narratives containing flashbacks: Evidence for temporally organized representations. *Journal of Experimental Psychology-Learning Memory and Cognition, 32*(5), 1031–1044.

Cleft Palate Foundation. (2006). Retrieved April 14, 2009, from http://www.cleftline.org/

Clostridium botulinum. (2009). Retrieved April 14, 2009, from http://en.wikipedia.org/wiki/Clostridium_botulinum

Collins, D. (2009). *Information for genetic professionals*. Retrieved April 14, 2009, from http://www.kumc.edu/gec/geneinfo.html

Columbia University. (2009). *The future role of functional MRI in medical applications*. Retrieved April 14, 2009, from http://www.fmri.org/fmri.htm

Comar, M., D'Agaro, P., Luzzati, R., Martini, F., Tognon, M., & Campello, C. (2007). SV40 and HIV sequences in the cerebrospinal fluid of a patient with AIDS dementia complex. *Current HIV Research, 5*(3), 345–347.

Computed tomography. (2009). Retrieved April 14, 2009, from http://en.wikipedia.org/wiki/Computed_tomography

Condon, W. S., & Sander, L. W. (1974). Synchrony demonstrated between movements of the neonate and adult speech. *Child Development, 45*, 456–462.

Connaghan, K. P., Moore, C. A., & Higashakawa, M. (2004). Respiratory kinematics during vocalization and nonspeech respiration in children from 9 to 48 months. *Journal of Speech Language and Hearing Research, 47*(1), 70–84.

Conti-Fine, B. M., Milani, M., & Kaminski, H. J. (2006). Myasthenia gravis: Past, present, and future. *Journal of Clinical Investigation, 116*(11), 2843–2854.

Corbera, S., Corral, M. J., Escera, C., & Idiazabal, M. A. (2005). Abnormal speech sound representation in persistent developmental stuttering. *Neurology, 65*(8), 1246–1252.

Cordes, A. K. (1994). The reliability of observational data. 1. theories and methods for speech-language pathology. *Journal of Speech Language and Hearing Research, 37*(2), 264–278.

Cordes, A. K. (2000). Individual and consensus judgments of disfluency types in the speech of persons who stutter. *Journal of Speech Language and Hearing Research, 43*(4), 951–964.

Cordes, A. K., & Ingham, R. J. (1995a). Judgments of stuttered and nonstuttered intervals by recognized authorities in stuttering research. *Journal of Speech and Hearing Research, 38*(1), 33–41.

Cordes, A. K., & Ingham, R. J. (1995b). Stuttering includes both within-word and between-word disfluencies. *Journal of Speech and Hearing Research, 38*(2), 382–386.

Cornell University Law School. (n.d.-a). *Amendment XIII*. Retrieved April 14, 2009, from http://www.law.cornell.edu/constitution/constitution.amendmentxiii.html .

Cornell University Law School. (n.d.-b). *Amendment XIV*. Retrieved April 14, 2009, from http://www.law.cornell.edu/constitution/constitution.amendmentxiv.html .

Cornell University Law School. (1857/2009). *Scott v. Sanford, 60 U.S. 393* (1857). Retrieved April 14, 2009, from http://www.law.cornell.edu/supct/html/historics/USSC_CR_0060_0393_ZS.html

Correll, C. U., Penzner, J. B., Frederickson, A. M., Richter, J. J., Auther, A. M., Smith, C. W., et al. (2007). Differentiation in the preonset phases of schizophrenia and mood disorders: Evidence in support of a bipolar mania prodrome. *Schizophrenia Bulletin, 33*(3), 703–714.

Costanzo, R. M., & Becker, D. P. (1986). Smell and taste disorders in head injury and neurosurgery patients. In H. L. Meiselman & R. S. Rivlin (Eds.), *Clinical measurements of taste and smell* (pp. 565–578). New York: Macmillan.

Counter, S. A., & Buchanan, L. H. (2004). Mercury exposure in children: A review. *Toxicology and Applied Pharmacology, 198*(2), 209–230.

Cousin, J. W. (1910). *A short biographical dictionary of English literature*. London: J. M. Dent & Sons; New York: E. P. Dutton.

Cox, C., Marsh, D., Myers, G. & Clarkson, T. (1995). Analysis of data on delayed development from the 1971–1972 outbreak of methyl mercury poisoning in Iraq: Assessment of influential points. *NeuroToxicology, 16*(4), 727–730.

Crick, F. (1981). *Life itself: Its origin and nature*. New York: Simon and Schuster.

Crossley, R., & Remington-Gurley, J. (1992). Getting the words out: Facilitated communication training. *Topics in Language Disorders, 12*, 29–45.

Crutcher, M. (2007, March). *The marketing of aborted baby parts*. Retrieved April 14, 2009, from http://lifedynamics.com/Abortion_Information/Baby_Body_Parts/index.cfm

Crystal, D. (1987). *The Cambridge encyclopedia of language*. Cambridge: Cambridge University Press.

Culotta, V. C., Yang, M., & O'Halloran, T. V. (2006). Activation of superoxide dismutases: Putting the metal to the pedal. *Biochimica et Biophysica Acta—Molecular Cell Research, 1763*(7), 747–758.

Cummins, J. (2003). *Language, power, and pedagogy: Bilingual children in the crossfire.* Clevedon, UK; Buffalo, NY: Multilingual Matters.

Cutler, A. (1994). Segmentation problems, rhythmic solutions. *Lingua, 92,* 81–104.

Daguerre, L. (1828). *History of photography.* Retrieved April 14, 2009, from http://inventors.about.com/library/inventors/blphotography.htm

Dallos, P., Zheng, J., & Cheatham, M. A. (2006). Prestin and the cochlear amplifier. *Journal of Physiology-London, 576*(1), 37–42.

Damasio, H. (2000). The lesion method in cognitive neuroscience. In F. Boller, J. Grafman, & G. Rizzolatti (Eds.), *Handbook of neuropsychology* (2nd ed., Vol. 1, pp. 77–102). Amsterdam: Elsevier Science.

Damasio, H., Tranel, D., Grabowski, T., Adolphs, R., & Damasio, A. (2004). Neural systems behind word and concept retrieval. *Cognition, 92*(1–2), 179–229.

Damico, J. S. (1985a). Clinical discourse analysis: A functional approach to language assessment. In C. S. Simon (Ed.), *Communication skills and classroom success* (pp. 165–204). London: Taylor and Francis.

Damico, J. S. (1985b). *The effectiveness of direct observation as a language assessment technique.* Unpublished doctoral dissertation, University of New Mexico, Albuquerque.

Damico, J. S. (1991). Descriptive assessment of communicative ability in LEP students. In E. V. Hamayan & J. S. Damico (Eds.), *Limiting bias in the assessment of bilingual students* (pp. 157–218). Austin, TX: Pro-Ed.

Damico, J. S. (2003). The role of theory in clinical practice: Reflections on model building. *Advances in Speech-Language Pathology, 5*(1), 57–60.

Damico, J. S., & Damico, S. K. (1993). Mapping a course over different roads: Language teaching with special populations. In J. W. Oller, Jr. (Ed.), *Methods that work: A smorgasbord of language teaching ideas* (2nd ed.). New York: Newbury House.

Damico, J. S., & Damico, S. K. (1997). The establishment of a dominant interpretive framework in language intervention. *Language Speech and Hearing Services in Schools, 28*(3), 288–296.

Damico, J. S., & Oller, J. W., Jr. (1980). Pragmatic versus morphological/syntactic criteria for language referrals. *Language, Speech, and Hearing Services in Schools, 11,* 85–94.

Damico, J. S., & Oller, J. W., Jr. (1985). *Spotting language problems.* San Diego, CA: Los Amigos Research Associates.

Damico, J. S., Oller, J. W., Jr., & Storey, M. E. (1983). The diagnosis of language disorders in bilingual children: Pragmatic and surface-oriented criteria. *Journal of Speech and Hearing Disorders, 48,* 385–394.

Damper, R. I., & Marchand, Y. (2006). Information fusion approaches to the automatic pronunciation of print by analogy. *Information Fusion, 7*(2), 207–220.

Damper, R. I., Marchand, Y. Adamson, M. J., & Gustafson, K. (1999). Evaluating the pronunciation component of text-to-speech systems for English: A performance comparison of different approaches. *Computer Speech and Language, 13*(2), 155–176.

Dang, X., Wuthrich, C., Axthelm, M. K., & Koralnik, I. J. (2008). Productive simian virus 40 infection of neurons in immunosuppressed rhesus monkeys. *Journal of Neuropathology and Experimental Neurology, 67*(8), 784–792.

Daniels, S. K., Corey, D. M., Fraychinaud, A., DePolo, A., & Foundas, A. L. (2006). Swallowing lateralization: The effects of modified dual-task interference. *Dysphagia, 21*(1), 21–27.

Dantzig, P. I. (2006). Parkinson's disease, macular degeneration and cutaneous signs of mercury toxicity. *Journal of Occupational and Environmental Medicine, 48*(7), 656.

Darley, F. L. (1967). Lacunae and research approaches to them. IV. In C. Milliken & F. L. Darley (Eds.), *Brain mechanisms underlying speech and language* (pp. 236–240). New York: Grune & Stratton.

Darley, F. L., Aronson, A. R., & Brown, J. R. (1975). *Motor speech disorders.* Philadelphia: W. B. Saunders.

Darwin, C. (1874). *The descent of man* (2nd ed.). New York: D. Appleton.

Daubert v. Merrell Dow Pharmaceuticals (92-102), 509 U.S. 579. (1993). Retrieved April 14, 2009, from http://en.wikipedia.org/wiki/Daubert_Standard also from http://straylight.law.cornell.edu/supct/html/92-102.ZS.html

Davidson, D. (1996). The folly of trying to define truth. *Journal of Philosophy, 93,* 263–278.

Davis, R. (2000, May 2). Hand of a fetus touched the world. *USA Today,* p. D8.

Day, J. J., Reed, M. N., & Newland, M. C. (2005). Neuromotor deficits and mercury concentrations in rats exposed to methyl mercury and fish oil. *Neurotoxicology and Teratology, 27*(4), 629–641.

de Jong, K. J., Lim, B. J., & Nagao, K. (2004). The perception of syllable affiliation of singleton stops in repetitive speech. *Language and Speech, 47*(3), 241–266.

De Nil, L., & Kroll, R. (2001). Searching for the neural basis of stuttering treatment outcome: Recent neuroimaging studies. *Clinical Linguistics and Phonetics, 15*(1), 163–168.

De Nil, L., Kroll, R., Kapur, S., & Houle, S. (2000). A positron emission tomography study of silent and oral single word reading in stuttering and nonstuttering adults. *Journal of Speech, Language and Hearing Research, 43*(4), 1038.

De Nil, L., Kroll, R., Lafaille, S., & Houle, S. (2003). A positron emission tomography study of short- and long-term treatment effects on functional brain activation in adults who stutter. *Journal of Fluency Disorders, 28*(4), 357.

de Saussure, F. (1959). *Course in general linguistics.* (C. Bally, A. Sechehaye, & A. Riedlinger, Eds.; W. Baskin, Trans.). New York: McGraw Hill Philosophical Library. (Original lectures ca. 1906).

Deafness—from birth to death. (2009). Retrieved April 14, 2009, from http://deafness.about.com/cs/earbasics/a/birthtodeath.htm

Declaration of Independence. (1776). Retrieved April 14, 2009, from http://www.ushistory.org/declaration/document/

Dehaene-Lambertz, G., & Pena, M. (2001). Electrophysiological evidence for automatic phonetic processing in neonates. *Neuroreport, 12,* 3155–3158.

Del Cul, A., Baillet, S., & Dehaene, S. (2007). Brain dynamics underlying the nonlinear threshold for access to consciousness. *PLOS Biology, 5*(10), 2408–2423.

DeLeon, J., Gottesman, R. F., Kleinman, J. T., Newhart, M., Davis, C., Heidler-Gary, J., et al. (2007). Neural regions essential for distinct cognitive processes underlying picture naming. *Brain, 130*(5), 1408–1422.

D'Entremont, B., & Muir, D. (1999). Infant responses to adult happy and sad vocal and facial expressions during face-to-face interactions. *Infant Behavior and Development, 22*(4), 527–539.

Derakhshan, I. (2003). Callosum and movement control: Case reports. *Neurological Research, 25*(5), 538–542.

Deth, R., Muratore, C., Benzecry, J., Power-Charnitsky, V. A., & Waly, M. (2008). How environmental and genetic factors combine to cause autism: A redox/methylation hypothesis. *Neurotoxicology, 29*(1), 190–201.

Deutsche Welle. (2005). *Young stutterers fight prejudices.* Retrieved April 14, 2009, from http://www.dw-world.de/dw/episode/0,1569,1683498,00.html

Dewey, J. (1925). *Experience and nature.* Chicago: Open Court.

Diana v. California State Board of Education. No. C-70 37 RFP, District Court of Northern California. (February, 1970).

Dickens, C. (1842). *American notes.* Retrieved April 14, 2009, from http://en.wikipedia.org/wiki/American_Notes

Didinium. (2003). Retrieved April 14, 2009, from http://www.microscope-microscope.org/applications/pond-critters/protozoans/ciliphora/didinium.htm

Digital Anatomist Project, University of Washington. (1995). Retrieved April 14, 2009, from http://www9.biostr.washington.edu:80/cgi-bin/DA/PageMaster?atlas:Neuroanatomy+ffpathIndex/3D^Pathways/Arcuate^Fasciculus+2

Dike, C. C., Baranoski, M., & Griffith, E. H. (2005). Pathological lying revisited, *Journal of the American Academy of Psychiatry and the Law, 33,* no. 3, 342–349.

DiLollo, A., Manning, W. H., & Neimeyer, R. A. (2003). Cognitive anxiety as a function of speaker role for fluent speakers and persons who stutter. *Journal of Fluency Disorders, 28,* 167–186.

DiLorenzo, T. J. (2003). *Politically correct history.* Retrieved April 14, 2009, from http://www.lewrockwell.com/dilorenzo/dilorenzo37.html

District Courts of the United States. (2007). Retrieved April 14, 2009, from http://www.uscourts.gov/images/CircuitMap.pdf

Doe v. Withers, Civil Action No. 92-C-92. Circuit Court of Taylor County, W. VA. (1993). Retrieved April 14, 2009, from http://www.wrightslaw.com/law/caselaw/case_Doe_Withers_Complaint.html

Domingo, J. L. (2006). Aluminum and other metals in Alzheimer's disease: A review of potential therapy with chelating agents. *Journal of Alzheimer's Disease, 10*(2–3), 331–341.

Drescher, M. J., Drescher, D. G., Khan, K. M., Hatfield, J. S., Ramakrishnan, N. A., Abu-Hamdan, M. D., et al. (2006). Pituitary adenylyl cyclase-activating polypeptide (PACAP) and its receptor (PAC1-R) are positioned to modulate afferent signaling in the cochlea. *Neuroscience, 142*(1), 139–164.

D'Souza, Y., Fombonne, E., & Ward, B. J. (2006). No evidence of persisting measles virus in peripheral blood mononuclear cells from children with autism spectrum disorder. *Pediatrics, 118*(4), 1664–1675.

Duda, J. E. (2007). History and prevalence of involuntary emotional expression disorder. *CNS Spectrums, 12*(4 Suppl. 5), 6–10.

Duffy, J. (1995). *Motor speech disorders: Substrates, differential diagnosis, and management.* St. Louis, MO: Mosby.

Dunlap, K. (1900). The effect of imperceptible shadows on the judgment of distance. *Psychological Review, 7,* 435–453.

Dunning, M. (2005). *The sign of the book.* New York: Simon and Schuster.

Dziewas, R., Soros, P., Ishii, R., Chau, W., Henningsen, H., Ringelstein, E. B., et al. (2003). Neuroimaging evidence for cortical involvement in the preparation and in the act of Swallowing. *Neuroimage, 20*(1), 135–144.

Easterling, C. S., & Mobbins, E. (2008). Dementia and dysphagia. *Geriatric Nursing, 2*(4), 275–285.

Edlich, R. F., Greene, J. A., Cochran, A. A., Kelley, A. R., Gubler, K. D., Olson, B. M., et al. (2008). Need for informed consent for dentists who use mercury amalgam restorative material as well as technical considerations in removal of dental amalgam restorations. *Journal of Environmental Pathology Toxicology and Oncology, 26*(4), 305–322.

Edlich, R. F., Son, D. M., Olson, B. M., Greene, J. A., Gubler, K. D., Winters, K. L., et al. (2007). Update on the national vaccine injury compensation program. *Journal of Emergency Medicine, 33*(2), 199–211.

Education of All Handicapped Children Act of 1975, Pub. L. 94-142 § 6. (November 29, 1975).

Education of the Handicapped Act Amendments of 1983, Pub. L. No. 98-199, 97 Stat. 1357 (20 U. S. C. §§ 1400–1461, 1994).

Education of the Handicapped Amendments of 1986, Pub. L. No. 99-457, 100 Stat. 1145. (1986).

Ehler, D. J., & McGhee, R. L. (2007). *Primary Test of Nonverbal Intelligence (PTONI)*. Austin, TX: Pro-Ed.

Eilers, R. E., & Oller, D. K. (1994). Infant vocalizations and the early diagnosis of severe hearing impairment. *Journal of Pediatrics, 124*(2), 199–203.

Einarsdóttir, E., & Ingham, R. J. (2005). Have disfluency-type measures contributed to the understanding and treatment of developmental stuttering? *American Journal of Speech-Language Pathology, 14,* 260–273.

Einstein, A. (1956). Physics and reality. In Author, *Out of my later years* (pp. 59–96). Secaucus, NJ: Citadel. (Originally published in 1936).

Einstein, A. (1956) The common language of science. In Author, *Out of my later years* (pp. 111–113). Secaucus, NJ: Citadel Press. (Originally produced as a radio broadcast in 1941).

Ejiri, K. (1998). Synchronization between preverbal vocalizations and motor actions in early infancy I: Precanonical babbling vocalizations synchronize with rhythmic body movements before the onset of canonical babbling. *Japanese Journal of Psychology, 68,* 433–440.

Ejiri, K., & Masataka, N. (2001). Co-occurrence of preverbal vocal behavior and motor action in early infancy. *Developmental Science, 4,* 40–48.

Ekman, P., & Friesen, W. V. (1974). Detecting deception from body or face. *Journal of Personality and Social Psychology, 29*(3), 288–298.

Ekman, P., & Friesen, W. V. (1975). *Unmasking the face: A guide to recognizing emotions from facial clues*. Englewood Cliffs, NJ: Prentice-Hall.

El-Imam, Y. A. (2004). Monetization of Arabic: Rules and algorithms. *Computer Speech and Language, 18*(4), 339–373.

El-Imam, Y. A. (2008). Synthesis of the intonation of neutrally spoken Modern Standard Arabic speech. *Signal Processing, 88*(9), 2206–2221.

El-Imam Y. A., & Don, Z. M. (2005). Rules and algorithms for phonetic transcription of Standard Malay. *IEICE Transactions on Information and Systems E88D, 10,* 2354–2372.

Elster, E. (2000). *What if Albert Einstein had been prescribed Ritalin?* Retrieved April 14, 2009, from http://www.erinelster.com/Articles/add_article_3_00.html

Emeril Lagasse. (2009). Retrieved April 14, 2009, from http://en.wikipedia.org/wiki/Emeril_Lagasse

Emmorey, K., Mehta, S. & Grabowski, T. J. (2007). The neural correlates of sign versus word production. *Neuroimage, 36*(1), 202–208.

Epinephrine. (2009). Retrieved April 14, 2009, from http://en.wikipedia.org/wiki/Epinephrine

Erdelyi, M. H. (1974). A new look at the new look: Perceptual defense and vigilance. *Psychological Review, 81*(1), 1–25.

Erdelyi, M. H. (2004). Subliminal perception and its cognates: Theory, indeterminacy, and time. *Consciousness and Cognition, 13,* 73–91.

Esiri, M. M. (2007). Ageing and the brain. *Journal of Pathology, 211*(2), 181–187.

Ethnologue. (2009). *An encyclopedic reference work cataloging all of the world's 6,912 known living languages*. Retrieved April 14, 2009, from http://www.ethnologue.com

Eugenics archive. (n.d.). *Agricultural genetics*. Retrieved September 24, 2008, from http://www.eugenicsarchive.org/html/eugenics/static/themes/28.html

Eugenics Movement. (2009). Retrieved April 14, 2009, from http://www.ferris.edu/isar/arcade/eugenics/movement.htm

Eugenics. (2009). Retrieved April 14, 2009, from http://en.wikipedia.org/wiki/Eugenics

Evans, M. (Director), & Pell, A. (Writer). (2006). *Snow Cake* [Motion picture]. United States: Revolution Films. Retrieved February 5, 2009, from http://www.youtube.com/watch?v=aqv5gmsikIQ&feature=related

Fauconnier, G. (1985). *Mental spaces*. Cambridge: Cambridge University Press.

Feinberg, D. (2007). Foreword. In J. McCarthy, *Louder than words: A mother's journey in healing autism*. New York: Dutton.

Feldman, R. (2007). Parent-infant synchrony and the construction of shared timing; physiological precursors, developmental outcomes, and risk conditions. *Journal of Child Psychology and Psychiatry, 48*(3–4), 329–354.

Felsenfeld, S., Kirk, K. M., Zhu, G., Statham, D. J., Neale, M. C., & Martin, N. G. (2000). A study of the genetic and environmental etiology of stuttering in a selected twin sample. *Behavior Genetics, 30*, 359–366.

Feng, L., Sun, Q. Gao, C., Dong, J., Wei, X. L., Xing, H., et al. (2007). Gene expression analysis of pancreatic cystic neoplasm in SV40Tag transgenic mice model. *World Journal of Gastroenterology, 13*(15), 2218–2222.

Ferdinand de Saussure. (1913/2008). Retrieved April 14, 2009, from http://en.wikipedia.org/wiki/Ferdinand_de_Saussure

Ferreira, S. T., Vieira, M. N. N., & De Felice, F. G. (2007). Soluble protein oligomers as emerging toxins in Alzheimer's and other amyloid diseases. *IUBMB LIFE 59*(4–5), 332–345.

Fetal Alcohol Syndrome. (2009). Retrieved April 14, 2009, from http://www.kidshealth.org/parent/medical/brain/fas.html

Field, F. (2005). *Essays in the design of language.* Santa Ana, CA: Calvary Chapel.

Film Scouts. (2006). Retrieved September 24, 2008, from http://www.filmscouts.com/scripts/matinee.cfm?Film=air-for&File=filmmkrs

Finegan, E., & Rickford, J. R. (2004). *Language in the USA: Themes for the twenty-first century.* Cambridge: Cambridge University Press.

Finn, P., Bothe, A. K., & Bramlett, R. E. (2005). Science and pseudoscience in communication disorders: Criteria and applications. *American Journal of Speech-Language Pathology, 14*, 172–186.

Fisch, M., Kloesel, C. J. W., Moore, E. C., Roberts, D. D., Ziegler, L. A., & Atkinson, N. P. (Eds.), (1982). *Writings of Charles S. Peirce: A chronological edition, Vol. 1 1857–1866.* Indianapolis: Indiana University Press. (Originally written or published in 1861).

Fitch, W. T. (2005). The evolution of language: A comparative review. *Biology and Philosophy, 20*(2–3), 193–230.

Fitch, W. T., Hauser, M. D., & Chomsky, N. A. (2005). The evolution of the language faculty: Clarifications and implications. *Cognition, 97*(2), 179–210.

Fodor, J. A. (1983). *The modularity of mind.* Cambridge, MA: Bradford Books, MIT Press.

Fombonne, E. (1999). The epidemiology of autism: A review. *Psychological Medicine, 29*, 769–786.

Fombonne, E. (2003). Epidemiological surveys of autism and other pervasive developmental disorders: An update. *Journal of Autism and Developmental Disorders, 33*, 365–382.

Fombonne, E. (2005). Epidemiology of autistic disorder and other pervasive developmental disorders. *Journal of Clinical Psychiatry, 66*(Suppl. 10), 3–8.

Fombonne, E. (2008). Thimerosal disappears but autism remains. *Archives of General Psychiatry, 65*, 15–16.

Food and Drug Administration. (2009). *Thimerosal in vaccines.* Retrieved April 14, 2009, from http://www.fda.gov/cber/vaccine/thimerosal.htm#pres

Food and Drug Administration & Centers for Disease Control. (2009). *Vaccine Adverse Event Report System (VAERS): Frequently asked questions.* Retrieved April 14, 2009, from http://www.fda.gov/cber/vaers/faq.htm

Food and Drug Administration & Centers for Disease Control. (n.d.). *VAERS table of reportable events following vaccination.* Retrieved April 14, 2009, from http://www.vaers.hhs.gov/pdf/ReportableEventsTable.pdf

Food and Drug Administration Center for Biologics Evaluation and Research. (2009). *What are the advantages to the public for regulation of biologics under the PHS Act?* Retrieved April 14, 2009, from http://www.fda.gov/cber/faq.htm#6

Foss, D. J., & Swinney, D. A. (1973). On the psychological reality of the phoneme: Perception, identification, and consciousness. *Journal of Verbal Learning and Verbal Behavior, 12*, 246–257. Retrieved September 25, 2008, from http://lcnl.ucsd.edu/LCNL main page/Publications_PDF/1973_Foss_Swinney.pdf

Foundas, A. L., Bollich, A. M., Feldman, J., Corey, D. M., Hurley, M., Lemen, L. C., et al. (2004). Aberrant auditory processing and atypical planum temporale in developmental stuttering. *Neurology, 63*(9), 1640–1646.

Fox, M. (2009, February 12). *U.S. Vaccine Court denies family's autism case.* Retrieved March 11, 2009, from http://www.newsdaily.com/stories/tre51b4an-us-us-vaccines-autism/

França, A. I. (2004). *Introduction to neurolinguistics.* Retrieved September 25, 2008, from http://mit.edu/kaitire/www/evelin2005/Neuro/RelatorioEvelin2004.pdf

Franco, J. L., Teixeira, A., Meotti, F. C., Ribas, C. M., Stringari, J., Pomblum, S. C. G., et al. (2006). Cerebellar thiol status and motor deficit after lactational exposure to methyl mercury. *Environmental Research, 102*(1), 22–28.

Franic, D. M., & Bothe, A. K. (2008). Psychometric evaluation of condition-specific instruments used to assess health-related, quality of life, attitudes, and related constructs in stuttering. *American Journal of Speech-Language Pathology, 17*(1), 60–80.

Franken, M. C. J., Kielstra-Van der Schalka, C. J., & Boelens, H. (2005). Experimental treatment of early stuttering: A preliminary study. *Journal of Fluency Disorders, 30*(3), 189–199.

Freeman, W. J. (2000). A neurobiological interpretation of semiotics: Meaning, representation, and information. *Information Sciences, 124*(1–4), 93–102.

Free and Appropriate Public Education. (1972). Definition from *PARC v. Pennsylvania* (1972). Retrieved April 14, 2009, from http://www.faculty.piercelaw.edu/redfield/library/Pdf/case-parc.pennsylvania.pdf

Frege, G. (1967). *Begriffsschrift*, a formula language, modeled upon that of arithmetic, for pure thought. In J. van Heijenoort (Ed.), *From Frege to Gödel: A sourcebook in mathematical logic* (pp. 5–82). Cambridge, Massachusetts: Harvard University Press. (Originally published 1879)

Frolenkov, G. I. (2006). Regulation of electromotility in the cochlear outer hair cell *Journal of Physiology—London, 576*(1), 43–48.

Frustaci, A., Magnavita, N., Chimenti, C., Caldarulo, M., Sabbioni, E., Pietra, R., et al. (1999). Marked elevation of myocardial trace elements in idiopathic dilated cardiomyopathy compared with secondary cardiac dysfunction. *Journal of the American College of Cardiology, 33*(6), 1578–1583.

Fukawa, T., Yoshioka, H., Ozawa, E., & Yoshida, S. (1988). Difference of susceptibility to delayed auditory feedback between stutterers and nonstutterers. *Journal of Speech and Hearing Research, 31*, 475–479.

Fuller, G. (1993). *Neurological examination made easy.* Edinburgh: Churchill Livingstone.

Gaasch, J. A., Lockman, P. R., Geldenhuys, W. J., Allen, D. D., & Van der Schyf, C. J. (2007). Brain iron toxicity: Differential responses of astrocytes, neurons, and endothelial cells. *Neurochemical Research, 32*(7), 1196–1208.

Gage, N., Roberts, T. P. L., & Hickok, G. (2006, January 19). Temporal resolution properties of human auditory cortex: Reflections in the neuromagnetic auditory evoked m100 component. *Brain Research, 1069*(1), 166–171.

Gainotti, G. (2007). Different patterns of famous people recognition disorders in patients with right and left anterior temporal lesions: A systematic review. *Neuropsychologia, 45*(8), 1591–1607.

Gallese, V. (2007). Before and below "theory of mind": Embodied simulation and the neural correlates of social cognition. *Philosophical Transactions of the Royal Society B-Biological Sciences, 362*(1480), 659–669.

Galton, F. (1869). *Hereditary genius: An inquiry into its laws and consequences.* London: Macmillan.

Gardner, E. J., & Snustadt, D. P. (1981). *Principles of genetics* (6th ed.). New York: Wiley.

Gardner, H. (1975). *The shattered mind.* New York: Knopf.

Garey, L. J. (1999). Brodmann's "Localisation in the cerebral cortex." Retrieved April 14, 2009, from http://www.worldscibooks.com/medsci/p151.html

Garg, A., Schwartz, D., & Stevens, A. A. (2007). Orienting auditory spatial attention engages frontal eye fields and medial occipital cortex in congenitally blind humans *Neuropsychologia, 45*(10), 2307–2321.

Gauss, J. C. F. (1855/2009). Retrieved April 14, 2009, from http://en.wikipedia.org/wiki/Carl_Friedrich_Gauss

Gazzaniga, M. S. (2000). Cerebral specialization and interhemispheric communication—Does the corpus callosum enable the human condition? *Brain, 123*(Pt. 7), 1293–1326.

Geier, D. A., & Geier, M. R. (2006a). An assessment of downward trends in neurodevelopmental disorders in the United States following removal of thimerosal from childhood vaccines. *Medical Science Monitor, 12*(6), CR231–CR239.

Geier, D. A., & Geier, M. R. (2006b). A clinical and laboratory evaluation of methionine cycle-transsulfuration and androgen pathway markers in children with autistic disorders. *Hormone Research, 66*(4), 182–188.

Geier, D. A., & Geier, M. R. (2006c). An evaluation of the effects of thimerosal on neurodevelopmental disorders reported following DTP and Hib vaccines in comparison to DTPH vaccine in the United States. *Journal of Toxicology and Environmental Health-Part A—Current Issues, 69*(15), 1481–1495.

Geier, D. A., & Geier, M. R. (2007a). A prospective study of mercury toxicity biomarkers in autistic spectrum disorders. *Journal of Toxicology and Environmental Health-Part A—Current Issues, 70*(20), 1723–1730.

Geier, D. A., & Geier, M. R. (2007b). A prospective study of thimerosal-containing Rho(D)-immune globulin administration as a risk factor for autistic disorders. *Journal of Maternal-Fetal and Neonatal Medicine, 20*(5), 385–390.

Geier, M. R., & Geier, D. A. (2008). *The biochemical basis of autistic disorders: The mercury, androgen (testosterone), and glutathione connection.* Silver Spring, MD: The Genetic Centers of America and the Institute of Chronic Illnesses. (PowerPoint presentation.) Retrieved September 25, 2008, from http://www.autismone.org/uploads/Geier%20Mark%20&%20Geier%20David%20AO%202008%20Biomed%20LaSalle%20BC.ppt

Genetics Education Center. (2008). *Genetic and rare conditions site.* Retrieved September 25, 2008, from http://www.kumc.edu/gec/support/index.html

George, G. N., Prince, R. C., Gailer, J., Buttigieg, G. A., Denton, M. B., Harris, H. H., et al. (2004). Mercury binding to the chelation therapy agents DMSA and DMPS and the rational design of custom chelators for mercury. *Chemical Research in Toxicology, 17*(8), 999–1006.

Gernsbacher, M. A., Dawson, M., & Goldsmith, H. H. (2005). Three reasons not to believe in an autism epidemic. *Current Directions in Psychological Science, 14*(2), 55–59.

Gettysburg Address. (1863). Abraham Lincoln on line: Speeches and writing. Retrieved April 14, 2009, from http://showcase.netins.net/web/creative/lincoln/speeches/gettysburg.htm

Ghosh, S. K., Chaudhuri, J., Gachhui, R., Mandal, A., & Ghosh, S. (2007). Effect of mercury and organomercurials on cellular glucose utilization: A study using resting mercury-resistant yeast cells. *Journal of Applied Microbiology, 102*(2), 375–383.

Gibbs, R. (2003). Embodied experience and linguistic meaning. *Brain and Language, 84*, 1–15.

Gibson, W. (1956). *The miracle worker.* New York: Doubleday.

Gillberg, C. (1999). Prevalence of disorders in the autism spectrum. *Infants and Young Children, 12*(2), 64–74.

Gillberg, C., Cederlund, M., Lamberg, K., & Zeijlon, L. (2006). Brief report: "The autism epidemic." The registered prevalence of autism in a Swedish urban area. *Journal of Autism and Developmental Disorders, 36*(3), 429–435.

Girard, M. (2007). When evidence-based medicine (EBM) fuels confusion: Multiple sclerosis after hepatitis B vaccine as a case in point. *Medical Veritas, 4*, 1436–1451.

Giummarra, M. J., Gibson, S. J., Georgiou-Karistianis, N., & Bradshaw, J. L. (2008). Mechanisms underlying embodiment, disembodiment and loss of embodiment. *Neuroscience and Biobehavioral Reviews, 32*(1), 143–160.

Givelberg, E., & Bunn, J. (n.d.). *Construction of a computational model of the cochlea.* Retrieved September 25, 2008, from http://pcbunn.cacr.caltech.edu/Cochlea/default.htm

Glattke, T. (2002). *Otoacoustic emissions in 2002: Some perspectives.* Retrieved September 25, 2008, from http://www.audiologyonline.com/articles/article_detail.asp?article_id=334

Glenberg, A. M. (1997). What memory is for. *Behavioral and Brain Sciences, 20*, 1–55.

Glutathione. (2008). Retrieved September 25, 2008, from http://en.wikipedia.org/wiki/Glutathione

Goldin-Meadow, S. (1996). Book review of *Kanzi: The Ape at the Brink of the Human Mind* by S. Savage-Rumbaugh & R. Lewin. *International Journal of Primatology, 17*, 145–148.

Gomase, V. S., & Tagore, S. (2008). Epigenomics. *Current Drug Metabolism, 9*(3), 232–237.

Gombrich, E. H. (1970). Standards of truth: The arrested image and the moving eye. *Critical Inquiry, 7*(2), 237–273.

Gombrich, E. H. (1972). The visual image. *Scientific American, 227*(3), 82–85.

Goodglass, H., & Geschwind, N. (1976). Language disorders. In E. Carterette & M. P. Friedman (Eds.), *Handbook of perception: Language and speech. Vol VII.* New York: Academic Press.

Goodglass, H., & Kaplan, E. (1983). *The assessment of aphasia and related disorders.* (2nd ed.). Philadelphia: Lea and Febiger.

Goodwin, C. (2003). Pointing as situated practice. In S. Kita (Ed.), *Pointing: Where language, culture and cognition meet* (pp. 217–241). Hillsdale, NJ: Lawrence Erlbaum.

Gorney, C. (2004, November). Gambling with abortion: Why both sides think they have everything to lose (*Harper's Magazine*). Retrieved September 25, 2008, from http://www.harpers.org/archive/2004/11/0080278

Gough, P. B., & Lee, C. H. (2007). A step toward early phonemic awareness: The effects of the turtle talk training. *Psychologia, 50*(1), 54–66.

Gould, S. J. (1981). *The mismeasure of man.* New York: Norton.

Gould, S. J. (1995). Mismeasure by any measure. In R. Jacoby & N. Glauberman (Eds.), *The bell curve debate: History, documents, opinions* (pp. 3–13). New York: Random House.

Graesser, A. C., Millis, K. K., & Zwaan, R. A. (1997). Discourse comprehension. *Annual Review of Psychology, 48*, 163–189.

Grandin, T. (2008). Web site. Retrieved September 25, 2008, from http://www.templegrandin.com/

Gray, H. (1918). *Anatomy of the human body.* Retrieved September 25, 2008, from http://www.bartleby.com/107/

Gross, J., & Strom, S. (June 18, 2007). *Autism debate strains a family and its charity.* Retrieved February 26, 2009, from http://www.nytimes.com/2007/06/18/us/18autism.html

Guardians Association v. Civil Service Commission of the City of New York 463 U.S. 582. (1983). Retrieved September 25, 2008, from http://supreme.justia.com/us/463/582/

Guimaraes, E. (2007). Feminist research practice: Using conversation analysis to explore the researcher's interaction with participants. *Feminism and Psychology, 17*(2), 149–161.

Guitar, B. (1996). From the 1996 Panel discussion on "recovery" ASHA Convention, Seattle, Washington. Retrieved April 14, 2009, from http://www.mnsu.edu/comdis/voices/voices.html

Guitar, B. (2006). *Stuttering: An integrated approach to its nature and treatment* (3rd ed.). New York: Lippincott Williams & Williams.

Gunderson, L., & Siegel, L. S. (2001). The evils of the use of IQ tests to define learning disabilities in first- and second-language learners. *Reading Teacher, 55*(1), 48–55.

Gupta, S. (March 6, 2008). *CNN's Dr. Sanjay Gupta interviews Dr. Jon Poling on 4-4-08.* Retrieved April 14, 2009, from http://www.youtube.com/watch?v=YxfgqsZ8BV0&NR=1.

Gupta, S. (April 1, 2008). *Vaccine-autism test case: Video of Michelle Cedillo.* Retrieved April 14, 2009, from http://www.cnn.com/2008/HEALTH/conditions/03/24/autism.vaccines/#cnnSTCVideo

Gutierrez, M., & Lopez, F. (2005). Mother-child verbal interaction: Responsiveness and intentionality. *Revista Mexicana de Psicologia, 22*(2), 491–503.

Haddon, M. (2003). *The curious case of the dog in the night-time.* New York: Doubleday.

Hagele, T. J., Mazerik, J. N., Gregory, A., Kaufman, B., Magalang, U., Kuppusamy, M. L., et al. (2007). Mercury activates vascular endothelial cell phospholipase D through thiols and oxidative stress. *International Journal of Toxicology, 26*(1), 57–69.

Hagler, D. J., Jr., Riecke, L., & Sereno, M. L. (2007). Parietal and superior frontal visuospatial maps activated by pointing and saccades. *Neuroimage, 35*(4), 1562–1577.

Hagoort, P., & van Berkum, J. (2007). Beyond the sentence given. *Philosophical Transactions of the Royal Society B-Biological Sciences, 362*(1481), 801–811.

Hair cells. (2009). Retrieved April 14, 2009, from http://www.uni-tuebingen.de/uni/khh/glossary.htm

Halassa, M. M., Fellin, T., Takano, H., Dong, J. H., & Haydon, P. G. (2007). Synaptic islands defined by the territory of a single astrocyte. *Journal of Neuroscience, 27*(24), 6473–6477.

Haller, J. S., Jr. (1971). *Outcasts from evolution: Scientific attitudes of racial inferiority, 1859–1900.* Urbana, IL: University of Illinois.

Handicapped Children's Protection Act of 1986, Public Law 99-372. (August 5, 1986).

Handley, J. B., & Handley, L. (2009). *Putchildrenfirst.org.* Retrieved March 11, 2009, from http://www.putchildrenfirst.org/intro.html

Hanna, P. R., Hanna, J. S., Hodges, R. E., & Rudorf, E. H. (1966). *Phoneme-grapheme correspondences as cues to spelling improvement.* Washington, DC: U.S. Department of Health, Education, and Welfare.

Hansen, G. H. A. (1874). Undersøgelser Angående Spedalskhedens Årsager Investigations concerning the etiology of leprosy [in Norwegian]. *Norsk Mag. Laegervidenskaben, 4*, 1–88.

Harlan, J. M. (1896). Dissent in *Plessy v. Ferguson, 163 U.S. 537 (1896).* Retrieved September 25, 2008, from http://laws.findlaw.com/us/163/537.html

Harman, D. (1956). Aging: A theory based on free radical and radiation chemistry. *Journal of Gerontology, 11*(3), 298–300.

Harman, D. (1972). The biologic clock: The mitochondria? *Journal of the American Geriatric Society, 20*(4), 145–147.

Harman, D. (1981). The aging process. *Proceedings of the National Academy of Sciences USA, 78*(11), 7124–7128.

Harris, S. B. (1998, January). *An interview with Dr. Denham Harman cancer and biopsy.* Retrieved April 14, 2009, from http://www.karlloren.com/biopsy/p61.htm

Harrison, E., Onslow, M., & Menzies, R. (2004). Dismantling the Lidcombe Program of early stuttering intervention: Verbal contingencies for stuttering and clinical measurement. *International Journal of Language and Communication Disorders, 39*(2), 257–267.

Harrison, J., & Howe, M. (1974). Anatomy of the descending auditory system (mammalian). In W. Keidel & W. Neff (Eds.), *Handbook of sensory physiology* (pp. 363–368). Berlin: Springer-Verlag.

Hart, N. W. M., Walker, R. F., & Gray, B. N. (1977). *The language of children: A key to literacy.* Reading, MA: Addison-Wesley.

Hashemian, A. (2006). *Attention and Achievement Center.* Retrieved April 14, 2009, from http://drugfreeadd.com/

Hatcher, J. M., Richardson, J. R., Guillot, T. S., McCormack, A. L., Di Monte, D. A., Jones, D. P., et al. (2007). Dieldrin exposure induces oxidative damage in the mouse nigrostriatal dopamine system. *Experimental Neurology, 204*(2), 619–630.

Haynes, J. D., & Rees, G. (2005). Predicting the orientation of invisible stimuli from activity in human primary visual cortex. *Nature Neuroscience, 8*(5), 686–691.

Healy, W., & Healy, M. T. (1926). *Pathological lying, accusation, and swindling.* Boston: Little, Brown.

Heinrich Hertz. (1894/2009). Retrieved April 14, 2009, from http://en.wikipedia.org/wiki/Heinrich_Hertz

Helen Keller. (1955/2009). Retrieved April 14, 2009, from http://en.wikipedia.org/wiki/Helen_Keller

Helicobacter pylori. (2009). Retrieved April 14, 2009, from http://en.wikipedia.org/wiki/Helicobacter_pylori

Hendler, T., Rotshtein, P., Yeshurun, Y., Weizmann, T., Kahn, I., Ben-Bashat, D., et al. (2003). Sensing the invisible: Differential sensitivity of visual cortex and amygdala to traumatic context. *Neuroimage, 19*(3), 587–600.

Henry Gray. (1861/2009). Retrieved April 14, 2009, from http://en.wikipedia.org/wiki/Henry_Gray

Herbert, M. R., Russo, J. P., Yang, S., Roohi, J., Blaxill, A., Kahler, S. G., et al. (2006). Autism and environmental genomics. *Neurotoxicology, 27*(5), 671–684.

Herrnstein, R. J. (1973). *IQ in the meritocracy*. Boston: Atlantic-little Brown.

Herrnstein, R. J., & Murray, C. (1994). *The bell curve: Intelligence and class structure in American life*. New York: Free Press.

Hespos, S. J. (2007). Language acquisition: When does the learning begin? *Current Biology, 17*(16), R628–R630.

Heubert, J. P., & Hauser, R. M. (1999). *High stakes testing for tracking, promotion, and graduation*. Washington, DC: National Research Council, National Academy Press. Retrieved April 14, 2009, from http://books.google.com/books?hl=en&lr=&id=YTNPwncyK18C&oi=fnd&pg=PA13&dq=%22Heubert%22+%22High+Stakes:+Testing+for+Tracking,+Promotion,+and+...%22+&ots=bUp5JnrRD-&sig=IeyONi4Wki6OALLv5wqZnaQvSrc#PPP2,M1

Hindmarsh, J., & Heath, C. (2000) Sharing the tools of the trade: The interactional constitution of workplace objects. *Journal of Contemporary Ethnography, 29*(5), 517–556.

Hippocrates (ca. 400 BC). *Hippocratic Oath*. Retrieved April 14, 2009, from http://www.cpforlife.org/id19.htm.

Hippocratic Oath. (2009). Retrieved April 14, 2009, from http://en.wikipedia.org/wiki/Hippocratic_Oath

Hirayasu, Y., McCarley, R. W., Salisbury, D. F., Tanaka, S., Kwon, J. S., Frumin, M., et al. (2000). Planum temporale and Heschl gyrus volume reduction in schizophrenia: A magnetic resonance imaging study of first-episode patients. *Archives of General Psychiatry, 57*(7), 692–699.

Hitzig, R. (Director), & O'Malley, J. (Writer/Director). (1990). *Backstreet Dreams* [Motion picture]. United States: Vidmark Entertainment.

Hobson v. Hansen, 265 F. Supp. 902 (D. D. C. 1967).

Hogan, J. A., & Bolhuis, J. J. (2005). The development of behavior: Trends since Tinbergen (1963). *Animal Biology, 55*(4), 371–398.

Hoit, J. (2006). Cross talking. *American Journal of Speech-Language Pathology, 15*, 102. Retrieved April 14, 2009, from http://www.asha.org/members/phd-faculty-research/interdis-collab/module1

Holland, J. G., & Skinner, B. F. (1961). *The analysis of behavior: A program for self instruction*. Retrieved April 14, 2009, from http://www.bfskinner.org/eductional.html

Hopkins, W. D., Taglialatela, J. P., & Leavens D. A. (2007). Chimpanzees differentially produce novel vocalizations to capture the attention of a human. *Animal Behavior, 73*(Pt. 2), 281–286.

Hornig, M., Chian, D., & Lipkin, W. I. (2004). Neurotoxic effects of postnatal thimerosal are mouse strain dependent. *Molecular Psychiatry, 9*(9), 833–845.

Hostetter, A. B., & Alibali, M. W. (2004). On the tip of the mind: Gesture as a key to conceptualization. In K. Forbus, D. Gentner, & T. Regier (Eds.), *Proceedings of the 26th annual meeting of the Cognitive Science Society* (pp. 589–594). Mahwah, NJ: Erlbaum.

Hostetter, A. B., & Alibali, M. W. (2008). Visible embodiment: Gestures as simulated action. *Psychonomic Bulletin and Review, 15*(3), 495–514.

Hostetter, A. B., Alibali, M. W., & Kita, S. (2007). I see it in my hands' eye: Representational gestures reflect conceptual demands. *Language and Cognitive Processes, 22*, 313–336.

How the Ear Works. (2009). Video retrieved February 25, 2009, from http://www.youtube.com/watch?v=skXQ6PuIc4s

Howard, R. (Director), Goldsman, A. (Screenplay), & Nasar, S. (2001). *A Beautiful Mind* [Motion picture]. United States: Universal Studios and Dreamworks. Retrieved March 7, 2009, from http://www.abeautifulmind.com/.

Howell, K., Selber, P., Graham, H. K., & Reddihough, D. (2007). Botulinum neurotoxin A: An unusual systemic effect. *Journal of Paediatrics and Child Health, 43*(6), 499–501.

Howell, P., Au-Yeung, J., & Sackin, S. (1999). Exchange of stuttering from function words to content words with age. *Journal of Speech, Language, and Hearing Research, 42*, 345–354.

Howell, P., Barry, W., & Vinson, D. (2006). Strength of British English accents in altered listening conditions. *Perception and Psychophysics, 68*(1), 139–153.

Howes D. H., & Solomon, R. L. (1951). Visual duration threshold as a function of probability. *Journal of Experimental Psychology, 41*, 401–410.

Hsu, H. C., & Fogel, A. (2003) Social regulatory effects of infant nondistress vocalization on maternal behavior. *Developmental Psychology, 39*(6), 976–991.

Hu, V. W., Frank, B. C., Heine, S. Lee, N. H., & Quackenbush, J. (2006, May 18). Gene expression profiling of lymphoblastoid cell lines from monozygotic twins discordant in severity of autism reveals differential regulation of neurologically relevant genes. *BMC Genomics, 7*, Art. No. 118.

Huang, Z. W., Luo, Y. Y., Wu, Z., Y., Tao, Z. Z., Jones, R. O., & Zhao, H. B. (2006). Paradoxical enhancement of active cochlear mechanics in long-term administration of salicylate. *Journal of Neurophysiology, 93*(4), 2053–2061.

Hunt, J. F., & Gaston, B. (2008). Airway acidification and gastroesophageal reflux. *Current Allergy and Asthma Reports, 8*(1), 79–84.

Hyman, L. M., & Katamba, F. X. (1993). A new approach to tone in Luganda. *Language, 69*(1), 34–67.

Ignatow, G. (2007). Theories of embodied knowledge: New directions for cultural and cognitive sociology? *Journal for the Theory of Social Behavior, 37*(2), 115.

Immune System. (2008). Retrieved April 14, 2009, from http://en.wikipedia.org/wiki/Immune_system

Improving America's Schools Act of 1994, Pub. L. 103-382 (20 U.S.C. 8001, October 20, 1994). Retrieved September 25, 2008, from http://www.ed.gov/legislation/ESEA/toc.html.

Inagaki, D., Miyaoka, Y., Ashida, I., Ueda, K., & Yamada, Y. (2007). Influences of body posture on duration of oral swallowing in normal young adults. *Journal of Oral Rehabilitation, 34*(6), 414–421.

Individuals with Disabilities Education Act of 1990. Pub. L. No. 101–476, 104 Stat. 1142. (1990).

Individuals with Disabilities Education Act of 1997. Pub. L. No. 105-17, 111 Stat. 37. (1997).

Individuals with Disabilities Education Improvement Act of 2004. (IDEA). Pub. L. No. 108-446, 118 Stat. 2647. (2004).

Ingham, R. J., & Cordes, A. K. (1992). Interclinic differences in stuttering-event counts. *Journal of Fluency Disorders, 17*(3), 171–176.

Institute of Medicine. (2008). *Projects and Reports*. Retrieved September 25, 2008, from http://www.iom.edu/?id=3740&redirect=0

Institute for Vaccine Safety. (2008). *Thimerosal content in some U. S. licensed vaccines*. Retrieved September 25, 2008, from http://www.vaccinesafety.edu/thi-table.htm

International Academy of Oral Medicine and Toxicology. (2009). *Safe removal of amalgam fillings*. Retrieved April 14, 2009, from http://www.iaomt.org/articles/category_view.asp?intReleaseID=288&catid=30

International Academy of Oral Medicine and Toxicology. (2009). *Smoking teeth*. Retrieved April 14, 2009, from http://www.iaomt.org/index.asp

International Academy of Oral Medicine and Toxicology. (n.d.). *The scientific case against amalgam*. Retrieved April 14, 2009, from http://www.iaomt.org/articles/files/files193/The%20Case%20Against%20Amalgam.pdf

International Civil Aviation Organization. (2004). *Manual on the implementation of ICAO language proficiency requirements*. Document 9835. Retrieved April 14, 2009, from www.icao.int/icao/en/ro/apac/2004/rasmag2/ip03.pdf

International Dyslexia Association. (2007). *Promoting literacy through research, education, and advocacy: Definition of dyslexia*. Retrieved April 14, 2009, from http://www.interdys.org/ewebeditpro5/upload/Definition_of_Dyslexia.pdf

International Phonetic Alphabet. (2009). Retrieved April 14, 2009, from http://en.wikipedia.org/wiki/International_Phonetic_Alphabet

International Phonetics Association. (1999). *Handbook of the International Phonetic Association: A guide to the use of the International Phonetic Alphabet*. Cambridge and New York: Cambridge University Press.

Jabberwocky. (1871/2009). A poem by Lewis Carroll. Retrieved April 14, 2009, from http://en.wikipedia.org/wiki/Jabberwocky

Jacoby, R., & Glauberman, N. (Eds.) (1995). *The bell curve debate: History, documents, opinions*. New York: Random House.

Jaffe, J., Beebe, B., Feldstein, S., Crown, C. L., & Jasnow, M. D. (2001). Rhythms of dialogue in infancy: Coordinated timing in development. *Monographs of the Society for Research in Child Development, 66*(2), 1–132.

James, S. J., Cutler, P., Melnyk, S., Jernigan, S., Janak, L., Gaylor, D. W., et al. (2004). Metabolic biomarkers of increased oxidative stress and impaired methylation capacity in children with autism. *American Journal of Clinical Nutrition, 80*(6), 1611–1617.

James, S. J., Slikker, W., Melnyk, S., New, E., Pogribna, M., & Jernigan, S. (2005). Thimerosal neurotoxicity is associated with glutathione depletion: Protection with glutathione precursors. *Neurotoxicology, 26*(1), 1–8.

Jarrett, C., & Barnes, G. (2005). The use of non-motion-based cues to pre-programme the timing of predictive velocity reversal in human smooth pursuit. *Experimental Brain Research, 164*(4), 423–430.

Jason McElwain autistic basketball player. (2009). *Unlikely hero*. YouTube, LLC. Retrieved April 14, 2009, from http://www.youtube.com/watch?v=1fw1CcxCUgg

Jax, P., & Vary, P. (2006). Bandwidth extension of speech signals: A catalyst for the introduction of wideband speech coding? *IEEE Communications Magazine, 44*(5), 106–111.

Jensen, A. R. (1969). How much can we boost IQ and scholastic achievement? *Harvard Educational Review, 39*, 1–123.

Jensen, A. R. (1980). *Bias in mental testing*. New York: Free Press.

Jepson, B., & Johnson, J. (2007). *Changing the course of autism: A scientific approach for parents and physicians*. Boulder, CO: Sentient Publications.

Jernigan, S., Melnyk, S. B., Janak, L., Cutler, P., & James, S. J. (2004, March 23). Impaired transsulfuration, oxidative stress, and genetic polymorphisms in children with autism. *FASEB Journal, 18*(4 Suppl. S), A105–A105.

Jezer, M. (1997). *Stuttering: A life bound up in words*. Brattleboro, VT: Small Pond Press.

John Wilkes Booth. (1865). Retrieved September 24, 2008, from http://en.wikipedia.org/wiki/John_Wilkes_Booth

Johnson, M. (1992). *The body in the mind: The bodily basis of meaning, imagination, and reason.* Chicago: University of Chicago Press.

Johnson, W., & Associates (1959). *The onset of stuttering.* Minneapolis: University of Minnesota Press.

Jones, J. A., & Munhall, K. G. (2000). Perceptual calibration of F0 production: Evidence from feedback perturbation. *Journal of the Acoustical Society of America, 108*(3, Pt. 1), 1246–1251.

Jim Crow laws. (1876–1965). Separate but equal. Retrieved April 14, 2009, from http://en.wikipedia.org/wiki/Jim_Crow_laws

Julia Ward Howe. (1910/2009). Retrieved April 14, 2009, from http://womenshistory.about.com/library/bio/blbio_howe_julia_ward.htm

Kako, E. (1999). Elements of syntax in the systems of three language-trained animals. *Animal Learning and Behavior, 27*(1), 1–14.

Kalinowski, J. S., & Saltuklaroglu, T. (2006). *Stuttering.* San Diego, CA: Plural.

Kalinowski, J., Saltuklaroglu, T., Stuart, A., & Guntupalli, V. K. (2007). On the importance of scientific rhetoric in stuttering: A reply to Finn, Bothe, and Bramlett (2005). *American Journal of Speech-Language Pathology, 16,* 69–76.

Kanai, R., Tsuchiya, N., & Verstraten, F. A. J. (2006). The scope and limits of top-down attention in unconscious visual processing. *Current Biology, 16*(23), 2332–2336.

Kane, R. (1998). *Slavery in Rhode Island: The economics of the Rhode Island slave trade 1709–1807.* Retrieved September 25, 2008, from http://www.providence.edu/afro/students/kane/slave_trade.htm

Kanner, L. (1943). Autistic disturbances of affective contact. *Nervous Child, 2,* 217–250.

Kanner, L. (1944). Early infantile autism. *Journal of Pediatrics, 25,* 211–217.

Kanner, L. (1946). Irrelevant and metaphorical language in early infantile autism. *American Journal of Psychiatry, 103,* 242–246.

Kanthasamy, A. G., Kitazawa, M., Kanthasamy, A., & Anantharam, V. (2005). Dieldrin-induced neurotoxicity: Relevance to Parkinson's disease pathogenesis. *Neurotoxicology, 26*(4), 701–719.

Kasahara, T., Toyokura, M., Shimoda, N., & Ishida, A. (2005). Cerebral hemorrhage restricted to the corpus callosum. *American Journal of Physical Medicine and Rehabilitation, 84*(5), 386–390.

Kastenholz, B. (2007). New hope for the diagnosis and therapy of Alzheimer's disease. *Protein and Peptide Letters, 14*(4), 389–393.

Katz, J., Stecker, N., & Henderson, D. (1992). *Central auditory processing: A transdisciplinary view.* St. Louis, MO: Mosby Yearbook.

Kaur, P., Aschner, M., & Syversen, T. (2006). Glutathione modulation influences methyl mercury induced neurotoxicity in primary cell cultures of neurons and astrocytes. *Neurotoxicology, 27*(4), 492–500.

Kaye, K. L., & Bower, T. G. R. (1994). Learning and intermodal transfer of information in newborns. *Psychological Science, 5,* 286–288.

Keenan, J. P., Thangaraj, V., Halpern, A. R., & Schlaug, G. (2001). Absolute pitch and planum temporale. *NeuroImage 14,* 1402–1408. Retrieved September 25, 2008, from http://www.musicianbrain.com/papers/Keenan_AP_2001.pdf

Keller, H. (1905). *The story of my life.* New York: Grosset & Dunlap.

Keller, H. (1955). *Teacher, Anne Sullivan Macy: A tribute by the foster-child of her mind.* Garden City, NY: Doubleday.

Keller, W. D. (1992). Auditory processing disorder or attention-deficit disorder? In J. Katz, N. Stecker, & D. Henderson (Eds.), *Central auditory processing: A transdisciplinary view* (pp. 107–114). St. Louis, MO: Mosby Yearbook.

Kelter, S., Kaup, B., & Claus, B. (2004). Representing a described sequence of events: A dynamic view of narrative comprehension. *Journal of Experimental Psychology—Learning Memory and Cognition, 30*(2), 451–464.

Kennedy, R. F., Jr. (2005, June 20). *Deadly immunity.* Retrieved September 25, 2008, from http://www.rollingstone.com/politics/story/7395411/deadly_immunity/

Kennedy, R. F., Jr., & Kirby, D. (2009, February 24). *Vaccine court: Autism debate continues.* HuffingtonPost.com. Retreived February 27, 2009, from http://news.yahoo.com/s/huffpost/20090225/cm_huffpost/169673

Kent, R. (1992). Auditory processing of speech. In J. Katz, N. Stecker, & D. Henderson (Eds.), *Central auditory processing: A transdisciplinary view* (pp. 93–105). St. Louis, MO: Mosby Yearbook.

Kent, R. (1997). *The speech sciences.* San Diego, CA: Singular.

Kern, J. K., Grannemann, B. D., Trivedi, M. H., & Adams J. B. (2007). Sulfhydryl-reactive metals in autism. *Journal of Toxicology and Environmental Health, 70*(8), 715–721.

Kern, J. K., & Jones, A. M. (2006). Evidence of toxicity, oxidative stress, and neuronal insult in autism. *Journal of Toxicology and Environmental Health, 9*(6), 485–499.

Khan, K. M., Drescher, M. J., Hatfield, J. S., Ramakrishnan, N. A., & Drescher, D. G. (2007). Immunohistochemical localization of adrenergic receptors in the rat organ of corti and spiral ganglion. *Journal of Neuroscience Research, 85*(13), 3000–3012.

Kharasch, M. S. (1932). *Stabilized bactericide and process of stabilizing it.* U.S. Patent 1,862,896.

Kharasch, M. S. (1935). *Stabilized organo-meruri-sulphur compounds.* U.S. Patent 2,012,820.

Kidd, P. M. (2005). Neurodegeneration from mitochondrial insufficiency: Nutrients, stem cells, growth factors, and prospects for brain rebuilding using integrative management. *Alternative Medicine Review, 10*(4), 268–293.

Kikkert, M. A., Ribbers, G. M., & Koudstaal, P. J. (2006). Alien hand syndrome in stroke: A report of 2 cases and review of the literature. *Archives of Physical Medicine and Rehabilitation, 87*(5), 728–732.

Kim, H. I., Lee, M. C., Lee, J. S., Kim, H. S., Kim, M. K., Woo, Y. J., et al. (2006). Bilateral perisylvian ulegyria: Clinicopathological study of patients presenting with pseudobulbar palsy and epilepsy. *Neuropathology, 26*(3), 236–242.

Kimbrough, P. (n.d.). *How Braille began.* Retrieved September 25, 2008, from http://www.brailler.com/braillehx.htm

Kimura, M. (1979). Neutral theory of molecular evolution. *Scientific American, 241*(5), 98.

Kimura, M., & Daibo, I. (2006). Interactional synchrony in conversations about emotional episodes: A measurement by "the between-participants pseudo-synchrony experimental paradigm." *Journal of Nonverbal Behavior, 30*(3), 115–126.

Kinesics. (2009). Retrieved April 14, 2009, from http://en.wikipedia.org/wiki/Kinesics

Kingston, M., Huber, A., Onslow, M., Jones, M., & Packman, A. (2003). Predicting treatment time with the Lidcombe Program: Replication and meta-analysis. *International Journal of Language and Communication Disorders/Royal College of Speech and Language Therapists, 38*(2), 165–177.

Kintsch, W. (1978). Toward a model of text comprehension and production. *Psychological Review, 85,* 363–394.

Kinzler, K. D., Dupoux, E., & Spelke, E. S. (2007). The native language of social cognition. *Proceedings of the National Academy of Sciences of the USA, 104*(30), 12577–12580.

Kirby, D. (2005). *Evidence of harm: Mercury in vaccines and the autism epidemic: A medical controversy.* New York: St. Martin's Press.

Kita, T., Wagner, G. C., & Nakashima, T. (2003). Current research on methamphetamine-induced neurotoxicity: Animal models of monoamine disruption. *Journal of Pharmacological Sciences, 92*(3), 178–195.

Klein, F. (2003). *About me.* Retrieved April 14, 2009 from http://home.att.net/~ascaris1/bio.html

Knight, K. (2009). Valentin Haüy. *New Advent, Catholic Encyclopedia.* Retrieved April 14, 2009, from http://www.newadvent.org/cathen/07152b.htm

Koch, M., & Trapp, R. (2006). Ethyl mercury poisoning during a protein A immunoadsorption treatment. *American Journal of Kidney Diseases, 47*(2), Art. No. E31.

Koger, S. M., Schettler, T., & Weiss, B. (2005). Enviromental toxicants and developmental disabilities: A challenge for psychologists. *American Psychologist, 60*(3), 243–255.

Kokayi, K., Altman, C. H., Callely, R. W., & Harrison, A. (2006, September-October). Findings of and treatment for high levels of mercury and lead toxicity in Ground Zero rescue and recovery workers and Lower Manhattan residents. *Explore—Journal of Science and Healing, 2*(5), 400–407.

Konturek, J. W. (2003, December). Discovery by Jaworski of Helicobacter pylori and its pathogenetic role in peptic ulcer, gastritis and gastric cancer. *Journal of Physiological Pharmacology, 54*(Suppl. 3), 23–41.

Koop, C. E. (1984). The slide to Auschwitz. In R. Reagan, *Abortion and the conscience of the nation* (pp. 40–73). Nashville, TN: Thomas Nelson.

Krashen, S. D. (1980). The input hypothesis. In J. E. Alatis (Ed.). *Current issues in bilingual education* (pp. 168–180). Washington, DC: Georgetown University.

Krashen, S. D. (2004). *The power of reading: Insights from the research* (2nd ed.). Portsmouth, NH: Heinemann.

Kratochvil, C. J., Michelson, D., Newcorn, J. H., Weiss, M. D., Busner, J. Moore, R. J., et al. (2007). High-dose atomoxetine treatment of ADHD in youths with limited response to standard doses. *Journal of the American Academy of Child and Adolescent Psychiatry, 46*(9), 1128–1137.

Kubo, T., Sakashita, T., Kusuki, M., Kyunai, K., Ueno. K., Hikawa, C., et al. (1998). Sound lateralization and speech discrimination in patients with sensorineural hearing loss. *Acta Otolaryngol Supplement, 538,* 63–69.

Kuhl, E. A. (2009, February 20). Get early look at *DSM-V* development process. *Psychiatric News, 44*(4), 13. Retrieved February 26, 2009, from http://www.pn.psychiatryonline.org/cgi/content/full/44/4/13

Kuhl, P. K., & Meltzoff, A. N. (1982). The bimodal perception of speech in infancy. *Science, 218*(4577), 1138–1141.

Kuhn, S., & Cruse, H. (2007). Static mental representations in recurrent neural networks for the control of dynamic behavioral sequences. *Connection Science, 17*(3–4), 343–360.

Kuroda, Y. (2007). Foix-Chavany-Marie syndrome: Case reports with literature review. *Journal of Medical Speech-Language Pathology, 15*(2), 137–147.

Kurt, T. L. (1998). Epidemiological association in U. S. veterans between Gulf War illness and exposures to anticholinesterases. *Toxicology Letters, 103*, 523–526.

Ladefoged, P. (2001). *A course in phonetics.* Stamford, CT: Heinle & Heinle.

Lakoff, G., & Johnson, M. (1980). *Metaphors we live by.* Chicago: University of Chicago Press.

Lane, H. L. (1976). *The wild boy of Aveyron.* Cambridge, MA: Harvard University Press.

Langleben, D. D., Schroeder, L., Maldjian, J. A., Gur, R. C., McDonald, S., Ragland, J. D., et al. (2002). Brain activity during simulated deception: An event-related functional magnetic resonance study. *Neuroimage, 15*, 727–732.

LaPointe, L., & Katz, R. C. (2002). Neurogenic disorders of speech in adults. *Human communication disorders: An introduction* (pp. 472–509). Boston: Allyn & Bacon.

Larry King Live. (March 7, 2008). *The autism vaccine debate.* Retrieved September 25, 2008, from http://www.cnn.com/video/#/video/bestoftv/2008/03/07/lkl.autism.vaccine.long.cnn?iref=videosearch.

Larry P. v. Riles, 793 F.2d 969 (9th Cir. 1984). Retrieved September 25, 2008, from http://wind.uwyo.edu/edec5250/assignments/Larry.pdf

Lash, J. P. (1980). *Helen and teacher: The story of Helen Keller and Anne Sullivan Macy.* New York: Delacorte Press.

Lateralization of brain function. (2008). Retrieved September 25, 2008, from http://en.wikipedia.org/wiki/Lateralization_of_brain_function

Lattermann, C., Shenker, R. C., & Thordardottir, E. (2005). Progression of language complexity during treatment with the Lidcombe Program for early stuttering intervention. *American Journal of Speech-Language Pathology, 14*(3), 242–253.

Lau v. Nichols, 414 U.S. 563. (1974). Retrieved September 25, 2008, from http://caselaw.lp.findlaw.com/scripts/getcase.pl?court=US&vol=414&invol=563

Laura Bridgman. (1889/2009). Retrieved April 14, 2009, from http://en.wikipedia.org/wiki/Laura_Bridgman

Law of Hippocrates. (ca. 350 BC/1993). Retrieved September 25, 2008, from http://www.cpforlife.org/id19.htm.

LD Online. (2009). *Dyslexia.* Retrieved September 25, 2008, from http://www.ldonline.org/glossary

Le Couteur, A., Bailey, A., Goode, S., Pickles, A., Robertson, S., Gottesman, I., et al. (1996). A broader phenotype of autism: The clinical spectrum in twins. *Journal of Child Psychology and Psychiatry and Allied Disciplines, 37*, 785–801.

Lederberg, J., & McCray, A.T. (2001). 'Ome sweet 'omics—a genealogical treasury of words. *Scientist, 15*, 8.

Lee, B. S. (1950a). Artificial stutter. *Journal of Speech and Hearing Disorders, 16*, 53–55.

Lee, B. S. (1950b). Effects of delayed speech feedback. *Journal of the Acoustical Society of America, 22*, 824–826.

Lee, B. S. (1950c). Some effects of side-tone delay. *Journal of the Acoustical Society of America, 22*, 639–640.

Lee, D. J., de Venecia, R. K., Guinan, J. J., & Brown, M. C. (2006). Central auditory pathways mediating the rat middle ear muscle reflexes. *Anatomical Record Part A-Discoveries in Molecular Cellular and Evolutionary Biology, 288a*(4), 358–369.

Leimbach, M. (2006). *Daniel isn't talking.* New York: Random House.

Lejeune, J. (1960). Le mongolisme: Trisomie degressive (Mongolism: Regressive trisomy). *Annales de Genetique, 2*, 1–34.

Lejeune, J., Gauthier, M., & Turpin, R. (1959). Les chromosomes humains en culture des tissus. (Human chromosomes in the culture of the tissues.) *Comptes rendus de l'Académie des sciences, 248*, 602–603.

Leong, C. C., Syed, N. I., & Lorscheider, F. L. (2001). Retrograde degeneration of neurite membrane structural integrity of nerve growth cones following in vitro exposure to mercury. *Neuroreport, 12*(4), 733–737.

Leprosy. (2009). Retrieved April 14, 2009, from http://en.wikipedia.org/wiki/Leprosy#_note-Heller_2003

Leprosy Mission Canada. (2009). *About leprosy.* Retrieved April 14, 2009, from http://www.leprosy.ca/site/

Leshin, L. (2003). *Trisomy 21: The story of Down syndrome.* Retrieved April 14, 2009, from http://www.ds-health.com/trisomy.htm

Levelt, W. J. M. (1983). Monitoring and self-repair in speech. *Cognition, 14*(1), 41–104.

Lewis, C., Packman, A., Onslow, M., Simpson, J. M., & Jones, M. (2008). A phase II trial of telehealth delivery of the Lidicombe Program of early, stuttering intervention. *American Journal of Speech-Language Pathology, 1*(2), 139–149.

Lewkowicz, D. J., & Marcovitch, S. (2006). Perception of audiovisual rhythm and its invariance in 4- to 10-month-old infants. *Developmental Psychobiology, 48*(7), 631–632.

Li, L., & Shao, F. (2003). Impaired auditory sensorimotor gating: An animal model of schizophrenia. *Chinese Science Bulletin, 48*(19), 2031–2037.

Lichtman, J. (2003, November 15). *Why a sparse synapse-resolution brain connectivity (SSRBC) atlas is needed?* Retrieved September 25, 2008, from http://www.extremeneuroanatomy.com/synapse_resolution.htm

Lichtheim, L. (1885, January). On aphasia. *Brain, 7*, 433–484. (Originally published in 1885 in German as *Ueber Aphasie. Aus der medicinischen Klinik in*

Bern. *Deutsches Archiv für klinische Medicin, Leipzig, 36,* 204–268).

Life Goes On. (2009). Retrieved April 14, 2009, from http://en.wikipedia.org/wiki/Life_Goes_On_(TV_series)

Lightman, A. (1993). *Einstein's dreams.* New York: Pantheon.

Lima, C. F., Fernandes-Ferreira, M., & Pereira-Wilson, C. (2006). Phenolic compounds protect HepG2 cells from oxidative damage: Relevance of glutathione levels. *Life Sciences, 79*(21), 2056–2068.

Lincoln, A. (June 16, 1858). *The "House Divided Speech" of 1858 in Springfield, Illinois.* Retrieved September 25, 2008, from http://www.nationalcenter.org/HouseDivided.html

Lincoln, A. (1861a). *Abraham Lincoln's State of the Union Address to Congress in 1861.* Retrieved September 25, 2008, from http://www.infoplease.com/t/hist/state-of-the-union/73.html

Lincoln, A. (1861b). *Abraham Lincoln's Inaugural Address.* Retrieved September 25, 2008, from http://everything2.com/index.pl?node_id=468294

Lincoln, A. (1862). *Letter to Horace Greeley.* Retrieved September 25, 2008, from http://showcase.netins.net/web/creative/lincoln/speeches/greeley.htm

Lincoln/Douglas Debates. (1858). Retrieved September 25, 2008, from http://www.nps.gov/archive/liho/debate1.htm

Linder, D. (2002). *The trial of the Lincoln assassination conspirators.* Retrieved September 25, 2008, from http://www.law.umkc.edu/faculty/projects/ftrials/lincolnconspiracy/lincolnaccount.html

Lindsay, R. L., Tomazic, T., Whitman, B. Y., & Accardo, P. J. (1999). Early ear problems and developmental problems at school age. *Clinical Pediatrics, 38*(3), 123–132.

Liu, L. L, & Franz, K. J. (2007). Phosphorylation-dependent metal binding by alpha-synuclein peptide fragments. *Journal of Biological Inorganic Chemistry, 12*(2), 234–247.

Locke, J. L. (2001). First communion: The emergence of vocal relationships. *Social Development, 10,* 294–308.

Loddenkemper, T., Holland, K. D., Stanford, L. D., Kotagal, P., Bingaman, W., & Wyllie, E. (2007). Developmental outcome after epilepsy surgery in infancy. *Pediatrics, 119*(5), 930–935.

Loftus, S. K., Dixon, J., Koprivnikar, K., Dixon, M. J., & Wasmuth J. J. (1992). Transcriptional map of the Treacher Collins: Candidate gene region. *Genome Research, 6,* 26–34.

Logan, K. J., & Conture, E. G. (1995). Length, grammatical complexity, and rate differences in stuttered and fluent conversational utterances of children who stutter. *Journal of Fluency Disorders, 20,* 35–61.

Lomen Abdo. (2006). *Lommen Abdo provides vaccine injury information.* Retrieved September 25, 2008, from http://www.lommen.com/news_detail.asp?RecordNumber=149

Lorenz, B., Lorenz, M., & Pulte, M. (1998). *Presidential deaths and misfortunes.* Retrieved September 25, 2008, from http://www.heptune.com/preslist.html#deaths

Lorenzo's Oil. (1992). 1992 drama film directed by George Miller. Retrieved September 25, 2008, from http://en.wikipedia.org/wiki/Lorenzo's_oil.

Loucks, T. M. J., Poletto, C. J., Simonyan, K., Reynolds, C. L., & Ludlow, C. L. (2007). Human brain activation during phonation and exhalation: Common volitional control for two upper airway functions. *Neuroimage, 36*(1), 131–143.

Louisiana HB 958. (July 16, 2008).

Louko, L. J., Conture, E. G., & Edwards, M. L. (1999). Treating children who exhibit cooccurring stuttering and disordered phonology. In R. Curlee (Ed.), *Stuttering and related disorders of fluency* (2nd ed., pp. 124–138). New York: Thieme Medical.

Lovely T. J., Levin, D. E., & Klekowski, E. (1982). Light-induced genetic toxicity of thimerosal and benzalkonium chloride in commercial contact-lens solutions. *Mutation Research, 101*(1), 11–18.

Ludlow, C. L., Hoit, J., Kent, R., Ramig, L. O., Shrivastav, R., Strand, E., et al. (2008). Translating principles of neural plasticity into research on speech motor control recovery and rehabilitation. *Journal of Speech Language and Hearing Research, 51*(1), S240–S258.

Luria, A. R. (1947). *Traumatic aphasia.* Moscow: Academy of Medical Sciences.

Luria, A. R. (1959). The directive function of speech in development and dissolution. *Word, 16,* 341–352.

Luria, A. R. (1966). *Higher cortical functions in man* (Basil Haigh, Trans.). New York: Basic Books.

Luria, A. R., & Yudovich, I. F. (1959). *Speech and the development of mental processes in the child: An experimental investigation.* London: Staples Press.

Lyon, G. R. (1997). *Difficulties with alphabetics.* Retrieved September 25, 2008, from http://www.readingrockets.org/article/221

Lyon, G. R., Shaywitz, S. E, & Shaywitz, B. A. (2003). A definition of dyslexia. *Annals of Dyslexia, 53,* 1–14.

Maaso, A. (2002). *The "McGurk effect."* Retrieved September 25, 2008, from http://www.media.uio.no/personer/arntm/McGurk_english.html

MacFabe, D. F., Cain, D. P., Rodriguez-Capote, K., Franklin, A. E., Hoffman, J. E., et al. (2007). Neurobiological effects of intraventricular propionic acid in rats: Possible role of short chain fatty acids on the pathogenesis and characteristics of autism spectrum disorders. *Behavioral Brain Research, 176*(1), 149–169.

Macknik, S. L. (2007). Visual masking approaches to visual awareness. *Spanish Journal of Psychology, 10*(2), 478–479.

Macnamara, J. (1972). Cognitive basis of language learning in infants. *Psychological Review, 79*(1), 1–13.

Magalhaes, M. H. C. G., da Silveira, C. B., Moreira, C. R., & Cavalcanti, M. G. P. (2007). Clinical and imaging correlations of Treacher Collins syndrome: Report of two cases. *Oral Surgery Oral Medicine Oral Pathology Oral Radiology and Endodontology, 103*(6), 836–842.

Magliano, J. P., Miller, J., & Zwaan R. A. (2001). Indexing space and time in film understanding. *Applied Cognitive Psychology, 15*(5), 533–545.

Magnetic Resonance Imaging. (2009). Retrieved April 14, 2009, from http://en.wikipedia.org/wiki/Magnetic _resonance_imaging

Maier, M. A., Bernier, A., Pekrun, R., Zimmermann, P., Strasser, K., & Grossmann, K. E. (2005). Attachment state of mind and perceptual processing of emotional stimuli. *Attachment and Human Development, 7*(1), 67–81.

Majerus, S., Amand, P., Boniver, V., Demanez, J. P., Demanez, L., & Van der Linden, M. (2005). A quantitative and qualitative assessment of verbal short-term memory and phonological processing in 8-year-olds with a history of repetitive otitis media. *Journal of Communication Disorders, 38*(6), 473–498.

Mandler, J. M., & Goodman, M. S. (1982). On the psychological validity of story structure. *Journal of Verbal Learning and Verbal Behavior, 21*(5), 507–523.

Manna, G., Hankeya, G. J., & Cameron, D. (2000). Swallowing disorders following acute stroke: prevalence and diagnostic accuracy. *Cerebrovascular Diseases, 10*, 380–386.

Manning, W. (1996). *From the 1996 Panel discussion on "recovery" ASHA Convention, Seattle, Washington.* Retrieved September 25, 2008, from http://www .mnsu.edu/comdis/voices/voices.html

Manning, W. H. (2001). *Clinical decision making in fluency disorders* (2nd ed.). San Diego, CA: Singular.

Manually Coded English. (2009). Retrieved April 14, 2009, from http://en.wikipedia.org/wiki/Manually_Coded _English

Manually Signed English. (2009). Retrieved April 14, 2009, from http://en.wikipedia.org/wiki/Signing_E xact_English

Marc Dax. (1836/2008). Retrieved September 24, 2008, from http://en.wikipedia.org/wiki/Marc_Dax

Marion, D. W. (1999). *Traumatic brain injury.* New York: Thieme Medical.

Markin, V. S., & Hudspeth, A. J. (1995). Modeling the active process of the cochlea: Phase relations, amplification, and spontaneous oscillation. *Biophysical Journal, 69*, 138–147.

Marn-Pernat, A., Buturovic-Ponikvar, J., Logar, M., Horvat, M., & Ponikvar, R. (2005). Increased ethyl mercury load in protein A immuno adsorption. *Therapeutic Apheresis and Dialysis, 9*(3), 254–257.

Marschark, M., Siple, P., Lillo-Martin, D., & Everhart, V. (1997). *Relations of language and thought.* New York: Oxford University Press.

Martin, R., Barr, A., MacIntosh, B., Smith, R., Stevens, T., Taves, D., et al. (2007). Cerebral cortical processing of swallowing in older adults. *Experimental Brain Research, 176*(1), 12–22.

Martineau, M., Baux, G., & Mothet, J. P. (2006). Gliotransmission at central glutamatergic synapses: D-serine on stage. *Journal of Physiology—Paris, 99*(2–3), 103–110.

Martinez-Conde, S., & Macknik, S. L. (2007, August). Windows on the mind. *Scientific American, 297*(2), 56–63.

Masataka, N. (1992). Early ontogeny of vocal behavior of Japanese infants in response to maternal speech. *Child Development, 63*, 1177–1185.

Masataka, N. (1995). The relation between index-finger extension and the acoustic quality of cooing in 3-month-old infants. *Journal of Child Language, 22*, 247–257.

Masataka, N. (2003). *The onset of language.* Cambridge: Cambridge University Press, Kyoto University.

Masataka, N., & Bloom, K. (1994). Acoustic properties that determine adults preferences for 3-month-old infant vocalizations. *Infant Behavior and Development, 17*(4), 461–464.

Mastropieri, D., & Turkewitz, G. (1999). Prenatal experience and neonatal responsiveness to vocal expressions of emotion. *Developmental Psychobiology, 35*(3), 204–214.

Mather, J. (n.d.). *Churchill's speech impediment was stuttering.* Retrieved April 14, 2009, from http://www .winstonchurchill.org/i4a/pages/index.cfm?page id=100

Mayer A. R., Xu, J., Pare-Blagoev, J., & Posse, S. (2006). Reproducibility of activation in Broca's area during covert generation of single words at high field: A single trial fMRI study at 4 T. *Neuroimage, 32*(1), 129–137.

McCaffrey, P. (2001). *Transcortical sensory aphasia.* Retrieved April 14, 2009, from http://www.csuchico .edu/~pmccaffrey//syllabi/SPPA336/336unit8.html

McCarthy, J. (2007). *Louder than words: A mother's journey in healing autism.* New York: Dutton.

McCarthy, J. (2008). *McCarthy's complete interview take the crap out.* Retrieved April 14, 2009, from http://www.youtube.com/watch?v=zLJ9ez3pJIg&feature=related

McGovern, C. (2006). *Eye contact.* New York: Penguin.

McGuigan, M. (2007). Hypothesis: Do homeopathic medicines exert their action in humans and animals via the vomeronasal system? *Homeopathy, 96*(2), 113–119.

McGurk, H. (1988). *Developmental psychology and the vision of speech: McGurk's Inaugural Lecture in 1988.* Retrieved April 14, 2009, from http://www.isca-speech.org/archive/archive_papers/avsp98/av98_003.pdf

McGurk, H., & MacDonald, J. (1976). Hearing lips and seeing voices. *Nature, 264,* 746–748.

McGurk Interactions. (1998, December 4–6). Conference *on Auditory-Visual Speech Processing, Terrigal - Sydney, Australia.* Retrieved April 14, 2009, from http://www.isca-speech.org/archive/avsp98/av98_003.html

McGurk Sentence Interactions. (1998). Retrieved April 14, 2009, from http://www.isca-speech.org/archive/avsp98/av98_003.html; download and play the MPEG file labeled av98_003_2.mpg (5494 KB) for the sentence interactions.

McGurk Syllable Interactions. (1998). Retrieved April 14, 2009, from http://www.isca-speech.org/archive/avsp98/av98_003.html; download and play the MPEG file labeled av98_003_1.mpg (7417 KB) for the syllable interactions.

McKeown, S. J., & Bronner-Fraser, M. (2008). Saving face: Rescuing a craniofacial birth defect. *Nature Medicine, 14*(2), 115–116.

Meek, L. R., Myren, K., Sturm, J., & Burau, D. (2007). Acute paternal alcohol use affects offspring development and adult behavior. *Physiology and Behavior, 91*(1), 154–160.

Mehler, B. (1988). *A history of the American Eugenics Society.* Unpublished doctoral dissertation, University of Illinois, Urbana-Champaign. Retrieved September 25, 2008, from http://www.ferris.edu/HTMLS/staff/webpages/site.cfm?LinkID=248&eventID=34

Melnick, K. S., Conture, E. G., & Ohde, R. N. (2003). Phonological priming in picture naming of young children who stutter. *Journal of Speech, Language, and Hearing Research, 46,* 1428–1443.

Meltzer, A. (1992). Horn stuttering. *Journal of Fluency Disorders, 17,* 257–264.

Meltzoff, A. N., & Borton, R. W. (1979). Inter-modal matching by human neonates. *Nature, 282*(5737), 403–404.

Meltzoff, A. N., & Moore, M. K. (1997). Explaining facial imitation: A theoretical model. *Early Development and Parenting, 6,* 179–192.

Mercer, J. R. (1973). *Labelling the retarded.* Berkeley: University of California Press.

Mercer, J. R. (1984). What is a racially and culturally nondiscriminatory test? In C. R. Reynolds & R. T. Brown (Eds.), *Perspectives on bias in mental testing* (pp. 293–356). New York: Plenum Press.

Michael Phelps. (2009). Retrieved April 14, 2009, from http://en.wikipedia.org/wiki/Michael_Phelps

Miles, E. (1995). Can there be a single definition of dyslexia? *Dyslexia, 1*(1), 37–45.

Miller, A. J. (2002). Pharyngeal reflexes in the mammalian nervous system: Their diverse range in complexity and the pivotal role of the tongue. *Critical Reviews in Oral Biology and Medicine, 13*(5), 409–425.

Miller, G. A. (1964). The psycholinguists: On the new scientists of language. *Encounter, 23,* 29–37.

Miller, G. M. (Director/Writer), & Enright, N. (Writer). (1992). *Lorenzo's oil* [Motion picture]. United States: Universal Pictures; article also retrieved January 26, 2009, from http://en.wikipedia.org/wiki/Lorenzo's_Oil

Miller, R. G., Anderson, F., Brooks, B. R., Mitsumoto, H., Bradley, W. G., & Ringel, S. P. (2009). Outcomes research in amyotrophic lateral sclerosis: Lessons learned from the amyotrophic aateral sclerosis clinical assessment, research, and education database. *Annals of Neurology, 6*(1), S24–S28.

Mills v. Board of Education of the District of Columbia, 348 F.Supp. 866. (DC 1972). Retrieved April 14, 2009, from http://www.faculty.piercelaw.edu/redfield/library/Pdf/case-mills.boe.pdf

Minamata disease. (2009). Retrieved April 14, 2009, from http://en.wikipedia.org/wiki/Minamata_disease

Ming, X., Stein, T. P., Brimacombe, M., Johnson, W. G., Lambert, G. H., & Wagner, G. C. (2005). Increased excretion of a lipid peroxidation Biomarkers in autism. *Prostaglandins Leukotrienes and Essential Fatty Acids, 73*(5), 379–384.

Miracle continues. (1984). Retrieved September 25, 2008, from http://movies2.nytimes.com/gst/movies/movie.html?v_id=126149

Miracle worker. (2009). Retrieved April 14, 2009, from http://en.wikipedia.org/wiki/The_Miracle_Worker

Mitchell, R. E. (2004). National profile of deaf and hard of hearing students in special education from weighted survey results. *American Annals of the Deaf, 149*(4), 336–349.

Mitchell, R. E. (2006). How many deaf people are there in the United States? Estimates from the survey of income and program participation. *Journal of Deaf Studies and Deaf Education, 11*(1), 112–119.

Mohammed Ali. (2009). Retrieved April 14, 2009, from http://en.wikipedia.org/wiki/Muhammad_Ali

Mohler, H. (2007). Molecular regulation of cognitive functions and developmental plasticity: Impact of GABA(A) receptors. *Journal of Neurochemistry, 102*(1), 1–12.

Monikowski, C. (1994). Required backgrounds, proficiencies and aptitudes for students entering an interpreter education program. In E. A. Winston (Ed.), *Conference of Interpreter Trainers Tenth National Convention, Mapping our course: A collaborative venture* (pp. 31–34). Washington, DC: Conference of Interpreter Trainers.

Moon, C., Cooper, R. P., & Fifer, W. P. (1993). 2-day-olds prefer their native language. *Infant Behavior and Development, 16*(4), 495–500.

Moore, C. A., & Ruark, J. L. (1996). Does speech emerge from earlier appearing oral motor behaviors? *Journal of Speech and Hearing Research, 39*(5), 1034–1047.

Moore, T. E. (1982). Subliminal advertising: What you see is what you get. *Journal of Marketing, 46*(2), 38–47.

Morata, T. C., Dunn, D. E., Kretschmer, L. W., Lemasters, G. K., & Keith, R. W. (1993). Effects of occupational exposure to organic-solvents and noise on hearing. *Scandinavian Journal of Work Environment and Health, 19*(4), 245–254.

More on UK abortion law. (2007, February). Retrieved April 14, 2009, from http://www.efc.org.uk/Foryou ngpeople/Factsaboutabortion/MoreonUKabortion law#1

Morford, J. P. (2006). How language originates: Linguistic acquisition with children with impaired and normal hearing. *Language, 82*(1), 179–182.

Morford, J. P., & Kegl, J. (2000). Gestural precursors to linguistic constructs: How input shapes the form of language. In D. McNeill (Ed.), *Language and gesture,* (pp. 358–387). Cambridge: Cambridge University Press.

Morford, J. P., Singleton, J. L., & Goldin-Meadow, S. (1995). The genesis of language: How much time is needed to generate arbitrary symbols in a sign system? In K. Emmorey, & J. S. Reilly (Eds.), *Language, gesture, and space* (pp. 313–332). Hillsdale, NJ: Lawrence Erlbaum.

Morgan, G., & Kegl, J. (2006). Nicaraguan sign language and theory of mind: The issue of critical periods and abilities. *Journal of Child Psychology and Psychiatry, 47*(8), 811–819.

Morris, C. W. (1958). Words without meaning: Review of B. F. Skinner's *Verbal Behavior. Contemporary Psychology, 3*, 212–214.

Moschitta, J. (2009). *World's fastest talker—John Moschitta.* Retrieved March 6, 2009, from http://www.v ideosift.com/video/Worlds-Fastest-Talker-John-M oschitta

Moses, L. J., Baldwin, D. A., Rosicky, J. G., & Tidball, G. (2001). Evidence for referential understanding in the emotions domain at twelve and eighteen months. *Child Development, 72*(3), 718–735.

Moskowitz, B. A. (1978, November). Acquisition of language. *Scientific American, 239*(5), 92–108.

Mostaghimi, A., Levison, J. H., Leffert, R., Ham, W., Nathoo, A., Halamka, J., et al. (2006). The doctor's new black bag: Instructional technology and the tools of the 21st century physician. *Medical Education Online, 11*. Retrieved September 25, 2008, from http://www.med-ed-online.org

Muhle, R., Trentacoste, S. V., & Rapin, I. (2004). The genetics of autism. *Pediatrics, 113*(5), E472–E486.

Muir, H. (April 30, 2003). *Einstein and Newton showed signs of autism.* Retrieved September 25, 2008, from http://www.newscientist.com/article.ns?id=dn3676

Muran, P. J. (2006). Mercury elimination with oral DMPS, DMSA, vitamin C, and glutathione: An observational clinical review. *Alternative Therapies in Health and Medicine, 12*(3), 70–75.

Musée Valentin Haüy. (2009). Retrieved April 14, 2009, from http://www.avh.asso.fr/rubriques/association /musee_avh.php

Musiek, F. E., & Lamb, L. (1992). Neuroanatomy and neurophysiology of central auditory processing. In J. Katz, N. Stecker, & D. Henderson (Eds.), *Central auditory processing: A transdisciplinary view* (pp. 11–38). St. Louis, MO: Mosby Yearbook.

Mutter, J., Naumann, J., Schneider, R., & Walach, H. (2007). Mercury and Alzheimer's disease. *Fortschritte Der Neurologie Psychiatrie, 75*(9), 528–540.

Mutter, J., Naumann, J., Schneider, R., Walach, H., & Haley, B. (2005). Mercury and autism: Accelerating evidence? *Neuroendocrinology Letters, 26*(5), 439–446.

Mutter, J., Naumann, J., Walach, H., & Daschner, F. (2005). Amalgam risk assessment with coverage of references up to 2005. *Gesundheitswesen, 67*(3), 204–216.

"The Myelin Project." (2009). Retrieved March 7, 2009, from http://www.myelin.org/en/cms/?14

Nagao, K., & de Jong, K. (2007). Perceptual rate normalization in naturally produced rate-varied speech. *Journal of the Acoustical Society of America, 121*(5), 2882–2898.

Nanotechnology. (2009). Retrieved April 14, 2009, from http://en.wikipedia.org/wiki/Nanotechnology

Naremore, R. C. (1985). Explorations of language use: Pragmatic mapping in L1 and L2. *Topics in Language Disorders, 5*(4), 66–79.

Nash, J. F. (2002). *Interview with John Nash: Misconceptions about mental illness.* Retrieved April 14, 2009, from http://www.pbs.org/wgbh/amex/nash/sfeature/sf_nash_07.html

Nash, J. F. (2009). Portrayal in *A Beautiful Mind* (film). Retrieved April 14, 2009, from http://en.wikipedia.org/wiki/A_Beautiful_Mind_(film)

Nash, R. A. (2009). Metals in medicine. *Alternative Therapies in Health and Medicine, 11*(4), 18–25.

National Center for Public Policy Research. (n.d.). *Brown v. Board of Education, 347 U.S. 483. (1954) (USSC+).* Retrieved April 14, 2009, from http://www.nationalcenter.org/brown.html

National Childhood Vaccine Injury Act (NCVIA) of 1986, Pub. L. 99-660 (42 U.S.C. §§ 300aa-1 to 300aa-34). Retrieved April 14, 2009, from http://en.wikipedia.org/wiki/National_Childhood_Vaccine_Injury_Act

National Federation for the Blind. (2009). Retrieved April 14, 2009, from http://www.nfb.org/

National Institute of Child Health and Human Development. (2006, August 18). *Facts about Down syndrome.* Retrieved September 25, 2008, from http://www.nichd.nih.gov/publications/pubs/downsyndrome.cfm#TheOccurrence

National Institute of Neurological Disorders and Stroke. (2007a). *What is agraphia?* Retrieved April 14, 2009, from http://www.ninds.nih.gov/disorders/dysgraphia/dysgraphia.htm

National Institute of Neurological Disorders and Stroke. (2007b). *What is dyslexia?* Retrieved April 14, 2009, from http://www.ninds.nih.gov/disorders/dyslexia/dyslexia.htm

National Institute of Neurological Disorders and Stroke. (2009). *Hydrocephalus fact sheet.* Retrieved April 14, 2009, from http://www.ninds.nih.gov/disorders/hydrocephalus/detail_hydrocephalus.htm

National Institute on Deafness and Other Communication Disorders. (1997). *Aphasia.* Retrieved April 14, 2009, from http://www.nidcd.nih.gov/health/voice/aphasia.htm

National Vaccine Injury Compensation Program. (n.d.). *Persons eligible to file a claim.* Retrieved April 14, 2009, from http://www.hrsa.gov/vaccinecompensation/persons_eligible.htm

Nazzi, T., Bertoncini, J., & Mehler, J. (1998). Language discrimination by newborns: Toward an understanding of the role of rhythm. *Journal of Experimental Psychology: Human Perception and Performance, 24*(3), 756–766.

Nazzi, T., & Ramus, F. (2003). Perception and acquisition of linguistic rhythm by infants. *Speech Communication, 41*(1), 233–243.

Ness, P. (Director), & Bass, R. (Writer). (2005). *Mozart and the Whale* [Motion Picture]. United States: Big City Pictures.

Neurons. (2009). Retrieved April 14, 2009, from http://en.wikipedia.org/wiki/Neurons

New York City's Riverside Church. (2008). *West por-tal (image).* Retrieved April 14, 2009, from http://www.einstein-website.de/images/WestPortal.jpg

Newland, M. C., & Rasmussen, E. B. (2003). Behavior in adulthood and during aging is affected by contaminant exposure in utero. *Current Directions in Psychological Science, 12*(6), 212–217.

Newschaffer, C. J. (2006). Diagnostic substitution and autism prevalence trends. *Pediatrics, 117*(4), 1436–1437.

Nicholls, M. E. R., & Searle, D. A. (2006). Asymmetries for the visual expression and perception of speech. *Brain and Language, 97*(3), 322–331.

Nickisch, A., Gross, M., Schonweiler, R., Uttenweiler, V., Zehnhoff-Dinnesen, A. A., Berger, R., et al. (2007). Auditory processing disorders. Consensus statement by the German Society for Phoniatrics and Pedaudiology. *HNO, 55*(1), 61–72.

Nieuwland, M. S., Otten, M., & Van Berkum, J. J. A. (2007). Who are you talking about? Tracking discourse-level referential processing with event-related brain potentials. *Journal of Cognitive Neuroscience, 19*(2), 228–236.

Nieuwland, M. S., & Van Berkum, J. J. A. (2006). Individual differences and contextual bias in pronoun resolution: Evidence from ERPs. *Brain Research, 1118,* 155–167.

Nishida, H., Kushida, M., Nakajima, Y., Ogawa, Y., Tatewaki, N., Sato, S., et al. (2007). Amyloid-beta-induced cytotoxicity of PC-12 cell was attenuated by Shengmai-san through redox regulation and outgrowth induction. *Journal of Pharmacological Sciences, 104*(1), 73–81.

Nishikawa, T., Okuda, J., Mizuta, I., Ohno, K., Jamshidi, J., Tokunaga, H., et al. (2001). Conflict of intentions due to callosal disconnection. *Journal of Neurology Neurosurgery and Psychiatry, 71*(4), 462–471.

No Child Left Behind Act of 2001. Pub. L. 107–110, 115 STAT. 1425. (January 8, 2002). Retrieved September 25, 2008, from http://www.ed.gov/policy/elsec/leg/esea02/107-110.pdf

Norris, D. (2006). The Bayesian reader: Explaining word recognition as an optimal Bayesian decision process. *Psychological Review, 113*(2), 327–357.

Norton, R. J. (1996). *Abraham Lincoln's assassination.* Retrieved September 25, 2008, from http://home.att.net/~rjnorton/Lincoln75.html

Nottet, J. B., Malawian, A., Brossard, N., Suc, B., & Job, A. (2006). Otoacoustic emissions and persistent tinnitus after acute acoustic trauma. *Laryngoscope, 116*(6), 970–975.

Obhi, S. S., Matkovich, S., & Gilbert, S. J. (2009). Modification of planned actions. *Experimental Brain Research, 1*(2), 265–274.

Odone, A. (2009). "*Lorenzo's Oil.*" Retrieved March 7, 2009, from http://en.wikipedia.org/wiki/Lorenzo's_oil

Office of Special Masters. (August 29, 2008). *Docket of Omnibus Autism Proceeding.* Retrieved April 14, 2009, from http://www.uscfc.uscourts.gov/docket-omnibus-autism-proceeding.

Offit, P. A. (2007). Thimerosal and vaccines—A cautionary tale. *New England Journal of Medicine, 357*(13), 1278–1279.

Offit, P. A., Quarles, J., Gerber, M. A., Hackett, C. J., Marcuse, E. K., Kollman, T. R., et al. (2002). Addressing parents' concerns: Do multiple vaccines overwhelm or weaken the infant's immune system? *Pediatrics, 109*(1), 124-129.

Olivieri, G., Novakovic, M., Savaskan, E., Meier, F., Baysang, G., Brockhaus, M., et al. (2002). The effects of beta-estradiol on SHSY5Y neuroblastoma cells during heavy metal induced oxidative stress, neurotoxicity and beta-amyloid secretion. *Neuroscience, 113*(4), 849–855.

Oller, D. K. (1975). Simplification as the goal of phonological processes in child speech. *Language Learning, 24,* 299–303.

Oller, D. K. (1980). The emergence of the sounds of speech in infancy. In G. Yeni-Komshian, J., Kavanaugh, & C. Ferguson (Eds.), *Child phonology* (pp. 93–112). New York: Academic Press.

Oller, D. K. (2000). *The emergence of the speech capacity.* Mahwah, NJ: Lawrence Erlbaum Associates.

Oller, D. K., Eilers, R. E., & Basinger, D. (2001). Intuitive identification of infant vocal sounds by parents. *Developmental Science, 4*(1), 49–60.

Oller, D. K., & Steffens, M. L. (1994). Syllables and segments in infant vocalizations and young child speech. In M. S. Yavas (Ed.), *First and second language phonology* (pp. 45–61). San Diego, CA: Singular.

Oller, J. W., Jr. (1970). Transformational theory and pragmatics. *Modern Language Journal, 54,* 504–507.

Oller, J. W., Jr. (1975). Pragmatic mappings. *Lingua, 35,* 333–344.

Oller, J. W., Jr. (1993). Reasons why some methods work. In J. W. Oller, Jr. (Ed.), *Methods that work: Ideas for literacy and language teachers* (pp. 374–385). Boston: Heinle & Heinle.

Oller, J. W., Jr. (1994). Cloze, discourse, and approximations to English. In J. W. Oller, Jr. & J. Jonz (Eds.), *Cloze and coherence* (pp. 119–134). Cranbury, NJ: Bucknell University Press.

Oller, J. W., Jr. (1997). Monoglottosis: What's wrong with the idea of the meritocracy and its racy cousins? *Applied Linguistics, 18*(4), 467–507.

Oller, J. W., Jr. (2002). Languages and genes: Can they be built up through random change and natural selection? *Journal of Psychology and Theology, 30*(1), 26–40.

Oller, J. W., Jr. (2005). Common ground between form and content: The pragmatic solution to the bootstrapping problem. *Modern Language Journal, 89,* 92–114.

Oller, J. W., Jr., & Chen, L. (2007). Episodic organization in discourse and valid measurement in the sciences. *Journal of Quantitative Linguistics, 14,* 127–144.

Oller, J. W., Jr., Chen, L., Oller, S. D., & Pan, N. (2005). Empirical predictions from a general theory of signs. *Discourse Processes, 40*(2), 115–144.

Oller, J. W., Jr., & Damico, J. S. (1980). Pragmatic versus morphological/syntactic criteria for language referrals. *Language Speech and Hearing Services in Schools, 11,* 85–94.

Oller, J. W., Jr., & Giardetti, J. R. (1999). *Images that work.* Westport, CT: Quorum Books.

Oller, J. W., Jr., Kim, K., & Choe, Y. (2001). Can instructions to nonverbal IQ tests be given in pantomime? Additional applications of a general theory of signs. *Semiotica, 133*(1/4), 15–44.

Oller, J. W., Jr., Kim, K., Choe, Y., & Hernandez-Jarvis, L. (2001). Testing verbal (language) and nonverbal abilities in children and adults acquiring a nonprimary language. *Language Testing, 18*(1), 33–54.

Oller, J. W., Jr., & Obrecht, D. H. (1969). The psycholinguistic principle of informational sequence: An experiment in second language learning. *International Review of Applied Linguistics, 7,* 165–174.

Oller, J. W., Jr., & Oller, S. D. (2009). *Autism: The diagnosis, treatment, and etiology of the undeniable epidemic.* Sudbury, MA: Jones and Bartlett.

Oller, J. W., Jr., Oller, S. D., & Badon, L. C. (2006). *Milestones: Normal speech and language development across the life span.* San Diego, CA: Plural.

Oller, J. W., Jr., & Perkins, K. (Eds.), (1978). *Language in education: Testing the tests.* Rowley, MA: Newbury House.

Oller, J. W., Jr., & Rascón, D. (1999). Applying sign theory to autism. *Clinical Linguistics and Phonetics, 13*(2), 77–112.

Oller, J. W., Jr., & Richard-Amato, P. (Eds.), (1983). *Methods that work.* Rowley, MA: Newbury House.

Oller, J. W., Jr., Harrington, R. V., & Sales, B. D. (1969). A basic circularity in traditional and current linguistic theory. *Lingua, 22,* 317–328.

Oller, J. W., Jr., Walker, R. F., & Rattanavich, S. (1993). Literacy in the third world for all the children. In J. W. Oller, Jr. (Ed.), *Methods that work: Ideas for literacy and language teachers* (pp. 163–180). Boston: Heinle & Heinle.

Oller, J. W., Sr. (1965). *El español por el mundo.* Chicago: Encyclopedia Britannica Films.

Oller, S. D. (2005). Meaning matters: A clinician's/student's guide to general sign theory and its applicability in clinical settings. *Journal of Communication Disorders, 38*, 359–373.

Oller, S.D. (in press). *Theory to practice: Language disorders in children.* Sudbury, MA: Jones and Bartlett.

Oller, S. D, Oller, J. W., Jr., Badon, L. C., & Arehole, S. (November, 2006). *Implications of the "McGurk effect" for assessment, diagnosis, and intervention.* A two-hour paper presented at the Annual meeting of the American Speech-Language-Hearing Association, Miami, Florida.

Omnibus Autism Proceeding. (2007). Retrieved April 14, 2009, from ftp://autism.uscfc.uscourts.gov/autism/transcripts/day01.pdf

Omnibus Autism Proceeding. (2008). Retrieved April 14, 2009, from http://www.uscfc.uscourts.gov/OSM/AutismDocket.htm

Onslow, M. (2006). Connecting stuttering management and measurement: V. Deduction and induction in the development of stuttering treatment outcome measures and stuttering treatments. *International Journal of Language and Communication Disorders, 41*(4), 407–421.

Onslow, M., Costa, L., & Rue, S. (1990). Direct early intervention with stuttering. *Journal of Speech and Hearing Disorders, 55*(3), 405–416.

Operation Smile. (2006). Retrieved April 14, 2009, from http://www.operationsmile.org/

Organ, L. E., & Raphael, R. M. (2007). Application of fluorescence recovery after photobleaching to study prestin lateral mobility in the human embryonic kidney cell. *Journal of Biomedical Optics, 12*(2), Art. No. 021003.

Ortiz, A. A. (1997). Learning disabilities occurring concomitantly with linguistic differences. *Journal of Learning Disabilities, 30*(3), 321–332.

Ortiz, G. G., Bitzer-Quintero, O. K., Zarate, C. B., Rodriguez-Reynoso, S., Larios-Arceo, F., Velazquez-Brizuela, I. E., et al. (2006). Monosodium glutamate-induced damage in liver and kidney: A morphological and biochemical approach. *Biomedicine and Pharmacotherapy, 60*(2), 86–91.

Ota Benga. (1916/2009). Retrieved April 14, 2009, from http://en.wikipedia.org/wiki/Ota_Benga

Oxford University Press. (1980). *Oxford English dictionary of quotations* (3rd ed.). Oxford: Oxford University.

Oxidative stress. (2008). Retrieved September 25, 2008, from http://en.wikipedia.org/wiki/Oxidative_stress

Ozyurek, A., & Kelly, S. D. (2007). Gesture, brain, and language. *Brain and Language, 101*(3), 181–184.

Ozyurek, A., Willems, R., Kita, S., & Hagoort, P. (2007). On-line integration of semantic information from speech and gesture. *Journal of Cognitive Neuroscience, 19*(4), 605–616.

Pabello, N. G., & Lawrence, D. A. (2006). Neuroimmunotoxicology: Modulation of neuroimmune networks by toxicants. *Clinical Neuroscience Research, 6*(1–2), 69–85.

Packman, A., Kingston, M., Huber, A., Onslow, M., & Jones, M. (2003). Predicting treatment time with the Lidcombe Program: Replication and meta-analysis. *International Journal of Language and Communication Disorders, 38*(2), 165.

Padhye, U. (2003). Excess dietary iron is the root cause for increase in childhood Autism and allergies. *Medical Hypotheses, 61*(2), 220–222.

Paiement, P., Champoux, F., Bacon, B. A., Lassonde, M., Gagne, J. P., Mensour, B., et al. (2008). Functional reorganization of the human auditory pathways following hemispherectomy: An fMRI demonstration. *Neuropsychologia, 46*(1), 2936–2942.

Palmer, J. B., Hiiemae, K. M., Matsuo, K., & Haishima, H. (2007). Volitional control of food transport and bolus formation during feeding. *Physiology and Behavior, 91*(1), 66–70.

Palmer, R. K. (2007). The pharmacology and signaling of bitter, sweet, and umami taste sensing. *Molecular Interventions, 7*(2), 87–98.

Palomo T., Beninger R. J., Kostrzewa, R. M., & Archer, T. (2003). Brain sites of movement disorder: Genetic and environmental agents in neurodevelopmental perturbations. *Neurotoxicity Research, 5*(1–2), 1–26.

Palop, J. J., Chin, J., & Mucke, L. (2006). A network dysfunction perspective on neurodegenerative diseases. *Nature, 443*(7113), 768–773.

Pan, N., & Chen, L. (2005). Phonological/phonemic awareness and reading: A crosslinguistic perspective. *Journal of Multilingual Communication Disorders, 3*(2), 145–152.

Parents in Action on Special Education (PASE) v. Joseph P. Hannon. (July, 1980). U.S. District Court, Northern district of Illinois, Eastern Division, No. 74 (3586). Retrieved April 14, 2009, from http://www.uwyo.edu/wind/edec5250/assignments/pase.pdf

Parran, D. K., Barker, A., & Ehrich, M. (2005). Effects of thimerosal on NGF signal transduction and cell death in neuroblastoma cells. *Toxicological Sciences, 86*(1), 132–140.

Partial birth abortion. (2009). Retrieved April 14, 2009, from http://en.wikipedia.org/wiki/Partial_birth_abortion

Partial-Birth Abortion Ban Act of 2003, 108th Cong. (2003, March 13). Retrieved April 14, 2009, from http://news.findlaw.com/hdocs/docs/abortion/2003s3.html

Pasca, S. P., Nemes, B., Vlase, L., Gagyi, C. E., Dronca, E., Miu, A. C., et al. (2006). High levels of homocysteine and low serum paraoxonase 1 arylesterase activity in children with autism. *Life Sciences, 78*(19), 2244–2248.

Patterson, F., & Linden, E. (1981). *The education of Koko.* New York: Holt.

Patterson, M. L., & Werker, J. F. (1999). Matching phonetic information in lips and voice is robust in 4.5-month-old infants. *Infant Behavior and Development, 22,* 237–247.

Patterson, M. L., & Werker, J. F. (2003). Two-month-old infants match phonetic information in lips and voice. *Developmental Science, 6*(2), 191–196.

Paulie. (1998). Retrieved September 25, 2008, from http://en.wikipedia.org/wiki/Paulie

Pearce, J. M. S. (2007). Corpus callosum. *European Neurology, 57,* 249–250.

Pearce, R. K. B., Owen, A., Daniel, S., Jenner, P., & Marsden, C. D. (1997). Iterations in the distribution of glutathione in the substantia nigra in Parkinson's disease. *Journal of Neural Transmission, 104*(6–7), 661–677.

Peirce, C. S. (1897). The logic of relatives. *The Monist, 7,* 161–217. Also In C. Hartshorne & P. Weiss (Eds.), (1932), *Collected papers of C. S. Peirce, Volume 2* (pp. 288–345). Cambridge, MA: Harvard University Press.

Peirce, C. S. (1908). A neglected argument for the reality of God. *Hibbert Journal, 7,* 90–112. Also in C. Hartshorne & P. Weiss (Eds.), (1935), *Collected papers of C. S. Peirce, Volume 6* (pp. 311–339). Cambridge, MA: Harvard University Press.

Peirce, C. S. (1982a). The logic notebook. In M. Fisch, C. J. W. Kloesel, E. C. Moore, D. D. Roberts, L. A. Ziegler, & N. P. Atkinson (Eds.), *Writings of Charles S. Peirce: A chronological edition, Volume 1, 1857–1866* (pp. 337–350). Indianapolis: Indiana University Press. (Originally written 1865).

Peirce, C. S. (1982b). [On a method of searching for the categories]. MS 133. In M. Fisch, C. J. W. Kloesel, E. C. Moore, D. D. Roberts, L. A. Ziegler, & N. P. Atkinson (Eds.), *Writings of Charles S. Peirce: A chronological edition, Volume 1 1857–1866* (pp. 515–528). Indianapolis: Indiana University Press. (Originally written in 1866).

Penfield, W., & Boldrey, E. (1937). Somatic motor and sensory representation in the cerebral cortex of man as studied by electrical stimulation. *Brain, 60,* 389.

Penn, D. C., & Povinelli, D. J. (2007). On the lack of evidence that non-human animals possess anything remotely resembling a "theory of mind." *Philosophical Transactions of the Royal Society B-Biological Sciences, 362*(1480), 731–744.

Pennisi, E. (1997). Haeckel's embryos: Fraud rediscovered. *Science, 277*(5331), 1435.

Pennsylvania Association of Retarded Children (PARC) v. Commonwealth of Pennsylvania, 334 F. Supp. 1257 (ED Pa. 1971), 343 F. Supp. 279 (ED Pa. 1972).

Pennycook, A. (1994). Incommensurable discourses? *Applied Linguistics, 15*(2), 131–138.

Pepperberg, I. M. (1999). Rethinking syntax: A commentary on E. Kako's "Elements of syntax in the systems of three language-trained animals." *Animal Learning and Behavior, 27*(1), 15–17.

Pepperberg, I. M., & Gordon, J. D. (2005). Number comprehension by a grey parrot (Psittacus erithacus), including a zero-like concept. *Journal of Comparative Psychology, 119*(2), 197–120.

Perez-Martinez, D. A., Puente-Munoz, A. I., Domenech, J., Baztan, J. J., Berbel-Garcia, A., et al. (2007). Unilateral apraxia of eyelid closure in ischemic stroke: Role of the right hemisphere in the emotional gesture communication. *Revista De Neurologia, 44*(7), 411–414.

Perkins, W. H. (1990). What is stuttering? *Journal of Speech and Hearing Disorders, 55,* 370–382.

Peryer, G., Noyes, J., Pleydell-Pearce, C. W., & Lieven, N. A. J. (2005). Auditory alert characteristics: A survey of pilot views. *International Journal of Aviation Psychology, 15*(3), 233–250.

Petersen, M. S., Halling, J., Bech, S., Wermuth, L., Weihe, P., Nielsen, F., et al. (2008). Impact of dietary exposure to food contaminants on the risk of Parkinson's disease. *Neurotoxicology, 29*(4), 584–590.

Petitto, L. A., & Marentette, P. F. (1991) Babbling in the manual mode: Evidence for the ontogeny of language. *Science, 251,* 1493–1496.

Petronis, A., Gottesman, I. L., Kan, P. X., Kennedy, J. L., Basile, V. S., Paterson, A. D., et al. (2003). Monozygotic twins exhibit numerous epigenetic differences: Clues to twin discordance? *Schizophrenia Bulletin, 29*(1), 169–178.

Phillips, D. (1997). Foreword. In G. D. Chermak & F. E. Musiek. *Central auditory processing disorders: New perspectives.* San Diego, CA: Singular.

Phineas Gage. (1860/2009). Retrieved April 14, 2009, from http://en.wikipedia.org/wiki/Phineas_Gage

Phonics basics. (2009). Retrieved April 15, 2009, from http://www.pbs.org/parents/readinglanguage/articles/phonics/pbasics.html

Piaget, J. (1950). *The psychology of intelligence.* London: Routledge and Kegan Paul.

Piaget, J. (1954). *The construction of reality in the child.* New York: Basic Books.

Pike, K. (1947). *Phonemics: A technique for reducing languages to writing.* Ann Arbor: University of Michigan Press.

Pioneer Fund. (n.d.). *Highlights of Pioneer Fund research and grantees.* Retrieved April 15, 2009, from http://www.pioneerfund.org/Grantees.html

Planum temporale. (2009). Retrieved April 15, 2009, from http://en.wikipedia.org/wiki/Planum_temporale

Platt, J. R. (1964). Strong inference. *Science, 146*(3642), 347–353.

Plessy v. Ferguson, 163 U.S. 537. (1896).

Poll shows little support for assisted suicide. (2000, March). Retrieved September 25, 2008, from http://www.nrlc.org/euthanasia/facts/suicideassistpoll.html

Poloni, C., Riquier, F., Zimmermann G., & Borgeat, F. (2003, December). Perceptual defense in anxiety disorders. *Perceptual and Motor Skills, 97*(3, Pt. 1), 971–978.

Popper, K. (1959). *The logic of scientific discovery.* New York: Harper.

Porky Pig. (2009). Retrieved April 15, 2009, from http://en.wikipedia.org/wiki/Porky_Pig

Portmanteau. (1871/2009). A term from Lewis Carroll. Retrieved April 15, 2009, from http://en.wikipedia.org/wiki/Portmanteau

Positron emission tomography. (2009). Retrieved April 15, 2009, from http://en.wikipedia.org/wiki/Positron_emission_tomography

Positron emission tomography: Applications. (2009). Retrieved April 15, 2009, from http://en.wikipedia.org/wiki/Positron_emission_tomography#_note-0

Posserud, M. B., Lundervold, A. J., & Gillberg, C. (2006). Autistic features in a total population of 7–9-year-old children assessed by the ASSQ (Autism Spectrum Screening Questionnaire). *Journal of Child Psychology and Psychiatry, 47*(2), 167–175.

Poto and Cabengo. (1979). Movie directed by Jean-Pierre Gorin. Information retrieved April 15, 2009, from http://vtap.com/topic/Poto+and+Cabengo/VM910480)

Poto and Cabengo. (2008). Retrieved September 25, 2008, from http://en.wikipedia.org/wiki/Poto_and_Cabengo

Povinelli, D. J. (1994). What chimpanzees (might) know about the mind. In Goodall, J., deWaal, F. B. M., & Wrangham, R., (Eds.), *Chimpanzee cultures* (pp. 285–300). Cambridge, MA: Harvard University Press.

Prasad, S., Kalra, N., & Shukla, Y. (2008). Modulatory effects of diallyl sulfide against testosterone-induced oxidative stress in Swiss albino mice. *Asian Journal of Andrology, 8*(6), 719–723.

Prasse, J. E., & Kikano, G. E. (2008). Stuttering: An overview. *American Family Physician, 77*(9), 1271–1276.

Pratkanis, A. R., & Aronson, E. (1992). *Age of propaganda: The everyday use and abuse of persuasion.* New York: W. H. Freeman.

Premack, D., & Woodruff, G. (1978). Does the chimpanzee have a theory of mind? *Behavioral and Brain Sciences, 1,* 515–526.

President Bush signs Partial Birth Abortion Ban Act. (2003, November). Retrieved September 25, 2008, from http://www.whitehouse.gov/news/releases/2003/11/20031105-1.html#

Previc, F. H. (2007). Prenatal influences on brain dopamine and their relevance to the rising incidence of autism. *Medical Hypotheses, 68*(1), 46–60.

Prieve, B. (2002). Otoacoustic emissions in neonatal hearing screening. In M. S. Robinette & T. J. Glattke (Eds.), *Otoacoustic emissions: Clinical applications* (2nd ed., pp. 348–374). New York: Thieme.

Probst, P. (2005). "Communication unbound—or unfound"?—An integrative review on the effectiveness of Facilitated Communication (FC) in non-verbal persons with autism and mental retardation. *Zeitschrift Fur Klinische Psychologie Psychiatrie Und Psychotherapie, 53*(2), 93–128.

Prosody (linguistics). (2009). Retrieved April 15, 2009, from http://en.wikipedia.org/wiki/Prosody_(linguistics)

Providence, Rhode Island. (n.d.) Narragansett Bay: Maritime commerce [= Slave traffic]. Retrieved April 15, 2009, from http://www.providenceri.com/NarragansettBay/maritime_commerce.html

Pseudobulbar palsy. (2009). *Encyclopedia of Neurological Disorders,* edited by S. L. Chamberlin & B. Narins. Gale Group, Inc., 2005. eNotes.com. 2006. Retrieved April 15, 2009, from http://www.enotes.com/neurological-disorders-encyclopedia/pseudobulbar-palsy

Public Law 94-142. (1975). Retrieved April 15, 2009, from http://users.rcn.com/peregrin.enteract/add/94-142.txt

Pylyshyn, Z. W. (2002). Mental imagery: In search of a theory. *Behavioral and Brain Sciences, 25,* 157–238.

Rachael Ray. (2009). Retrieved April 15, 2009, from https://www.rachaelraymag.com/

Radvansky, G., Zwaan, R. A., Federico, T., & Franklin, N. (1998). Retrieval from temporally organized situation models. *Journal of Experimental Psychology—Learning Memory and Cognition, 24*(5), 1224–1237.

Ramig, P. (1996). *From the 1996 Panel discussion on "recovery" ASHA Convention, Seattle, Washington.* Retrieved April 15, 2009, from http://www.mnsu.edu/comdis/voices/voices.html

Ramón y Cajal, S. (1933). *Histology* (10th ed.). Baltimore: Wood.

Ramus, F., & Mehler, J. (1999). Language identification with suprasegmental cues: A study based on speech resynthesis. *Journal of the Acoustical Society of America, 105*(1), 512–521.

Raphael, Y., & Altschuler, R. A. (2003). Structure and innervation of the cochlea. *Brain Research Bulletin, 60*(5–6), 397–422.

Rattanavich, S., Walker, R. F., & Oller, J. W., Jr. (1992). *Teaching all the children to read.* London: Open University Press.

Raymond Herbert Stetson. (1950/2009). Retrieved April 15, 2009, from http://fr.wikipedia.org/wiki/Raymond_Herbert_Stetson

Razagui, I. B. A., & Haswell, S. J. (2001). Mercury and selenium concentrations in maternal and neonatal scalp hair—Relationship to amalgam-based dental treatment received during pregnancy. *Biological Trace Element Research, 81*(1), 1–19.

Reagan, R. (1984). *Abortion and the conscience of the nation.* Nashville, TN: Thomas Nelson.

Redman, T. A., Finn, J. C., Bremner, A. P., & Valentine, J. (2008). Effect of upper limb botulinum toxin-A therapy on health-related quality of life in children with hemiplegic cerebral palsy. *Journal of Paediatrics and Child Health, 44*(7–8), 409–414.

Redox. (2009). *Oxidation.* Retrieved April 15, 2009, from http://en.wikipedia.org/wiki/Oxidation

Redstone, F. (2005). Seating position and length of utterance of preschoolers with cerebral palsy. *Perceptual and Motor Skills, 101*(3), 961–962.

Reggia, J. A., Goodall, S. M., Shkuro, Y., & Glezer, M. (2001). The callosal dilemma: Explaining diaschisis in the context of hemispheric rivalry via a neural network model. *Neurological Research, 23*(5), 465–471.

Rehabilitation Act of 1973, Pub. L. 93-112. (U. S. C. § 791, 1973).

Reybrouck, M. (2004). Music cognition, semiotics and the experience of time: Ontosemantical and epistemological claims. *Journal of New Music Research, 33*(4), 411–428.

Rescue dawn: The truth. (n.d.) A family member's critique of Werner Herzog's *Rescue Dawn* (film). Retrieved April 15, 2009, from http://www.rescuedawnthetruth.com/

Rice, T. D. (1828). *Jump Jim Crow* (song). Retrieved April 15, 2009, from http://en.wikipedia.org/wiki/Jump_Jim_Crow

Richard-Amato, P. (2003). *Making it happen: From interactive to participatory language teaching theory and practice* (3rd ed.). London: Longman.

Richardson, D. C., Dale, R., & Kirkham, N. Z. (2007). The art of conversation is coordination—Common ground and the coupling of eye movements during dialogue. *Psychological Science, 18*(5), 407–413.

Rigamonti, M. M., Custance, D. M., Previde, E. P., & Spiezio, C. (2005). Testing for localized stimulus enhancement and object movement reenactment in pig-tailed macaques (Macaca nemestrina) and young children (Homo sapiens). *Journal of Comparative Psychology, 119*(3), 257–272.

Rillos, L. (February 22, 2006). *Michelle Nunez-Fields Mother sentenced in drowning death of her son.* Retrieved April 15, 2009, from http://www.topix.net/forum/city/dateland-az/TQBL1KS5GGSAEVSLR

Ritter, J. (1996, January 9). Transcript of crash shows controller error/Review reveals poor English "Over and Over." *USA Today*, p. 7A.

Ritvo, R. A., Ritvo, E. R., Guthrie, D., & Ritvo, M. J. (2008). Clinical evidence that Asperger's disorder is a mild form of autism. *Comprehensive Psychiatry, 49*(1), 1–5.

Ritvo, R. A., Ritvo, E. R., Guthrie, D., Yuwiler, A., Ritvo, M. J., & Weisbender, L. (2008). A scale to assist the diagnosis of autism and Asperger's Disorder in adults (RAADS): A pilot study. *Journal of Autism and Developmental Disorders, 38*(2), 213–223.

Rivera, S. M., & Zawaydeh, A. N. (2007). Word comprehension facilitates object individuation in 10- and 11-month-old infants. *Brain Research, 1146,* 146–157.

Roger Bannister. (2009). Retrieved April 15, 2009, from http://en.wikipedia.org/wiki/Roger_Bannister

Rohyans, J., Walson, P. D., Wood G. A., & Macdonald, W. A. (1984). Mercury toxicity following merthiolate ear irrigations. *Journal of Pediatrics, 104*(2), 311–313.

Roman, K. G. (1959) Handwriting and speech. *Logos, 2,* 29–39.

Röntgen, W. C. (1901). *The Nobel Prize in Physics 1901.* Retrieved April 15, 2009, from http://nobelprize.org/nobel_prizes/physics/laureates/1901/rontgen-bio.html

Rosenblum, L. D. (n.d.). *The McGurk effect.* Retrieved April 15, 2009, from http://www.faculty.ucr.edu/~rosenblu/VSMcGurk.html

Rosenblum, L. D., Schmuckler, M.A., & Johnson, J. A. (1997). The McGurk effect in infants. *Perception and Psychophysics, 59*(3), 347–357.

Ross, D. S., & Bever, T. G. (2004). The time course for language acquisition in biologically distinct populations: Evidence from deaf individuals. *Brain and Language, 89*(1), 115–121.

Rossignol, D. A., & Rossignol, L. W. (2006). Hyperbaric oxygen therapy may improve symptoms in autistic children. *Medical Hypotheses, 67*(2), 216–228.

Rotary Lighthouse Literacy Programs. (2009). Retrieved April 15, 2009, from http://www.cleliteracy.org/

Rouas, J. L. (2007). Automatic prosodic variations modeling for language and dialect discrimination. *IEEE Transactions on Audio Speech and Language Processing, 15*(6), 1904–1911.

Royal National Institute of Blind People. (2009). *The life of Louis Braille.* Retrieved April 15, 2009, from http://www.rnib.org.uk/xpedio/groups/public/documents/publicwebsite/public_braille.hcsp

Ruark, J. L., & Moore, C. A. (1997). Coordination of lip muscle activity by 2-year-old children during speech and nonspeech tasks. *Journal of Speech Language and Hearing Research, 40*(6), 1373–1385.

Russo, R. N., Crotty, M., Miller, M. D., Murchland, S., Flett, P., & Haan, E. (2007). Upper-limb botulinum toxin A injection and occupational therapy in children with hemiplegic cerebral palsy identified from a population register: A single-blind, randomized, controlled trial. *Pediatrics, 119*(5), E1149–E1158.

Rutter, M. (1978). Diagnosis and definition of childhood autism. *Journal of Autism and Developmental Disorders, 8,* 139–161.

Ryan, K. J., & Ray, C. G. (Eds.), (2004). *Sherris medical microbiology* (4th ed.). New York: McGraw Hill.

Rybicki, B. A., Johnson, C. C., Uman, J., & Gorell, J. M. (1993). Parkinson's disease mortality and the industrial use of heavy-metals in Michigan. *Movement Disorders, 8*(1), 87–89.

Sacks, H., Schegloff, E. A., & Jefferson, G. (1974). A simplest systematic for organization of turn taking in conversation. *Language, 50,* 696–735.

Safe removal of amalgam fillings. (2007). *International Academy of Oral Medicine and Toxicology.* Retrieved April 14, 2009, from http://www.iaomt.org/articles/category_view.asp?intReleaseID=288&catid=30

Sai, F. Z. (2005). The role of the mother's voice in developing mother's face preference: Evidence for intermodal perception at birth. *Infant and Child Development, 14*(1), 1–29.

Samuel A. Foote. (ca. 1797). Retrieved September 25, 2008, from http://en.wikipedia.org/wiki/Samuel_A._Foot

Samuel Gridley Howe. (2009). Retrieved April 15, 2009, from http://en.wikipedia.org/wiki/Samuel_Gridley_Howe

Sanford, J. (2005). *Genetic entropy and the mystery of the genome.* San Diego, CA: Ivan Press.

Sandhi. (2009). Retrieved April 15, 2009, from http://en.wikipedia.org/wiki/Sandhi

Santos-Sacchi, J. (2003). New tunes from Corti's organ: The outer hair cell boogie rules. *Current Opinion in Neurobiology, 13*(4), 459–468.

Santos-Sacchi, J., Song, L., Zheng, J. F., & Nuttall, A. L. (2006). Control of mammalian cochlear amplification by chloride anions. *Journal of Neuroscience, 26*(15), 3992–3998.

Sapir, E. (1933). The psychological reality of the phoneme. *Journal de Psychologie Normale et Patholoique, 30,* 247–265. Reprinted in D. G. Mandelbaum (Ed.), (1949) *Selected writings of Edward Sapir in language, culture and personality.* Berkeley: University of California Press.

Sarrazin, J. C., Cleeremans, A., & Haggard, P. (2008). How do we know what we are doing? Time, intention and awareness of action. *Consciousness and Cognition, 17*(3), 602–615.

Sarton, G. (1952). *A history of science.* Cambridge, MA: Harvard University Press.

Sasaki, S., Takeshita, F., Okuda, K., & Ishii, N. (2001). Mycobacterium leprae and leprosy: A compendium. *Microbiological Immunology, 45*(11), 729–736.

Sato, Y. (1993). The durations of syllable-final nasals and the mora hypothesis in Japanese. *Phonetica, 50*(1), 44–67.

Saul, R., & Sperry, R. W. (1968). Absence of commissurotomy symptoms with agenesis of the corpus callosum. *Neurology, 18,* 307.

Savage-Rumbaugh, S., & Lewin, R. (1994). *Kanzi: The ape at the brink of the human mind.* Toronto: John Wiley and Sons.

Schizophrenia.com. (2004). *Schizophrenia symptoms and diagnosis.* Retrieved April 15, 2009, from http://www.schizophrenia.com/diag.php#diagnosis

Schmidt, K. L., Cohn, J. F., & Tian, Y. L. (2003). Signal characteristics of spontaneous facial expressions: Automatic movement in solitary and social smiles. *Biological Psychology, 65*(1), 49–66.

Schmithorst, V. J., & Holland, S. K. (2006). Functional MRI evidence for disparate developmental processes underlying intelligence in boys and girls. *Neuroimage, 31*(3), 1366–1379.

Schneider, P. (2004). *Transcending stuttering—the inside story.* Retrieved September 25, 2008, from http://www.onlineceus.com/continuingeducation/fluency/stutteringvideo.html

Scott v. Sanford, 60 U.S. 393. (1857).

Scripture, E. W. (1909). Penmanship stuttering. *Journal of the American Medical Association, 52,* 1480–1481.

Sebeok, T. A., & Umiker-Sebeok, J. (Eds.). (1980). *Speaking of apes: A critical anthology of two-way communication with man.* New York: Plenum.

Sedgwick, J. (1995). Inside the Pioneer fund. In R. Jacobi & N. Glauberman (Eds.), *The bell curve debate* (pp. 144–161). New York: Times Books.

Segura-Aguilar, J., & Kostrzewa, R. M. (2006). Neurotoxins and neurotoxicity mechanisms. An overview. *Neurotoxicity Research, 10*(3–4), 263–287.

Sell, J. Z. (2003). *Vaccine litigation.* Retrieved April 15, 2009, from http://www.jzslaw.com/vaccinelitigation.html

Senghas, A. (2003). Intergenerational influence and ontogenetic development in the emergence of spatial grammar in Nicaraguan Sign Language. *Cognitive Development, 18*(4), 511–531.

Senghas, A. (2005). Language emergence: Clues from a new Bedouin sign language. *Current Biology, 15*(12), R463–R465.

Senghas, A., & Coppola, M. (2001). Children creating language: How Nicaraguan sign language acquir-ed a spatial grammar. *Psychological Science, 12*(4), 323–328.

Senghas A., Kita, S., & Ozyurek, A. (2004). Children creating core properties of language: Evidence from an emerging sign language in Nicaragua. *Science, 305*(5691), 1779–1782.

Sensory aphasia. (2009). Retrieved April 15, 2009, from http://en.wikipedia.org/wiki/Alexia_%28disorder%29

September 11, 2001. (2009). Video of September 11, 2001. Retrieved February 25, 2009, from http://www.metacafe.com/watch/684526/september_11/

Sequoyah. (n.d.). Retrieved April 15, 2009, from http://www.manataka.org/page81.html

Sequoyah. (2009). Retrieved April 15, 2009, from http://en.wikipedia.org/wiki/Sequoyah

Seymour, P. K. H. (1986). *Cognitive analysis of dyslexia.* London: Routledge & Kegan Paul.

Shakespeare, W. (ca. 1601). *Hamlet.* Retrieved September 25, 2008, from http://en.wikipedia.org/wiki/Speak_the_speech

Shames, G. H., & Anderson, N. B. (Eds.). (2002). *Human communication disorders* (6th ed.). Boston: Allyn & Bacon.

Shanker, S. G., Savage-Rumbaugh, E. S., & Taylor, T. J. (1999). Kanzi: A new beginning. *Animal Learning and Behavior, 27*(1), 24–25.

Sharif v. New York State Education Department, 709 F.Supp. 345 (S.D.N.Y. 1989). Retrieved September 25, 2008, from http://www.faculty.piercelaw.edu/redfield/library/case-sharif.htm

Shaywitz, S. E., Escobar, M. D., Shaywitz, B. A., Fletcher, J. M., & Makuch, R. (1992). Evidence that dyslexia may represent the lower tail of a normal distribution of reading ability. *New England Journal of Medicine, 326*(3), 145–150.

Shenker, R. C. (2006). Connecting stuttering management and measurement: I. Core speech measures of clinical process and outcome. *International Journal of Language and Communication Disorders, 41*(4), 355–364.

Shestack, J. (2003). *Presentation: The face of autism.* Presented at the Autism Summit Conference: Developing a national agenda. Retrieved September 25, 2008, from http://www.tvworldwide.com/events/nimh/031119/agenda.cfm

Shi, X. B., Xue, L. R., Tepper, C. G., Gandour-Edwards, R., Ghosh, P., Kung, H. J., et al (2007). The oncogenic potential of a prostate cancer-derived androgen receptor mutant. *Prostate, 67*(6), 591–602.

Shigemitsu, H., & Afshar, K. (2007). Aspiration pneumonias: Under-diagnosed and under-treated. *Current Opinion in Pulmonary Medicine, 13*(3), 192–198.

Shuster, L. I., & Lemieux, S. K. (2005). An fMRI investigation of covertly and overtly produced mono- and multisyllabic words. *Brain and Language, 93*(1), 20–31.

Sickle cell disease. (2009). Retrieved April 15, 2009, from http://en.wikipedia.org/wiki/Sickle-cell_disease

Silbert, N., & de Jong, K. (2008). Focus, prosodic context, and phonological feature specification: Patterns of variation in fricative production *Journal of the Acoustical Society of America, 12*(5), 2769–1277.

Silver, J. A. (2003). *Movie day at the Supreme Court or "I know it when I see it": A History of the definition of obscenity.* Retrieved September 25, 2008, from http://library.findlaw.com/2003/May/15/132747.html

Silverman, F. H. (2004). *Stuttering and other fluency disorders* (3rd ed.). Long Grove, IL: Waveland Press.

Silverman, F. H., & Bohlman, P. (1988). Flute stuttering. *Journal of Fluency Disorders, 13,* 427–428.

Silverman, F. H., & Silverman, E. M. (1971). Stutter-like behavior in the manual communication of the deaf. *Perceptual and Motor Skills, 33,* 45–46.

Silverman, M. (2007). Musical interpretation: Philosophical and practical issues. *International Journal of Music Education, 25*(2), 101–117.

Silverstein, A. E. (2009). *Innovative therapies.* Retrieved April 15, 2009, from http://www.innovative-therapies.com/aboutus_resume_aes.htm

Simmons, R. J. (April 30, 2003). Letter from the Office of the President, Ruth J. Simmons, Brown University, Providence Rhode Island, commissioning the *Slavery and Justice Report.* Retrieved April 15, 2009, from http://www.brown.edu/Research/Slavery_Justice/about/charge.html

Simon, C. (2009). *Let the River Run* (song), main song in sound track for the movie, *Working Girl.* Retrieved April 15, 2009, from http://video.yahoo.com/watch/2033746/v2164490

Simpson, L. L. (2000, September-October). Identification of the characteristics that underlie botulinum toxin potency: Implications for designing novel drugs. *Biochimie, 82*(9–10), 943–953. Retrieved April 15, 2009, from http://www.ncbi.nlm.nih.gov/sites/entrez?cmd=Retrieve&db=PubMed&list_uids=11086224&dopt=AbstractPlus

Skinner, B. F. (1957). *Verbal behavior*. New York: Appleton-Century-Crofts.

Slavery and Justice Report. (2006). Retrieved September 25, 2008, from http://www.brown.edu/Research/Slavery_Justice/report

Slotkin, T. A., Oliver, C. A., & Seidler, F. J. (2005). Critical periods for the role of oxidative stress in the developmental neurotoxicity of chlorpyrifos and terbutaline, alone or in combination. *Developmental Brain Research, 157*(2), 172–180.

Smith, A. (1966). Speech and other functions after left (dominant) hemispherectomy. *Journal of Neurology, Neurosurgery and Psychiatry, 29,* 467–471.

Smith, A., & Sugar, O. (1975). Development of above normal language and intelligence 21 years after left hemispherectomy. *Neurology, 25*(9), 813–818.

Smith, D. (2009). *Lichtheim 1885 "On aphasia."* Retrieved April 15, 2009, from http://www.smithsrisca.demon.co.uk/PSYlichtheim1885.html

Smith-Magenis syndrome. (2009). Retrieved April 15, 2009, from http://www.smithmagenis.org/WhatisSMS/overview_ssynd.htm

Smith v. Robinson, 468 U.S. 992. (1979/1984). Retrieved April 15, 2009, from http://caselaw.lp.findlaw.com/cgi-bin/getcase.pl?court=US&vol=468&invol=992

Snow, C., Burns, M. S., & Griffin, P. (Eds.). (1998). *Preventing reading difficulties in young children*. Washington, DC: National Academy Press.

Snyder, G. (2006, September 18). *The existence of stuttering in sign language and other forms of expressive communication: Sufficient cause for the emergence of a new stuttering paradigm?* Paper presented at the International Stuttering Awareness Day Online Conference, 2006. Retrieved April 15, 2009, from http://www.mnsu.edu/comdis/isad9/papers/snyder9.html

Soderstrom, M., & Morgan, J. L. (2007). Twenty-two-month-olds discriminate fluent from disfluent adult-directed speech. *Developmental Science, 10*(5), 641–653.

Sogut, S., Zoroglu, S. S., Ozyurt, H., Yilmaz, H. R., Ozugurlu, F., Sivasli, E., et al. (2003). Changes in nitric oxide levels and antioxidant enzyme activities may have a role in the pathophysiological mechanisms involved in autism. *Clinica Chimica Acta, 331*(1–2), 111–117.

Sparks, N. (1996). *The notebook*. New York: Warner.

Speer, N. K., & Zacks, J. A. (2005). Temporal changes as event boundaries: Processing and memory conse-quences of narrative time shifts. *Journal of Memory and Language, 53*(1), 125–140.

Speer, N. K., Zacks, J. M., & Reynolds, J. R. (2007). Human brain activity time-locked to narrative event boundaries. *Psychological Science, 18*(5), 449–455.

Spence, S. A., Kaylor-Hughes, C. J., Brook, M. L., Lankappa, S. T., & Wilkinson, I. D. (2008). "Munchausen's syndrome by proxy" or a "miscarriage of justice"? An initial application of functional neuroimaging to the question of guilt versus innocence. *European Psychiatry, 23*(4), 309–314.

Spencer, K. A., & Slocomb, D. L. (2007). The neural basis of ataxic dysarthria. *Cerebellum, 6*(1), 58–65.

Sperry, R. W. (1968). Plasticity of neural maturation. *Developmental Biology Supplement, 2,* 306–327.

Sperry, R. W. (1981). *Nobel lecture: Some effects of disconnecting the cerebral hemispheres.* Retrieved September 25, 2008, from http://nobelprize.org/nobel_prizes/medicine/laureates/1981/sperry-lecture.html

Squire, L. R., Bloom, F. E., McConnell, S. K., Roberts, J. L., Spitzer, N. C., Zigmond, M. J., et al. (Eds.). (2003). *Fundamental neuroscience*. Amsterdam: Academic Press.

St. Louis, K., Myers, F., Faragasso, K., Townsend, P., & Gallaher, A. (2004). Perceptual aspects of cluttered speech. *Journal of Fluency Disorders, 29*(3), 213–235.

St. Louis, K. O., Raphael, L. J., Myers, F. L., & Bakker, K. (2003, Nov. 18). Cluttering updated. *ASHA Leader* (pp. 4–5, 20–22).

Stacy Keach Official Web site. (2009). Retrieved April 15, 2009, from http://www.stacykeach.com/

Stan Kurtz. (2009). Retrieved April 15, 2009, from http://www.stankurtz.com/

Starkweather, C. W. (1987). *Fluency and stuttering*. Englewood Cliffs, NJ: Prentice-Hall.

State, M. W. (2006). A surprising METamorphosis: Autism genetics finds a common functional variant. *Proceedings of the National Academy of Sciences of the USA, 103*(45), 16621–16622.

Statistics about accidental death. (2008). Retrieved September 25, 2008, from http://www.wrongdiagnosis.com/a/accidental_death/stats.htm

Statistics by country for cleft palate. (2008). Retrieved September 25, 2008, from http://www.wrongdiagnosis.com/c/cleft_palate/stats-country.htm

Stetson, R. H. (1945). *The bases of phonology*. Oberlin, OH: Oberlin College.

Stetson, R. H. (1951). *Motor phonetics, a study of speech movements in action* (2nd ed.). Amsterdam: Published for Oberlin College by North-Holland Publishers.

Stidham, K. R., Olson, L., Hillbratt, M., & Sinopoli, T. (2006). A new antistuttering device: Treatment of stuttering using bone conduction stimulation with delayed temporal feedback. *Laryngoscope, 116*(11), 1951–1955.

Stip, E., Lecours, A. R., Chertkow, H., Elie, R., & O'Connor, K. (1994). Influence of affective words on lexical decision tasks in major depression. *Journal of Psychiatry and Neuroscience, 19*(3), 202–207.

Stone, O. (2006). *World Trade Center* (film). Retrieved September 25, 2008, from http://en.wikipedia.org/wiki/World_Trade_Center_(film)

Strauss, L. T., Gamble, S. B., Parker, W. Y., Cook, D. A., Zane, S. B., & Hamdan, S. (November 24, 2006). Abortion surveillance—United States, 2003. *Morbidity and Mortality Weekly Report (MMWR), 55*(SS11), 1–32.

Streissguth, A. (2007). Offspring effects of prenatal alcohol exposure from birth to 25 years: The Seattle prospective longitudinal study. *Journal of Clinical Psychology in Medical Settings, 14*(2), 81–101.

Strickland, E. A. (2001). The relationship between frequency selectivity and overshoot. *Journal of the Acoustical Society of America, 109*, 2062–2073.

Strohmayer, W. (1902). Subcortical sensory aphasia. *Journal of Nervous and Mental Disease, 21*, 163–164.

Stroke. (2009). *National Institute of Neurological Disorders and Stroke: Stroke information page*. Retrieved April 15, 2009, from http://www.ninds.nih.gov/disorders/stroke/stroke.htm

Strong, M. J. (2008). The syndromes of frontotemporal dysfunction in amyotrophic lateral sclerosis. *Amyotrophic Lateral Sclerosis, 9*(6), 323–338.

Strong, T. (2005). Constructivist ethics? Let's talk about them: An introduction to the special issue on ethics and constructivist psychology. *Journal of Constructivist Psychology, 18*(2), 89–102.

Stuart, A., Frazier, C. L., Kalinowski, J., & Vos, P. W. (2008). The effect of frequency altered feedback on stuttering duration and type. *Journal of Speech Language and Hearing Research, 51*(4), 889–897.

Stuart, A., Jones, S. M., & Walker, L. J. (2006). Insights into elevated distortion product otoacoustic emissions in sickle cell disease: Comparisons of hydroxyurea-treated and non-treated young children. *Hearing Research, 212*(1–2), 83–89.

Stuart, A., Kalinowski, J., Rastatter, M., Saltuklaroglu, T., & Dayalu, V. (2004). Investigations of the impact of altered auditory feedback in-the-ear devices on the speech of people who stutter: Initial fitting and 4-month follow-up. *International Journal of Language and Communication Disorders, 39*(1), 93–113.

Stump, T. (1978). Cloze and dictation tasks as predictors of intelligence and achievement scores. In J. W. Oller, Jr. & K. Perkins (Eds.), *Language in education:*

Testing the tests (pp. 36–63). Rowley, MA: Newbury House.

Stuttering Foundation. (2008, December 28). Retrieved April 15, 2009, from http://www.stutteringhelp.org/

Suga, N., Gao, E., Zhang, E., Ma, X., & Olsen, J. F. (2000). The corticofugal system for hearing: Recent progress. *Proceedings of the National Academy of Sciences, 97*(22), 11807–11814.

Sullivan, M. W., & Lewis, M. (2003). Emotional expressions of young infants and children: A practitioner's primer. *Infants and Young Children, 16*(2), 120–142.

Suzuki, K., Yamadori, A., Endo, K., Fujii, T., Ezura, M., & Takahashi, A. (1998). Dissociation of letter and picture naming resulting from callosal disconnection. *Neurology, 51*(5), 1390–1394.

Swain, M. K. (1972). *Bilingualism as a first language*. Unpublished Ph.D. dissertation, University of California, Irvine.

Sweet, B. H., & Hilleman, M. R. (1960, November). The vacuolating virus, S.V. 40. *Proceedings of the Society of Experimental Biological Medicine, 105*, 420–427.

Sweet, L. I., Passino-Reader, D. R., Meier, P. G., & Omann G. A. (2006). Effects of polychlorinated biphenyls, hexachlorocyclohexanes, and mercury on human neutrophil apoptosis, actin cytoskelton, and oxidative state. *Environmental Toxicology and Pharmacology, 22*(2), 179–188.

Swerdlow, N. R., Braff, D. L., & Geyer, M. A. (2000). Animal models of deficient sensorimotor gating: What we know, what we think we know, and what we hope to know soon. *Behavioral Pharmacology, 11*(3–4), 185–204.

Taber, K. H., & Hurley, R. A. (2007). Traumatic axonal injury: Atlas of major pathways. *Journal of Neuropsychiatry and Clinical Neurosciences, 19*(2), 100–104.

Taglialatela, J. P., Savage-Rumbaugh, S., & Baker, L. A. (2003). Vocal production by a language-competent Pan paniscus. *International Journal of Primatology, 24*(1), 1–17.

Tajima, A. (2004). Fatal miscommunications: English in aviation safety. *World Englishes, 23*, 451–470.

Takeshita, F., Takase, K., Tozuka, M., Saha, S., Okuda, K., Ishii, N., et al. (2007). Muscle creatine kinase/SV40 hybrid promoter for muscle-targeted long-term transgene expression. *International Journal of Molecular Medicine, 19*(2), 309–315.

Tallal, P. (1998). *Language learning impairment: Integrating research and remediation*. Retrieved September 25, 2008, from http://www.newhorizons.org/neuro/tallal.htm

Tallal, P. (n.d.). *Tallal Laboratory*. Retrieved September 25, 2008, from http://cmbn.rutgers.edu/research/tallal.aspx

Taney, R. B. (1864/2009). *Roger Brooke Taney.* Retrieved April 15, 2009, from http://en.wikipedia.org/wiki/Roger_Taney

Tarski, A. (1949). The semantic conception of truth. In H. Feigl & W. Sellars (Eds. and Trans.), *Readings in philosophical analysis* (pp. 341–374). New York: Appleton. (Original work published 1944).

Tarski, A. (1956). The concept of truth in formalized languages. In J. J. Woodger (Ed. and Trans.), *Logic, semantics, and metamathematics* (pp. 152–278). Oxford: Oxford University Press. (Original work published 1936)

Tennyson, A. L. (1870). *The charge of the light brigade* (poem). Retrieved April 15, 2009, from http://poetry.eserver.org/light-brigade.html

Terao, Y., Ugawa, Y., Yamamoto, T., Sakurai, Y., Masumoto, T., Abe, O., et al. (2007). Primary face motor area as the motor representation of articulation. *Journal of Neurology, 254*(4), 442–447.

Terpstra, F. G., van't Wout, A. B., Schuitemaker, H., van Engelenburg, F. A. C., Dekkers, D. W. C., Verhaar, R., et al. (2008). Potential and limitation of UVC irradiation for the inactivation of pathogens in platelet concentrates. *Transfusion, 48*(2), 304–313.

Terre, R., & Mearin, F. (2007). Videofluoroscopy quantification of laryngotracheal aspiration outcome in traumatic brain injury-related oropharyngeal dysphagia. *Revista Espanola de Enfermedades Digestivas, 99*(1), 7–12.

Tetanus. (2009). Retrieved April 15, 2009, from http://en.wikipedia.org/wiki/Tetanus

Thackray, R. I., & Touchstone, R. M. (1970). Recovery of motor performance following startle. *Perception and Motor Skills, 30,* 279–292.

Thorndike, R. M. (1997). *Measurement and evaluation in psychology and education* (6th ed.). New York: Prentice-Hall.

Thorndyke, P. W. (1977). Cognitive structures in comprehension and memory of narrative discourse. *Cognitive Psychology, 9,* 77–110.

Throneburg, R. N., Yairi, E., & Paden, E. (1994). Relation between phonologic difficulty and the occurrence of disfluencies in the early stage of stuttering. *Journal of Speech and Hearing Research, 37,* 504–509.

Tillery, K. L. (1998). Central auditory processing assessment and therapeutic strategies for children with attention deficit hyperactivity disorder. In M. G. Masters, N. A. Stecker, & J. Katz (Eds.), *Central auditory processing disorders: Mostly management* (pp. 175–194). Boston: Allyn & Bacon.

Titzer, R. C. (1997). *Infants' understanding of transparency: A reinterpretation of studies using the object retrieval task and visual cliff.* Ph.D. dissertation, Indiana University, Bloomington.

Titzer, R. C. (2009). *Your baby can read.* Retrieved April 15, 2009, from http://www.yourbabycanread.com/ce-y-about.aspx

Tocopherol. (2009). Retrieved April 15, 2009, from http://en.wikipedia.org/wiki/Tocopherol

Torppa, M., Poikkeus, A. M., Laakso, M. L., Tolvanen, A., Leskinen, E., Leppanen, P. H. T., et al. (2007) Modeling the early paths of phonological awareness and factors supporting its development in children with and without familial risk of dyslexia. *Scientific Studies of Reading, 11*(2), 73–103.

Tosteson, D. C., Adelstein, S. J., & Carver, S. T. (1994). *New pathways to medical education.* Cambridge, MA: Harvard University Press.

Trabasso, T., van den Broek, P., & Suh, S. (1989). Logical necessity and transitivity of causal relations in stories. *Discourse Processes, 12,* 1–25.

Transcortical motor aphasia. (2009). Retrieved April 15, 2009, from http://en.wikipedia.org/wiki/Transcortical_motor_aphasia

Tremblay, S., Shiller, D. M., & Ostry, D. J. (2003). Somatosensory basis of speech production. *Nature, 423*(6942), 866–869.

Tresilian, J. R., & Plooy, A. M. (2006). Effects of acoustic startle stimuli on interceptive action. *Neuroscience, 142*(2), 579–594.

Troncoso, X. G., Macknik, S. L., Otero-Milian, J., & Martinez-Conde, S. (2008). Microsaccades drive illusory motion in the Enigma illusion. *Proceedings of the National Academy of Sciences of the United States of America, 105*(41), 16033–16038.

Truffaut, F. (Director/Screenplay), & Itard, J. (Novel). (1969). *L'enfant sauvage* [Motion picture]. France: Les Films du Carrosse.

Turpin, G., Schaefer, F., & Boucsein, W. (1999). Effects of stimulus intensity, risetime, and duration on autonomic and behavioral responding: Implications for the differentiation of orienting, startle, and defense responses. *Psychophysiology, 36,* 453–463.

Umami. (2009). Retrieved April 15, 2009, from http://en.wikipedia.org/wiki/Umami

U.S. Court of Federal Claims. (n.d.). *Brochure with images and history.* Retrieved April 15, 2009, from http://www.uscfc.uscourts.gov/sites/default/files/court_info/Court_History_Brochure.pdf

U.S. Department of Justice Civil Rights Division. (n.d.). Retrieved April 15, 2009, from http://www.usdoj.gov/crt/ada/5yearadarpt/i_introduction.htm

U.S. Environmental Protection Agency. (2000). *Mercury compounds.* Retrieved April 15, 2009, from http://www.epa.gov/ttn/atw/hlthef/mercury.html

U.S. Holocaust Memorial Museum. (n.d.). *Mentally and physically handicapped: Victims of the Nazi era.* Retrieved April 15, 2009, from http://www.ushmm.org/education/resource/handic/handicapped.php?menu=/export/home/www/doc_root/education/foreducators/include/menu.txt&bgcolor=CD9544

U.S. Public Health Services (USPHS) and American Academy of Pediatrics (AAP). (1999, September). Joint Statement of the American Academy of Pediatrics (AAP) and the United States Public Health Service (USPHS). *Pediatrics, 104*(3), 568–569. Retrieved April 15, 2009, from http://www.putchildrenfirst.org/media/1.1.pdf

United States v. Fordice, 505 U.S. 717. (1992). Retrieved April 15, 2009, from http://www.law.cornell.edu/supct/html/historics/USSC_CR_0505_0717_ZS.html

University of California Regents v. Bakke, 438 U.S. 265. (1978). Retrieved April 15, 2009, from http://caselaw.lp.findlaw.com/scripts/getcase.pl?court=US&vol=438&invol=265

University of Maryland Medical Center. (2008). *Beta-carotene.* Retrieved September 25, 2008, from http://www.umm.edu/altmed/ConsSupplements/BetaCarotenecs.html#Dietary

University of Minnesota. (n.d.). *Mercury risk assessment.* Retrieved April 15, 2009, from http://enhs.umn.edu/hazards/hazardssite/mercury/mercriskassess.html

Urnovitz, H. B. (1996). *Summary of paper at the 8th Annual Houston Conference on AIDS.* Retrieved April 15, 2009, from http://www.whale.to/vaccines/sweet.html

Uversky, V. N., Li, J., & Fink, A. L. (2001). Metal-triggered structural transformations, aggregation, and fibrillation of human alpha-synuclein—A possible molecular link between Parkinson's disease and heavy metal exposure. *Journal of Biological Chemistry, 276*(47), 44284–44296.

Vaccine Adverse Event Reporting System. (1988). Retrieved April 15, 2009, from http://www.fda.gov/cber/vaers/faq.htm

VAERS. (1993–present). *Download the VAERS Database.* Retrieved April 15, 2009, from http://www.medalerts.org/vaersdb/access.html

Valette, R. M. (1967). *Modern language testing.* New York: Harcourt, Brace, and World.

Valicenti-McDermott, M., McVicar, K., Rapin, I., Wershil, B. K., Cohen, H., & Shinnar, S. (2006). Frequency of gastrointestinal symptoms in children with autistic spectrum disorders and association with family history of autoimmune disease. *Journal of Developmental and Behavioral Pediatrics, 27*(2, Suppl. S.), S128–S136.

Vallant, B., Deutsch, J., Muntean, M., & Goessler, W. (2008). Intravenous injection of metallic mercury: case report and course of mercury during chelation therapy with DMPS. *Clinical Toxicology, 46*(6), 566–569.

Valli, C., Lucas, C., & Mulrooney, K. (2005). *The linguistics of American Sign Language: An introduction* (4th ed.). Washington, DC: Gallaudet University.

Van Borsel, J., Reunes, G., & Van den Bergh, N. (2003). Delayed auditory feedback in the treatment of stuttering: Clients as consumers. *International Journal of Language and Communication Disorders, 38*(2), 119–129.

Van Borsel, J., Sunaert, R., & Engelen, S. (2005). Speech disruption under delayed auditory feedback in multilingual speakers. *Journal of Fluency Disorders, 30*(3), 201–217.

Van den Berg, J. W. (1958). Myoelastic-aerodynamic theory of voice production. *Journal of Speech and Hearing Research, 1*, 227–244.

Van Riper, C. (1957). *Voices past and present: Charles van Riper from the 1957 Panel discussion on "recovery," ASHA Convention—Cincinnati, Ohio.* Retrieved April 15, 2009, from http://www.mnsu.edu/comdis/voices/voices.html

Van Riper, C. (1973). *The treatment of stuttering.* Englewood Cliffs, NJ: Prentice-Hall.

Van Riper, C. (1991). A personal message. *Letting Go, 11*, 19–21. Retrieved April 15, 2009, from http://www.mnsu.edu/comdis/isad7/papers/bridgebuilders7/vanriper7.html

Venclikova, Z., Benada, O., Bartova, J., Joska, L., Mrklas, L., Prochazkova, J., et al. (2006, December). In vivo effects of dental casting alloys. *Neuroendocrinology Letters, 27*(Suppl. 1), 61–68.

Verstichel, P., Cambier, J., Masson, C., Masson, M., & Robine, B. (1994). Apraxia and autopoagnosia, without aphasia nor agraphia, and compulsive linguistic productions after a right-hemispheric lesion. *Revue Neurologique, 150*(4), 274–281.

Visetti Y. M., & Rosenthal, V. (2002). Human expression and experience: What does it mean to have language? *Behavioral and Brain Sciences, 25*(5), 643–644.

Vitamin C. (2009). Retrieved April 15, 2009, from http://en.wikipedia.org/wiki/Vitamin_C

Vocal hygiene. (2004). Retrieved April 15, 2009, from http://pvcrp.com/vocal_hygiene.php

Voelker, E. S., & Voelker, C. H. (1937). Spasmophemia in dyslalia cophotica. *Annals of Otology, Rhinology, and Laryngology, 46*, 740–743.

Vojdani, A., Pangborn, J. B., Vojdani, E., & Cooper, E. L. (2003). Infections, toxic chemicals and dietary peptides binding to lymphocyte receptors and tissue enzymes are major instigators of autoimmunity in autism. *International Journal of Immunopathology and Pharmacology, 16*(3), 189–199.

Vokshoor, A., & McGregor, J. (2006). *Anatomy of the olfactory system.* Retrieved April 15, 2009, from http://www.emedicine.com/ent/topic564.htm

Volz, T. J., Fleckenstein, A. E., & Hanson, G. R. (2007). Methamphetamine-induced alterations in monoamine transport: Implications for neurotoxicity, neuroprotection and treatment. *Addiction, 102*(Suppl. 1), 44–48.

von Békésy, G. (1960). *Experiments in hearing.* New York: McGraw-Hill.

von Tetzchner, S. (1997). Historical issues in intervention research: Hidden knowledge and facilitating techniques in Denmark. *European Journal of Disorders of Communication, 32*(1), 1–18.

Vygotsky, L. S. (1962). *Language and thought* (Ed. and Trans. by E. Hanfmann & G. Vakar). Cambridge, MA: Harvard University Press. (Original work in Russian published in 1934).

Vygotsky, L. S. (1978). *Mind in society: The development of higher psychological processes.* (Eds. and trans. from Russian by M. Cole, V. John-Steiner, S. Scribner, & E. Souberman). Cambridge, MA: Harvard University Press. (Original works published in Russian between 1930 and 1935).

Walton, G. E., & Bower, T. G. R. (1993). Amodal representation of speech in infants. *Infant Behavior and Development, 16*, 233–243.

Ward, G. (2004). Equatives and deferred reference. *Language, 80*(2), 262–289.

Warren, E. (1954). *Brown v. Board of Education, 347 U.S. 483 (1954).* Retrieved April 15, 2009, from http://www.nationalcenter.org/brown.html

Weems, S. A., & Reggia, J. A. (2006). Simulating single word processing in the classic aphasia syndromes based on the Wernicke-Lichtheim-Geschwind theory. *Brain and Language, 98*(3), 291–309.

Weigl, D. M., Arbel, N., Katz, K., Becker, T., & Bar-On, E. (2007). Botulinum toxin for the treatment of spasticity in children: attainment of treatment goals. *Journal of Pediatric Orthopaedics—Part B, 16*(4), 293–296.

Weiss, B., Clarkson, T. W., & Simon, W. (2002). Silent latency periods in methyl mercury poisoning and in neurodegenerative disease. *Environmental Health Perspectives, 110*(Suppl. 5), 851–854.

Weiss, D. (1964). *Cluttering.* Englewood Cliffs, NJ: Prentice-Hall.

Werker, J. F., & Tees, R. C. (1999). Influences on infant speech processing: Toward a new synthesis. *Annual Review of Psychology, 50*, 509–535.

Wernicke, C. (1977). *Wernicke's works on aphasia: A sourcebook and review* (G. H. Eggert, Ed. & Trans., pp. 87–283). The Hague: Mouton. (Original work published in German in 1874).

White, M. K., Gordon, J., Reiss, K., Del Valle, L., Croul, S., Giordano, A., et al. (2005). Human polyomaviruses and brain tumors. *Brain Research Reviews, 50*(1), 69–85.

Whitebread, G. (2004). *Stuck on the tip of my thumb: Stuttering in American Sign Language.* Unpublished honors thesis, Gallaudet University.

Wiener, N. (1948). *Cybernetics or control and communication in the animal and the machine.* Paris: Hermann et Cie; and Cambridge, MA: MIT Press.

Wilcox, S., & Wilcox, P. P. (1997) *Learning to see: Teaching American sign language as a second language* (2nd ed.). Washington, DC: Gallaudet University Press.

Wilcox, S. E., Scheibman, J., Wood, D., Cokely, D., & Stokoe, W. C. (2009). *Multimedia dictionary of American Sign Language.* Retrieved April 15, 2009, from http://portal.acm.org/citation.cfm?id=191031&coll=portal&dl=ACM&CFID=44481895&CFTOKEN=83467642

Wilkins, P. A. (1982). Effects of noise on people. In R. G. White & J. G. Walker (Eds.), *Noise and vibration.* New York: Wiley.

Willems, R. M., & Hagoort, P. (2007). Neural evidence for the interplay between language, gesture, and action: A review. *Brain and Language, 101*(3), 278–289.

Wills, G. F. (1979, April 16). As I was saying. *Newsweek,* 100.

Wiltshire, S. (2009a). *Beautiful minds: Stephen Wiltshire.* Retrieved April 15, 2009, from http://video.stumbleupon.com/#p=0k4lsi1dql.

Wiltshire, S. (2009b). *About Stephen.* Retrieved April 15, from http://www.stephenwiltshire.co.uk/

Windham, G. C., Zhang, L., Gunier, R., Croen, L. A., & Grether, J. K. (2006). Autism spectrum disorders in relation to distribution of hazardous air pollutants in the San Francisco Bay area. *Environmental Health Perspectives, 114*(9), 1438–1444.

Wingate, M. E. (1964). A standard definition of stuttering. *Journal of Speech and Hearing Research, 2*, 326–335.

Wingate, M. E. (1970). Effect on stuttering of changes in audition. *Journal of Speech and Hearing Research, 13*, 861–873.

Winstein, C. J. (1983). Neurogenic dysphagia: Frequency, progression, and outcome in adults following head injury. *Physical Therapy, 63*(12), 1992–1997.

Winston Churchill. (1965/2009). Retrieved April 15, 2009, from http://en.wikipedia.org/wiki/Winston_Churchill

Wojcik, D. P., Godfrey, M. E., Christie, D., & Haley, B. E. (2006). Mercury toxicity presenting as chronic fatigue, memory impairment and depression: Diagnosis, treatment, susceptibility, and outcomes in a New Zealand general practice setting (1994–2006). *Neuroendocrinology Letters, 27*(4), 415–423.

Wolman, C., van den Broek, P., & Lorch, R. (1997). Effects of causal structure on immediate and delayed story recall by children with mild mental retardation, children with learning disabilities, and children without disabilities. *Journal of Special Education, 30,* 439–455.

Woo, E. J., Ball, R., Landa, R., & Zimmerman, A. W. (2007). Developmental regression and autism reported to the vaccine adverse event reporting system. *Autism, 11*(4), 301–310.

Wood, E. (2007). *Evelyn Wood reading dynamics.* Retrieved April 15, 2009, from http://www.evelynwood.com.au/

Woods, S., Shearsby, J., Onslow, M., & Burnham, D. (2002). Psychological impact of the Lidcombe Program of early stuttering intervention. *International Journal of Language and Communication Disorders, 37*(1), 31–40.

World Health Organization. (n.d.). *Mercury in health care: Policy paper.* Retrieved April 15, 2009, from http://www.who.int/water_sanitation_health/medicalwaste/mercurypolpaper.pdf

World Health Organization. (2003). *Elemental mercury and inorganic mercury compounds: Human health aspects.* Retrieved April 15, 2009, from http://www.who.int/ipcs/publications/cicad/en/cicad50.pdf

World Health Organization. (2009). About the *International Classification of Diseases, Tenth Revision, Clinical Modification (ICD-10-CM).* Retrieved April 15, 2009, from http://www.cdc.gov/nchs/about/otheract/icd9/abticd10.htm

World Health Organization. (2009). *ICD-10-CM.* Retrieved April 15, 2009, from http://www.who.int/classifications/icd/en/

Wright, K. (2007). Foreword. In B. Jepson, B., & J. Johnson, *Changing the course of autism: A scientific approach for parents and physicians* (pp. xiii–xx). Boulder, CO: Sentient.

Wright, P. W. D., & Wright, P. D. (2009). Your child's IEP: Practical and legal guidance for parents. Retrieved April 15, 2009, from http://www.wrightslaw.com/advoc/articles/iep_guidance.html

Wright, P. W. D., Wright, P. D., & Heath, S. W. (2008). No Child Left Behind—Wrightslaw. Retrieved April 15, 2009, from http://www.wrightslaw.com/nclb/

Wu, J. C., Maguire, G., Riley, G., Fallon, J., Lacasse, L., Chin, S., et al. (1995). A positron emission tomography [f-18] deoxyglucose study of developmental stuttering. *Neuroreport, 6*(3), 501–505.

Wu, J. C., Maguire, G., Riley, G., Lee, A., Keator, D., Tang, C., et al. (1997). Increased dopamine activity associated with stuttering. *Neuroreport, 8*(3), 767–770.

Wu, Y. C., & Coulson, S. (2007). Iconic gestures prime related concepts: An ERP study. *Psychonomic Bulletin and Review, 14*(1), 57–63.

Yairi, E., & Ambrose, N. G. (2005). *Early childhood stuttering: For clinicians by clinicians.* Austin, TX: Pro-Ed.

Yan, J., Zhang, Y., & Ehret, G. (2005). Corticofugal shaping of frequency tuning curves in the central nucleus of the inferior colliculus of mice. *Journal of Neurophysiology, 93*(1), 71–83.

Yan, R. (2007). *Assessing English language proficiency in international aviation: Issues of reliability, validity, and aviation safety.* Unpublished doctoral dissertation, University of Louisiana at Lafayette.

Yan, R., & Oller, J. W., Jr. (2007). "Processing-Dependent Measures" as a failed solution to the assessment of individuals from language and dialect minorities. *Communication Disorders Review, 1*(3), 201–213.

Yang, Y., Raine, A., Narr, K. L., Lencz, T., LaCasse, L., Colletti, P., et al. (2007). Localization of increased prefrontal white matter in pathological liars. *British Journal of Psychiatry, 190,* 174–175.

Yao, Y. M., Walsh, W. J., McGinnis, W. R., & Pratico, D. (2006). Altered vascular phenotype in autism: Correlation with oxidative stress. *Archives of Neurology, 63*(8), 1161–1164.

Yaruss, J. S. (1998). Describing the consequences of disorders: Stuttering and the international classification of impairments, disabilities, and handicaps. *Journal of Speech, Language, and Hearing Research, 41,* 249–257.

Yaruss, J. S. (2006). What causes stuttering, and is there a cure? *Scientific American, 294*(3), 104.

Yauk, C. L., Berndt, L., Williams, A., Rowan-Carroll, A., Douglas, G. R., & Stampfli, M. R. (2007). Mainstream tobacco smoke causes paternal germ-line DNA mutation. *Cancer Research, 67*(11), 5103–5106.

Yerkes, R. M. (Ed.). (1921). *Psychological testing in the United States Army. National Academy of Sciences, Volume XV.* Washington, DC: Government Printing Office.

Yoakum, C. S., & Yerkes, R. M. (Eds.), (1920). *Army mental tests.* New York: Henry Holt and Company.

Yogi Berra. (2009). Official Web site. Retrieved April 15, 2009, from http://www.yogiberra.com/yogi-isms.html

Yokel, R. A. (2006). Blood-brain barrier flux of aluminum, manganese, iron and other metals suspected to contribute to metal-induced neurodegeneration. *Journal of Alzheimer's Disease, 10*(2–3), 223–253.

Yole, M., Wickstrom, M., & Blakley, B. (2007). Cell death and cytotoxic effects in YAC-1 lymphoma cells following exposure to various forms of mercury. *Toxicology, 231*(1), 40–57.

York, M. W. (2005, June). Comment on perceptual defense in anxiety disorders. *Perceptual and Motor Skills, 100*(3, Pt. 1), 839–840.

York, M. W., Rabinowitz, J. A., Burdick, K., Coffey, S., & Tongul, E. (1996). Predicting perceptual defense. *Perceptual and Motor Skills, 82*(1), 185–186.

Young stutterers fight prejudices. (2005, August 20). Retrieved April 15, 2009, from http://www.dw-world.de/dw/episode/0,1569,1683498,00.html

Zackheim, C. T., & Conture, E. G. (2003). Childhood stuttering and speech disfluencies in relation to children's mean length of utterance: A preliminary study. *Journal of Fluency Disorders, 28*, 115–142.

Zacks, J. M., Speer, N. K., Swallow, K. M., Braver, T. S., & Reynolds, J. R. (2007). Event perception: A mind-brain perspective. *Psychological Bulletin, 133*(2), 273–293.

Zahir, F., Rizwi, S. J., Haq, S. K., & Khan, R. H. (2005). Low dose mercury toxicity and human health. *Environmental Toxicology and Pharmacology, 20*(2), 351–360.

Zak, O. (2005). *Methods of communication with the Deaf.* Retrieved April 15, 2009, from http://www.zak.co.il/deaf-info/old/methods.html

Zapawa, J. E., & Alcantara, A. L. (n.d.). *Radiologic anatomy: Welcome to the brain module.* Retrieved April 15, 2009, from http://www.med.wayne.edu/diag Radiology/Anatomy_Modules/brain/brain.html

Zarei, M., Johansen-Berg, H., Smith, S., Ciccarelli, O., Thompson, A. J., & Matthews, P. M. (2006). Functional anatomy of interhemispheric cortical connections in the human brain. *Journal of Anatomy, 209*(3), 311–320.

Zemeckis, R. (Director), Groom, W. (Screenplay), & Roth, E. (Screenplay). (1994). *Forrest Gump* [Motion picture]. United States: Paramount Pictures.

Zentz, R. (2006, September 6). *Comments of Dr. Ronald R. Zentz.* Retrieved April 15, 2009, from http://www.ada.org/public/media/presskits/fillings/testimony_zentz.pdf

Zhang, Q., & Haydon, P. G. (2005). Roles for gliotransmission in the nervous system. *Journal of Neural Transmission, 112*(1), 121–125.

Zifan, A., Gharibzadeh, S., & Moradi, M. H. (2007). Could dynamic attractors explain associative prosopagnosia? *Medical Hypotheses, 68*(6), 1399–1405.

Zimmerman, E. K., Eslinger, P. J., Simmons, Z., & Barrett, A. M. (2007). Emotional perception deficits in amyotrophic lateral sclerosis. *Cognitive and Behavioral Neurology, 2*(2), 79–82.

Zoroglu, S. S., Armutcu, F., Ozen, S., Gurel, A., Sivasli, E., Yetkin, O., & Meram, I. (2004). Increased oxidative stress and altered activities of erythrocyte free radical scavenging enzymes in autism. *European Archives of Psychiatry and Clinical Neuroscience, 254*(3), 143–147.

Zwaan, R. A. (1994). Effect of genre expectations on text comprehension. *Journal of Experimental Psychology: Learning, Memory, and Cognition, 20*, 920–933.

Index

A

Abdesslem, H. 622, 703
abducted 252, 274, 671
Abe, N. 41, 508, 703
Abe, O. 737
Abell, R. B. 209, 653, 654, 703
ability tracking system 594, 609, 671
abortion 52, 69, 73, 76, 77, 80, 81, 596, 662, 670, 686, 691, 703, 708, 711, 717, 722, 727, 730, 732, 733, 736
Abraham Lincoln 110, 118, 130, 352, 449, 595, 598–602, 604, 637, 680, 716, 724, 728
absolute pitch 368, 387, 671, 692, 721
abstractness 2, 20, 338, 511, 537, 557, 558, 671
Accardo, P. J. 358, 724
acetylcholine 142, 187, 224, 252, 296, 303, 304, 671, 689
acid reflux 252, 284, 310, 671
acoustic phonetics 312, 317, 363, 671, 675, 695
acquired disorder 671
acquired dyslexia 424, 439, 522, 671
acquired immune deficiency syndrome 476, 545, 671, 672, 689

acute disseminated encephalomyelitis 198, 199
Ad Hoc Committee on Scope of Practice 667, 703, 704
Adams, J. B. 220, 224, 662, 721
Adamson, M. J. 448, 712
adducted 252, 274, 276, 671
Adelstein, S. J. 46, 738
Adolf Hitler 531, 573, 575, 596–598, 684
Adolphs, R. 500, 712
adrenoleukodystrophy 2, 476, 478, 543, 671
adverse impact 594, 641, 672
afferent nerve fibers 142, 186, 672
afferent nerves 2, 29, 181, 672
Afshar, K. 259, 735
agnosias 98, 476, 518, 521–523, 525, 526, 529, 536, 539, 541, 550, 551, 672
AIDS 198, 223, 284, 448, 476, 545, 546, 548, 615, 633, 672, 684, 689, 695, 711, 739
Ainswort, W. A. 447, 448, 703
Aitken, J. E. 642, 703
Akyol, O. 736
Alcantara, A. L. 489, 533, 742
Aldersley, S. 623, 624, 630, 703
Aldridge, M. A. 151, 703
Aleka Titzer 11, 425, 429–433, 442, 443, 466, 473, 518, 703
Alexander, L. 69, 70, 88, 100, 703

alexia 424, 439, 462, 476, 513, 522, 672, 696, 698, 735
Alibali, M. W. 255, 525, 719
alien hand syndrome 252, 265, 672, 678, 707, 722
Alimonti, A. 707
Allen, A. J. 722
Allen, D. D. 716
Allen, G. E. 573, 703, 704
allophones 424, 451, 672
alphabetic principle 312, 345, 346, 424, 430, 451–453, 456, 672
alphabetic writing system 128, 344, 672
Alsop, D. 706
Alter, W. 705
Altman, C. H. 239, 722
Altschuler, R. A. 191, 732
alveolar ridge 312, 327, 672
Alzheimer's disease 6, 202, 223–225, 294, 297, 546, 672, 689, 696, 704, 707, 713, 721, 727, 741
Amand, P. 725
Ambrose, N. G. 704, 741
Amedi, A. 706
American Academy of Audiology 662, 704
American Academy of Pediatrics 120, 208, 230, 249, 704, 738
American Academy of Special Education Professionals 663, 704

American Counseling Association 663, 665, 667, 704

American Dental Association 226, 230, 237, 249, 250, 543, 704

American Diabetes Association 64, 704

American Medical Association 388, 658, 664, 704, 734

American Psychiatric Association 205, 609, 646, 658, 664, 695, 704

American Psychological Association 657, 659, 663, 665, 704

American School for the Deaf 129, 704

American Sign Language (ASL) 104, 122, 124, 341, 342, 672, 704, 739, 740

American Speech-Language-Hearing Association 47, 657, 658, 675, 703, 704

American Stroke Association 705

Americans with Disabilities Act of 1990 594, 614, 640, 704, 705

amino acids 198, 219, 671, 672, 674, 680

amniocentesis 142, 147, 672

amplitude 142, 167, 178, 182, 187, 279, 321, 322, 672, 677, 678, 698

amyloid plaques 224, 225, 705

amyotrophic lateral sclerosis 198, 202, 294, 543, 546, 672, 687, 726, 737, 742

Anaki, D. 531, 705

Anantharam, V. 721

Andersen, D. H. 65, 705

Anderson, F. 203, 710, 726, 735

anosmia 52, 88, 672

antioxidants 198, 222, 672

anxiety disorder 142, 672

Aoki, S. 737

aphasic jargon 476, 485, 672

apoplexy 476, 672

Aposhian, H. V. 227, 705

Aposhian, M. M. 227, 705

applied behavior analysis 198, 211, 236, 243, 671, 672

apraxia 93, 94, 98, 99, 264, 265, 286, 299, 300, 359, 518, 536, 537, 539, 541, 551, 672, 698, 710, 731, 739

Arbel, N. 740

Archer, T. 546, 730

Arehole, S. 149, 729

Arky, R. A. 727

Armstrong, D. F. 317, 318, 341, 705

Armutcu, F. 742

Arnoux, Y. V. 707

Arons, B. 705, 414, 705

Aronson, A. R. 286, 712

Aronson, E. 184, 732

arrhythmia 476, 543, 672

articulator 142, 313, 327, 673

articulatory phonetics 312, 316, 321, 332, 673

Aschner, M. 229, 237, 239, 550, 721, 727

Ashida, I. 719

ASL 104, 122, 124–129, 177, 316, 397, 672, 704

Asperger syndrome 198, 211, 212, 214, 424, 673, 691

Asperger's disorder 198, 211, 673

aspiration pneumonia 252, 259, 260, 673, 735

assimilation 312, 337, 338, 673, 695

assistive technology 594, 642, 673

asymmetry 368, 387, 673

asymptomatic 476, 544, 673

ataxic dysarthria 298, 673, 736

Atianjoh, F. E. 479, 705

Atkinson, N. P. 715

atrophy 252, 290, 673, 684, 692

attention deficit disorder 142, 206, 671, 673

attention deficit hyperactivity disorder 671, 673, 738

audible electronic text 104, 121, 673

audiologists 71, 175, 198, 203, 323, 657, 658, 663, 665, 673

audition 142, 165, 673, 740

auditory discrimination 142, 165, 167, 673

auditory illusions 476, 503, 673

auditory pattern recognition 142, 165, 167, 673

auditory phonetics 312, 317, 673

auditory processing 142, 162, 165, 172, 175, 176, 186, 188, 191, 195, 673, 698, 704, 710, 715, 721, 727, 728, 731, 738

auditory recognition 142, 168, 673

Auther, A. M. 711

autism 2, 3, 5, 6, 32, 43, 46, 48, 49, 60, 68, 88, 99, 104, 107, 120, 131, 140, 143, 174, 195, 197–218, 220–223, 225, 227–236, 238–242, 245, 248–250, 307, 309, 332, 354, 358, 359, 375, 424, 428, 455, 478, 505, 548, 556, 560, 594, 596, 632, 633, 639, 643, 647, 651–655, 669, 670, 673, 674, 681, 683–686, 691, 704–706, 708–710, 713–730, 732–736, 739–742

Autism Developmental Disabilities Monitoring Network 705

Autism Society of America 705

Autism Speaks 48, 211, 705

autism spectrum disorders 198, 201–203, 206, 213, 216, 217, 225, 229, 358, 673, 705, 708, 724, 740

autoimmune disease 303, 476, 547, 674, 739

autoimmunity 198, 220, 223, 547, 674, 739

autonomic nervous system 2, 23, 25, 91, 92, 266, 269, 287, 671, 674

autopsy 476, 481, 483, 674

aversive stimuli 198, 244, 674

axial 476, 490–492, 496, 532, 534, 674–677

axon 252, 288, 674, 685, 737

Axthelm, M. K. 545, 712

Azar, B. 705

B

Backlund, H. 520, 705

Bacon, B. A. 730

Badon, L. C. 14, 31, 34, 37, 39, 40, 52, 61, 132, 143, 146, 149, 185, 319, 323, 332, 354, 356, 361, 392, 398, 524, 573, 622, 705, 729

Bailey 209, 544, 653, 703, 705, 723

Bailey, A. 723

Bailey, D. M. 705

Baillet, S. 185, 713

Bairros, A. V. 715

Bajaj, A. 405, 410, 705

Baker J. 705

Baker, L. A. 737

Bakker, K. 419, 736

Balasubramanian, V. 418, 706

Baldwin, D. A. 213, 342, 727

Baler, R. D. 280, 706

Ball, M. J. 315, 430, 706
Ball, R. 740
Ballard, D. H. 62, 706
Banerjee, S. 29, 706
Bannister, R. xv, 230, 233, 564, 565, 706, 733
Baranoski, M. 41, 506–508, 713
Baratz, J. 177, 706
Barbeau, E. 264, 706
Barden, D. 239, 709
Bargh, J. A. 17, 710
Barker, A. 227, 228, 730
Barlow, B. K. 297, 706
Barnes, G. 266, 268, 720
Barnhart, C. L. 430, 431, 441, 443, 707
Barr, A. 725
Barr, L. 6, 226, 227, 706
Barregard, L. 706
Barrett, A. M. 742
Barry, W. 386, 416, 719
Barsalou, L. W. 62, 706
Barshatzky, M. 710
Bartova, J. 739
Bartsch, P. 705
Barwise, J. 355, 706
basal ganglia 252, 295–298, 394, 674, 698, 699
Basile, V. S. 731
Basinger, D. 15, 729
Battle Hymn of the Republic 706
Bauer, A. 214, 706
Baux, G. 181, 725
Baysang, G. 729
Baztan, J. J. 731
BBC News Channel 706
Bech, S. 731
Becker, D. P. 88, 711
Becker, H. 706
Becker, T. 306, 740
Bedrossian, C. W. M. 545, 709
Beebe, B. 148, 336, 720
behaviorism 198, 244, 674, 681, 685, 692, 695
Bellinger, D. C. 226, 706
Bell's palsy 252, 292, 294, 674
Benada, O. 739
Beninger R. J. 730
Bennett, M. V. L. 708
Benson, J. D. 19, 706
Bentivoglio, M. 181, 706
Benveniste, H. 280, 706

Benzecry, J. 332, 713
Bergmann, C. 358, 706
Bermpohl, F. 183, 706
Bernard, S. 22, 229, 231, 383, 706
Berndt, L. 741
Bernier, A. 725
Bernoulli effect 252, 276, 674
Bernstein-Ratner, N. 706
Bersoff, D. N. 597, 659, 706
Bertoncini, J. 16, 35, 323, 728
beta amyloid 674
beta-carotene 222, 674, 739
Bever, T. G. 122, 733
Bhat, M. A. 29, 706
Bickerton, D. 333, 706
Biklen, D. 120, 706
bilabial 312, 326, 335, 358, 674
Bill of Rights xii, 80, 578, 595, 607, 656, 657, 706
bimoraic 312, 322, 674
binaural hearing 142, 166, 674
Binet, A. 579, 618, 646, 706
Bingaman, W. 724
Binstock, T. 229, 706
Biran, I. 265, 707
Birdwhistell, R. 350, 707
Birnholz, J. 147, 707
Björk, E. A. 193, 707
Black, J. P. 710
Black, J. W. 383–385, 387, 391, 707
Blair, Tony 531
Blakley, B. 228, 741
Blass, E. M. 35, 707
Blaxill, A. 718
Blaxill, M. 229, 706
Bleich, A. 718
Bloodstein, O. 386, 391, 392, 396, 404, 707
Bloom 17, 631, 707, 725, 736
Bloom, A. S. 631, 707
Bloom, F. E. 736
Bloom, K. 17, 725
Bloomfield, L. 349, 351, 352, 356, 430–432, 441–443, 452, 524, 698, 707
Blotcky, A. J. 297, 707
Blume, H. 598, 708
Bobes, M. A. 530, 707
Bocca, B. 546, 707
Bocca, E. 174, 707
Bodaghi, B. 227, 228, 234, 707
Boeing 7, 707

Boelens, H. 409, 715
Bohland, J. W. 254, 707
Bohrer, D. 715
Boldrey, E. 490, 731
Bolhuis, J. J. 12, 18, 707, 719
Bollich, A. M. 715
Bomboi, G. 707
Boniver, V. 725
Boon, F. 130, 724
Boorstin, J. 342, 707
Booth, J. W. 600, 601, 707
Borgeat, F. 182, 707, 732
Bornstein, H. 125, 708
Borton, R. W. 726
Bosshardt, H. 393, 708
Boswell, J. 597, 708
Bothe, A. K. 386, 401, 402, 715, 721
Botox 252, 305, 308, 674, 708
bottom-up processing 164, 674
botulinum neurotoxin 252, 306, 674, 676, 719
botulism 252, 305, 480, 674
Boucsein, W. 738
Bower, T. G. R. xi, xiii, 35, 145–147, 151, 703, 708, 721, 740
Bradford, P. V. 708
Bradley, W. G. 726
Bradshaw, J. L. 265, 717
Braff, D. L. 194, 737
Braille, L. 87, 90, 95, 104, 109–121, 124, 128, 129, 135, 137–140, 438, 562, 563, 574, 588, 594, 651, 683, 694, 708, 718, 722, 733
Braille writing 111, 438, 588, 708
brain-stem 142, 186, 188, 194, 292, 295, 518, 674, 675, 677, 687, 688, 701
Bramlett, R. E. 386, 715, 721
branchial arch syndromes 52, 66, 674
Branigan, E. 342, 708
Bransfield, R. C. 200, 708
Bravaccio, C. 709
Braver, T. S. 470, 741
breath group 674, 702
Bremner, A. P. 306, 733
Bridgeman Art Library v. Corel Corp. 708
Brigham, C. C. 580, 708
Brimacombe, M. 726
British Broadcasting Company 34, 708

British Dyslexia Association 435, 708

Britt, L. D. 714

broadened criteria theory of autism 198, 211–213, 674

Broca, P. P. 312, 359, 476, 481–484, 487, 489, 498, 509, 512, 514–516, 536, 672, 674, 699, 708, 725

Broca's aphasia 312, 359, 481, 512, 536, 674, 708

Broca's area 476, 481, 483, 514–516, 672, 674, 699, 725

Brockhaus, M. 729

Brodman, K. 489, 708

Brodmann's areas xiv, 488, 489, 515, 708

Brook, M. L. 508, 736

Brooks, B. R. 726

Brooks, R. B. 659, 708

Brookshire, R. H. 515, 700, 708

Brossard, N. 728

Brown v. Board of Education 606, 607, 612, 708, 740

Brown, A. M. 708

Brown, J. R. 712

Brown, M. C. 723

Brown, W. T. 710

Bruce Willis 213, 370, 708

Bruce, D. C. 705

Bruner, 132, 356, 708

Bruner, Joseph 38, 71, 72, 75, 708

Bruner, Jerome S. 708

Brunotto, M. 285, 708

Buchanan, L. H. 227, 711

bulbar palsy 252, 292–295, 675, 694, 722, 732

bulbar region 252, 294, 675

Bullock, T. H. 181, 708

Burau, D. 68, 726

Burbacher, T. M. 233, 708

Burchfiel, C. M. 710

Burdick, K. 182, 741

Burghaus L. 708

Burman, C. xiv, 517, 521, 530, 708

Burnham, D. 409, 740

Burns, M. S. 451, 736

Burr, C. W. 513, 708

Bush, George W. 77, 214, 531, 732

Bushnell, I. W. R. 35, 520, 705, 708

Bushnell, M. C. 705

Busner, J. 722

Butler, S. R. 262, 708

Butovskaya, M. L. 709

Buttigieg, G. A. 716

Buxbaum, L. 265, 707

Buyske, S. 709

C

C. Everett Koop 71, 82, 100, 709

Cabrera, S. 239, 709

Cadet, J. L. 479, 705

Cadwell, S. 741

Cain, D. P. 724

Caldarulo, M. 716

Calearo, C. 174, 707

Cally, R. W. 239, 722

calligrapher 104, 109, 675

Cambier, J. 739

Cameron, D. 301, 725

Camp, C. A. 35, 707

Campbell, D. B. 5, 206, 216, 218, 250, 709

Campbell, S. xi, xii, 12, 34, 709

Campbell, T. 177, 569–572, 574, 578, 653, 709

Campbell-Smith, P. 653

Campello, C. 711

Cannell, S. J. 328, 330, 424, 425, 438, 457–459, 658, 709

canonical babble 424, 425, 428, 560, 675, 701

Caputi, F. 27, 709

Carbon, C. C. 281, 530, 531, 709

Carbone, M. 545, 709

Carbone, V. 245–248

carcinogenic qualities 252, 280, 675

Carlsen, W. 545, 709

Carpi, A. 220, 709

Carroll, J. B. 581, 709

Carroll, L. 485, 486, 692, 709, 720, 732, 741

Carver, S. T. 46, 738

Carvey, P. M. 297, 709

case law 594, 612, 640, 675, 686

case studies 554, 584, 675

Cassinari, V. 174, 707

Cavalcanti, M. G. P. 66, 725

Cave, S. 208, 216, 223, 226, 227, 231, 233, 409, 633, 635, 644, 709

CDC 198, 201–210, 213, 215, 217, 225, 227, 230, 233, 261, 596, 632–636, 643, 647, 653, 654, 670, 675, 703, 705, 709, 740

Cederlund, M. 211, 717

Cedrola, S. 227, 709

Cellini, C. 716

Center for Biologics Evaluation and Research 715

Centers for Disease Control 198, 201, 205, 233, 249, 281, 634, 643, 675, 703, 709, 715

central auditory processes 142, 165, 675

central nervous system (CNS) 675

central sulcus 2, 27, 675, 681, 689, 690, 696

cerebellar ataxia 198, 240, 675

cerebellum 2, 27, 188, 290, 295, 296, 298, 675, 736

cerebral palsy 2, 48, 270, 297, 305, 306, 384, 625, 626, 630, 675, 733

cerebrum 142, 188, 295, 298, 675, 677, 686

Cernichiari, E. 706, 708

Certificate of Clinical Competence in Speech-Language Pathology 667, 675, 704

cesarean section 52, 71, 675

ceteris paribus principle 554, 585, 586, 588–590, 675, 677

Chadwick, R. S. 180, 709

Chamberlain, D. 78, 710

Chambon, M. 628, 710

Champoux, F. 730

Chandrashekar, D. J. J. 88, 710

Charles, L. E. 710

Chartrand, T. L. 17, 710

Chatterjee, A. 265, 707

Chau, W. 713

Chaudhuri, J. 716

Chauhan, A. 218–220, 710

Chauhan, V. 218–220, 710

Cheatham, M. A. 187, 712

chelation therapy 198, 238, 308, 675, 716, 739

Chen, C. S. 306, 710

Chen, L. xii, 37, 39, 62, 157, 161, 313, 348, 362, 400, 460, 470, 471, 524, 590, 710, 723, 729, 730

Chen, R. T. 633, 710

Chermak, G. D. 163, 165, 710, 731

Cherokee 347, 710

Cherry, S. R. 491, 710

Chertkow, H. 182, 736

Chian, D. 228, 719

Chiat, S. 432, 710

childhood aphasia 476, 536, 675
childhood apraxia 536, 710
Childress, A. R. 723
Chimenti, C. 716
Chin, J. 224, 730
Chin, S. 741
Choe, Y. 577, 581, 582, 729
Choisser, B. 710
Chomsky, N. A. 19, 24, 47, 61, 105, 146, 156, 244, 315, 337, 338, 356, 379, 393, 396, 430, 451, 692, 710, 715
Christ, S. 705
Christie, D. 237, 740
Christopher Burke 478, 710
chromosome 2, 59, 65, 66, 216, 358, 675, 679, 682
chronological narrative order 424, 469, 675
Churchill, Winston 369, 418, 424, 531, 595, 596, 725, 740, 741
Ciccarelli, O. 741
Cicilline, D. N. 628, 710
Cismondi, I. A. 708
civil litigation 594, 655, 675
Civil Rights Act of 1964 561, 607, 613, 616–619, 641, 644, 648, 710
Claassen, J. P. 297, 707
Clancy, M. xi, xiii, 71, 72, 74, 76, 77, 79, 710
Clarkson, T. W. 230, 231, 636, 708, 711, 740
Claus, B. 134, 470, 711, 721
Cleeremans, A. 185, 734
cleft palate 48, 51, 52, 56, 68, 80, 82, 85, 358, 360, 676, 684, 703, 711, 736
Cleft Palate Foundation 711
clinical neurology 252, 304, 676
cloning 476, 548, 549, 676
Clostridium botulinum 252, 305, 306, 674, 676, 711
Clostridium tetani 252, 304, 676, 700
cluster reduction 312, 336, 676
cluttering xii, 368, 417–419, 676, 699, 736, 740
coarticulation 312, 336, 337, 676
cochlear implant 142, 175, 711
cochlear nuclei vi, 142, 188, 190–194, 676
Cochran, A. A. 713
Code of Ethics 594, 662–668, 676, 680, 684, 704

codon 2, 676
Coffey, S. 182, 741
cognitive momentum 142, 159, 160, 676
Cohen, H. 739
Cohen, I. L. 220, 710
Cohn, J. F. 13, 734
Cokely, D. 128, 740
Cole, M. 740
Colin, J. 604, 707
Colletti, P. 741
Collins, D. F. 193, 544, 708, 711
Comar, M. 546, 711
commissure 476, 510, 676, 698
commissurotomy 476, 536, 537, 676, 682, 698, 734
communication disorder 2, 4, 64, 370, 411, 613, 662, 676
comorbidity iii, 52, 60, 62, 100, 174, 299, 515, 676
competing acoustic signals 142, 165, 676
computed axial tomography 476, 490, 675–677
computed tomography 490, 677, 711
concordance rates 198, 216, 676
Condon, W. S. 16, 37, 79, 148, 332, 333, 711
conduction aphasia 476, 513, 676
congenital anomalies 52, 71, 676
congenital disorders 476, 478, 676
Connaghan, K. P. 271, 711
consent decree 594, 610, 676
consistency requirement 554, 589, 590, 676, 693
consonant cluster 252, 271, 676
consonants 85, 86, 158, 170, 312, 323, 324, 326, 327, 444, 566, 673, 676, 677, 687, 692, 695, 696, 699
contact ulcer 677
content words 368, 392, 481, 677, 682, 699, 719
continuous reinforcement 198, 244, 677
contralateral 252, 264, 290, 476, 517, 677
contralateral pathways 476, 517, 677
control group 393, 554, 585, 586, 677, 679, 701
Conture, E. G. 392, 396, 724, 726, 741

conventional 2, 10, 39, 323, 356, 363, 557, 558, 677, 699
conventions 10, 11, 104, 116
conversation analysis ix, 312, 330, 677, 717
Cook, D. A. 115, 731, 736
Cooper, E. L. 220, 739
Cooper, R. P. 35, 727
Coppola, M. 122, 734
Corbera, S. 389, 711
Cordes, A. K. 401, 402, 711, 720
Corey, D. M. 712, 715
Cornblatt, B. A. 711
coronal 476, 533, 534, 677
corpus callosum 252, 262, 264, 265, 268, 295, 308, 476, 500, 501, 517, 518, 523, 535–539, 550, 676, 677, 698, 706, 716, 721, 731, 734
Corral, M. J. 389, 711, 730
Correll, C. U. 294, 711
cortical deafness 142, 174, 513, 677, 707
cortical functions 2, 29, 302, 677, 695, 724
corticospinal tract 252, 287, 677, 681, 686, 694
Costa, L. 88, 407, 711, 730
Costanzo, R. M. 88, 711
Coulson, S. 342, 741
Council on Professional Standards 704
Counter, S. A. 128, 170, 172, 222, 227, 245, 264, 284, 463, 539, 625, 630, 643, 711, 726
Cousin, J. W. 130, 461, 486, 711
covert repair hypothesis 368, 394, 395, 399, 677
Cox, C. 122, 124, 128, 129, 231, 317, 318, 341, 705, 711, 740
cranial nerves xiv, 252, 290–293, 675, 677, 690, 694
craniofacial anomalies iii, iv, 51, 52, 54, 56, 68, 82, 677
craniosynostosis 52, 58, 677
cranium 52, 57, 73, 677
Cremer, L. 718
Crick, F. 711
Croen, L. A. 740
Crohn's disease 252, 284, 677
Crossley, R. 120, 711
Crotty, M. 733
Croul, S. 740
Crown, C. L. 148, 336, 720

Cruse, H. 355, 722
Crutcher, M. 76, 711
Crystal, D. 62, 444, 711
Culotta, V. C. 546, 711
Cummins, J. 568, 577, 581, 622, 647, 712
Custance, D. M. 12, 733
Cutler 220, 333, 712, 720
Cutler, A. 333, 712
Cutler, P. 220, 720
cybernetics 368, 385, 677, 740
cycle of abstraction 424, 427, 677
cystic fibrosis 52, 63–65, 677, 705
cytoarchitecture 476, 489, 677

D

D'Agaro, P. 711
da Silveira, C. B. 66, 725
DAF 368, 383–387, 389–391, 399, 420, 677
Dafre, A. L. 715
Daguerre, L. 489, 712
Daibo, I. 37, 722
Dale, R. 330, 733
Dallos, P. 187, 712
Damasio, A. 524, 531, 534, 712
Damasio, H. 494, 500, 524, 531, 712
Damico, J. S. 37, 362, 363, 459, 712, 729
Damico, S. K. 712
damp 142, 167, 677
Damper, R. I. 447, 448, 452, 712
Dang, X. 545, 712
Daniel, D. 706
Daniel, S. 297, 731
Dantzig, P. I. 546, 712
Darbinyan, A. 740
Darley, F. L. 254, 286, 299, 380, 712
Dart, R. C. 705
Darwin, C. 130, 598, 712
Daschner, F. 229, 237, 550, 727
Daubert v. Merrell Dow Pharmaceuticals 647, 712
David, H. 707
Davidson, D. 39, 712
Davis, C. 713
Davis, R. 74, 712
Davis, R. L. 710
Dawson, M. 48, 716
Dax, M. 481–483, 725
Day, J. J. 712
Dayalu, V. 386, 737

de Divitiis, E. 27, 709
De Felice, F. G. 224, 715
De Gelfo, A. M. Z. 708
De Halac, R. I. N. 708
de Jong, K. 315, 316, 334, 335, 712, 727, 735
de Korte, D. 738
De Nil, L. 394, 712, 713
de Saussure, F. 177, 318, 319, 337, 713, 715
de Venecia, R. K. 190, 723
Debashish, M. 706
decoding 348, 424, 434, 453, 677, 705
decussation of pyramids 252, 290, 677
degenerate 316, 476, 502, 524, 678
degraded acoustic signals 142, 678
Dehaene, S. 79, 185, 713
Dekkers, D. W. C. 738
Del Cul, A. 185, 713
Del Valle, L. 740
delay technique 198, 247, 248, 678
delayed auditory feedback 368, 383, 384, 399, 411, 420, 421, 677, 678, 716, 739
delayed side-tone 383, 678, 707
DeLeon 38, 713
DeLeon, J. 713
delusional pathology 2, 41, 508, 678
Demanez, J. P. 725
Demanez, L. 725
dementia pugilistica 476, 479, 678, 688
dendrites 252, 288, 678
dental amalgam 2, 6, 60, 223, 225–229, 233, 236, 237, 240, 249, 308, 543, 545, 547, 550, 596, 678, 704–706, 714
Denton, M. B. 716
Derakhshan, I. 713
derived signed languages 104, 124, 678
Deth, R. 332, 713
detoxification systems 2, 23, 678
Deutsch, J. 239, 739
Deutsche Welle 713
developmental regression 2, 4, 678, 740
developmental stuttering 368, 391, 392, 411, 418–421, 678, 685, 691, 711, 714, 715, 741

Dewey, J. 2, 713
Di Monte, D. A. 718
diabetes mellitus 52, 63, 64, 678
diacritic 312, 327, 346, 678
diadochokinesis 312, 335, 678
diagonistic dyspraxia 252, 264, 678, 706
Diana v. California State Board of Education 609, 620, 713
Dickens, C. 105, 106, 131, 669, 713
Dickson, R. 722
Dickson, S. V. 450, 710
Didinium nasutum 713
Digital Anatomist Project xiv, 514, 713
digital text 104, 121, 673, 678
Dike, C. C. 41, 505–508, 713
DiLollo, A. 369, 403, 713
DiLorenzo, T. J. 601, 713
dimercaptuosuccinic acid 198, 239, 678, 679
discourse processing 355, 364, 368, 411, 453, 456, 459, 460, 465, 511, 524, 527, 678
discrepancy approach 424, 436, 437, 449, 473, 678
discriminated symbol 424, 428, 679
disfluencies 368, 377, 378, 380, 382, 390, 395, 396, 401–403, 407, 409, 415, 417–419, 679, 698, 711, 738, 741
disproportionate representation problem 554, 555, 572, 591, 679
dissimilation 312, 337, 338, 679, 695
distributed neural networks 142, 679
distributed processing 142, 164, 679
District Courts of the United States 713
Dixon, J. 66, 724
Dixon, M. J. 66, 724
dizygotic twins 198, 216, 368, 375, 679
DMSA 198, 239, 679, 716, 727
Doe v. Withers 618, 645, 713
Dollaghan, C. 177, 709
Domenech, J. 731
Domingo J. L. 713
Don Z. M. 714
Dong, J. 714, 718
Dong, J. H. 718

dopamine 252, 296, 297, 368, 394, 679, 699, 705, 709, 718, 732, 741

Douglas, G. R. 741

Douglas, Stephen A. 598, 599, 604, 613, 724

Down syndrome 52, 63, 65, 66, 210, 354, 478, 546, 679, 723, 728

Dred Scott decision 594, 599, 601, 605, 606, 679

Drescher, D. G. 191, 713, 721

Drescher, M. J. 191, 713, 721

Dronca, E. 730

Dronca, M. 730

dual–tasks 393, 679

Duda, J. E. 294, 713

Duffy, J. 286, 713

Dumont, M. 182, 707

Dunlap, K. 184, 713, 721

Dunn, D. E. 190, 727

Dunning, M. 214, 713

Dupoux, E. 336, 722

dysarthria 92, 252, 286, 290, 292, 293, 295, 297–300, 310, 364, 673, 679, 681, 684, 688, 697, 698, 701, 736

dysfluencies 97, 254, 368, 377, 679

dysgraphia 424, 439, 679, 728

dysosmia 52, 88, 672, 679

dysostosis 52, 58, 66, 679, 687

dyspraxia 252, 264, 265, 678, 679, 706

Dziewas, R. 263, 269, 713

D'Entremont, B. 16, 713

D'Souza, Y. 241, 713

E

Easterling, C. S. 302, 713

Ebert, P. J. 709

Edlich, R. F. 199, 203, 223, 234, 309, 654, 713, 714

Education of All Handicapped Children Act of 1975 714

Education of the Handicapped Act Amendments of 1983 714

Education of the Handicapped Amendments of 1986 714

Edwards, M. L. 396, 724, 735

effect size 554, 586, 679

efferent nerve fibers 2, 29, 142, 186, 679

Ehler, D. J. 577, 714

Ehrich, M. 227, 228, 730

Eilers, R. E. 15, 122, 714, 729

Einarsdttir, E. 370, 714

Einstein, A. 7, 11, 29, 50, 52, 96, 424, 425, 473, 595, 714, 727, 728

Ejiri, K. 333, 426, 714

Ekman, P. 350, 714

electromyography 368, 394, 679

electron 198, 220, 221, 285, 288, 491, 546, 679, 692–694

Elia, M. 530, 697, 705, 709

elicited imitation 142, 177, 679

Elie, R. 182, 736

El-Imam, Y. A. 447, 448, 452

elision 312, 336, 679

ellipsis 312, 336, 679, 680

Elster, E. 424, 714

Emancipation Proclamation 594, 595, 602–604, 606, 680

embodiment 312, 355, 356, 680, 706, 717, 719

embryological development 52, 54, 57, 79, 80, 680

embryologist 52, 680

Emmorey, K. 263, 714, 727

emphysema 2, 18, 280, 281, 680

Enayati, A. 229, 706

Endo, K. 275, 737

Engelen, S. 386, 737, 738

entrainment 2, 16, 52, 80, 148, 680

epenthesis 312, 338, 594, 680, 695

epidemic 48, 49, 198–200, 206, 207, 210–213, 215, 217, 218, 250, 309, 653, 680, 716, 717, 722, 729

epidemiologists 198, 200, 230, 680

epidemiology 2, 46, 680, 715

epigenetic disorder 63

epigenetic systems 52, 55, 680

epiglottis 252, 259, 260, 292, 305, 309, 680

epileptic seizures 476, 519, 680, 698

epinephrine 193, 252, 258, 671, 680, 714

Equal Protection Clause 561, 616, 640, 644, 680

Erdelyi, M. H. 182, 183, 714

Escera, C. 389, 711

Escobar, M. D. 436, 735

Esiri, M. M. 546, 714

Eslinger, P. J. 742

esophagus 252, 259, 270, 284, 680

Essa, M. M. 710

ethical conduct 594, 657, 658, 665, 680

Ethnologue 348, 567, 710, 714

etiology 2, 9, 302, 386, 390, 419, 421, 548, 680, 714, 718, 729

eugenics 1, 104, 129–131, 475, 545, 548, 549, 553, 567, 573, 575, 578, 592, 597, 598, 670, 680, 703, 704, 714, 726

eugenics movement 129–131, 573, 575, 578, 597, 714

euthanasia movement 52, 69, 680

Evans, M. 714

Everhart, V. 317, 725

expiratory reserve volume 252, 273, 681

expressive aphasia 476, 481, 681

extinction 198, 244, 246, 407, 681

extralinguistic elements 312, 351, 681

extrapyramidal tract xiv, 287, 296, 681

extrinsic factors 424, 440, 543, 681

Ezura, M. 737

F

facilitated communication 104, 120, 681, 704, 711, 732

facilitating context 368, 380, 681

Factura, M. F. 709

Fallon, J. 741

false representation 476, 521, 681

FAPE 594, 610, 611, 613, 614, 626, 629–631, 642, 650, 681

Faragasso, K. 419, 736

Faria, M. 147, 707

Farina, M. 715

fasciculation 252, 290, 681

fast speech 312, 334, 418, 681, 690, 699

Fauconnier, G. 356, 714

Federico, T. 470, 732

Feinberg, D. 14, 714

Fekedulegn,, R. J. 37, 714, 715

Feldstein, S. 148, 336, 720

Fellin, T. 718

Felsenfeld, S. 376, 714

Feng, L. 545, 714

Fernandes-Ferreira, M. 238, 724

Ferrari, D. 709

Ferreira, S. T. 224, 238, 715, 723

fetal alcohol syndrome 52, 63, 66, 67, 681, 715

fictional representation 356, 476, 521, 681

Field, F. 597, 715
Fields R. D. 708
Fifer, W. P. 35, 727
filtering effects 142, 167, 172, 681
Finegan, E. 575, 715
Fink, A. L. 546, 739
Finn, J. C. 306, 733
Finn, P. 386, 715, 721
Fisch, M. 357, 715, 731
fissure of Rolando 2, 27, 675, 681, 689
Fitch, W. T. 17, 24, 715
fixed-ratio schedule of reinforcement 244, 681
flaccid dysarthrias 252, 286, 292, 681
Fleckenstein, A. E. 479, 739
Fletcher, J. M. 436, 735
Flett, P. 733
floppy child syndrome 236, 312, 359, 681
fluency shaping 368, 412–416, 681
fMRI 142, 146, 184, 394, 476, 496, 497, 506, 508, 551, 681, 682, 707, 711, 725, 730, 735
Fodor, J. A. 393, 396, 710, 715
Fogel, A. 148, 719
Fombonne, E. 200, 209–211, 216, 241, 713, 715
fontanel (fontanelle) 52, 58, 681
Food and Drug Administration 634, 715
Foote, S. A. 486, 734
foreign accent syndrome 252, 681, 707
formants 142, 171, 172, 681
Forte, G. 707
Foss, D.J. 453, 715
Foundas, A. L. 387, 389, 712, 715
Fowler, J. S. 280, 706
Fox, M. 654, 715
França, A. I. 509, 715
Franceschetti syndrome 52, 66, 681
Franco, J. L. 239, 715
Franic, D. M. 401, 402, 715
Frank, B. C. 216, 719
Franken, M. C. J. 409, 715
Franklin, A. E. 724
Franklin, N. 470, 732
Franz, K. J. 546, 724
Frazier, C. L. 369, 386, 737
Frede, S. 708
Frederickson, A. M. 711

Free and Appropriate Public Education 610, 681, 685, 715
free radical 198, 221, 549, 681, 705, 710, 718, 742
Freedman, M. 531, 705
Freeman, W. J. 398, 715, 732
Frege, G. 356, 715
Fregni, F. 706
fricative sounds 252, 278, 682
fricatives 312, 326, 682
Friesen, W. V. 350, 714
Frolenkov, G. I. 716
frontal lobes 2, 27, 30, 294, 540, 675, 681, 682, 689, 690, 699
Frumin, M. 719
Frustaci, A. 543, 716
Fujii, T. 41, 508, 703, 737
Fukawa, T. 389, 716
Fuller, G. 450, 510, 716
function words 368, 392, 481, 677, 682, 699, 719
functional disorders 252, 281, 682
functional hemispherectomy 476, 519, 682
functional Magnetic Resonance Imaging 142, 184, 497, 681, 682
functional MRI 476, 496, 682, 711, 734
fundamental frequency 142, 170, 277, 682
Fung, Y. K. 202, 241, 297, 359, 707

G

Gaab, N. 706
Gaasch, J. A. 546, 716
GABA 252, 296, 682, 690, 700, 726
Gachhui, R. 716
Gage, Phineas 293, 540–542, 731
Gage, N. 172, 716
Gagne, J. P. 730
Gagyi, C. E. 730
Gahr, M. 18, 707
Gailer, J. 716
Gallaher, A. 419, 736
Galldiks, N. 708
Gallese, V. 354, 355, 716
Galton, F. 130, 716
Gamble, S. B. 561, 736
gamma amino butyric acid 252, 296, 682, 690
Gantwerk, B. F. 392, 707
Gao, C. 714

Gao, E. 737
Gardner, E. J. 55, 544, 716
Gardner, H. 484, 716
Gardner, P. 718
Garey, L. J. 489, 708, 716
Garg, A. 95, 716
gas theory of smiling 2, 14, 15, 78, 682
Gaston, B. 259, 719
gastroesophageal reflux disease 682, 683
Gati, J. 725
gauss 476, 495, 682, 716
Gauss, J. C. F. 716
Gauthier, M. xii, 65, 723
Gaylor, D. W. 720
gaze 682, 695
Gazzaniga, M. S. 499, 500, 509, 518, 525, 716
Geier, D. A. 218, 220, 228, 233, 238, 239, 643, 655, 716
Geier, M. R. 218, 220, 228, 233, 238, 239, 643, 655, 716
Geldenhuys, W. J. 716
Gellin, B. G. 729
gene pool 104, 130, 131, 682
General American English 142, 171, 271, 326, 327, 437, 452, 453, 556, 560, 567, 569–572, 575, 576, 582, 619, 682
generality 2, 20, 338, 511, 682
genes plus toxins theory 198, 218, 682
genetic disorders 52, 55, 56, 59, 299, 438, 440, 478, 479, 682
genetic theory 198, 217, 682
Genetics Education Center 716
geniculate fibers 252, 290, 682
Genius, J. 136, 705, 716
genome 2, 20, 23–26, 32, 59, 61, 130, 143, 280, 375, 376, 545, 549, 657, 676, 682, 683, 695, 724, 734
genotoxic 228, 252, 280, 682
genotoxin 52, 59, 249, 683
George, G. N. 239, 716
Gerber, M. A. 729
GERD 252, 284, 683
germ cells 52, 59, 476, 479, 683
Gernsbacher, M. A. 48, 716
Geschwind, N. 481, 525, 717, 740
gestational period 52, 71, 72, 683
Geyer, M. A. 194, 737
Gharibzadeh, S. 530, 742

Ghosh, P. 735
Ghosh, S. 716
Ghosh, S. K. 716
Giardetti, J. R. 342, 659, 729
Gibbs, R. 62, 355, 717
Gibson, S. J. 265, 717
Gibson, W. xiii, 133, 717
Gilbert, S. J. 265, 728
Gillberg, C. 211, 717, 732
Giordano, A. 740
Giovannetti, T. 265, 707
Girard, M. 223, 717
Giubilei, F. 707
Giummarra, M. J. 265, 717
give-me-the-money theory 210, 683
Glattke, T. 187, 717, 732
Glenberg, A. M. 355, 717
Glezer, M. 500, 733
glial cells 2, 29, 181, 227, 288, 683, 685
glides 312, 324, 364, 683, 696
gliotransmissions 252, 288, 683
global agnosia 476, 525, 683
global aphasia 476, 522, 683
glottal plosive 312, 326, 683
glottal stop 312, 326, 683
glottis 683
glutamate 88, 252, 288, 683, 690, 730
glutathione 198, 238, 239, 683, 716, 717, 720, 721, 724, 727, 731
Godfrey, M. E. 237, 490, 740
Goessler, W. 239, 739
Golden Rule 594, 658, 659, 683
Goldin-Meadow, S. 727
Goldsmith, H. H. 48, 716
Gomase, V. S. D. 710
Gombrich, E. H. 342, 717
Goodall, S. M. 500, 732, 733
Goode, S. 723
Goodglass, H. 481, 516, 700, 717
Goodman, M. S. 470, 725
Goodwin, C. 330, 717
Gordon, J. D. J. 18, 731, 740
Gorell, J. M. 297, 734
Gorin, Jean-Pierre 123
Gorney, C. 76, 717
Gottesman, I. L. 713, 723, 731
Gottesman, R. F. 713
Gough, P. B. 315, 430, 432, 717
Gould, S. J. 130, 573, 717
Grabowski, T. 263, 500, 712, 714

grade point average 562, 594, 640, 683
Graham 88, 129, 130, 137, 306, 333, 594, 702, 719
Graham, H. K. 306, 719
grammar 2, 19, 104, 341, 352, 353, 365, 678, 683, 685, 692, 699, 734
Grandin, T. 107, 109, 478, 717
Grandjean, P. 731
Grannemann, B. D. 220, 721
Grant, K. S. xi, 598, 708
granulomas 252, 284, 285, 683
Gray, B. N. 718
Gray, H. 57, 58, 60, 179, 189, 256, 257, 287, 293, 468, 596, 677, 685, 717
Greaves, W.S. 706
Greene, J. A. 713, 714
Gregory, A. 718
Grether, J. K. 740
Griffin, P. 451, 736
Griffith, E. H. 41, 369, 506–508, 713
Gritti, A. 709
Gross, J. 717
Gross, M. 728
Grossman, H. 391, 707, 717
Grossman, M. 707
Grossmann, K. E. 725
GSH 198, 238, 239, 683
Gubler, K. D. 713, 714
Guenther, F. H. 254, 707
Guillot, T. S. 718
Guimaraes, E. 328, 665, 717
Guinan, J. J. 190, 723
Guitar, B. 380, 393, 401, 402, 407, 416, 717
Gulf War syndrome 252, 298, 683
Gunderson, L. 622, 717
Gunier, R. 740
Guntupalli, V. K. 386, 721
Gupta, S. 203, 209, 225, 653, 717
Gur, R. C. 723
Gurel, A. 742
Gustafson, K. 448, 712
gustatory 476, 526, 683
Guthrie, D. 212, 733
Gutierrez, M. 17, 718
Guzzi, G. 709

H

Haan, E. 733
Hachinski, V. 725

Hackett, C. J. 729, 735
Haddon, M. 214, 718
Haemophilus influenzae B 594, 683
Hagele, T. J. 543, 718
Haggard, P. 185, 734
Hagler, D. J. xiv, 263, 266–268, 718
Hagoort, P. 342, 354, 718, 730, 740
hair cells 142, 180, 187, 189–191, 685, 690, 693, 718
Haishima, H. 269, 730
Halamka, J. 727
Halassa, M. M. 29, 288, 718
Haley, B. 233, 237, 238, 727, 740
Haley, B. E. 740
Halle, M. 315, 430, 451, 710
Haller, J. S. 130, 718
Halling, J. 731
hallucinations 2, 40, 504, 683, 695
Ham, W. 727
Hamdan, S. 713, 736
Handicapped Children's Protection Act of 1986 630, 641, 657, 718
Handley, J. B. 655, 718
Handley, L. 655, 718
hand-eye coordination 143, 683
hand flapping 16, 199, 215, 232, 235, 236, 674, 683, 685
Hankeya, G. J. 301, 725
Hanna, J. S. 203, 209, 446–448, 452, 718
Hanna, P. R. 203, 209, 446–448, 452, 718
Hansen, G. H. A. 89, 437, 609, 718, 719
Hanson, G. R. 479, 622, 739
Haq, S. K. 546, 741
hard glottal attack 252, 283, 683
hard of hearing 104, 123, 153, 684, 726
Harlan, J. M. 605, 606, 718
Harman, D. 222, 479, 544, 545, 718
Harrington, R. V. 38, 524, 729
Harris 1, 222, 572, 617, 619, 707, 716, 718
Harris, H. H. 716
Harris, S. B. 222, 718
Harrison 186, 239, 369, 408, 718, 722
Harrison, A. 239, 722
Harrison, E. 408, 718
Harrison Ford 369
Harrison, J. 186, 718

Hart, N. W. M. 324–327, 468, 718
Harvey, W. T. 200, 708
Hashemian, A. 143, 718
Haswell, S. J. 227, 732
Hatcher, J. M. 297, 718
Hatchwell, E. 718
Hatfield, J. S. 713, 721
Hauser, R. M. M. D. 24, 561, 644,
    715, 718
Haydon, P. G. 718, 742
Hayhoe, M. M. 62, 706
Haynes, J. D. 184, 185, 718
Healy, M. T. 507, 718
Healy, W. 718
Heath, C. 354, 355, 719
Heath, S. W. 206, 741
Hedges, P. 718
Heilman, K. M. 715
Heine, S. 216, 719
Heinrich Hertz 718
Heiss, W. D. 708
Helen Keller xiii, 87, 106, 131–140,
    175, 242, 333, 423, 465, 498, 557,
    574, 588, 594, 669, 718, 721, 723
Helicobacter pylori 284, 285, 718
Heller, H. C. 89, 723, 732
hemispherectomy 476, 519, 551,
    682, 684, 705, 730, 735
hemoglobin 52, 63, 684
hemorrhagic strokes 476, 542, 684
Henderson, D. 186, 721, 727
Hendler, T. 183, 718
Henningsen, H. 713
Herbert, M. R. 220, 230, 313, 718,
    732
heritability 368, 375, 684
Hernandez-Jarvis, L. 577, 581
Herrnstein, R. J. 574, 718
hertz 142, 169, 684, 718
hesitation phenomena 368, 379,
    380, 420, 684
Hespos, S. J. 336, 718
Hess, K. 501, 705
Heubert, J. P. 561, 644, 718, 719
HFA 104, 107, 198, 212, 214, 684
HiB 207, 594, 633, 634, 654, 684,
    716, 731
Hickok, G. 172, 716
Higashakawa, M. 271, 711
high functioning autism 104, 107,
    198, 212, 478, 673, 684
Hiiemae, K. M. 269, 730
Hikawa, C. 722

Hilker, R. 708
Hillbratt, M. 389, 736
Hilleman, M. R. 545, 737
Hillis, A. E. 713
Hindmarsh, J. 354, 355, 719
Hippocrates 72, 77, 78, 660, 662,
    664, 665, 668, 719, 723
Hippocratic Oath 594, 660, 661,
    665, 684, 719
Hirayasu, Y. xiv, 388, 719
Hitler, Adolf 531, 573, 575,
    596–598, 684
Hitzig, R. 719
HIV 476, 545, 546, 633, 684, 695,
    706, 711, 723
Hliba, E. 708
Hobson v. Hansen 437, 609, 719
Hodges, R. E. 446, 718
Hodson, B. 410, 705
Hoffman, J. E. 199, 724
Hogan, J. A. 12, 719
Hoit, J. 405, 719, 724
Holland, J. G. 244, 719
Holland, K. D. 724
Holland, S. K. 501, 734
Holocaust 594, 597, 598, 684, 738
homeopathic effect 142, 188, 196,
    684
Hoon, M. A. 88, 710
Hopkins, D. B. 713
Hopkins, W. D. 19, 719
Hornig, M. 228, 719
Hornstein, N. 451, 710
Horvat, M. 725
Hostetter, A. B. 255, 525, 719
Houle, S. 394, 712, 713
Howard, R. 41, 130, 503, 545, 605,
    719
Howe, Samuel Gridley 106–109,
    131, 132, 134, 138, 242, 243, 498,
    595, 734
Howe, Julia Ward 721
Howe, M. 186, 719
Howell, K. 306, 719
Howell, P. 386, 392, 719
Howes, D. H. 182, 719
HPV 252, 285, 684
Hsu, H. C. 148, 719
Hu, V. W. 216, 719
Huang, Z. W. 188, 719
Huber, A. 409, 722
Hudson, M. A. 713
Hudspeth, A. J. 180, 725

human immunodeficiency virus
    476, 545, 684
human papilloma virus 252, 285,
    684
Hunt, J. F. 259, 719
Huntington's (disease) chorea 252,
    296, 684
Hurlbut, K. M. 705
Hurley, M. 517, 715, 737
Hurley, R. A. 737
hydrocephalus 52, 73, 74, 83, 684,
    728
Hyman, L. M. 322, 719
hyperactivity 142, 174, 198, 206,
    671, 673, 680, 684, 738
hyperfunction disorders 252, 281,
    684
hypernasality 52, 85, 86, 684
hypertonia 252, 304, 310, 684
hypokinetic dysarthria 252, 297,
    684
hyposmia 52, 88, 684
hypostasis 424, 427, 429, 677, 684
hypostatic symbols 349, 424, 429,
    684
hypotonia 198, 240, 252, 303, 304,
    310, 359, 684

I

icon 185, 266, 344, 433, 518, 521,
    525, 685
IDEA 1990 642, 645, 649, 720
IDEA 1997 644, 649, 652, 720
IDEA 2004 644, 649, 652, 720
ideographic writing 312, 348, 365,
    685
Idiazabal, M. A. 389, 711
IEP 594, 614, 681, 685
Ignatow, G. 355, 719
Ikejiri, Y. 728
illusion 40, 150, 154, 156, 173, 210,
    211, 250, 332, 685, 709, 738
immune systems ix, 2, 23, 91, 92,
    685
imperforate anus 52, 71, 82, 685
Improving America's Schools Act
    of 1994 594, 648, 685, 719
Inagaki, D. 270, 719
incipient stuttering 368, 391–393,
    404, 406, 417, 418, 421, 685, 691
indexes 268, 313, 332, 343, 427, 499,
    521, 522, 524, 577

individualized education program (IEP) 594, 614, 681, 685
infantile autism 198, 200, 240, 359, 685, 686, 721
infantile paralysis 70, 685
inflammatory bowel disease 198, 685
infrasystems 2, 3, 5, 685
Ingham, R. J. 370, 401, 402, 711, 714, 720
innate intelligence 554, 574, 577, 685, 698
inner hair cells 142, 180, 685
inspiratory reserve volume 252, 272, 685
Institute for Vaccine Safety 227, 720
Institute of Medicine (IOM) 635, 716, 720, 726
instructional dyslexia 312, 329, 339, 440–442, 449, 450, 456–459, 461, 472, 524, 685
instructional utility 2, 45, 563, 564, 685
integration training 142, 143, 685, 704, 705
intermittent schedule of reinforcement 198, 244, 245, 685
internal capsule 252, 290, 685, 698
International Academy of Oral Medicine and Toxicology 6, 720, 734, 736
International Civil Aviation Organization 8, 720
International Dyslexia Association 434, 720
International Phonetic Alphabet 112, 312, 324, 325, 345, 430, 685, 720
International Phonetics Association 720
interneurons 2, 29, 181, 190, 193, 196, 288, 685
inter-rater reliability 401, 685
intonation 2, 327, 379, 686, 693, 699, 714
intracerebral hemorrhage 476, 542, 686
intrarater reliability 686
intrinsic factors 424, 440, 686
intubation 252, 283, 686
IOM 635, 716, 720, 726
ipsilateral 252, 290, 476, 518, 686

ipsilateral pathways 476, 518, 686
ischemic stroke 476, 541, 686, 731
Ishida, A. 265, 721
Ishii, N. 89, 734, 737
Ishii, R. 713
isomorphic 198, 229, 432, 465, 686
Itoh, M. 41, 508, 703
Jabberwocky 485, 486, 692, 720

J

Jacoby, R. 703, 704
Jaffe, J. 148, 336, 720
James, S. J. 220, 224, 228, 238, 297, 369, 379, 690, 720
Jamshidi, J. 728
Janak, L. 220, 720
Janosky, J. 177, 709
jargon 3, 424, 439, 476, 485, 486, 672, 686
Jarrett, C. 266, 268, 720
Jasnow, M. D. 148, 336, 720
Jason McElwain 214, 720
Jaulerry, S. D. 707
Jax, P. 170, 720
Jefferson, G. 330, 734
Jenner, P. 297, 731
Jensen, A. R. 575, 580, 720
Jepson, B. xiii, 5, 6, 46, 48, 60, 81, 82, 88, 100, 199, 200, 202, 204, 211, 220, 235, 236, 240, 241, 309, 687, 720, 741
Jernigan, S. 220, 720
Jezer, M. 368, 370, 379, 403, 720
Jim Crow laws 594, 605, 607, 644, 686, 721
Job, A. 728
Johnson
Johnson, C. C. 297, 734
Johnson, J. 5, 46, 60, 88, 199, 200, 202, 204, 211, 220, 236, 240, 241, 309, 392, 404, 709, 720, 741
Johnson, J. A. 150, 733
Johnson, M. 62, 355, 720, 723
Johnson, W. 404, 392, 709, 720
Johnson, W. G. 709, 726
Johnston, D. 708
John-Steiner, V. 740
Jolesz, F. A. 719
Jones, A. M. 218, 220, 222, 721
Jones, D. P. 718
Jones, J. A. 196, 720
Jones, M. 407, 409, 722, 723, 730

Jones, R. O. 719
Jones, S. M. 737
Jorgensen, P. J. 731
Josephson, R. 708
Joska, L. 739
Julia Ward Howe 721
Jung, S. 722
jurisprudence 594, 612, 675, 686

K

Kahler, S. G. 718
Kahn, I. 718
Kako, E. 17, 18, 721
Kalinowski, J. S. 369, 386, 389, 403, 407, 413, 415, 721, 737
Kallenberg, K. 705
Kalra, N. 239, 732
Kaminski, H. J. 24, 303, 711
Kan, P. X. 185, 721, 731, 738
Kanai, R. 185, 721
Kane, J. M. 711
Kane, R. 628, 721
Kanner, L. 198, 200, 211, 215, 233, 240, 241, 683, 685, 686, 721
Kanner-type autism 200, 683, 685, 686
Kanthasamy, A. G. 297, 721
Kaplan, E. 516, 700, 717
Kapur, S. 394, 712
Kasahara, T. 265, 721
Kashon, M. L. 710
Kastenholz, B. 546, 721
Katamba, F. X. 322, 719
Katz, J. 186, 235, 242, 254, 275, 380, 727, 738
Katz, K. 306, 740
Katz, R. C. 721, 723
Kaufman, B. 718
Kaufman, Y. 531, 705
Kaup, B. 470, 721
Kaur, P. 239, 721
Kavaliers, M. 724
Kaye, K. L. xiii, 35, 145, 146, 721
Keator, D. 741
Kegl, J. 122, 123, 333, 727
Keith, R. W. 190, 727
Keller, H. xiii, 87, 106, 131–140, 175, 242, 333, 423, 465, 498, 557, 574, 588, 594, 669, 718, 721, 723
Keller, W. D. 174, 721
Kelley, A. R. 213, 713, 714
Kelly, S. D. 342, 730

Kelter, S. 470, 711, 721
Kennedy, J. F. 339, 531
Kennedy, J. L. 731
Kennedy, R. F., Jr. 123, 199, 204, 209, 280, 339, 531, 595, 596, 654, 721
Kent, R. 175, 274, 721, 724
Kenwell, Z. R. 193, 708
Kern, J. K. 218, 220, 222, 721
Khalili, K. 740
Khan, K. M. 191, 713, 721
Khan, R. H. 546, 741
Kharasch, M. S. 227, 722
Kidd, P. M. 546, 722
Kikano, G. E. 373, 732
Kikinis, R. 719
Kim, H. I. 190, 293, 722
Kim, H. S. 190, 293, 722
Kim, J. H. 190, 293, 722
Kim, K. 109, 110, 112, 114, 577, 581, 582, 729
Kim, M. K. 190, 293, 722
Kim, S. U. 190, 293, 722
Kimbrough, P. 109, 110, 112, 114, 722
Kimura, M. 37, 544, 722
kinesics 312, 350, 686, 707, 722
kinesthetic feedback 142, 156, 382, 390, 686
Kingston, M. 409, 722, 730
Kintsch, W. 470, 722
Kinzler, K. D. 722
Kirby, D. 199, 204, 205, 209, 218, 228, 234, 643, 721, 722
Kirk, K. M. 714
Kirkham, N. Z. 330, 733
Kita, S. 122, 717, 719, 730, 734
Kita, T. 220, 354, 719, 722
Kitazawa, M. 297, 721
Klein F. 722
Klein, E. 741
Kleinman, J. T. 713
Klekowski, E. 228, 724
Kloesel, C. J. W. 715, 731
Knauth, M. 705
Knecht, S. 713
Knight, K. 109, 110, 722
Koch, M. 228, 722
Koger, S. M. 548, 550, 722
Kokayi, K. 239, 722
Kollman, T. R. 729
Konishi, T. 728
Konturek, J. W. 284, 722
Koop, C. E. 71, 82, 100, 709, 722

Koprivnikar, K. 66, 724
Koralnik, I. J. 545, 712
Kostrzewa 219, 223, 546, 730, 734
Kostrzewa, R. M. 730, 734
Kotagal, P. 724
Krashen, S. D. 37, 459, 722
Krasnova, I. N. 479, 705
Kratochvil, C. J. 294, 722
Kretschmer, L. W. 190, 727
Kroll, R. 394, 712, 713
Kubo, T. 166, 722
Kuhl 205, 426, 722
Kuhl, E. A. 205, 722
Kuhl, P. K. 426, 722
Kuhn, S. 722
Kuhn, T. S. 355, 397, 722
Kung, H. J. 735
Kuppusamy, M. L. 718
Kuppusamy, P. 718
Kuroda, Y. 293, 722
Kurt, T. L. 298, 722
Kushida, M. 728
Kusuki, M. 722
Kwon, J. S. 719
Kyunai, K. 722

L

La Porta, C. A. M. 709
Laakso, M. L. 738
lability 252, 293, 294, 686
Lacasse, L. 741
Ladenheim, B. 479, 705
Lafaille, S. 394, 713
Lakoff, G. 355, 723
Lamb, L. 192, 727
Lamberg, K. 211, 717
Lambert, G. H. 709, 726
Landa, R. 740
Landry, S. xi, 729
Lane, H. L. 213, 723
Langleben, D. D. 506, 508, 723
language disorder theory 368, 391, 686
language learning impaired 424, 686, 687
Lankappa, S. T. 508, 736
LaPointe, L. 235, 242, 254, 275, 380, 723
Larry King Live 203, 604, 723
Larry P. v. Riles 437, 561, 618–622, 645, 646, 723

laryngeal webbing 252, 285, 686
larynx 252, 259, 260, 270, 272, 274–277, 279, 283, 284, 292, 303, 341, 379, 682, 686, 691, 698, 702
Lash, J. P. 105, 106, 108, 109, 129, 131–138, 723
Lassonde, M. 730
lateral cerebrospinal fasciculus 252, 290, 686
lateral progress 554, 557, 686
lateralization 142, 165, 166, 476, 482–484, 523, 532, 550, 551, 686, 712, 722, 723
lateralization hypothesis 476, 482–484, 686
late-term abortion 686
Lattermann, C. 409, 723
Lau v. Nichols 568, 583, 612, 613, 620–622, 723
Laura Bridgman 87, 107, 723
Law of Hippocrates. 723
Lawrence, D. A. 730
Le Couteur, A. 216, 723
Le Hoang, P. 707
learning disability 424, 434, 436, 437, 556, 619, 678, 686
least restrictive environment 594, 615, 624, 686, 703
Leavens D. A. 719
Lecours, A. R. 182, 736
Lee, A. 713, 741
Lee, B. S. 383–387, 389, 391, 723
Lee, C. H. 220, 228, 315, 430, 432, 717
Lee, D. J. 190, 239, 723
Lee, J. S. 722
Lee, M. C. 722
Lee, N. H. 216, 719
Leffert, R. 727
legal discovery 594, 655, 686
legal injunction 594, 630, 687
legal precedent 594, 607, 610, 687
legal sanity 476, 508, 687
Lehnhardt, F. G. 708
Leimbach, M. 214, 723
Lejeune, J. 65, 679, 723
Lemasters, G. K. 190, 727
Lemen, L. C. 715
Lemieux, S. K. 263, 735
Lemonnier, L. A. 713
Lencz, T. 741
Leon, I. 707
Leong, C. C. 6, 60, 224, 227, 543, 723

Lepore, F. 730
Leppanen, P. H. T. 738
leprosy xiii, 89–91, 284, 683, 718, 723, 734
Leprosy Mission Canada xiii, 89–91, 723
Leroux, J. M. 730
Leshin, L. 65, 723
Leskinen, E. 738
Lessac, M. 723
Levelt, W. J. M. 385, 386, 723
Levin, D. E. 228, 724
Levinson, B. 723
Levison, J. H. 727
Levitt, P. 709
Lewin, R. 18, 19, 717, 734
Lewis, C. 407, 723
Lewis, M. 14, 737
Lewkowicz, D. J. 336, 723
Li, H.-D. 714
Li, J. 546, 739
Li, L. 193, 723
Liberato, N. 708
Lichtheim, L. 509–513, 522, 694, 723, 736
Lichtman, J. 488, 723
Lidcombe Program 367, 368, 407–409, 687, 718, 722, 723, 740
Lieven, N. A. J. 193, 731
Lightman, A. 527, 723
Lim, B. J. 315, 316, 335, 712
Lima, C. F. 238, 625, 724
Lincoln, Abraham 110, 118, 130, 352, 449, 595, 598–602, 604, 637, 680, 716, 724, 728
Linden, E. 19, 725, 730
Linder, D. 601, 724
Lindsay, R. L. 358, 724
linear processing 142, 164, 687
linguistic expectations 142, 161, 687
Lipkin, W. I. 228, 719
lip-reading 95, 153, 687
liquids 258, 261, 312, 324, 364, 687
literacy modality 424, 434, 687
Liu, L. 546, 724
LMN 252, 286, 288, 290, 296, 298, 302, 687
Lobner, D. 239, 709
local educational agencies 594, 614, 687
localization 142, 165, 166, 476, 481, 483, 484, 550, 551, 667, 687, 708, 721, 741

localization hypothesis 476, 483, 484, 550, 551, 687
Locke, J. L. 9, 724
Lockman, P. R. 716
Loddenkemper, T. 520, 724
Loftus, S. K. 66, 724
Logan, K. J. 392, 724
Logar, M. 725
logographic writing 312, 348, 687
Lomen Abdo 724
Long, W. B. 713, 714
Lopez, F. 17, 718
Lorch, R. 470, 740
Lorenz, B. 596, 724
Lorenz, M. 596, 724
Lorenzo's Oil 46, 479, 724, 726
Lorscheider, F. L. 6, 60, 224, 227, 543, 723
Lottenberg, S. 741
Lou Gehrig's disease 198, 202, 294, 476, 543, 672, 687
Loucks, T. M. J. 263, 724
Louisiana HB 958 724
Louko, L. J. 396, 724
Lovely, T. J. 228, 724
lower motor neurons (LMN) 252, 286, 288, 290, 296, 298, 302, 687
Luber, S. 722
Lucas, C. 342, 739
Ludlow, C. L. 286, 724
Lukas, J. 706
Lundervold, A. J. 211, 732
Luo, Y. Y. 719
Luria, A. R. 29, 515, 522, 540, 724
Luzzati, R. 711
Lyon, G. R. 425, 444, 455, 724
Lyytinen, H. 738

M

Ma, X. 738
Maaso, A. 149, 724
Macdonald 149, 150, 228, 383, 726, 733
MacDonald, J. 149, 150, 726
Macdonald, W. A. 228, 733
MacFabe, D. F. 218, 724
MacIntosh, B. 725
Macklin, Charles 486, 710
Macknik, S. L. 146, 158, 185, 343, 724, 725, 738
Macnamara, J. 38, 132, 725
macrophages 198, 223, 687

Magalang, U. 718
Magalhaes, M. H. C. G. 66, 725
Magliano, J. P. 470, 725
Magnavita, N. 716
magnetic resonance imaging xiv, 142, 184, 295, 388, 476, 494, 497, 681, 682, 687, 689, 719, 725
Magos, L. 230, 711
Maguire, G. 741
Maier, M. A. 183, 725
mainstreaming principle 594, 615, 687
Majerus, S. 358, 725
Makuch, R. 436, 735
Malach, R. 718
Malawian, A. 728
Maldjian, J. A. 723
Mandal 716
Mandal, A. 716
mandibulofacial dysostosis 52, 66, 687
Mandler, J. M. 470, 725
Manna, G. 301, 725
manner, of articulation 312, 324, 687
Manning, W. H. 369, 370, 380, 403, 404, 413, 416, 417, 713, 725
manual babbling 104, 122, 687
manual modality 104, 125, 316, 687
Manually Coded English 725
Manually Signed English 104, 124, 688, 725
Maraj, B. K. V. 193, 708
Marchand, Y. 447, 448, 712
Marcovitch, S. 336, 723
Marcuse, E. K. 729
Marder, E. 708
Marentette, P. F. 16, 122, 426, 731
Marion, D. W. 480, 541, 725
Markin, V. S. 180, 725
Mars, A. E. 317, 709, 725
Marschark, M. 317, 725
Marsden, C. D. 297, 731
Marsh, C. B. 718
Marsh, D. 231, 711
Martin, N. G. 714
Martin, R. 269, 725
Martineau, M. 181, 725
Martinez-Conde, S. 146, 343, 725
Martini, F. 711
Masataka, N. 16, 17, 37, 143, 426, 714, 725
Maseri, A. 716

masking effects 142, 172, 688
Masters, M. G. 738
Masson, M. C. 739
Mastropieri, D. 35, 725
Masumoto, T. 737
Masutani, Y. 737
Mather, J. 725
Matkovich, S. 265, 728
Matsuo, K. 269, 730
Matthews, P. M. 741
Max, L. 418, 706
Mayer, A. R. 497, 725
Mazerik, J. N. 718
McCaffrey, P. 515, 700, 725
McCarley, R. W. 719
McCarthy, J. 5, 14, 46, 199, 200, 202, 203, 241, 359, 714, 725
McConnell, S. K. 736
McCormack, A. L. 718
McDonald, S. 723
McEneny, J. 705
McGhee, R. L. 577, 714
McGinnis, W. R. 218, 220, 741
McGovern, C. 214, 725
McGregor, J. 88, 739
McGregor, W. 713
McGuigan, M. 189, 725
McGurk, H. 94, 142, 143, 149–155, 157–162, 164, 165, 173, 174, 176, 183, 185, 186, 191, 194, 195, 266, 315–317, 333, 334, 383, 411, 524, 534, 685, 688, 724, 726, 733
McGurk effect 142, 149, 150, 688, 733
McGurk interactions 142, 149, 150, 152–155, 158, 159, 164, 165, 173, 174, 176, 183, 185, 186, 194, 195, 315–317, 333, 383, 411, 524, 534, 685, 688, 726
McGurk Sentence Interactions 155, 160, 726
McGurk Syllable Interactions 153, 154, 726
McKeown, S. J. 66, 726
McKinlay, S. 706
McVicar, K. 739
Meade, A. G. 297, 707
meaningful sequence 424, 471, 485, 486, 497, 688, 696
Mearin, F. 301, 738
measurement error 376, 554, 560, 688, 701
mechanical injuries 476, 480, 688

median canal 142, 179, 688
medulla oblongata 189, 252, 290, 675, 685, 688
Meek, L. R. 68, 726
Mehler, J. 16, 35, 323, 335, 726, 728, 732
Mehler, B. 131, 726
Mehta 263, 714
Mehta, P. 710
Mehta, S. 714
Meier, F. 220, 729
Meier, P. G. 737
Meisel, F. 705
Melanie Griffith 369
Melmed, R. 709
Melnick, K. S. 392, 726
Melnyk, S. B. 220, 720
Meltzer, A. 397, 726
Meltzoff, A. N. 16, 147, 426, 722, 726
Menon, R. 725
Mensour, B. 730
Menzies, R. 408, 718
Meotti, F. C. 715
Merabet, L. B. 706
Meram, I. 742
Mercer, J. R. 575, 582, 726
mercury 6, 59, 60, 207, 208, 213, 217, 223–234, 236–240, 249, 250, 294, 297, 543, 546–548, 550, 551, 596, 633, 634, 636, 653, 654, 670, 678, 688, 695, 703, 705, 706, 708, 709, 711, 712, 714–716, 718, 721–723, 725, 727, 732, 733, 737–741
merthiolate 198, 227, 688, 700, 733
mesothelioma 476, 545, 688, 709
metabolism ix, 2, 5, 21, 23, 24, 26, 27, 55, 61, 64, 68, 197, 220, 235, 678, 680, 688, 705, 717
metathesis 312, 338, 688, 695
Michael Douglas 531
Michael Phelps 491, 564, 726
Michelson, D. 722
microglia 198, 223, 688
Migliavacca 174, 707
Migliavacca, F. 707
Milani 24, 303, 711
Milani, M. 711
Miles 6, 76, 88, 368, 434–436, 635, 655, 726
Miles, E. 726

Militerni 709
Militerni, R. 709
Miller 138, 256, 294, 306, 371, 470, 479, 710, 718, 724–726, 733
Miller, A. J. 726
Miller, G. A. 726
Miller, G. W. 718
Miller, J. 725
Miller, M. D. 733
Miller, N. R. 710
Miller, R. G. 726
Minamata Disease. 726
Ming, S. X. 709
Ming, X. 726
minimal pair 312, 345, 361, 688
Miracle Continues 133, 726
Miracle Worker xiii, 133, 717, 726
Mitchell, R. E. 123, 213, 726
Mitsumoto, H. 726
Miu, A. C. 730
mixed dysarthrias 252, 299, 688
Miyaoka, Y. 719
Mizuta, I. 728
Mobbins, E. 302, 713
modular 368, 393, 398, 688
modules 368, 393, 394, 396, 398, 489, 533, 688, 742
Mohammed Ali 479, 726
Mohler, H. 29, 298, 726
Mohr, A. 705
Monikowski, C. 342, 726
monitoring functions 368, 394, 688
monolingual/monodialectal assessment 554, 567, 568, 591, 688
monomoraic 312, 322, 688
monosyllabic word 252, 271, 688
monotone 368, 414, 415, 688
monozygotes 368, 376, 688
monozygotic 198, 216, 368, 375, 688, 719, 731
Moon, C. 35, 727
Moore, C. A. 16, 147, 271, 711, 727, 733
Moore, E. C. 715
Moore, M. K. 147, 726
Moore, R. J. 722
Moore, T. E. 448, 727
mora timed 312, 322, 688
Moradi, M. H. 530, 742

Morata, T. C. 190, 727
Moreira, C. R. 66, 725
Morford, J. P. 123, 333, 727
Morgan, G. 122, 123, 727
Morgan, J. L. 370, 736
Mori, E. 41, 508, 703
Morin, C. 520, 705
Morlot, S. 358, 706
Moro, A. M. 715
Morris, C. W. 244, 727
mortality vii, 3, 198, 201, 222, 545, 689, 709, 734, 736
Moschitta, J. 414, 418, 444, 727
Moscovitch, M. 531, 705
Moses, L. J. 342, 627, 727
Moskowitz, B. A. 727
Mostaghimi, A. 46, 727
Mothet, J. P. 181, 725
motor cortex 2, 28, 29, 288, 675, 681, 685, 689
motor phonetics 312, 313, 689, 736
motor strip 2, 27, 29, 300, 689
MRI 388, 476, 494–496, 517, 533, 539, 682, 689, 711, 734
Mrklas, L. 739
Mucke, L. 224, 730
Muir, D. 16, 713
Muir, H. 424, 727
Muller, N. 706, 729
Mullin, J. T. 35, 708
Mulrooney, K. 342, 739
multimodal 142, 143, 146, 689
multimodal integration 142, 146, 689
multiple sclerosis 2, 48, 70, 199, 223, 294, 476, 543, 546, 548, 689, 717
Munhall, K. G. 358, 720
Muntean, M. 239, 739
Muran, P. J. 238, 727
Muratore, C. 332, 713
Murchland, S. 733
Murray, C. 574, 718
Musée Valentin Haüy 727
Musiek, F. E. 163, 165, 192, 710, 727, 731
Muthaiyah, B. 219, 710
Mutter, J. 229, 233, 237, 238, 550, 727
myasthenia gravis 252, 303, 689, 711
myelin 46, 476, 479, 671, 689, 701, 727

Myers, F. L. 419, 736
Myers, G. 231, 711
myoelastic aerodynamic theory of phonation 252, 276, 689
Myren, K. 68, 726
mythomania 2, 41, 505, 689, 691, 694

N

Nagao, K. 315, 316, 335, 712, 727
Najafi, A. 741
Nakagawa, Y. 728
Nakai, Y. 722
Nakajima, Y. 728
Nakashima, T. 220, 722
nanotechnology 476, 544, 689, 727
Naremore, R. C. 37, 727
Narr, K. L. 741
nasalized 52, 85, 684, 689
Nash, R. A. 543, 550, 727
Nash, J. F. 26, 41, 154, 330, 503–505, 508, 727
Nashold, B. S. 27, 709
Nathoo, A. 727
National Center for Public Policy Research 607, 727
National Childhood Vaccine Injury Act 594, 631, 728
National Federation for the Blind 728
native models 104, 122, 123, 333, 467, 689
natural signed languages 104, 124, 127, 689
Naumann, J. 229, 233, 237, 238, 550, 727
Nazzi, T. 16, 35, 323, 336, 728
Neale, M. C. 714
Needleman, H. 177, 709
negative inertia 424, 457, 461, 689
negative reinforcement 198, 244, 408, 415, 689, 694
Neimeyer, R.A. 369, 403, 713
Nemes, B. 730
neologisms 476, 485, 689
Ness, P. 136, 728
Neubrander, J. A. 720
neuroAIDS 198, 223, 546, 548, 689, 695
neurofibrillary tangles 198, 224, 225, 689, 705
neurogenic disorders 52, 60, 223, 689, 723

neurogenic stuttering 368, 417–419, 689
neurolinguistics 424, 451, 689, 707, 715
neurotoxicity 198, 220, 223, 230, 237, 238, 240, 243, 547, 548, 689, 720–722, 729, 730, 734, 735, 739
neurotransmitter 2, 24, 88, 187, 224, 288, 296, 297, 303, 394, 671, 679, 680, 682, 689
New, E. 720
Newcorn, J. H. 722
Newhart, M. 713
Newland, M. C. 548, 636, 712, 728
Newman, M. B. 297, 709
Newschaffer, C. J. 210, 728
Nicholls, M. E. R. 95, 266, 728
Nielsen, F. 731
Nieuwland, M. S. 354, 355, 728
Nishida, H. 223, 550, 728
Nishikawa, T. 264, 728
No Child Left Behind Act of 2001 728
nonverbal/performance assessment procedures 554, 567, 578–580, 582, 590, 591, 690
normal speech 44, 170, 200, 272, 312, 334, 387, 400, 463, 506, 585, 684, 690, 692, 695, 711, 729
normative expectations 554, 584, 585, 591, 690
Norris, D. 183, 728
Northoff, G. 706
Norton, R. J. 600, 708, 717, 728
Nottet, J. B. 188, 728
Novakovic, M. 729
Noyes, J. 193, 731
nuclei of the cranial nerves 252, 290, 292, 293, 690
Nuremberg 69, 80, 703
Nuttall, A. L. 187, 734
NVPAP 554, 567, 579, 580, 582, 590, 591, 690

O

Obhi, S. S. 265, 728
Obrecht, D. H. 470, 729
Odone, A. 46, 479, 728
Offit, P. A. 208, 633, 728, 729
Ogawa, Y. 728
Ohde, R. N. 392, 726
Ohno, K. 728

Okuda, J. 89, 734, 737
Okuda, K. 728
Olausson, H. 520, 705
olfactory 290, 476, 526, 690, 705, 739
Oliver, C. A. 129, 220, 227, 391, 587, 735
Olivieri, G. 239, 729
Oller, D. K. 15, 122, 353–355, 426, 714, 729
Oller, J. W., Jr. 14, 31, 34, 37, 39, 40, 52, 61, 132, 143, 146, 185, 319, 323, 332, 356, 392, 398, 573, 622, 705, 729, 732, 741
Oller, J. W., Sr. 467, 729
Oller, S. D. 14, 31, 34, 37, 39, 40, 52, 61, 132, 143, 146, 185, 319, 323, 332, 356, 392, 398, 573, 622, 705, 729
Olsen, J. F. 737
Olson, B. M. 713, 714
Olson, L. 389, 736
Omann, G. A. 737
Omnibus Autism Proceeding 199, 204, 209, 594, 596, 632, 639, 643, 647, 652, 654, 670, 728, 730
onset 4, 205, 216, 225, 346, 391, 392, 418, 424, 450, 456, 639, 678, 683, 690, 714, 720, 725
Onslow, M. 407–409, 718, 722, 723, 730, 740
operant conditioning 198, 244, 246, 247, 407, 408, 690
Operation Smile 730
oral babbling 104, 122, 690
organ of Corti 142, 178–180, 191, 688, 690, 693, 721
Organ, L. E. 187, 730
Orians, G. H. 732
Ortiz, A. A. 567, 568, 622, 647, 730
Ortiz, G. G. 88, 730
Ossenkopp, K. P. 724
ossification 52, 58, 690
Ostry, D. J. 738
Ota Benga 598, 730
Otero-Milian 146, 738
otitis media 312, 358, 690, 725
otoacoustic emission (OAE) 142, 187, 690
Otten, M. 354, 355, 728
outer hair cells 142, 180, 187, 189–191, 690, 693
Owen, A. 297, 731

Oxford University Press. 725, 730, 737
oxidation 198, 220, 221, 672, 690, 694, 733
oxidative stress 198, 219–223, 235, 239, 249, 250, 544–546, 549, 550, 552, 674, 682, 690, 700, 710, 718, 720, 721, 729, 730, 732, 735, 741, 742
Ozawa, E. 389, 716
Ozen, S. 742
Ozugurlu, F. 736
Ozyurek, A. 122, 342, 354, 730, 734
Ozyurt, H. 736
O'Brien, C. P. 723
O'Connor, K. 182, 736
O'Halloran, T. V. 546, 711

P

Pabello, N. G. 219, 547, 730
Packman, A. 407, 409, 722, 723, 730
Paden, E. 392, 738
Padhye, U. 220, 730
Paiement, P. 520, 730
Palmer, A. 722
Palmer, C. E. xi
Palmer, J. B. 262, 269, 730
Palomo T. R. K. 88, 730
Palop, J. J. 224, 730
Pan, N. 729, 730
pancreas 52, 64, 690, 705
Pangborn, J. B. 220, 739
Pantev, C. 713
paralinguistic devices 312, 350, 351, 690
parallel neural networks 142, 690
parallel processing 142, 164, 690
parallel universes 312, 356, 690
paranormal phenomena 52, 63, 560, 690
Parents in Action on Special Education 437, 617, 730
parietal lobes 2, 27, 263, 675, 681, 690, 696
Parinandi, N. L. 718
Parker, W. Y. 736
Parkinson's disease 6, 199, 252, 294, 297, 394, 479, 544, 546, 547, 551, 679, 690, 691, 706, 708, 709, 712, 721, 731, 734, 739
parosmia 52, 88, 690

parotid salivary gland 252, 292, 690
Parran, D. K. 227, 228, 730
partial birth abortion 52, 76, 77, 670, 686, 691, 730, 732
Partial Birth Abortion Ban Act 77, 732
Pasca, S. P. 218, 220, 730
Paterson, A. D. 731
pathological lying 2, 41, 505–508, 689, 691, 713, 718
Patterson, F. 18, 730
Patterson, M. L. 426, 730
Paulie 332, 731
PDD 198, 204, 205, 215, 227, 231, 235, 691
PDD-NOS 205, 691
Pearce, J. M. S. 193, 223, 500, 731
Pearce, R. K. B. 297, 731
pediatric surgeon 691
pediatricians 14, 215, 223, 234, 420, 425, 461, 556, 592, 594, 631, 634, 682, 691
Peirce, C. S. 7, 52, 157, 158, 332, 355–357, 471, 498, 526, 528, 529, 715, 731
Pekrun, M. R. 725
Pendergrass, J. C. 709
Penfield, W. 490, 731
Penn, D. C. 12, 19, 213, 731
Pennell, K. D. 718
Pennisi, E. 79, 731
Pennsylvania Association of Retarded Children 610, 731
Pennycook, A. 115, 731
Penzner, J. B. 711
Pepperberg, I. M. 17, 18, 332, 731
peptic ulcers 252, 284, 691
perceptual defense 142, 182, 183, 196, 691, 693, 707, 714, 732, 741
perceptual vigilance vi, xxii, xxxix, 142, 182, 183, 191, 194, 195, 691, 693
Pereira-Wilson, C. 238, 724
Perez, J. 298, 707, 731
peritoneum 476, 480, 691
peritonitis 476, 480, 691
Perkins Institute for the Blind 107, 131, 134, 135
Perkins, K. 107, 575, 729, 737
Perkins, W. H. 378, 402, 731
Perry, J. 355, 706
Persico, A. M. 709

persistent developmental stuttering 391, 419, 420, 685, 691, 711

pervasive developmental disorders (PDD) 52, 60, 96, 198, 204, 205, 248, 354, 556, 691, 715

pervasive developmental disorders not otherwise specified (PDD-NOS) 198, 205, 691

Peryer, G. 193, 731

PET 368, 382, 391, 394, 476, 491–494, 691

Petersen, M. S. 297, 731

petition for certiorare 594, 618, 691

petitioner 594, 637, 691

Petitto, L. A. 16, 122, 426, 731

Petronis, A. 216, 731

Petrovitch, H. 710

pharyngeal cavity 252, 259, 284, 691

pharynx 85, 86, 252, 259, 277, 292, 341, 691, 698

Phelps, M. E. 491, 564, 565, 710, 726

Phillips, D. 163, 731

philtrum 52, 68, 691

Phineas Gage 293, 540–542, 731

phonation 252, 274, 276, 281, 299, 668, 689, 691, 724

phoneme 312, 346, 385, 386, 420, 451–456, 472, 672, 685, 691, 715, 718, 734

phonemic awareness 424, 432, 444, 450, 691, 692, 717, 730

phonemic segments 312, 345, 691

phones 168, 424, 451, 672, 691

phonetic code 104, 112, 691

phonetic features 312, 346, 691

phonetic segments 312, 345, 692, 696, 699

phonetic transcription 424, 447, 448, 692, 714

phonetician 328, 692

phonics 424, 430–432, 441–450, 452, 456, 457, 459, 462, 466, 469, 472, 473, 521, 692, 702, 731

phonological awareness 424, 432, 450, 454–456, 466, 472, 691, 692, 710, 738

phonotactics 312, 322, 326, 680, 683, 692

phylogenetic speculation 2, 24, 692

Piaget, J. 29, 52, 143, 710, 731

Pickering, I. J. 716

Pickles, A. 723

Pietra, R. 716

Pike, 692

Pioneer Fund 315, 430, 731

pitch 142, 170, 245, 277, 279, 281, 298, 313, 321, 322, 350, 368, 381, 384, 386, 387, 389, 414, 671, 678, 688, 692, 693, 698, 702, 721

place of articulation 312, 324, 326, 337, 362, 692

plagiarism 104, 137, 692

plaintiff 609, 610, 637, 645, 675, 678, 692

planum temporale 368, 387, 388, 692, 694, 715, 719, 721, 731

plaques 198, 224, 225, 674, 692, 705

Platt 230, 731

Platt, J. R. 731

Plessy v. Ferguson 604–607, 644, 718, 731

Plooy, A. M. 193, 738

plosive 312, 326, 337, 338, 673, 683, 692, 698

Podzimek, S. 739

Pogribna, M. 720

Poikkeus, A. M. 738

point of articulation 312, 337, 692, 701

Poletto, C. J. 724

polio 204, 545, 547, 633, 635, 636, 685, 692, 697, 709

poliomyelitis 685, 692

Poloni, C. 182, 732

polyp 692

Pomblum, S. C. G. 715

Poncet, M. 264, 706

Ponikvar, R. 725

Pook, P. K. 62, 706

Popendikyte, V. 731

Popper, K. 230, 732

Porky Pig 732

portmanteau 476, 485, 496, 682, 692, 732

positions of discourse 252, 253, 308, 314, 315, 317, 364, 373, 420, 692

positive reinforcement 198, 244, 692

positron 368, 394, 476, 491–493, 691–693, 712, 713, 732, 741

positron emission tomography 368, 394, 476, 491, 691, 692, 712, 713, 732, 741

Possati, G. F. 716

Posse, S. 497, 725

Posserud, M. B. 211, 732

possible worlds 312, 356, 693

post hoc ergo propter hoc fallacy 554, 584, 592, 693

postmodernism 104, 115, 693

post-traumatic stress syndrome 693

Poto and Cabengo 123, 333, 732

Povinelli, D. J. 12, 19, 731, 732

pragmatic isomorphism 424, 432, 693

pragmatic mapping 2, 37–39, 98, 99, 104, 108, 109, 111, 132, 138, 139, 148, 168, 247, 268, 300, 313, 319, 338, 340, 352, 353, 357, 365, 423, 427–429, 433, 442, 443, 445, 465, 466, 469, 498–500, 504, 509, 517, 518, 521, 523, 524, 530, 531, 535, 550, 693, 727

Prasad, S. 239, 732

Prasse, J. E. 373, 732

Pratico, D. 218, 220, 741

Pratkanis, A. R. 184, 732

precipitating factors 368, 376, 693

Premack, D. 19, 732

preparatory set 368, 416, 693

prescinded symbol 424, 428, 693

prescinding 424, 427, 693

prestin 142, 187, 693, 712, 730

prevalence 198, 199, 201, 204, 213, 216, 248, 548, 693, 705, 713, 717, 725, 728

Previc, F. H. 218, 249, 732

Previde, E. P. 12, 733

Prieve, B. 187, 732

prima facie evidence 240, 594, 617, 693

Prince, R. C. 716

principle of consistency 554, 589, 693

Probst, P. 120, 732

processing malfunction models 368, 394, 395, 693

Prochazkova, J. 739

profound deafness 104, 123, 139, 693

prognosis 202, 235, 252, 302, 417, 462, 693

progressive palsy 252, 292, 693
proposition 111, 142, 160, 165, 449, 595, 598, 599, 669, 670, 693
prosodic elements 321, 686, 693
prosody 52, 79, 94, 298, 299, 310, 313, 336, 398, 414, 448, 693, 732
prosopagnosia xiv, 98, 476, 517, 529–531, 537, 693, 708, 742
prospective study 198, 241, 693, 716
proton 198, 220, 221, 694
Prout, C. 727
Providence, Rhode Island 575, 627, 628, 721, 732, 735
pseudobulbar palsy 252, 292–294, 694, 722, 732
pseudologia fantastica 2, 41, 505, 506, 508, 689, 694
pseudologue 2, 41, 507, 508, 694
psychogenic stuttering 368, 417–419, 694
psycholinguistics 424, 451, 694
psychosis 694
Ptito, A. 520, 705
Ptok, M. 358, 706, 728
public awareness theory 198, 213–215, 694
Public Law 94-142 616, 619, 623, 624, 626, 629–631, 649
pull-out 415, 611, 621, 694
pull-out programs 694
Pulte, M. 596, 724
Punati, A. 297, 709
punishment 198, 244, 415, 620, 657, 689, 694
Puolakanaho, A. 738
Purves, W. K. 732
Pylyshyn, Z. W. 62, 355, 732
pyramidal tract xiv, 252, 287, 288, 296, 297, 677, 681, 686, 694

Q

Quackenbush, J. 216, 719
Quarles, J. 729
Quattrochi, J. 727
QuiÒonez, I. 707

R

Rabinowitz, J. A. 182, 741
Rachael Ray 471, 732
Rack, E. P. 297, 361, 707

radioactive tracers 476, 492, 694
Radvansky, G. 470, 732
Ragland, J. D. 723
Raine, A. 741
raised print 104, 108–112, 114, 124, 132, 137, 139, 498, 694
Ramakrishnan, N. A. 713, 721
Ramig, L. O. 724
Ramig, P. 413, 732
Ramón y Cajal, S. 181, 706, 732
Ramsey, J. 722
Ramus, F. 335, 336, 728, 732
Rao, R. P. N. 62, 706
Raphael, L. J. 419, 736
Raphael, R. M. 197, 730
Raphael, Y. 191, 732
Rapin 206, 727, 739
Rapin, I. 727, 739
Rascón, D. 202, 729
Rasmussen, E. B. 636, 728
Rastatter, M. 386, 737
Rattanavich, S. 468, 729, 732
Ray, C. G. 734
Rayca, K. O. 418, 706
Razagui, I. B. A. 227, 732
reading readiness 424, 426, 429–431, 694
Reagan, Ronald 68, 69, 202, 595, 596, 722, 733
real-time processing 694
receptive aphasia 476, 484, 694, 696, 702
receptive repertoire 424, 429, 432, 434, 694
recurrence risk 198, 216, 694
Reddihough, D. 306, 719
Reddy, C. 709
Redman, T. A. 306, 733
redox 198, 220, 694, 713, 728, 733
Redstone, F. 270, 733
reduction (*also see* redox) 88, 198, 220, 221, 244, 292, 312, 336, 358, 359, 388, 403, 408, 676, 681, 694, 706, 719
Redwood, L. 229, 348, 706
Reed, M. N. 276, 548, 712
Rees, G. 184, 185, 718
referential content 142, 159, 694
referring term 37, 104, 132, 340, 429, 499, 557, 694
reflex 2, 15, 190, 192, 254, 291, 476, 510, 694
reflex arc 476, 510, 694

Reggia, J. A. 500, 510, 536, 733, 740
Rehabilitation Act of 1973 594, 612, 619, 641, 733
reinforcing stimuli 198, 244, 695
Reiss, K. 740
reliability 2, 8, 45, 279, 368, 401–403, 563, 577, 665, 666, 685, 686, 695, 711, 741
Remington-Gurley, J. 120, 711
replication requirement 554, 589, 693, 695
Rescue Dawn: The Truth 733
residual volume 252, 274, 695, 702
resin composite 198, 236, 695
resonance 142, 171, 184, 278, 286, 295, 388, 476, 494–497, 668, 681, 682, 687, 689, 695, 719, 723, 725
respondent 594, 637, 655, 695
retrotransposons 476, 545, 695
Rett syndrome 198, 212, 691, 695
Reunes, G. 389, 739
reversion principle 554, 558, 559, 695
Reybrouck, M. 398, 733
Reynolds, J. R. C. L. 470, 724, 726, 736, 741
Ribas, C. M. 715
Ribbers, G. M. 722
Rice, T.D. 605, 733
Richardson, D. 418, 706
Richardson, D. C. 330, 733
Richardson, J. R. , 718, 733
Richard-Amato, P. 38, 132, 363
Richfield, E. K. 297, 706
Richter, J. J. 711
Rickford, J. R. 715
Riecke, L. 263, 266–268, 718
Rigamonti, M. M. 12, 733
rigid transliteration 104, 125, 127, 695
Riley, G. 741
Rillos, L. 505, 733
rime 232, 424, 450, 620, 657, 695
Ringel, S. P. 726
Ringelstein, E. B. 713
Riquier, F. 732
Ritter, J. 8, 733
Ritvo, E. R. 212, 733
Ritvo, M. J. 212, 733
Ritvo, R. A. 212, 733
Rivera, S. M. 432, 733
Rizwi, S. J. 546, 741
Roberts, Julia 529, 715, 716, 731, 736

Roberts, D. D. 715
Roberts, J. L. 736
Roberts, T. P. L. 172, 716
Robertson, S. 723
Robine, B. 739
Roger, H. 229, 706
Rohyans, J. 228, 733
Roman, K. G. 113, 346, 397, 597, 661, 733
Ronald Reagan 68, 69, 202, 595, 596, 722, 733
Röntgen, W.C. 489, 490, 733
Roohi, J. 718
Rosenblum, L. D. 150, 733
Rosenthal, V. 19, 739
Rosicky, J. G. 342, 727
Ross, D. S. 122, 733
Ross, G. W. 710
Rossignol, D. A. 218, 220, 733
Rossignol, L. W. 218, 220, 733
Rotary Lighthouse Literacy Programs 468, 733
Rotshtein, P. 718
Rouas, J. L. 336, 733
Roukens, R. 705
rounded 151, 312, 327, 695
Roy, P. 432, 710
Royal National Institute of Blind People 111, 112, 733
Ruark, J. L. 271, 727, 733
Rudorf, E. H. 446, 718
Rue, S. 407, 730
Ruff, D. D. 722
Russo, J. P. 718
Russo, R. N. 306, 733
Rutter, M. 211, 723, 734
Ryan, K. J. 5, 46, 216, 217, 224, 235, 305, 734
Ryba, N. J. P. 88, 710
Rybicki, B. A. 297, 734

S

Sabbioni, E. 716
saccades 263, 266–268, 342, 682, 695, 718
Sacco, R. 709
Sackin, S. 392, 719
Sacks, H. 330, 688, 734
Sadava, D. 732
Saepoff, J. 713
Safe removal of amalgam fillings 734

sagittal 257, 476, 532, 695, 698
Saha, S. 265, 721, 737
Sai, F. Z. 36, 146, 333, 708, 734
Sakashita, T. 722
Sakurai, Y. 737
Sales, B. D. 38, 524, 729
Salisbury, D. F. 719
Saltuklaroglu, T. 369, 386, 403, 407, 408, 413, 415, 721, 737
Sander, L. W. 16, 37, 80, 148, 332, 333, 711
Sanderson, W. T. 710
sandhi 312, 338, 695, 734
Sanford, J. 25, 61, 130, 376, 544, 549, 711, 734
Santos, A. R. S. 180, 186, 187, 453, 715, 734
Santos-Sacchi, J. 186, 187, 453
Sapienza, C. M. 724
Sapir, E. 453, 734
Sarrazin, J. C. 185, 734
Sarton, G. 664, 734
Sasaki, S. 89, 734, 737
Sato, S. 728
Sato, Y. 322, 734
Saucier, J. F. 182, 707
Saul, R. 734
Sauvageau, I. 182, 707
Savage-Rumbaugh, S. 17–19, 706, 717, 734, 735, 737
Savas, H. A. 736
Savaskan, E. 729
Saylor, K. E. 722
scale of development 554, 557, 559, 560, 565, 567, 695, 702
Schaefer, F. 193, 738
schedule of reinforcement 198, 244, 245, 681, 685, 695
Schegloff, E. A. 330, 734
Scheibman, J. 128, 740
Schettler, T. 548, 550, 722
schizophrenia 294, 388, 476, 504, 597, 694, 695, 711, 719, 723, 731, 734
schizophrenic 69, 695
Schlaug, G. 387, 706, 721
Schmidt, K. L. 13, 734
Schmithorst, V. J. 501, 734
Schmuckler, M. A. 150, 733
Schneider, C. 371, 709
Schneider, P. 371, 734
Schneider, R. 233, 238, 727
Schroeder, L. 723

Schuitemaker, H. 738
Schwartz, D. 95, 716
Scott v. Sanford 711, 734
Scribner, S. 740
Scripture, E. W. 397, 734
Searle, D. A. 95, 266, 728
Sebeok, T. A. 19, 734
secondary behaviors (also known as "secondaries") 97, 368, 402, 405, 406, 410, 411, 413, 420, 695, 698
secondary injury 476, 480, 695
Sedgwick, J. 573, 574, 734
segmental sounds 312, 349, 364, 696
Segura-Aguilar, J. 219, 223, 734
Seidler, F. J. 220, 227, 735
Selber, P. 306, 719
self-contradiction 118, 578, 696
Sell, J. Z. 639, 654, 734
semantic aphasia 476, 484, 511, 696, 702
semantic function 2, 19, 696
semiotics 405, 424, 451, 696, 715, 733
semivowels 312, 324, 696
Senghas, A. 122, 734
senile dementia 198, 223, 696
sensorineural hearing loss 142, 187, 696, 722
sensory alexia 476, 513, 696
sensory aphasia 424, 439, 476, 513, 515, 516, 696, 698, 700, 702, 725, 734, 737
sensory asignia 476, 513, 696
sensory cortex 2, 29, 516, 675, 681, 696, 697
sensory dyslexia 476, 513, 696
sensory prejudices 104, 113, 696
sensory strip 2, 27, 696
sensory systems 2, 20, 27, 28, 61, 152, 174, 195, 517, 676, 696, 697
separate but equal 594, 605, 696, 721
September 11, 2001 153, 231, 239, 587, 735
sequential (episodic) organization 471, 696
Sequoia (also spelled "Sequoyah") 312, 347, 348, 696
Sereno, M. L. 263, 266–268, 718
serial neural networks 142, 696
serial processing 142, 164, 696

Seymour, P. K. H. 436, 735

Shakespeare, W. 379, 735

Shanker, S. G. 17, 735

Shao, F. 194, 723

Sharif v. New York State Education Department 640, 735

Shaywitz, B. A. 425, 436, 724, 735

Shaywitz, S. E. 425, 436, 724, 735

Shearsby, J. 409, 740

Shen, D. D. 37, 459, 708, 722

Shenker, R. C. 396, 409, 723, 735

Shenton, M. E. 719

Shestack, J. 5, 46, 48, 49, 200–203, 217, 307, 555, 735

Shi, X. B. 545, 722, 735, 737

Shibata, T. 722

Shigemitsu, H. 259, 735

Shiller, D. M. 358, 738

Shimoda, N. 265, 721

Shinnar, S. 739

Shkuro, Y. 500, 733

short-term memory 389, 425, 480, 696

Shrivastav, R. 724

Shukla, Y. 239, 732

Shuster, L. I. 263, 735

Shyer, C. 735

sibilant 312, 337, 696

sickle cell anemia 52, 63, 64, 190, 696, 697

Siegel, L. S. 622, 717

signal detection 142, 174, 696

Signed Exact English (SEE) 104, 124, 696

Silbert, N. 335, 735

Silver, J. A. 62, 223, 348, 370, 704, 716, 735

Silverman, E. M. 397, 735

Silverman, F. H. 379, 380, 394, 397, 401, 402, 419, 735

Silverman, M. 398, 735

Silverstein, A. E. 143, 735

Simian virus 40 (SV40) 476, 545, 633, 697, 699, 712

Simmons, R. J. 627, 735

Simmons, Z. 742

Simon, Carly 369, 381, 735

Simon, C. S. 712

Simon, T. 579, 706

Simon, W. 636, 740

Simonyan, K. 724

simple frequency theory 142, 182, 183, 196, 697

Simpson, L. L. 306, 407, 723, 735

simultaneous interpretation 104, 125, 697

singer's nodes 252, 282, 697

single nucleotide polymorphism (sn) 697

Singleton, J. L. 333, 712, 727

Sinopoli, T. 389, 736

Siple, P. 317, 725

situation based 697

Sivasli, E. 736, 742

Skinner, B. F. 244, 245, 407, 719, 735

slavery 105, 106, 130, 575, 595, 597–602, 604, 606, 620, 627–629, 657, 670, 680, 686, 710, 721, 735

Slavery and Justice Report 627, 628, 710, 735

Slikker, W. 720

Slocomb, D. L. 298, 736

Slotkin, T. A. 220, 227, 735

slow speech 312, 334, 336, 337, 384, 415, 690, 697

Smith v. Robinson 612, 625, 626, 629, 630, 657, 736

Smith, A. 579, 735

Smith, C. W. 711

Smith, D. xiv, 509, 511, 736

Smith, R. 725

Smith, S. 741

Smith-Magenis syndrome 312, 358, 697

Smoking teeth 736

smooth pursuit 266, 268, 342, 682, 695, 697, 720

Snow, C. 451, 736

Snustadt, D. P. 55, 544, 716

Snyder, G. 396–398, 405, 736

Snyderman, D. 719

social Darwinism 104, 130, 553, 573, 575, 592, 597, 598, 670, 697

sociolinguistics 424, 451, 697

Soderstrom, M. 336, 370, 736

Sogut, S. 220, 238, 736

solar plexus 252, 273, 697

Solomon, R. L. 182, 719

somatic (bodily) systems 2, 697

somatosensory cortex 2, 27, 696, 697

somnambulism 476, 503, 697

Son, D. M. 714

Song, L. 734

Sorenson, J. A. 491, 710

Soros, P. 713

Souberman, E. 740

Sparks, N. 224, 736

spastic dysphonia 252, 297, 697

Spaziante, R. 27, 709

special education 66, 71, 198, 199, 203, 425, 436, 437, 609, 614, 615, 617–619, 630, 645, 646, 650, 651, 660, 663, 665, 697, 704, 726, 730, 740

Special Masters 204, 209, 594, 611, 637, 653, 697, 703, 728

spectral properties 142, 168, 171, 172, 697

spectrogram 142, 171, 697

speech to text (STT) 341, 424, 446, 697

speech-language pathology 4, 163, 254, 255, 335, 665, 667, 675, 682, 697, 704, 714

Speer, N. K. 470, 736, 741

Spelke, E. S. 336, 722

Spence, S. A. 508, 736

Spencer, K. A. 298, 736

Sperry, R. W. 21, 61, 313, 518, 519, 525, 534, 535, 537, 538, 551, 734, 736

sphere of reference 142, 167, 697

Spiezio, C. 12, 733

spina bifida 51, 52, 56, 71, 72, 76–78, 674, 697

spinal cord 27, 56, 142, 181, 186, 477, 674, 675, 687–689, 697

Spitzer, N. C. 736

splenium of the corpus callosum 476, 538, 698

split-brain experiments 519, 698

spondee 312, 322, 698

Squire, L. R. 267, 736

Sreenath, M. 709

St. Louis, K. O. 419, 708, 713, 721, 727, 736

Stacy Keach 82, 86, 100, 736

Stampfli, M. R. 741

Stan Kurtz 5, 46, 236, 241, 710, 736

standardized IQ tests 554, 574, 645, 698

Stanford, L. D. 446, 618, 646, 724

Starkweather, C. W. 390, 391, 736

startle response vi, xxii, xxxix, 2, 15, 192, 193, 698

State, M. W. 216, 736

Statham, D. J. 714

statute of limitations 594, 637, 639, 654, 698

Stecker, N. 186, 721, 727, 738

Steffens, M. L. 122, 729

Stein, T. P. 726

Steiner, T. 705, 740

Stejskal, V. 739

Stenroos, E. S. 709

Stephens, J. C. 147, 707

stereotyped movements 198, 199, 685, 698

Stetson, R. H. 313, 315, 316, 331–335, 342, 732, 736

Stevens, A. A. 95, 716

Stevens, T. 725

Stidham, K. R. 389, 736

Stillman, R. D. 151, 703

Stip, E. 182, 736

Stokoe, W. C. 128, 317, 318, 341, 705, 740

Stone, O. 587, 595, 736

stop consonant 337, 683, 698

Storey, M. E. 712

Strand, E. 724

Strasser, K. 725

Strauss, L. T. 76, 736

Streissguth, A. 67, 736

stress pattern 312, 322, 698, 701

stress timed language 312, 322, 698

Strickland, E. A. 187, 737

stridor 252, 283, 698

Stringari, J. 715

Strohmayer, W. 516, 737

stroke 513, 542, 549, 672, 722, 728, 737

Strom, S. 204, 717

Strong, M. J. 249, 737

Strong, T. 328, 737

structural linguistics 312, 349, 698

Stuart, A. 721, 737

Stump, T. 327, 575, 737

Sturm, J. 68, 726

Sturm, V. 708

stuttering block 368, 379, 395, 698

stuttering events 368, 370, 372, 373, 377, 379, 381, 382, 386, 390, 391, 396–399, 403, 405–408, 411–413, 415, 417, 419–421, 698

Stuttering Foundation 737

stuttering modification 368, 412, 415–417, 698

stuttering severity index 368, 401, 698

stylopharyngeus 252, 292, 698

subarachnoid hemorrhage 476, 542, 698

subcortical motor aphasia 476, 515, 698

subcortical sensory aphasia 476, 516, 698, 702, 737

subliminal messages 142, 183–185, 698

substantia nigra 252, 297, 699, 731

Suc, B. 728

Suga, N. 186, 737

Sugar, O. 519, 735

Sullivan, Annie xiii, 14, 132–138, 465, 498, 705, 718, 721, 723

Sullivan, M. W. 14, 737

Sun, Q. 714

Sunaert, R. 386, 739

supplementary motor area 476, 515, 699

suprasegmental elements 312, 350, 699

Sutcliffe, J. S. 709

Suzuki, K. 538, 737

Suzuki, M. 41, 508, 703

SV40 476, 545–547, 633–635, 699, 711, 714, 737

Swain, M. K. 465, 467, 737

Swallow, K. M. 470, 741

Sweet 88, 220, 222, 545, 674, 707, 730, 737, 738

Sweet, B. H. 545, 737

Sweet, L. I. 220, 737

Swerdlow, N. R. 194, 737

Swinney, D. A. 453, 715

Syed, N. I. 6, 60, 224, 227, 543, 723

syllabary 347, 348, 696, 699

syllabic writing 312, 347, 699

syllable timed 312, 322, 699

symptomology 2, 9, 699

synapses 142, 180, 181, 188, 193, 309, 699, 725

synostosis 52, 58, 699

syntax 2, 19, 98, 341, 377, 392, 442, 443, 448, 451, 459, 463, 487, 583, 668, 683, 699, 710, 721, 731

synthesized speech 104, 121, 699

syphilis 284, 476, 481, 484, 699

syphilis lesion 476, 481, 484, 699

Syversen, T. 239, 721

T

Taber, K. H. 517, 737

tachyphemia 368, 418, 419, 676, 699

Taeda, M. 728

Taglialatela, J. P. 19, 706, 719, 737

Tagore, S. 216–218, 717

Tajima, A. 8, 737

Takahashi, A. 737

Takano, H. 718

Takase, K. 737

Takeshita, F. 89, 633, 734, 737

Tallal, P. 454, 455, 737

Tanabe, H. 728

Tanaka, S. 719

Taney, R. B. 600, 601, 604, 679, 737

Tang, C. 741

Tao, Z. Z. 719

Tarakcioglu, M. 736

Tarski, A. 158, 355, 356, 471, 737

Tatewaki, N. 728

Tavares, M. 706

Taves, D. 725

Taylor, A. R. 17, 735

Taylor, T. J. 724

Tees, R. C. 426, 428, 740

Teixeira, A. 715

telegraphic 476, 481, 699

temporal integration threshold (hypothetical) 142, 165, 424, 454, 699

temporal lobes 2, 27, 295, 530, 699

temporal ordering 142, 165, 699

temporal resolution 142, 165, 172, 699, 716

Tennyson, A. L. 464, 737

Tepper, C. G. 735

Terao, Y. 298, 737

teratology 52, 68, 69, 699, 712

Terpstra, F. G. 546, 738

Terre, R. 301, 738

testosterone 198, 239, 700, 716, 732

tetanospasmin 252, 304, 305, 700

Tetnowksi, J. 706

text to speech (TTS) 104, 128, 431, 446–448, 452, 456, 472, 700, 701

Thackray, R. I. 193, 738

The Myelin Project 727

theory of abstraction 142, 146, 149, 158, 159, 172, 185, 427–429, 432, 464, 465, 511, 700

theory of the meritocracy 554, 574, 700

Thiel, A. 708

thimerosal 198, 207–210, 216, 225–228, 233, 234, 249, 280, 543, 545, 596, 632, 634, 639, 653, 654, 688, 700, 706, 708, 715, 716, 719, 720, 724, 728, 730

Thiruchelvam, M. 297, 706

Thompson, A. J. 741
Thordardottir, E. 409, 723
Thorndike, R. M. 667, 738
Thorndyke, P. W. 470, 738
threshold of coherence 476, 526–529, 700
threshold of insanity 476, 700
Throneburg, R. N. 392, 738
Tian, Y. L. 14, 734
Tidball, G. 342, 727
Tillery, K. L. 174, 738
tinnitus 142, 188–190, 194, 700, 728
tip of the mind 476, 525, 700, 719
tip of the tongue 312, 327, 476, 511, 525, 700
Titzer, A. 11, 425, 429–433, 442, 443, 466, 473, 518, 703
Titzer, R. C. 430, 433, 466, 738
Tocopherol 738
Toga, A. W. 741
Tognon, M. 711
Tokunaga, H. 728
Tolvanen, A. 738
Tomazic, T. 358, 724
Tongul, E. 182, 741
Tony Blair 531
top-down processing 164, 674, 700
Torppa, M. 432, 738
Tosteson, D. C. 727, 738
Touchstone, R. M. 193, 718, 738
Townsend, P. 419, 736
Toyokura, M. 265, 721
Tozuka, M. 737
trachea 252, 259, 272, 277, 283, 305, 680, 700
tracheostomy 252, 283, 700
Trachtenberg, F. 706
Tranel, D. 500, 712
transcortical motor aphasia 476, 515, 700, 738
transcortical sensory aphasia 476, 515, 516, 696, 700, 725
transitive relations 142, 157, 158, 355, 471, 531, 590, 700
translation 104, 118, 125–127, 146, 348, 425, 571, 658, 695, 697, 700
Trapp, R. 228, 722
traumatic brain injury (TBI) 301, 310, 476, 540, 541, 651, 688, 699, 700, 725, 738
traumatic injury 2, 23, 303, 700

treatment effect 554, 586, 592, 701
treatment group 554, 585, 701
Tremblay, S. 738
Tresilian, J. R. 193, 738
triangulate 142, 166, 701
trigeminal neuralgia 252, 305, 701
trilingualism 424, 467, 701
Trillo, S. 709
trimoraic 312, 322, 701
Trivedi, M. H. 220, 721
trochee 312, 322, 701
Troncoso, X. G. 146, 738
true narrative representation 476, 521, 701
Truffaut, F. 738
Tsuchiya, N. 185, 721
Tsuji, S. 737
Turgay, A. 722
Turkewitz, G. 35, 725
Turpin, R. G. 65, 193, 723, 738
Tutkun, H. 736

U

U.S. Court of Federal Claims 203, 596, 632, 636, 637, 653, 655, 670, 689, 738
Ueda, K. 184, 719, 733
Ueno, K. 722
Ugawa, Y. 737
Umami 683, 738
Uman, J. 297, 734
UMN 231, 252, 286, 287, 290, 292, 295–298, 300, 302, 701, 739
unilateral motor neuron dysarthria 252, 298, 701
United States v. Fordice 561, 640, 644, 738
unity of conception 476, 526, 528, 529, 701
universal quantifiers 554, 577, 701
University of California Regents v. Bakke 616, 739
unreliability 554, 560, 562, 591, 688, 701
unrounded 312, 327, 701
unvoiced 312, 326, 701, 702
upper motor neuron (UMN system) 231, 252, 286, 287, 290, 292, 295–298, 300, 302, 701, 738
Urnovitz, H. B. 545, 633, 739
Usman, A. I. 200, 708
Uversky, V. N. 546, 739

V

Vaccine Adverse Event Reporting System (VAERS) 594, 634–637, 643, 655, 701, 715, 739, 740
Vaccine Safety Datalink 643, 709
VAERS 594, 634–637, 643, 655, 701, 715, 739, 740
Valentine 306, 733
Valentine, J. 733
Valette, R. M. 177, 739
Valicenti-McDermott, M. 241, 739
validity 2, 45, 74, 154, 279, 330, 401–403, 408, 434, 500, 558, 563, 565, 577, 591, 665, 666, 701, 725, 741
Vallant, B. 238, 239, 739
Valli, C. 342, 739
Van Berkum, J. J. A. 354, 355, 718, 728
Van Borsel, J. 386, 389, 418, 706, 739
Van den Berg, J. W. 276, 689, 739
Van den Bergh, N. 389, 739
van den Broek, P. 470, 738, 740
Van der Linden, M. 725
Van der Schyf , C. J. 716
van Engelenburg, F. A. C. 738
Van Riper, C. 415–417, 739
van't Wout, A. B. 738
variegated babble 424, 428, 701
Vary, P. 170, 720
Vaughan, B. 722
vegetative (sounds) 2, 18, 253, 254, 271, 701
vegetative movements 253, 254, 701
velar 312, 326, 335–337, 362, 363, 684, 701
velopharyngeal insufficiency 52, 85, 701
Venclikova, Z. 547, 739
verbal behavior 198, 244, 701, 710, 715, 725, 727, 735
Verhaar, R. 738
Verhoeven, A. J. 738
Verstichel, P. 265, 739
Verstraten, F. A. J. 185, 721
vertical progress 554, 557, 701
Vescovi, A. L. 709
vestibular canal 142, 179, 688, 702
vestibular system 142, 179, 702
VICP 594, 636, 637, 639, 702

Vieira, M. N. N. 224, 715
Vinson, D. 386, 719
Visetti, Y. M. 739
visible speech 104, 129, 702
visuocentricity 104, 113, 139, 702
vital capacity 253, 274, 702
vitamin C 198, 222, 702, 727, 739
vitamin E 198, 222, 702
Vlase, L. 730
vocal folds xiv, 142, 169, 170, 259, 274–277, 279, 282–285, 297, 320, 671, 682, 683, 686, 697, 701, 702
vocal hygiene 253, 279, 702, 739
vocal nodules 253, 282, 284, 285, 307, 310, 702
vocal timbre 253, 279, 702
vocal tract 142, 170–172, 256, 257, 259, 321, 326, 673, 682, 702
vocalic center 253, 271, 702
Voelker, C. H. 397, 739
Voelker, E. S. 397, 739
voice disorder 253, 272, 281, 302, 303, 702
voiced 249, 253, 312, 326, 337, 409, 683, 702
voiceless 312, 326, 701, 702
voicing 255, 271, 274, 276, 279, 312, 323, 324, 671, 689, 702
Vojdani, A. 220, 739
Vojdani, E. 220, 739
Vokshoor, A. 88, 739
volitional control 2, 21, 22, 40, 92, 93, 254, 255, 265, 266, 269, 300, 313, 379, 433, 500, 689, 694, 700, 702, 724, 730
Volkow, N. D. 280, 706
Volz, T. J. 479, 739
von Békésy, G. 739
von Tetzchner, S. 120, 739
Vos, P. W. 369, 386, 737
vowels 142, 170, 271, 323, 324, 327, 452, 453, 566, 570, 687, 695, 701, 702
Vygotsky, L. S. 29, 242, 243, 247, 357, 740

W

Wada, T. 722
Wagner, G. C. 220, 722, 726
Wakefield, A. 60, 633
Walach, H. 229, 233, 237, 238, 550, 727

Walker, L. J. 190, 737
Walker, J. G. 740
Walker, R. F. 468, 640, 718, 729, 732, 737
Walsh, W. J. 218, 220, 741
Walson, P. D. 228, 733
Walton, G. E. 35, 740
Waly, M. 332, 713
Wang, R. 709
Ward, B. J. 241, 713
Ward, G. 38, 740
Ward, J. I. 710
Warren, E. 606, 607, 644, 740
Wasmuth, J. J. 724
wavelength 171, 277, 278, 702
Weber, M. E. 707, 708
Weems, S. A. 510, 740
Wei, X. L. 714
Weigl, D. M. 306, 740
Weihe, P. 731
Weisbender, L. 733
Weiss, B. 548, 550, 636, 722, 740
Weiss, D. 418, 740
Weiss, M. D. 722
Weiss, P. 731
Weisskopf, B. 631, 707
Weizmann, T. 718
Werker, J. F. 426, 428, 730, 740
Wermuth, L. 731
Wernicke, C. 482, 484–487, 489, 498, 509, 512, 513, 516, 686, 702, 740
Wernicke's aphasia 94, 476, 484–487, 512, 513, 696, 702
Wernicke's area 368, 387, 388, 514, 515, 672, 702
Wershil, B. K. 739
Westby, C. 410, 705
white noise 253, 278, 382, 702
White, M. K. 545, 740
White, R. W. D. 735
Whitebread, G. 397, 740
Whitman, B. Y. 358, 724
Wickstrom, M. 228, 741
Wiener, N. 385, 386, 740
Wilcox, P. P. 122, 124, 129, 740
Wilcox, S. E. 122, 124, 128, 129, 317, 318, 341, 705, 740
Wilkins, P. A. 193, 740
Wilkinson, I. D. 508, 736
Willems, R. M. 342, 354, 730, 740
Williams, A. 741
Williams, T. A. 709

Wills, G. F. 484, 740
Wiltshire, S. 32, 36, 740
Windham, G. C. 228, 740
Wingate, M. E. 397, 402, 740
Winstein, C. J. 301, 740
Winston Churchill 369, 418, 424, 531, 595, 596, 725, 740, 741
Winters, K. L. 714
Wojcik, D. P. 237, 740
Wolf, M. 239, 709
Wolman, C. 470, 740
Woo, E. J. 5, 740
Woo, Y. J. 722
Wood G. A. 228, 733
Wood, D. 128, 740
Wood, E. 339, 740
Woode, D. R. 713
Woodruff, G. 19, 390, 732
Woods, S. 213, 409, 740
Wooley, R. S. 736
word deafness 476, 516, 698, 702
word recognition 424, 434, 702, 705, 728
Wright, K. 5, 204–206, 213, 218, 234, 741
Wright, P. D. 206, 623, 645, 741
Wright, P. W. D. 206, 623, 645, 741
Wright, Judge Skelly 609
Wu 342, 394, 719, 741
Wu, J. C. 741
Wu, Y. C. 741
Wu, Z. 719
Wulfman, J. S. 200, 708
Wuthrich, C. 545, 712
Wyllie, E. 724

X

xenobiotic 198, 228, 249, 688, 702
Xing, H. 274, 674, 714
Xu, J. 497, 725
Xue, L. R. 735

Y

Yairi, E. 391, 392, 396, 404, 704, 738, 741
Yamada, Y. 719
Yamadori, A. 737
Yamamoto, T. 737
Yan, R. xii, 8, 45, 176, 177, 186, 437, 568, 581, 622, 712, 741
Yang, M. 546, 711

Yang, S. 718
Yang, Y. 41, 741
Yanik, M. 736
Yao, Y. M. 218, 220, 741
Yaruss, J. S. 372, 373, 401, 420, 741
Yauk, C. L. 280, 741
Yerkes, R. M. 576, 741
Yeshurun, Y. 718
Yetkin, O. 736, 742
Yilmaz, H. R. 736
Yoakum, C. S. 576, 741
Yoder, C. 713
Yogi Berra. 741
Yokel, R. A. 546, 741
Yole, M. 228, 741
York, M. W. 182, 741
Yorkston, K. 724
Yoshida, S. 389, 716
Yoshimine, T. 728
Yoshioka, H. 389, 716

Young, I. S. 705
Yudovich, I. F. 724
Yuwiler, A. 733

Z

Zackheim, C. T. 392, 741
Zacks, J. A. 470, 736, 741
Zacks, J. M. 736, 741
Zahir, F. 546, 741
Zak, O. 125, 741
Zane, S. B. 736
Zapawa, J. E. xv, 489, 533, 742
Zarate, C. B. 730
Zarei, M. 517, 741
Zawaydeh, A. N. 432, 733
Zeijlon, L. 211, 717
Zemeckis, R. 742
Zentz, R. 543, 742
Zhang, E. 737
Zhang, L. 288, 740

Zhang, Q. 186, 742
Zhao, H. B. 719
Zheng, J. 187, 712, 734
Zhu, G. 86, 714
Ziegler, L. A. 715, 731
Zifan, A. 530, 742
Zigmond, M. J. 736
Zimmerman, A. W. 740
Zimmerman, E. K. 294, 742
Zimmermann, G. 732
Zimmermann, P. 182, 725, 732
zone of proximal development
    (ZPD) 198, 243, 247, 248, 426,
    429, 460, 559, 702
Zoroglu, S. S. 220, 736, 742
ZPD 198, 243, 247, 248, 426, 429,
    460, 559, 702
Zuker, C. S. 88, 710
Zwaan, R. A. 470, 527, 717, 725,
    732, 742